Functional Foods and Cardiovascular Disease

Edited by
Mohammed H. Moghadasian
N. A. Michael Eskin

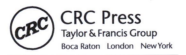

CRC Press
Taylor & Francis Group
Boca Raton   London   New York

CRC Press is an imprint of the
Taylor & Francis Group, an **informa** business

CRC Press
Taylor & Francis Group
6000 Broken Sound Parkway NW, Suite 300
Boca Raton, FL 33487-2742

Version Date: 20111207

International Standard Book Number: 978-1-4200-7110-8 (Hardback)

Library of Congress Cataloging-in-Publication Data

Functional foods and cardiovascular disease / editors, Mohammed H. Moghadasian, N.A. Michael Eskin.
    p. cm.
  Includes bibliographical references and index.
  ISBN 978-1-4200-7110-8 (hardback)
  1. Cardiovascular system--Diseases--Diet therapy. 2. Functional foods. I. Moghadasian, Mohammed H. II. Eskin, N. A. M. (Neason Akivah Michael)

RC684.D5F857 2012
616.1'0654--dc23   2011037593

Visit the Taylor & Francis Web site at
http://www.taylorandfrancis.com

and the CRC Press Web site at
http://www.crcpress.com

Contents

Preface

Coronary heart disease (CHD) is the leading cause of death in developed countries. Although there have been great improvements in treating CHD through surgery and medications, these interventions are very expensive in countries where budgets are severely strained. An alternative approach, however, is to prevent the development of cardiovascular disease through a combination of diet and exercise. This book focuses on the use of functional foods defined as foods with physiological benefits that can reduce the risk of chronic diseases such as cardiovascular disease. Over the last decade, researchers around the world have focused on identifying and developing functional foods that will enhance the health and well-being of an aging population. This book brings together important information on the benefits that a selected group of functional foods have on cardiovascular disease.

Each chapter in this book provides a critical discussion on the bioactive components responsible for the cardiovascular benefits of selected functional foods. These bioactive components are referred to as nutraceuticals. The opening chapter, Chapter 1, provides a detailed overview of the pathogenesis of coronary artery disease. Chapter 2 discusses genetic methods for enhancing bioactives in foods as well as new and improved techniques for extracting bioactive components for developing functional foods. The remaining chapters focus on particular functional foods and/or their bioactive components. Chapter 3 covers the clinical and experimental evidence for the cardiovascular benefits of fish oils. Chapter 4 discusses the cardiovascular benefits of plant oils, focusing on flaxseed oil. The importance of folic acid in homocysteine metabolisms and its impact on cardiovascular disease is presented in Chapter 5. The clinical and experimental evidence for the cardiovascular benefits of plant sterols is covered in Chapter 6. The ability of wine to prevent cardiovascular disease is the subject of Chapter 7. The role of garlic products in the management of cardiovascular disease is discussed in Chapter 8. Chapter 9 deals with the controversy surrounding the impact of egg consumption by presenting evidence showing the beneficial effects on cardiovascular disease. The importance of fiber for the treatment of cardiovascular disease is clearly described in Chapter 10. The beneficial effects of cocoa and chocolate on heart health are covered in Chapter 11. The last chapter, Chapter 12, focuses on the growing scientific evidence that points to the beneficial effects of beverages such as coffee and tea, with particular emphasis on their effects on cardiovascular disease.

We hope that this book will provide useful information to nutritionists, food scientists, as well as those working in the health or health-related industry. We believe that this book will enhance our understanding of the potential role of functional foods in combating cardiovascular disease. We are most appreciative of the contributions by all the authors in making this a valuable and timely publication on an important topic that affects us all directly or indirectly. We also appreciate the support provided by the editorial staff of Taylor & Francis.

Editors

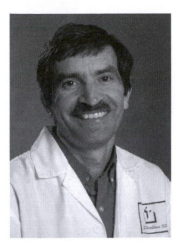

Dr. Mohammed H. Moghadasian is currently a professor in the Department of Human Nutritional Sciences, Faculty of Human Ecology at the University of Manitoba, Winnipeg, Canada. He is also a principal investigator at the Canadian Centre for Agri-food Research in Health and Medicine (CCARM) at the St. Boniface Hospital Research Centre, Winnipeg, Canada. He obtained his PhD in the discipline of pathology and laboratory medicine from the University of British Columbia, Vancouver, Canada in 1998. After extensive postdoctoral training in the area of functional foods and nutraceuticals, Dr. Moghadasian joined the University of Manitoba in 2003. Dr. Moghadasian's research program is well funded through a number of major grant agencies. His research activities have extensively contributed to advancing the applications of functional foods and nutraceuticals in the prevention and treatment of cardiovascular diseases. Dr. Moghadasian is the primary author on numerous scientific articles plus several book chapters. Dr. Moghadasian is a recipient of a number of research and teaching excellence awards including the Canadian Nutrition Society Centrum Foundation New Scientist Award. He serves several scientific journals as a member of the editorial board.

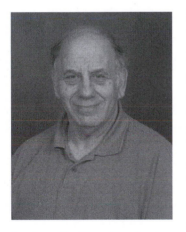

Dr. N. A. Michael Eskin is currently a professor in the Department of Human Nutritional Sciences and associate dean, Faculty of Human Ecology at the University of Manitoba, Winnipeg, Canada. He obtained his PhD in physiological chemistry at Birmingham University, United Kingdom, where he conducted research on toxicology focusing on mercapturic acid. Dr. Eskin holds several patents and has published 25 chapters and over 115 scientific papers related to edible oils and mustard gum. He has authored and edited 10 books, several of which were translated into German and Japanese. Dr. Eskin is the recipient of a number of awards including the Timothy Mounts Award by the American Oil Chemists' Society and the W. J. Eva Award by the Canadian Institute of Food Science and Technology for his outstanding contributions to research and service. He is a fellow of the American Oil Chemists' Society, the Canadian Institute of Food Science and Technology, and the Institute of Food Science and Technology of the United Kingdom. Dr. Eskin sits on the board of five international journals and was recently appointed co-editor of *Lipid Technology*.

Contributors

Ayyappan Appukuttan Aachary
Department of Human Nutritional Sciences
University of Manitoba
Winnipeg, Manitoba, Canada

Michel Aliani
Department of Human Nutritional Sciences
University of Manitoba
Winnipeg, Manitoba, Canada

Atif B. Awad
Department of Exercise and Nutritional Sciences
State University of New York
Buffalo, New York

Chantal M. C. Bassett
Department of Physiology
University of Manitoba
Winnipeg, Manitoba, Canada

Peter G. Bradford
Department of Pharmacology and Toxicology
State University of New York
Buffalo, New York

Mirna N. Chahine
Department of Physiology
University of Manitoba
Winnipeg, Manitoba, Canada

Justin F. Deniset
Department of Physiology
University of Manitoba
Winnipeg, Manitoba, Canada

Andrea L. Edel
Department of Physiology
University of Manitoba
Winnipeg, Manitoba, Canada

N. A. Michael Eskin
Department of Human Nutritional Sciences
University of Manitoba
Winnipeg, Manitoba, Canada

Kelley C. Fitzpatrick
Flax Canada
Winnipeg, Manitoba, Canada

Andrew Francis
Department of Physiology
University of Manitoba
Winnipeg, Manitoba, Canada

James D. House
Department of Human Nutritional
  Sciences
University of Manitoba
Winnipeg, Manitoba, Canada

Sun-Young Hwang
Department of Animal Science
University of Manitoba
Winnipeg, Manitoba, Canada

Mingyan Jing
Department of Human Nutritional
  Sciences
University of Manitoba
Winnipeg, Manitoba, Canada

Tabitha Marshall
Department of Human Nutritional
  Sciences
University of Manitoba
Winnipeg, Manitoba, Canada

Giuseppe Mazza
Mazza Innovation Ltd.
Penticton, British Columbia, Canada

Richelle S. McCullough
Department of Physiology
University of Manitoba
Winnipeg, Manitoba, Canada

Donald J. McNamara
Eggs for Health Consulting
Laurel, Maryland

Mohammed H. Moghadasian
Department of Human Nutritional Sciences
University of Manitoba
Winnipeg, Manitoba, Canada

Amy Noto
Department of Human Nutritional Sciences
University of Manitoba
Winnipeg, Manitoba, Canada

Karmin O
Departments of Animal Science and
    Physiology
University of Manitoba
Winnipeg, Manitoba, Canada

Rgia A. Othman
Department of Nutritional Sciences
University of Manitoba
Winnipeg, Manitoba, Canada

Grant N. Pierce
Department of Physiology
University of Manitoba
Winnipeg, Manitoba, Canada

Curtis Rempel
Richardson Centre for Functional Foods and
    Nutriceuticals
University of Manitoba
Winnipeg, Manitoba, Canada

Natalie D. Riediger
Department of Community Health Sciences
University of Manitoba
Winnipeg, Manitoba, Canada

Delfin Rodriguez-Leyva
Institute of Cardiovascular Sciences
St. Boniface Hospital Research Centre
and
Department of Physiology
University of Manitoba
Winnipeg, Manitoba, Canada

Carla Taylor
Department of Human Nutritional Sciences
University of Manitoba
Winnipeg, Manitoba, Canada

Usha Thiyam
Department of Human Nutritional Sciences
University of Manitoba
Winnipeg, Manitoba, Canada

Peter Zahradka
Department of Physiology
University of Manitoba
Winnipeg, Manitoba, Canada

1 The Pathophysiology of Coronary Artery Disease

Chantal M. C. Bassett, Richelle S. McCullough,
Justin F. Deniset, Andrea L. Edel, Andrew Francis,
Delfin Rodriguez-Leyva, Mirna N. Chahine, and
Grant N. Pierce
University of Manitoba

CONTENTS

1.1   INTRODUCTION

Coronary artery atherosclerosis is the principle cause of cardiovascular morbidity and mortality in North America (Yusuf et al., 2004; Rosamond et al., 2007). Atherosclerosis is a progressive degenerative disease which involves a chronic inflammatory response and an accumulation of macrophages and LDL cholesterol in the walls of arteries. This results in the narrowing and stenosis of blood vessels. Atheromatous plaques develop in the subendothelial space of arteries and consist of soft, yellowish differentiated macrophages that have engulfed cholesterol and lipids, referred to as foam cells, and areas of cholesterol crystal formation and/or calcification in advanced fibrous plaques. Atherosclerosis induces two significant pathological processes: an ischemic event due to blood flow obstruction and vascular contractile dysfunction.

Elevated circulating cholesterol levels have long been associated with the development of atherosclerosis and cardiovascular risk. The lipid hypothesis, first proposed in the mid-nineteenth century by the German pathologist Virchow, suggested that the accumulation of blood lipids causes atherosclerosis (Virchow, 1856). This belief was supported by several studies demonstrating that feeding rabbits cholesterol induces atherosclerosis (Anitschkow, 1913; Schwenke and Carew, 1988; Kinscherf et al., 2003). Further evidence demonstrating that cardiovascular risk can be reduced by either limiting dietary cholesterol intake or inhibiting endogenous cholesterol production by cholesterol-lowering drugs has contributed to our current understanding of the role of cholesterol and lipids in atherosclerotic disease. However, cardiovascular risk is not entirely dependent on circulating cholesterol levels. Many cardiovascular events occur in individuals with cholesterol concentrations below the National Cholesterol Education Program thresholds of 200 mg/dL for total cholesterol (TC) and 130 mg/dL for low-density lipoprotein (LDL) cholesterol (Packard and Libby, 2008). Therefore, other contributing factors have been implicated in atherosclerotic development.

1.2   PATHOGENESIS OF ATHEROSCLEROSIS

According to the "Response to Injury" model, Ross postulates that atherosclerosis is an inflammatory condition preceded by endothelial cell (EC) dysfunction (Ross, 1993a,b). This "injury" to the arterial endothelium results from the alteration in cell attachment to the arterial lining, so that shear blood flow causes desquamation of the endothelium. Adherence and aggregation of platelets ensue at the site of injury. The endothelium becomes dysfunctional and susceptible to atherogenesis in response to stress or injury. The following key processes are involved during atherogenesis: (1) endothelial injury, (2) inflammation, (3) accumulation of cholesterol and lipids and the infiltration of monocytes into the subendothelial space, (4) macrophage differentiation and foam cell formation, (5) migration and proliferation of smooth muscle cells (SMCs), (6) local thrombus formation, (7) calcification and/or plaque rupture, and (8) final occlusion due to plaque rupture/thrombus formation (Hanke et al., 2001).

1.3   ENDOTHELIAL DYSFUNCTION AND CARDIOVASCULAR DISEASE

Damage to the endothelial lining of arteries upsets the balance between vasoconstriction and vasodilation and initiates a number of processes that promote or exacerbate atherosclerosis; these include increased endothelial permeability, platelet aggregation, leukocyte adhesion, and generation of cytokines (Ross, 1999; Davignon and Ganz, 2004). The hallmark of endothelial dysfunction is impaired endothelium-dependent vasodilation, which is mediated by nitric oxide (NO). Decreased production or activity of NO, manifested as impaired vasodilation, may be one of the earliest signs of atherosclerosis (Celermajer, 1997). Under normal healthy conditions, eNOS generates low concentrations of NO which protects against atherosclerosis and contributes to vessel homeostasis by regulating vascular tone and blood pressure, preventing platelet aggregation and adherence, and by inhibiting vascular smooth muscle cells (VSMC) contraction and proliferation (Cooke, 2003;

Moncada and Higgs, 2006). Paradoxically, higher concentrations of NO generated by iNOS contributes to atherosclerosis by LDL oxidation and activating macrophages, among other mechanisms (De Caterina and Massaro, 1999).

Following endothelial injury, the endothelial lining of arteries loses its ability to normally act as a barrier to blood constituents, control vascular responses, and inhibit platelet aggregation. The endothelium becomes pro-adhesive through cytokine-induced endothelial activation, which is important for the initiation and progression of atherosclerosis since it enables surface expression of endothelial leukocyte adhesion molecules and secretion of soluble proinflammatory products, such as interleukins-1 and -6 (IL-1 and IL-6), tumor necrosis factor-alpha (TNF-α), vascular cell adhesion molecule-1 (VCAM-1), platelet-derived growth factors (PDGFs), and monocyte chemoattractant proteins (MCP) (De Caterina et al., 2000). Because most adhesion molecules and inflammatory products are not expressed under basal conditions, cytokine-induced endothelial activation requires initiation of gene transcription. Nuclear factor NF-κB, a gene regulatory protein implicated in the development of atherosclerosis, can activate gene transcription and expression of adhesion molecules (De Caterina et al., 2000). Thus, damage to the endothelial lining, due to factors such as hypertension, hypercholesterolemia, and systemic inflammation causes an infiltration of monocytes and lipoproteins, including LDL and oxidized LDL (oxLDL), into the subendothelial space of the arterial wall. Two adhesion molecules expressed following endothelial activation aid in the infiltration of substrates into the subendothelial space. Selectins cause monocytes to loosely adhere and roll along the inflammation-activated ECs and integrins mediate firm attachment which enables monocytes to infiltrate into the subendothelial space (Packard and Libby, 2008). There, monocytes differentiate into macrophages which engulf lipids and cholesterol to become foam cells. Macrophages secrete cytokines that encourage further infiltration of monocytes into the subendothelial space and promote the differentiation and migration of smooth muscles cells into the lesion area. As the lesion progresses, the foam cells accumulate and apoptose to form the necrotic lipid core of the atherosclerotic lesion.

Atherosclerotic lesions can eventually become large, calcified, fibrous plaques that limit or occlude blood flow, or unstable plaques that rupture to form a thrombus, resulting in clinical symptoms (angina) and cardiovascular complications, such as arrhythmias, ischemic heart disease, peripheral vascular disease, myocardial infarction, and cerebrovascular disease (stroke). Atherosclerosis involves multiple processes including inflammation, oxidation, vascular proliferation and migration, and endothelial dysfunction.

1.4 INVOLVEMENT OF INFLAMMATION AND INFECTIOUS DISEASE IN CARDIOVASCULAR DISEASE

1.4.1 INNATE IMMUNITY AND ATHEROSCLEROSIS

The innate immune system, comprised of a network of specialized cells, is responsible for mediating the initial inflammatory actions in response to tissue damage and foreign particles within the body. Monocyte-derived macrophages were the first immune cells to be identified within atherosclerotic lesions (Gerrity et al., 1979) and represent a major component of the innate immune network during atherosclerotic development. They are involved in disease progression through their involvement in lipid metabolism and initial immune mediation (Glass and Witztum, 2001). Pattern-recognition receptors which include scavenger receptors (SRs) and toll-like receptors (TLRs) expressed on the cell surface are important components for both of these functions. SRs bind and mediate the uptake of modified LDL found within the vessel wall. During normal lipid loading, macrophages mediate reverse cholesterol transport by expressing proteins involved in cholesterol efflux (Wang et al., 2007). However, under conditions of constant lipid loading this mechanism is overwhelmed and excessive lipid storing leads to foam cell formation and subsequent production and release of proinflammatory molecules such as cytokines and reactive oxygen species (Shibata and Glass, 2009). TLRs recognize a broad range of targets that not only include pathogen-derived antigens such as lipopolysaccharide (LPS) but also endogenous molecules such as heat-shock proteins (HSPs). Upon binding to TLRs, these molecules will stimulate downstream signaling cascades leading to activation of transcription factors such as nuclear factor kappa-light-chain-enhancer of activated B cells (NF-κB) that are involved in the production of inflammatory mediators. TLRs appear to play an important role in atherosclerosis. Their expression is not limited to macrophages within the vessel wall and multiple members of its family are upregulated during human atherosclerosis (Edfeklt et al., 2002). Furthermore, a deficiency in TLR2 and/or TLR4 signaling reduces atherosclerotic development in atherogenic-prone mice (Bjorkbacka et al., 2004; Mullick et al., 2005).

Other members of the innate immune system have also been localized within atherosclerotic lesions. Mast cells have been found in the adventitia and shoulder regions of atherosclerotic plaque (Lindstedt et al., 2007). Once activated, mast cells may contribute to atherothrombosis through the release of proinflammatory cytokines and proteolytic enzymes. Atherogenic-prone mice deficient in mast cells display decreased atherosclerosis with a reduction in leukocyte population, apoptosis, and necrosis within the plaque (Sun et al., 2007). In addition, an increase in fibrous cap formation and collagen production was found. These effects were dependent upon interferon (IFN)-γ and interleukin (IL)-6 release. Mast cells are also involved in lipid metabolism (Heikkila et al., 2010) and cholesterol efflux (Lee et al., 2002). Dendritic cells, which can be localized in the intimal region of normal vessels, increase in number upon lesion progression (Galkina and Ley, 2009) and their recruitment appears to be VCAM-1 dependent (Jongstra-Bilen et al., 2006). They have the potential to prime naive T lymphocytes through antigen presentation and thereby provide a link between the innate and adaptive immune system.

1.4.2 ADAPTIVE IMMUNITY AND ATHEROSCLEROSIS

The adaptive immune system offers the body a more refined network to fight pathogens and foreign molecules. It differs from the innate immune system because it is initially slower, is dependent on past exposure and provides more specificity. T lymphocytes, the key mediators of the adaptive response, are recruited to the lesion during early and late atherosclerotic development where they undergo activation (Hansson et al., 1989). Additionally, the presence of oxLDL- (Paulsson et al., 2000), HSP60- (Rossmann et al., 2008), and *Chlamydia pneumoniae* (Cpn)-specific (Mosorin et al., 2000) T cells provide evidence of clonal expansion within the vessel wall. There exist two major subtypes of helper T (Th) cells involved in plaque development, Th1 and Th2. Th1 cells are the predominant form within the plaque (Bui et al., 2009) and promote atherogenesis by secreting proinflammation cytokines, inducing macrophage activation and driving cell-mediated responses (Romagnani, 2000). Th2 cells appear more antiatherogenic by secreting cytokines such as IL-4, -5, and -10 that drive antibody production, and inhibit Th1 responses. Regulatory T (Treg) lymphocytes, mediators of immune tolerance within the body, play an important role in controlling Th1/Th2 switching (Sakaguchi et al., 2006). Induction of Treg cells in atherosclerotic-prone mice lead to inhibition of Th1 responses and reduced atherosclerotic development. These changes were accompanied by decreased IFN-γ levels and increased IL-10 levels (Mallat et al., 2003). B cells, effector cells of the humoral immune response, produce antibodies that recognize specific antigens. Recent findings have suggested that natural antibodies against oxLDL (oxLDL IgM) may play a protective role in preventing atherosclerosis (Caligiuri et al., 2002; Major et al., 2002). These natural antibodies act by binding oxLDL molecules to prevent their uptake by macrophages, and block the subsequent inflammatory response and potential presentation of self-antigen to T lymphocytes (Binder et al., 2005).

1.4.3 INFECTION AND ATHEROSCLEROSIS

The important involvement of a host immune response in the development of atherosclerosis has prompted interest in infectious agents as potential triggers for the disease. Initial work in this field was pioneered by Fabricant et al. in the late 1970s when they showed that an avian herpes virus (Marek's disease virus) is able to promote atherosclerotic lesions in chickens (Fabricant et al., 1978). Since then, numerous investigations have established an association between coronary artery disease (CAD) and human pathogens such as *Chlamydia pneumoniae* (Cpn), *Cytomegalovirus* (CMV), Herpes simplex virus (HSV), *Helicobacter pylori* (*H. pylori*), periodontal pathogens, and more recently human immunodeficiency virus (HIV) (Adam et al., 1987; Saikku et al., 1988: Thom et al., 1992; Mendall et al., 1994; Sorlie et al., 1994; Bruggeman, 2000; Moutsopoulos and Madianos, 2006; Lo et al., 2010).

Various mechanisms have been proposed to describe the involvement of these microorganisms. First, invasion of vascular cells can stimulate cellular changes that can lead to vascular remodeling. Cpn and CMV have been recovered from human atheromas (Gyorkey et al., 1984; Hendricks et al., 1990; Grayston et al., 1995; Ramirez, 1996) and are proposed to be transported to these areas via monocytes from the lungs and bone marrow, respectively (Epstein et al., 1999). Both can reside in ECs and SMCs of the vessel wall and are able to initiate pro-atherogenic effects such as adhesion molecule expression, SMC proliferation, cytokine production, and matrix metalloprotease production (Span et al., 1991; Kaukoranta-Tolvanen et al., 1996; Speir et al., 1998; Dechend et al., 1999; Hirono et al., 2003; Rodel et al., 2003). Pathogens have the ability to initiate inflammatory responses through activation of TLRs on macrophages, ECs, and VSMCs. Their ligands include membrane components of bacteria and bacterial HSPs. Cellular components (i.e., LPS, HSP) of Cpn, *H. pylori*, and *Porphyromonas gingivalis* can stimulate atherogenic effects in these cell types via TLR binding (Sasu et al., 2001; Triantafilou et al., 2007; Chen et al., 2008; Jiang et al., 2008). In addition to their ability to stimulate TLR signaling, HSPs may play a role in autoimmune responses during atherosclerosis. HSPs are highly conserved between species and as such, immune responses directed to bacterial HSPs may cross react with self-HSP antigens (Young and Elliott, 1989). Antibodies against human HSP60 correlate with the incidence and severity of atherosclerotic development (Zhu et al., 2001). Infectious agents may also play more of an indirect role by stimulating systemic responses. Periodontal pathogens have been shown to induce acute phase reactants (Slade et al., 2000).

There is considerable evidence to support the involvement of infectious disease in the development of atherosclerosis. However, it remains debatable whether pathogens are causal agents for the progression of the disease. As such, further research is needed to better understand the role of both the immune system and these pathogens.

1.4.4 Oxidized LDL and Atherosclerosis

Atherosclerosis has long been regarded as a state of heightened oxidation stress.

Numerous studies report elevated levels of oxLDL in the plasma of patients with demonstrated atherosclerotic disease, and that these high levels can be used to predict the patients' risk of myocardial infarction (Ehara et al., 2001; Inoue et al., 2001; Tsimikas et al., 2003). In addition, autoantibodies to oxLDL have also been reported in atherosclerotic lesions of cardiac patient (Ehara et al., 2001). Oxidized LDL demonstrates many atherogenic actions; oxLDL is involved in foam cell formation, it is cytotoxic for ECs in culture, it acts as a chemoattractant for monocyte–macrophages and it inhibits the vasodilatative effect of NO (Hessler et al., 1983; Quinn et al., 1987; Albertini et al., 2002). LDL oxidation is a free radical-driven chain reaction where polyunsaturated fatty acids are converted into lipid peroxides, which decompose to biologically active products, such as aldehydes (Albertini et al., 2002). Oxidation of LDL enhances the accumulation of cholesterol in macrophages, leading to foam cell formation and initiation of atherosclerotic process. Unlike native LDL, oxLDL binds to receptors on the cellular membrane of macrophages, such as scavenger receptor A and CD36, which are not downregulated by intracellular cholesterol concentration (Boullier et al., 2001). There is therefore no negative-feedback loop for the accumulation of oxLDL in lipid-laden foam cells. The evidence that oxidants contribute to atherosclerotic disease is further supported by research in experimental animals that report that various antioxidant compounds (probucol, vitamin E) can prevent atherosclerosis (Albertini et al., 2002). Additionally, oxidized lipids may act as early mediators of a chronic inflammatory reaction through activation of transcription factors, such as nuclear factor-κB (NF-κB) or alternate pathways that induce the expression of genes which instigates fatty streak development (Berliner et al., 1995). oxLDL initiates a chain of molecular events leading to the transmigration of monocytes into the subendothelial space and their differentiation into macrophages. Mature macrophages in the subendothelial space further potentiate the degree of LDL oxidation and subsequent uptake, in addition to the progressive inflammatory response in the atheroma (Kutuk and Basaga, 2003).

1.4.5 ROLE OF CELL PROLIFERATION IN ATHEROSCLEROSIS

Another key atherogenic process involves the focal accumulation and proliferation of VSMCs into the neointimal space of arteries. Vascular proliferation is associated with other cellular processes such as inflammation, apoptosis, and matrix alterations (Dzau et al., 2002). VSMCs contribute to the development of atherosclerotic lesions via the production of proinflammatory mediators such as VCAM-1 and MCP-1 and matrix molecules required for the retention of lipoproteins (Dzau et al., 2002). In turn, inflammatory mediators, growth factors, and both LDL and mildly oxLDL further induce VSMC proliferation (Koba et al., 1999). VSMC proliferation and migration is also important in maintaining the stability of the atherosclerotic plaque, as VSMCs, fibroblasts, and extracellular calcification are the main constituents of the fibrocalcific cap enclosing advanced atherosclerotic lesions (Dzau et al., 2002). The fibrous cap surrounding lipid-laden lesions is often thin and weak, due to inflammatory processes which induce the expression of collagenase and proteolytic inhibitors resulting in extracellular matrix degradation and VSMC apoptosis (Dzau et al., 2002; Libby et al., 2002). VSMC proliferation and migration is an ongoing process during atherogenesis that provides an essential fibrous cap that could prevent plaque rupture. However, excessive and uncontrolled VSMC proliferation and migration can prove detrimental. Loss of growth-inhibitory factors, occurring as a result of either endothelial dysfunction which decreases EC secretion of NO, or by the inactivation of NO by reactive oxygen species, may contribute to excessive migration and proliferation of VSMCs and to an increased inflammatory response, resulting in unstable plaques and increased risk of myocardial infarctions and stroke (Dzau et al., 2002).

1.4.6 ADIPOKINES AND CORONARY ARTERY DISEASE

Adipocytes, the cells that store lipids and make up the bulk of adipose tissue stores in the body, are now known to have an important physiological role beyond their lipid storage capacity. Adipocytes, as well as stromal–vascular cells, including macrophages, in adipose tissue, secrete a number of important cellular signaling molecules, termed adipokines. These adipokines have consequences ranging from autocrine and paracrine effects, to systemic endocrine actions. Adipokines also vary widely in both their function and mechanisms of control. One such mechanism of control is the fatty acid composition of adipose tissue, which can affect cellular signaling, fatty acid trafficking, gene expression and, consequently, metabolism (Gertow et al., 2006). Adipose tissue composition varies based on three main effectors: energy balance, which regulates the metabolism of free fatty acids (FFAs) within the adipose tissue, and diet, which will alter the fatty acid profile of the adipose tissue, and physical location, as local factors can influence fatty acid storage and lipolysis. When an individual consumes more calories than they can immediately metabolize, lipids are stored as energy in the adipose tissue. A person who is consistently in a state of caloric excess will gain fat tissue, and consequently become obese. During obesity, the adipokine profile shifts dramatically from an anti-inflammatory state to a proinflammatory state. Although these changes with caloric intake are well documented, the effects of the variations in dietary composition on the endocrine function of adipose tissue have only recently begun to be investigated.

1.5 ADIPOSE TISSUE SOURCES AND THEIR ROLES

Adipokines are expressed in both brown and white adipose tissue, however, brown adipose tissue's impact on systemic adipokine activity is believed to be negligible in most cases (Cannon and Nedergaard, 2004). White adipose tissue is the primary source of adipokines in circulation

(Wajchenberg, 2000; Trayhurn and Wood, 2004). White adipose tissue is deposited both subcutaneously and viscerally, and these two types of deposits have differential expression of adipokines (Wajchenberg, 2000). Subcutaneous white adipose tissue is located beneath the derma, and primarily functions for thermoregulation, expressing uncoupling proteins and preventing heat loss through the skin. Generally, it expresses low levels of most adipokines, having little effect on systemic levels of these adipokines, although it may have important paracrine effects on insulin sensitivity in skeletal muscle. Subcutaneous adipose tissue is also the primary source of the beneficial, anti-inflammatory adipokine, adiponectin (Lihn et al., 2004). Visceral adipose tissue is located in the abdomen, and in adult humans, by mass, consists mainly of retroperitoneal, perirenal, mesenteric, and omental tissue. Smaller visceral sources such as epicardial adipose tissue have special significance for cardiovascular disease due to the close proximity to the myocardium as well as the coronary left anterior descending artery (Sacks and Fain, 2007). Perivascular adipose tissue also surrounds most vessels. From this location, adipocytes may infiltrate into the adventitia, where they can have paracrine actions on endothelial and VSMC without affecting circulating adipokine levels (Henrichot et al., 2005; Sacks and Fain, 2007). In general, visceral sources of adipose tissue highly express both anti- and proinflammatory adipokines, while thermoregulatory activities play a minor role in their function.

1.5.1 Fatty Acid Metabolism

After being consumed, fatty acids cross the intestinal wall in lipid-rich chylomicrons, which are then taken up by the lymphatic system and shunted into the blood stream (Large et al., 2004). Once in the blood, FFAs bind to albumin or circulate in lipoproteins, and can be used to provide for immediate energy needs. However, over 95% of consumed fatty acids are stored for later use (Large et al., 2004). In addition to the consumption of fats, the adipose tissue can produce many required fatty acids de novo from carbohydrates. However, animals cannot create omega-3 or omega-6 fatty acids, and therefore, these key polyunsaturated fatty acids are termed essential fatty acids, as they must originate from the diet.

In the adipose tissue, chylomicrons and very low-density lipoproteins (VLDLs) have the lipids extracted by lipoprotein lipase (Large et al., 2004). The fats are then transferred into the adipocytes by one of two methods. The fatty acids can insert into the lipid bilayer of the adipocyte cell membrane, where they can be flipped across the bilayer to the intracellular side of the membrane. Although long believed to be the primary means of entry into the cell, the efficiency of this process is subject to debate. Lipids may also be transferred into cells enzymatically, a much more rapid and chemically favorable situation than a lipid "flip-flop." Adipocytes produce numerous proteins to facilitate the uptake of lipids. Fatty acid transport protein (FATP) and fatty acid translocase (FAT) are responsible for the transfer of the lipids from the external environment to the cytoplasm, while fatty acid binding proteins (FABP) bind lipids in order to shuttle them to the translocators. Once inside the cell, the fatty acids are then stored in the form of triacylglycerols—a three-carbon chain with three fatty acid ester groups. Changes in the quantity as well as the type of lipids stored in adipocytes can dramatically affect the cell's function and thus the signal it secretes.

The release of FFAs from the adipose into the plasma is a highly regulated event under normal conditions (Koutsari and Jensen, 2006). This process ensures fatty acids are systemically available for β-oxidation, a major energy source for most tissues, including the heart. However, high BMI has been associated with increased FFA levels as lipolysis in the adipose increases. High FFA levels are an independent risk factor for atherosclerosis, hypertension, and sudden cardiac death (Fagot-Campagna et al., 1998; Jouven et al., 2001; Sarafidis and Bakris, 2007). Increased levels of FFAs are also known to directly contribute to hepatic steatosis and insulin resistance, through inhibition of glucose uptake (Bays et al., 2004; Roden, 2004). It is also important to note, however, that FFAs are in a continuous state of flux within the body, and vary based on hormones, activity, fitness levels, and diet (Roden, 2004). Therefore, changes in FFA levels without establishment of baseline fluctuations should be interpreted with caution.

1.5.2 ADIPONECTIN

Adiponectin (Acrp30) is the most highly expressed and secreted adipokine, with beneficial effects on metabolism, inflammation, and vascular function (Scherer et al., 1995). The sole source of circulating adiponectin is the adipose tissue. In healthy individuals, adiponectin acts as an insulin-sensitizing agent and antioxidant, suppresses proinflammatory cytokines such as TNF-α and IL-6, and increases eNOS activation, causing vasodilation. However, adiponectin has a paradoxical expression—as adiposity increases, adiponectin expression and secretion decreases within the adipose tissue (Arita et al., 1999). This dichotomy is a function of the inhibitory effects of TNF-α on adiponectin expression (Sowers, 2008). Adiponectin suppresses TNF-α expression in the adipose tissue, but if TNF-α upregulation signals are stronger than adiponectin's downregulative effects, as in obesity, the system can rapidly switch to a proinflammatory phenotype (Figure 1.1). It is believed that these changes play an important role in the initiation of pathological obesity, and are symptomatic of dysfunctional adipose tissue. Adiponectin also has roles in inhibiting LDL oxidation, and increasing fatty acid catabolism. Thus, hypoadiponectinemia is of interest as a biomarker of cardiovascular disease and metabolic syndrome.

Polyunsaturated fats have diverse impacts on adiponectin production in the adipose tissue. Omega-3 fatty acid accumulation in the adipose tissue can increase levels of adiponectin in the healthy children of type-II diabetes patients, as well as in obese humans, mice, and rats (Duque-Guimaraes et al., 2009; Gonzalez-Periz et al., 2009; Kuda et al., 2009; Rizza et al., 2009). Omega-3 fatty acids inhibit TNF-α production through enzymatic competition with arachidonic acid, a precursor to the proinflammatory eicosanoid. Thus, the consumption of omega-3 polyunsaturates can ameliorate the downregulation of adiponectin production, leading to a recovery of adiponectin levels in the plasma (Gonzalez-Periz et al., 2009). Conversely, adiponectin expression may be suppressed by the same pathway, through the bioconversion of omega-6 fatty acids into proinflammatory eicosanoids, leading to TNF-α production. In this way, a diet rich in omega-3 fatty acids may

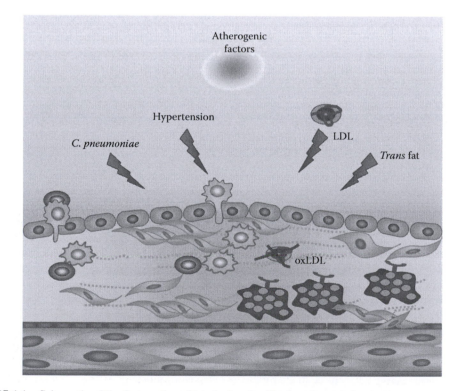

FIGURE 1.1 Schematic of the factors thought to be involved in the atherogenic process.

suppress adiponectin production. Other polyunsaturates which affect adiponectin include the numerous isomers of conjugated linoleic acid, such as *trans*-10, *cis*-12-CLA. CLA has variable effects on adiponectin production. In one human study looking at a population of healthy postmenopausal women, CLA suppressed adiponectin via unknown mechanisms, despite its other beneficial effects on the cardiovascular function and obesity (Raff et al., 2009). However, in hypertensive patients, CLA had the opposite effect on adiponectin expression, while still showing cardiovascular benefits (Zhao et al., 2009). In rats, dietary CLA alternatively increased or did not affect adiponectin production (Lopes et al., 2008; Raff et al., 2009). As the effects of dietary supplementation of CLA are variable, its mechanism for adiponectin regulation should be identified.

1.5.3 LEPTIN

Leptin was first discovered by Zhang et al. in 1994 as the protein encoded by the *obese* gene, named for the phenotype of the double knockout mouse (Zhang et al., 1994). These mice experience no satiety, and thus eat continuously when fed ad libidum, leading to severe diet-induced obesity. After a meal, the body metabolizes the nutrients that were consumed in order to meet its current energy needs. Once these needs have been met, excess calories are stored in the form of lipids in the adipose tissue. This storage process induces the release of leptin to the blood stream, where it can cross the blood–brain barrier to the hypothalamus and suppresses hunger. In humans, genetic or metabolic leptin deficiencies have been implicated in cases of morbid obesity, especially in children (Gibson et al., 2004). Leptin's canonical role of hypothalamic appetite suppression in response to caloric intake, however, is not its only function. It is expressed in numerous other tissues, although the only other source of leptin in circulation is the placenta, where it plays a role in the suppression of uterine contraction and is vital for early pregnancy maintenance (Moynihan et al., 2006; Toth et al., 2009).

Leptin receptors are present in the brain, liver, lung, heart, skeletal muscle, spleen, kidney, and testes (Kawachi et al., 2007). Plasma leptin levels have clinically been associated with body fat and short-term energy balance, due to its important roles in hunger suppression. However, chronic leptin expression may also be important in modulation of T-cell activity in the early stages of atherosclerotic development, as well as other immune cells (Taleb et al., 2007). Obesity can affect leptin in one of two ways: leptin may be under-expressed by the adipose in response to a consistent high-caloric diet, or, more commonly, leptin receptors in the periphery may be downregulated, leading to elevated plasma leptin and leptin resistance (Dubey and Hesong, 2006). Leptin resistance is widespread in obesity-associated cardiovascular diseases, such as hypertension, atherosclerosis, myocardial infarction, and heart failure (Phillips et al., 2010). *Ex vivo*, leptin treatments at pathophysiologically high levels have been shown to induce endothelial dysfunction through the suppression of endothelial nitric oxide synthase (eNOS) (Procopio et al., 2009). Although in general, leptin appears to exacerbate cardiovascular issues in disease-state individuals, it is important to note that this adipokine is still highly expressed in the healthy state.

The effects of consumption of polyunsaturated fatty acids on leptin expression are not well understood. When evaluating changes in leptin, a key point to consider is that leptin expression is also affected by caloric intake. Therefore, the effects of dietary components in the absence of an isocaloric control should be interpreted with caution. Early work on nutritional effects on adipokine expression indicated that the addition of fish oils (EPA and DHA) to the diet had no effect on leptin (Flachs et al., 2006). Recent evidence indicates that in animals fed a regular diet supplemented with an omega-3 PUFA found in flaxseed, α-linolenic acid, leptin expression increases independently of caloric intake (McCullough et al., 2010). In diet-induced obese rats, addition of conjugated linoleic acid (CLA) to a diet high in saturated fats decreased leptin expression in both brown and white visceral adipose tissue (Gudbrandsen et al., 2009). Clinical investigations have identified a leptin receptor polymorphism which puts individuals most at risk for insulin resistance and metabolic syndrome (Phillips et al., 2010). In individuals with this leptin receptor polymorphism, a low omega-3, high omega-6 diet increases their risk for insulin resistance. However, when these individuals ate a high omega-3, low omega-6 diet, there was an apparent masking of the deleterious genotype. Consumption of monounsaturated fatty acids, in contrast, had no effect on risk of metabolic syndrome. Although the specific role of polyunsaturated fatty acids in regulation of leptin expression and signaling has not been fully elucidated, it is clear that omega-3 PUFAs have an important role in leptin expression and signaling.

1.5.4 RESISTIN

Resistin was first identified in 2001 in a screen for adipocytes genes that were downregulated after treatment with antidiabetic drugs (Steppan et al., 2001). It is an important obesity-related adipokine in rodents, although in humans it is expressed primarily in the macrophages and may or may not be related to insulin resistance (Nogueiras et al., 2010). In mice and rats, it is expressed robustly and almost exclusively in visceral white adipose tissue, and serum concentrations correlate positively with insulin resistance and obesity (Steppan et al., 2001). It is important for the maintenance of hyperglycemia and insulin resistance in diabetic individuals, acting as an insulin antagonist in circulation. Furthermore, resistin promotes the activation of vascular ECs through VCAM-1 and MCP-1 upregulation, and has been associated with increased severity of atherosclerosis (Verma et al., 2003). In human adipose tissue, resistin is produced in lympho-cytes, monocytes, and macrophages, but not primary adipocytes (Nagaev et al., 2006). Although some evidence indicates that resistin may be of use as a biomarker for obesity in human beings (Pischon, 2009; Wang et al., 2009), clinical data generally do not support a direct role for resistin in insulin resistance or cardiovascular disease in human beings (Lee et al., 2003; Aeberli et al., 2009; Won et al., 2009).

In culture, exposure of murine adipocytes to both short- and long-chain omega-3 and omega-6 polyunsaturated fatty acids reduced resistin expression (Haugen et al., 2005). However, in animal models, no effects on resistin have been observed with either type of dietary PUFA (Duque-Guimaraes et al., 2009; Gonzalez-Periz et al., 2009). Despite the effects of PUFAs on insulin resistance, there appears to be no *in vivo* correlation with resistin. However, dietary interventions that assess resistin are limited, and therefore it may be premature to assert that they are unrelated.

1.5.5 TUMOR NECROSIS FACTOR-ALPHA

Tumor necrosis factor-alpha (TNF-α) is most notable for its roles in inflammation. TNF-α is acutely secreted in large quantities by macrophages as a key mediator of local immune response to infection (McKellar et al., 2009). However, it is also produced in low doses by numerous tissues, including the adipose. The production of TNF-α can lead to a chronic low-grade state of inflammation, one of the hallmarks of obesity, and a key player in the progression of atherosclerosis. In adipose, TNF-α plays a major role in obesity through its autocrine and paracrine actions. TNF-α leads to the activation of the MAPK pathway, and downstream second messenger NF-κB, which directly opposes the benefi-cial effects of adiponectin (Zhao et al., 2005). Furthermore, as discussed previously, TNF-α inhibits the production of adiponectin, exacerbating the proinflammatory state of the adipose tissue (Figure 1.2). It is hypothesized that this shift from anti-inflammatory to proinflammatory endocrine activi-ties leads to the pathogenesis of obesity. Although TNF-α has clinical importance for numerous reasons, it is notable in the context of obesity, diet, and cytokines for its associations with endothe-lial dysfunction, insulin resistance, and macrophage infiltration.

Omega-3 PUFAs inhibit the production of inflammatory cytokines, including TNF-α (Rudkowska et al., 2010). Numerous studies have associated dietary omega-3 fatty acids with reductions in plasma TNF-α (Zeitlin et al., 2003), and omega-3 treatment of macrophages with decreases in TNF-α secretion. *In vitro*, adipocytes treated with docosahexaenoic acid (DHA), one of the major

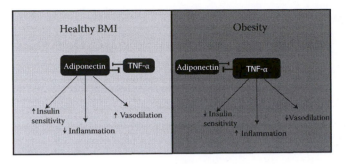

FIGURE 1.2 The adiponectin paradox. When individuals are healthy weight, the adipose tissue produces enough adiponectin to suppress the expression of the TNF-α. This suppression of TNF-α leads to a predominance of adiponectin production. This causes a decrease in systemic inflammation and ultimately results in increases in insulin sensitivity and the vasodilation capacity of the blood vessels. During obesity, TNF-α is upregulated causing increased suppression of adiponectin. Consequently, the adipose tissue of an obese individual produces far less adiponectin, shifting to a proinflammatory, damaging cytokine profile. (Adapted from Sowers, J. R. 2008. *Clin. Cornerstone.* **9**(1): 32–38.)

omega-3s in fish, did not exhibit any changes in TNF-α secretion. Furthermore, TNF-α has been correlated with changes in BMI after PUFA supplementation (Mehra et al., 2006).

1.5.6 C-Reactive Protein

Like TNF-α, C-reactive protein (CRP) is an important biomarker for inflammation, mainly secreted from the liver, but also from adipocytes (Du Clos et al., 2004). CRP production is stimulated by interleukin-6 production by macrophages and adipocytes. It has roles in innate immunity, binding foreign or damaged cells and targeting them for phagocytosis. It is dramatically upregulated in response to acute infection, but it is a current marker of interest due to its use as a cardiovascular risk factor. In a healthy population, chronically elevated CRP levels predict future metabolic syndrome and cardiovascular disease, from stroke to peripheral artery disease to myocardial infarction (Ridker et al., 2003). Furthermore, its predictive value is independent of other well-established biomarkers. In animal research, CRP appears to play an active role in atherosclerosis. CRP treatment reduces NO production by the ECs, upregulates monocyte infiltration, increases the production of reactive oxygen species, and stimulates VSMC proliferation and migration within the vessel walls (Venugopal et al., 2005). Elevated CRP levels also have been shown to be associated with cancer risk in healthy individuals and with increased mortality after cancer diagnosis, especially in nonmetastatic cancers (Allin et al., 2009).

As CRP is an inflammatory marker, and omega-3 PUFAs act in an anti-inflammatory fashion, it can be predicted that omega-3s will reduce CRP levels. This is usually but not always the case. Several human and animal trials showed a significant reduction of circulating CRP with the addition of fish oil to the diet (Saifullah et al., 2007; Zhang et al., 2009). In other clinical trials, CRP did not appear to vary as a direct result of the addition of fatty acids to the diet (Pischon et al., 2003; St-Onge et al., 2009). Instead, starting CRP concentrations predicted the benefits of a high PUFA diet. Individuals with high CRP levels (i.e., those most at risk for cardiovascular disease) gain more benefit from the lipid-lowering effects of omega-3 polyunsaturates (St-Onge et al., 2009). The disparity between these trials, which gave similar levels of omega-3 fatty acids, can be explained by the omega-3/omega-6 ratio (Simopoulos, 2008). If the experimental diet provided a high omega-6 content in conjunction with the omega-3s, emulating the ratio of a Western Diet (16 omega-6:1 omega-3), no effects on CRP were seen. However, if the relative omega-6 content was reduced to 4:1 or less, plasma CRP decreased (Zampelas et al., 2003). Whether this change is due to a decrease in omega-6 content, or the relative increase in omega-3 content has not yet been elucidated. Furthermore, the source of the plasma CRP in these studies—the hepatocytes or adipocytes—is unclear.

1.6 BIOMARKERS OF CORONARY ARTERY DISEASE

The progression of atherosclerosis in humans is the result of a complex myriad of events that are regulated by a number of factors (Libby, 2002). In response to this "silently" progressing disease, the vascular endothelium and vessel lumen produce a number of inflammatory markers and mediators that in turn yield a cascade of other signaling molecules. Soluble forms of these molecules then enter the circulatory system at various stages throughout the development of the disease. At certain stages of disease progression, levels of specific signaling molecules are more elevated than others. The first few stages observed in the pathogenesis of atherosclerosis, referred to as the acute phase reactants, comprise plaque formation and progression, plaque destabilization and rupture followed by thrombus formation. Cardiac ischemia and necrosis are the final stages. Significant interest lies in isolating which markers are most prevalent at specific stages during atherogenesis so that therapeutic interventions can be implemented prior to the onset of possible irreversible cardiac damage brought on by an ischemic event.

By definition, a biomarker is a quantifiable biological parameter which provides information regarding ones health status, that is, it helps in elucidating disease risk, disease status (preclinical or clinical), or the rate at which the disease progresses (Sharrett et al., 2001; Vasan, 2006). A number of invasive and noninvasive methods for obtaining biomarkers of coronary heart disease (CHD) are available to clinicians. These include (1) biological tests involving blood, urine, or tissue samples, (2) medical imaging tests such as cardiac catheterization, positron emission tomography, intravascular ultrasound, cardiac ECHOs, computed tomography angiography, and magnetic resonance imaging, and (3) physiological and electrophysiological tests such as blood pressure, electrocardiographs (ECGs), events and Holter monitoring and cardiac stress testing, which provide extensive information regarding blood, arterial, or myocardial status. The focus of this section is to provide a brief overview of some of the principal circulating biomarkers that have demonstrated promising clinical relevance as biomarkers in the pathogenesis of CHD (Myers et al., 2004; Apple et al., 2005; Vasan, 2006; Dotsenko et al., 2008; Howie-Esquivel and White, 2008; Martin-Ventura et al., 2009; Rizvi, 2009; Zakynthinos and Pappa, 2009). Figure 1.3 provides an overview of some of the target circulating biomarkers and their place of reference in the pathogenesis of atherosclerosis. The following section will discuss how each biomarker is linked to CHD, whether or not the marker concentration increases as a result of injury, and the feasibility of using this marker within a clinical setting.

Although a wide range of circulating inflammatory markers is present during the development of atherosclerosis, only a few have found application in clinical settings. Several factors have influenced this. The simplicity in obtaining the biomarker for both the patient and clinician, analyte stability, effectiveness of the analyte as a biomarker (i.e., is the biomarker predictive of a specific pathological condition independent of other biomarkers; is it cardiac specific, etc.), ease of analytical methodologies, the cost of analysis, and the availability of a suitable reference standard are all important translational factors (Dotsenko et al., 2008).

1.6.1 BIOMARKERS OF PLAQUE FORMATION AND PROGRESSION

Abnormal lipid profiling is a key indicator for cardiovascular risk assessment. Individuals with abnormally high fasting levels of low-density lipoprotein-cholesterol (LDL-C) (>160 mg/dL), TC (>240 mg/dL), and triacylglycerides (TAGs) (>400 mg/dL) are assessed as high-risk patients in terms of their potential to develop CHD (Stein and Myers, 1995; Bachorik and Ross, 2001). Excessive levels of cholesterol that cannot be utilized and stored within the cell lead to the formation within the vessel lumen of a toxic form of cholesterol known as oxLDL (Meisinger et al., 2005). Generation of oxLDL leads to the production of a number of proinflammatory responses that are released at various stages during plaque formation. Cytokines [i.e., interleukin-1 (IL-1), IL-6, IL-18, TNF-α, soluble CD40 ligand, (sCD40L)], chemokines [i.e., monocyte chemoattractant protein-1 (MCP-1), interleukin-8 (IL-8)], C-reactive protein (CRP), apolipoprotein-B100 (apo-B100), lipoprotein-associated phospholipase A2 (LP-PLA2), and serum amyloid A (SAA), are just a few of these regulating molecules that

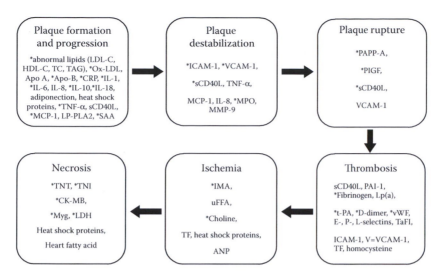

FIGURE 1.3 Biomarkers of cardiovascular disease. Markers with "*" in front of it are discussed within this section. Definitions: Apo A, apolipoprotein A; Apo B, apolipoprotein B; ANP, atrial natriuretic peptide; CK-MB, creatine kinase-MB fraction; CRP, C-reactive protein; IL, interleukin; ICAM-1, intercellular adhesion molecule-1; IMA, ischemia-modified albumin; LDL-C, low-density lipoprotein cholesterol; HDL-C, high-density lipoprotein cholesterol; LDH, lactate dehydrogenase; Lp(a), lipoprotein (a); LP = PLA2, lipoprotein-associated phospholipase A2; MCP-1, monocyte chemoattractant protein-1; MIP-1, macrophage inflammatory protein-1; MMP-9, matrix metalloproteinase-9; MPO, myeloperoxidase; Myg, myoglobin; ox-LDL, oxidized low-density lipoprotein PAI-1, plasminogen activator inhibitor-1; PAPP-A, pregnancy-associated plasma protein-A; PIGF, placental growth factor; SAA, serum amyloid A; sCD40L, soluble CD40 ligand; TAFI, thrombin activatable fibrinolysis inhibitor; TAG, triacylglycerides; TC, total cholesterol; TF, tissue factors, TNF-α, tumor necrosis factor; TNI, troponin I; TNT, troponin T; t-PA, tissue-type plasminogen activator; uFFA, unbound free fatty acids; VCAM-1, vascular cell adhesion molecule-1; and vWF, von Willebrand factor. (Adapted from Apple, F.S. et al. 2005. *Clin. Chem.* **51**(5): 810–824; Dotsenko, O. et al. *Curr. Pharm. Des.* **14**(24): 2445–2461.)

are turned on during this acute phase (Myers et al., 2004; Dotsenko et al., 2008; Rizvi, 2009; Zakynthinos and Pappa, 2009).

Of the markers of inflammation produced during plaque formation and progression in CHD, CRP has been the most studied. It is a marker of systemic inflammation and demonstrates increased circulating levels (several hundred fold) in response to tissue damage, infection, and inflammatory stimuli (Myers et al., 2004). CRP aids in macrophage uptake of LDL, signals the onset of LDL oxidation, minimizes vascular relaxation through the attenuation of NO, recruits monocytes into the vessel wall, and triggers the onset of tissue factor (TF) production in monocytes (Zwaka et al., 2001; Verma et al., 2002; Bassuk et al., 2004). A characteristic of CRP, which makes it unique and highly favorable in a clinical laboratory setting, is its stability in plasma or serum. Measurement of CRP is accomplished using commercial assays; however, chronic inflammatory levels appear at much lower concentrations than individuals who have acute inflammation. This has led to the design of high-sensitivity CRP (hsCRP) assays which offer lower limits of detection, thus enabling the prediction of CHD risk in apparently normal, healthy subjects, which is essential for early diagnosis and treatment (Hamwi et al., 2001). The American Heart Association (AHA) has defined baseline levels of hsCRP as <1 mg/L and levels >3 mg/L for high inflammation and bacterial infection. Although CRP is a valuable marker for identifying cardiovascular risk, it is advisable to screen patients using both CRP and cholesterol results as these associated values offer greater predictive power in cardiovascular disease risk assessment.

A number of cytokines and chemokines have been implicated in the pathogenesis of early atherosclerotic development. The major proteins that comprise this group are the interleukins (IL), some of which include IL-1, IL-6 and IL-10, TNF-α, and MCP-1 (Vasan, 2006; Dotsenko et al., 2008). IL-1 and IL-6, produced by hepatocytes, are precursors of CRP production. IL-6 promotes the expression of matrix metalloproteinases (MMPs), TNF-α, and MCP-1, which are all proinflammatory markers (Ridker et al., 2000; Blankenberg et al., 2002, 2003; Cesari et al., 2003; Pai et al., 2004). IL-10 is protective against proinflammatory mediators, whereas TNF-α promotes cellular apoptosis and induces inflammation (Ridker et al., 2000; Heeschen et al., 2003). Increased levels of the chemokine MCP-1 have been correlated with increased risk of death or myocardial infarction (MI). Its role in atherosclerosis is to recruit monocytes into the vessel lumen (Gu et al., 1998). These proteins are typically measured using enzyme-linked immunosorbent assay (ELISA) techniques, however, analyte instability and low levels of quantitation limit their use in clinical settings.

Controversy surrounds the role of SAA in the pathogenesis of atherosclerosis (Johnson et al., 2004; Jylhava et al., 2009). Increased production of SAA within the liver is the result of a direct response to inflammation, injury, infection, or stress (Uhlar and Whitehead, 1999). Inflammation due to atherosclerosis has been linked to elevated levels of SAA in cardiovascular disease (Song et al., 2009). Quantitation of SAA is not readily available at the clinical level yet, however, a nephelometric assay has been developed for research use only.

1.6.2 BIOMARKERS OF PLAQUE DESTABILIZATION AND RUPTURE

Plaque destabilization has been associated with increased levels of intracellular adhesion molecule-1 (ICAM-1), vascular adhesion molecule-1 (VCAM-1), soluble CD40 ligand (sCD40L), myeloperoxidase (MPO), pregnancy-associated plasma protein-A (PAPP-A), and placental growth factor (PlGF), amongst others. The soluble adhesion molecules sICAM-1 and sVCAM-1 play a role in the interaction between white blood cells, platelets, and the vascular wall, which is a key preliminary step in the atherosclerotic process (Blankenberg et al., 2001; Luc et al., 2003). These markers of inflammation offer no additional information than some of the better, more established markers (i.e., CRP), rendering them poor analytes in disease prognosis (Malik et al., 2001).

Soluble CD40L is another proinflammatory marker that has been identified in plaque instability. Elevated levels of sCD40L have been positively correlated with atherosclerotic progression and destabilization of the fibrous cap (Varo et al., 2003; Yan et al., 2004). Binding of sCD40L with its receptor results in the activation of platelets. As a consequence of this action, MMPs within the plaques are turned on which then signal the release of TF, thus increasing sCD40L concentrations within the blood and creating a pro-thrombotic environment. Clotting factors must be present at the time of blood collection to insure the accuracy of the measurement. This minimizes the activation of platelets that would otherwise continue to release sCD40L and alter actual levels. The use of this marker in clinical laboratories requires further research as it is not cardiac specific. Myeloperoxidase (MPO), an enzyme primarily found in monocytes and neutrophils, also demonstrates pro-atherogenic behavior (Meuwese et al., 2007). Catalytic modification of LDL to the more toxic ox-LDL is accomplished via MPO along with a reduction of NO levels, which interferes with normal endothelial functioning within the vasculature. Elevated concentrations of MPO have been positively correlated with CHD, independent of troponin levels, CRP and sCD40L, suggesting that MPO might independently be associated with cardiovascular risk assessment (Baldus et al., 2003). MPO risk was also identified in presumably healthy individuals as early serum MPO levels correlated with future risk of disease (Meuwese et al., 2007). Despite these positive trends observed in clinical cardiovascular models, MPO is not unique to vascular injury as monocytes and neutrophils respond to any pathological injury or infection.

Plaque rupture is identified by the presence of elevated circulating levels of pregnancy-associated plasma protein-A (PAPP-A) and PlGF (Bayes-Genis et al., 2001; Khosravi et al., 2002; Kaski and Holt, 2006; Lund et al., 2006; Sangiorgi et al., 2006). PAPP-A, an insulin-like growth factor, specifically binds metalloproteinase, which has previously been linked with plaque instability (Bayes-Genis et al., 2001). Elevated levels of PAPP-A significantly correlate with a future ischemic event (Lund et al., 2006). Its use as an independent marker of CHD is possible as increased levels of

PAPP-A do not correlate with either creatinine kinase-MB (CK-MB) or troponin-I, which are well-defined markers of cardiac necrosis (Bayes-Genis et al., 2001; Khosravi et al., 2002). Analysis of PAPP-A is accomplished using immunoassays with serum only, as anticoagulants have been found to skew results. Its relevance as a cardiac marker is also not well defined in that most immunoassays have been designed for use with pregnancy serum, which may behave differently from serum in patients with coronary disease.

PlGF levels correlate highly with negative outcomes in patients with suspected cardiovascular illness (Tarnow et al., 2005; Lenderink et al., 2006). A trial by Hattori and colleagues demonstrated that PlGF can inhibit plaque instability, thus reducing the progression of atherosclerosis (Hattori et al., 2002). This reflects PlGF's potential in risk assessment, disease identification, and therapeutic intervention. As this marker has also demonstrated elevated levels relative to those of cardiac troponin, it has potential importance as an independent marker in the onset of CHD (Heeschen et al., 2004). Unlike PAPP-A, PlGF can be measured in either serum or plasma using ELISA techniques, with detection limits as low as 7 ng/L.

1.6.3 Biomarkers of Thrombosis

Thrombosis involves the formation of a blood clot within the vessel lumen that either reduces or prevents blood flow to the remainder of the tissue. Plaque formation, a consequence of this process, results from the deposition of platelets and fibrins that are recruited by signaling molecules to the site of vascular injury. A positive association with elevated levels of thrombotic markers, such as fibrinogen, hsCRP, IL-6, D-dimer, tissue-type plasminogen activator (t-PA), lipoprotein (a) [Lp(a)] and von Willebrand factor (vWf) to mention a few, has been significantly correlated to CHD as determined in the Edinburgh Artery Study (Tzoulaki et al., 2007).

Fibrinogen, a glycoprotein produced in the liver, is an independent marker of thrombosis (Kannel et al., 1987; Thompson et al., 1995; Danesh et al., 1998, 2005). It can be cleaved into the fibrin adduct which is a key component in platelet adhesion and aggregation. Increased levels of fibrinogen were shown in the Framingham Study to correlate significantly with a high incidence of CHD in both males and females (Kannel et al., 1987). An earlier study found that reduced levels of fibrinogen were associated with a low risk of developing CHD even though serum cholesterol levels were elevated (Thompson et al., 1995). Immunoassay-based measurements of fibrinogen in EDTA plasma are currently available, however, despite its outstanding potential as a risk marker for CHD, it is not yet a suitable marker for use in a clinical setting.

Tissue-type plasminogen activator (t-PA) and lipoprotein (a) [Lp(a)] represent a clear, definite association with CHD and their levels increase as disease state progresses (Danesh et al., 2000; Lowe et al., 2004; Bennet et al., 2008; Erqou et al., 2009). D-dimer and vWf also display a positive association with CHD risk, however, all of these groups require more research as not enough clinical evidence is yet available (Whincup et al., 2002).

1.6.4 Biomarkers of Ischemic Heart Disease

Following thrombus formation, the next stage in cardiovascular disease progression is myocardial ischemia. Ischemic conditions can be detected within the circulatory system by a number of signaling molecules. A few of these markers include: ischemia-modified albumin (IMA), FFAs, and choline (Anwaruddin et al., 2005; Pilz et al., 2007; Bali et al., 2008; LeLeiko et al., 2009). Epidemiological studies have shown that during ischemia, the N-terminus of serum albumin becomes altered such that it has a lower binding affinity for cobalt. As a result, the Food and Drug Administration (FDA) has approved the albumin cobalt binding (ACB) test, which enables the quantitation of albumin in serum (Bar-Or et al., 2000). However, elevated levels of IMA in the serum are not cardiac specific as similar levels have been detected in other tissues suffering injury.

Choline is another signaling molecule that has been linked to advanced coronary plaque instability or myocardial ischemia (Danne et al., 2003; LeLeiko et al., 2009). Ischemia is associated with the phospholipase A (PLA)-mediated cleavage of membrane phospholipids, which results in increased levels of whole blood choline (WBC) and plasma choline (PC). The mechanism of choline uptake occurs first into the plasma and then through a secondary pathway into blood cells. Plaque destabilization is only associated with WBC, not PC (Danne et al., 2003). This is because the activation of platelets and white blood cells stimulates an elevation in intracellular choline that cannot be observed in plasma. However, PC levels are extremely useful within the first 24 h following chest pains as the arrhythmias that usually ensue liberate choline first into the plasma and much later into the blood cells. Once again, more clinical evidence and a standardized method of analysis is required.

1.6.5 Biomarkers of Necrosis

Cardiac tissue death, a result of myocardial ischemia, is now being successfully monitored at the clinical level through the use of two critical markers: cardiac Troponin-T and -I (cTNT and cTNI) and creatine kinase MB (CK-MB) (Bassand et al., 2007). Myoglobin (Myg) and lactate dehydrogenase (LDH) have both shown potential as biomarkers of necrosis as well; however, they have been far less studied (Savory and Pryce, 1980; Karacalioglu et al., 2007; Szymanski et al., 2008).

Troponin has been used in a number of clinical trials as both a prognostic and diagnostic tool (Heidenreich et al., 2001; Scirica and Morrow, 2004; Szymanski et al., 2008; Sundstrom et al., 2009). It is unique in that it is highly selective for cardiac tissue. Increased levels of troponin correlate highly with infarct size and thus with the severity of the disease. Similarly, the longer troponin remains in the blood, the more severe the outcome of the ischemia will be (Babuin and Jaffe, 2005). At 4–12 h following an ischemic event, troponin levels start to become detectable with maximum levels being achieved within 12–48 h. Despite the accuracy with which troponin detects necrosis, it suffers in that it is unable to detect any additional infarcts and is only detectable in the circulation once the necrotic process is already underway, rendering it inadequate in preventative measures.

CK-MB is a highly sensitive marker of necrosis, however, its use is not as favored as troponin due to its inability to distinguish cardiac muscle from skeletal muscle. Alternatively, when it is used in conjunction with troponin, CK-MB has the ability to identify secondary infarcts, which troponin is unable to do (Rajappa and Sharma, 2005).

1.7 PREVENTION AND REGRESSION OF ATHEROSCLEROSIS

Reverse cholesterol transport, the return of extrahepatic cholesterol to the liver and its subsequent secretion into bile and removal as feces, is regulated by two processes: (1) cholesterol influx, mediated by LDL-cholesterol (LDL-C), and (2) cholesterol efflux, mediated by Apo-AI/HDL-cholesterol (HDL-C). Generally, an imbalance between cholesterol removal and deposition can induce disease conditions such as atherosclerosis. Since elevated LDL-C and decreased HDL-C are important independent risk factors for cardiovascular disease, an increase in plasma HDL-C levels or a decrease in LDL-C plasma levels are two possible approaches to reestablish a balance between cholesterol deposition and removal (Mereno et al., 2009).

The beneficial role of HDL is based on cholesterol efflux to HDL particles, either passively or through its association with ATP-binding cassette (ABC) transporters and SR class B, type-I (SR-BI) receptors (Mereno et al., 2009). Despite the number of ABC transporters involved in cholesterol efflux, type AI is responsible for 50% of the overall efflux of cholesterol from macrophage to the lipid-poor HDL-C (Ibanez et al., 2007; Mereno et al., 2009). Following this increase in lipid content, the mature HDL-C is transported to the liver where it binds to SR-BI receptors, which facilitates the discharge of cholesterol into the liver for bile acid synthesis (Ibanez et al., 2007).

This instrumental role of plasma HDL-C levels in plaque regression was first reported by Badimon et al. (1989). The addition of exogenous HDL-C caused a significant reduction of aortic plaque cholesterol and esterified cholesterol in rabbits (Badimon et al., 1989). Since then, other studies have also demonstrated that atherosclerotic plaque regression can be achieved through injection of HDL or HDL-like apolipoprotein A-I (Williams et al., 2008). HDL infusion was also found to induce a more stable atheroma phenotype. It is known that human populations with high HDL-C levels, such as Inuit, premenopausal women, and athletes, are protected from developing cardiovascular disease.

Currently, two drugs are commonly utilized to increase plasma HDL-C levels: fibrates and niacin. Fibrates regulate the transcription of lipoprotein lipase (LPL), apolipoprotein C-II, and apolipoprotien A-I (apoA-I) through the activation of the nuclear transcription factor peroxisome proliferators activated receptor alpha (PPAPα). Fibrates also mediate a myriad of anti-inflammatory and antiatherogenic effects. This includes increased hepatic β-oxidation, decreased triglyceride (TG) secretion, increased clearance of plasma VLDL, increased plasma HDL, and a decrease in inflammatory biomarkers. Niacin (also known as nicotinic acid or vitamin B_3) also raises HDL-C levels. It is one of the most powerful and reliable HDL-C elevating agents. Similar to fibrates, niacin also exhibits anti-inflammatory and antiatherogenic actions. However, this is achieved through a different mechanism than fibrates. Niacin decreases hepatic secretion of VLDL and the mobilization of peripheral FFAs, and it increases apoA-I availability (Venkatesh et al., 2008).

Therapies which modulate LDL-C biosynthesis are currently used more frequently to regress plaques than strategies that are aimed at HDL. LDL-C regulation has been extensively studied because of its implications in atheroma cholesterol dynamics. Cholesterol, TG, and apolipoproteins (C, B-100, and E) are packaged within the liver and secreted into the bloodstream as VLDLs. The TG within VLDL are cleaved by lipoprotein lipase-producing intermediate density lipoproteins. With the loss of apolipoproteins C and E, IDL is converted into LDL. LDL binds to the hepatic LDL receptor and is cleared by the liver or it can remain within the circulation where it can transport cholesterol to peripheral tissues. During hyperlipidemic or hypercholesterolemic conditions, LDL is significantly elevated, leading to an accelerated release and deposition of extrahepatic cholesterol into peripheral tissues. Thus, an elevation of circulating LDL-C correlates well with an increased incidence of atherosclerosis.

Lowering LDL-C has become an important research focus. Currently, the main agents used to lower LDL-levels are statins. Statins are 3-hydroxy-3-methylglutaryl-coenzyme A (HMG-CoA) reductase inhibitors and decrease the formation of mevalonate, the rate-limiting step of sterol synthesis. By reducing plasma LDL-C levels, statins create a tissue:blood LDL-C concentration gradient causing the preferential removal of LDL-C from atherosclerotic plaques back into the systemic circulation where it can be cleared. In addition to lowering LDL-C levels, statins have many antiatherogenic and anti-inflammatory effects including ameliorating endothelial function, reducing the levels of C-reactive protein, altering the collagen content of atheromas, decreasing the inflammatory component of plaques, and lowering plasma Apo-B lipoproteins concentrations (Williams et al., 2008; Riccioni, 2009).

Although agents which lower LDL-C levels have largely overshadowed the effectiveness of HDL-C raising therapies, animal and human studies now focus on combination therapies which aim to enhance atherosclerotic regression by increasing reverse cholesterol transport and significantly reducing cholesterol levels.

Omega-3 fatty acids are powerful agents in the decrease of hepatic and circulating TG and VLDL levels (Biscione et al., 2007). These decreases in TG and VLDL are not limited to patients with abnormal lipid profile but to normal subjects as well (Goodnight, 1989). The type of omega-3 fatty acids also influences the extent of TG lowering. For instance, both EPA and DHA lower TG levels to a similar extent. α-Linolenic acid, on the other hand, has not been shown to reduce TG levels to the same extent as EPA and DHA when comparable amounts have been consumed. Omega-3 fatty acids are also able to modestly increase HDL-C levels (Biscione et al., 2007; Bays et al., 2008).

Interestingly, dietary intake of omega-3 fatty acids has no influence or variable effects on LDL concentrations (Goodnight, 1989; Biscione et al., 2007). Although intake of omega-3 fatty acids (~8 g/day) has the potential to decrease total and LDL cholesterol, this concentration causes a high incidence of adverse effects. On the other hand, the acceptable dose (4 g/day) has not been shown to decrease LDL-C concentrations in neither normal nor hyperplipidemic subjects (Biscione et al., 2007).

Although the mechanism by which omega-3 fatty acids lower TG levels is not completely understood, several mechanisms have been proposed. These include (1) inhibiting VLDL synthesis through the reduction of TGs integration into VLDL particles; (2) the targeting of genes and transcription factors which are responsible for cellular TG synthesis; (3) an increase in the β-oxidation of fatty acids which reduces the availability of TG for VLDL incorporation; and (4) the inhibition and degradation of apo-B100 (Biscione et al., 2007; Bays et al., 2008). Likely, all of the proposed mechanisms are active simultaneously. However, irrespective of the mechanism, omega-3 fatty acids decrease the half-life of circulating TG (Bays et al., 2008). The conundrum of having a constant LDL level in the face of decreasing VLDL levels is yet to be fully understood.

ACKNOWLEDGMENTS

This work was supported by a grant from the Canadian Institutes for Health Research (CIHR) to G. Pierce. J. Deniset, A. Edel, and A. Francis were recipients of CIHR studentship awards. R. McCullough was supported by a Manitoba Health Research Council Studentship. M. Chahine was supported by a Heart and Stroke Foundation of Canada Postdoctoral Fellowship.

REFERENCES

Adam, E., Melnick, J.L., Probtsfield, J.L., Petrie, B.L., Burek, J., Bailey, K.R., McCollum, C.H., and DeBakey, M.E. 1987. High levels of cytomegalovirus antibody in patients requiring vascular surgery for atherosclerosis. *Lancet* **2**(8554): 291–293.

Aeberli, I., Spinas, G.A., Lehmann, R., l'Allemand, D., Molinari, L., and Zimmermann, M.B. 2009. Diet determines features of the metabolic syndrome in 6- to 14-year-old children. *Int. J. Vitam. Nutr. Res.* **79**(1): 14–23.

Albertini, R., Moratti, R., and De Luca, G. 2002. Oxidation of low-density lipoprotein in atherosclerosis from basic biochemistry to clinical studies. *Curr. Mol. Med.* **2**(6): 579–592.

Allin, K.H., Bojesen, S.E., and Nordestgaard, B.G. 2009. Baseline C-reactive protein is associated with incident cancer and survival in patients with cancer. *J. Clin. Oncol.* **27**(13): 2217–2224.

Anitschkow, N., C.S. 1913. Uber experimentelle Cholesterinsteatose und ihre Bedeutung fur die Entstehung einiger pathologischer Prozesse. *Zentbl. Allg. Pathol. Pathol. Anat.* **24**: 1–9.

Anwaruddin, S., Januzzi Jr., J.L., Baggish, A.L., Lewandrowski, E.L., and Lewandrowski, K.B. 2005. Ischemia-modified albumin improves the usefulness of standard cardiac biomarkers for the diagnosis of myocardial ischemia in the emergency department setting. *Am. J. Clin. Pathol.* **123**(1): 140–145.

Apple, F.S., Wu, A.H.B., Mair, J., Ravkilde, J., Panteghini, M., Tate, J., Pagani, F. et al. 2005. Future biomarkers for detection of ischemia and risk stratification in acute coronary syndrome. *Clin. Chem.* **51**(5): 810–824.

Arita, Y., Kihara, S., Ouchi, N., Takahashi, M., Maeda, K., Miyagawa, J., Hotta, K. et al. 1999. Paradoxical decrease of an adipose-specific protein, adiponectin, in obesity. *Biochem. Biophys. Res. Commun.* **257**(1): 79–83.

Babuin, L. and Jaffe, A.S. 2005. Troponin: The biomarker of choice for the detection of cardiac injury. *CMAJ* **173**(10): 1191–1202.

Bachorik, P. and Ross, J.W. 2001. Executive summary of the third report of The National Cholesterol Education Program (NCEP) expert panel on detection, evaluation, and treatment of high blood cholesterol in adults (adult treatment panel III). *JAMA* **285**(19): 2486–2497.

Badimon, J.J., Badimon, L., Galvez, A., Dische, R., and Fuster, V. 1989. High density lipoprotein plasma fractions inhibit tic fatty streaks in cholesterol-fed rabbits. *Lab. Invest.* **60**: 455–461.

Baldus, S., Heeschen, C., Meinertz, T., Zeiher, A.M., Eiserich, J.P., Munzel, T., Simoons, M.L., and Hamm, C.W, 2003. Myeloperoxidase serum levels predict risk in patients with acute coronary syndromes. *Circulation* **108**(12): 1440–1445.

Bali, L., Cuisset, T., Giorgi, R., Monserrat, C., Quillici, J., Correga, L., Mouret, J-P. et al. 2008. Prognostic value of ischaemia-modified albumin in patients with non-ST-segment elevation acute coronary syndromes. *Arch. Cardiovasc. Dis*. **101**(10): 645–651.

Bar-Or, D., Lau, E., and Winkler, J.V. 2000. A novel assay for cobalt–albumin binding and its potential as a marker for myocardial ischemia—A preliminary report. *J. Emerg. Med*. **19**(4): 311–315.

Bassuk, S.S., Rifai, N., and Ridker, P.M. 2004. High-sensitivity C-reactive protein: Clinical importance. *Curr. Probl. Cardiol*. **29**(8): 439–493.

Bassand, J.P., Hamm, C.W., Ardissino, D., Boersma, E., Buday, A. et al. 2007. Guidelines for the diagnosis and treatment of non-ST-segment elevation acute coronary syndromes. *Eur. Heart. J*. **28**(13): 1598–1660.

Bayes-Genis, A., Conover, C.A., Overgaard, M.T., Bailey, K.R., Christiansen, M., Holmes, Jr., D.R., Virmani, R., Oxvig, C., and Schwartz, R.S. 2001. Pregnancy-associated plasma protein A as a marker of acute coronary syndromes. *N. Engl. J. Med*. **345**(14): 1022–1029.

Bays, H., Mandarino, L., and DeFronzo, R.A. 2004. Role of the adipocyte, free fatty acids, and ectopic fat in pathogenesis of type 2 diabetes mellitus: Peroxisomal proliferator-activated receptor agonists provide a rational therapeutic approach. *J. Clin. Endocrinol. Metab*. **89**(2): 463–478.

Bays, H.E., Tighe, A.P., Sadovsky, R., and Davidson, M.H. 2008. Prescription omega-3 fatty acid and their lipid effects: Physiologic mechanisms of action and clinical implications. *Expert Rev. Cardiovasc. Ther*. **6**(3): 391–409.

Bennet, A., Angelantonio, E.D., Erqou, S., Eriksdottir, G., Sigurdsson, D., Woodward, M., Rumley, A., Lowe, G.D.O., Danesh, J., and Gudnason, V. 2008. Lipoprotein (a) levels and risk of future coronary heart disease: Large-scale prospective data. *Arch. Intern. Med*. **168**(6): 598–608.

Berliner, J.A., Navab, M., Fogelman, A.M., Frank, J.S., Demer, L.L., Edwards, P.A., Watson, A.D., and Lusis, A.J. 1995. Atherosclerosis: Basic mechanisms. Oxidation, inflammation, and genetics. *Circulation* **91**(9): 2488–2496.

Binder, C.J., Shaw, P.X., Chang, M.K., Boullier, A., Hartvigsen, K., Horkko, S., Miller, Y.I., Woelkers, D.A., Corr, M., and Witztum, J.L. 2005. The role of natural antibodies in atherogenesis. *J. Lipid Res*. **46**(7): 1353–1363.

Biscione, F., Pignalberi, C., Totteri, A., Messina, F., and Altamura, G. 2007. Cardiovascular effects of omega-3 free fatty acids. *Curr. Vasc. Pharmacol*. **5**: 163–172.

Bjorkbacka, H., Kunjathoor, V.V., Moore, K.J., Koehn, S., Ordija, C.M., Lee, M.A., Means, T. et al. 2004. Reduced atherosclerosis in MyD88-null mice links elevated serum cholesterol levels to activation of innate immunity signaling pathways. *Nat. Med*. 2**10**(4): 416–421.

Blankenberg, S., Rupprecht, H.G., Bickel, C., Peetz, D., Hafner, G., Tiret, L., and Meyer, J. 2001. Circulating cell adhesion molecules and death in patients with coronary artery disease. *Circulation* **104**(12): 1336–1342.

Blankenberg, S., Tiret, L., Bickel, C., Peetz, D., Cambien, F., Meyer, J., and Rupprecht, H.J. 2002. Interleukin-18 is a strong predictor of cardiovascular death in stable and unstable angina. *Circulation* **106**(1): 24–30.

Blankenberg, S., Luc, G., Ducimetiere, P., Arveiler, D., Ferrieres, J., Amouyel, P., Evans, A., Cambien, F., and Tiret, L. 2003. Interleukin-18 and the risk of coronary heart disease in European men: The prospective epidemiological study of myocardial infarction (PRIME). *Circulation* **108**(20): 2453–2459.

Boullier, A., Bird, D.A., Chang, M-K., Dennis, A.D., Friedman, P., Gillotte-Taylor, K., Horkko, S. et al. 2001. Scavenger receptors, oxidized LDL, and atherosclerosis. *Ann. N. Y. Acad. Sci*. **947**: 214–222; discussion 222–223.

Bruggeman, C.A. 2000. Does cytomegalovirus play a role in atherosclerosis? *Herpes*. **7**(2): 51–54.

Bui, Q.T., Prempeh, M., and Wilensky, R.L. 2009. Atherosclerotic plaque development. *Int. J. Biochem. Cell Biol*. **41**(11): 2109–2113.

Caligiuri, G., Nicoletti, A., Poirier, B., and Hansson, G.K. 2002. Protective immunity against atherosclerosis carried by B cells of hypercholesterolemic mice. *J. Clin. Invest*.**109**(6): 745–753.

Cannon, B. and Nedergaard, J. 2004. Brown adipose tissue: Function and physiological significance. *Physiol. Rev*. **84**(1): 277–359.

Celermajer, D.S. 1997. Endothelial dysfunction: Does it matter? Is it reversible? *J. Am. Coll. Cardiol*. **30**(2): 325–333.

Cesari, M., Penninx, B.W.J.H., Newman, A.B., Kritchevsky, S.B., Niklas, B.J., Sutton-Tyrrell, K.S., Rubin, S.M. et al. 2003. Inflammatory markers and onset of cardiovascular events: Results from the Health ABC study. *Circulation* **108**(19): 2317–2322.

Chen, S., Sorrentino, R., Shimada, K., Bulut, Y., Doherty, T.M., Crother, T.R., and Arditi, M. 2008. *Chlamydia pneumoniae*-induced foam cell formation requires MyD88-dependent and -independent signaling and is reciprocally modulated by liver X receptor activation. *J. Immunol*. **181**(10): 7186–7193.

Cooke, J.P. 2003. Flow, NO, and atherogenesis. *Proc. Natl. Acad. Sci.* USA **100**(3): 768–770.

Danesh, J., Collins, R., Appleby, P., and Peto, R. 1998. Association of fibrinogen, C-reactive protein, albumin, or leukocyte count with coronary heart disease: Meta-analyses of prospective studies. *JAMA* **279**(18): 1477–1482.

Danesh, J., Collins, R., and Peto, R. 2000. Lipoprotein(a) and coronary heart disease. Meta-analysis of prospective studies. *Circulation* **102**(10): 1082–1085.

Danesh, J., Whincup, P., Walker, M., Lennon, L., Thomson, A., Apleby, P., Rumley, A., and Lowe, G.D.O. 2001. Fibrin D-dimer and coronary heart disease: Prospective study and meta-analysis. *Circulation* **103**(19): 2323–2327.

Danesh, J., Lewington, S., Thompson, S.G. et al. 2005. Plasma fibrinogen level and the risk of major cardiovascular diseases and nonvascular mortality: An individual participant meta-analysis. *JAMA* **294**(14): 1799–1809.

Danne, O., Mockel, M., Lueders, C., Zachunke, G.A., Lufft, H., Muller, C., and Frei, U. 2003. Prognostic implications of elevated whole blood choline levels in acute coronary syndromes. *Am. J. Cardiol.* **91**(9): 1060–1067.

Davignon, J. and Ganz, P. 2004. Role of endothelial dysfunction in atherosclerosis. *Circulation* **109**(23 Suppl 1): III27–III32.

De Caterina, R. and Massaro, M. 1999. Effects of diet and of dietary components on endothelial leukocyte adhesion molecules. *Curr. Atheroscler. Rep.* **1**(3): 188–195.

De Caterina, R., Liao, J.K., and Libby, P. 2000. Fatty acid modulation of endothelial activation. *Am. J. Clin. Nutr.* **71**(1 Suppl): 213S–223S.

Dechend, R., Maass, M., Gieffers, J., Dietz, R., Scheidereit, C., Leutz, A., and Gulba, D.C. 1999. *Chlamydia pneumoniae* infection of vascular smooth muscle and endothelial cells activates NF-kappaB and induces tissue factor and PAI-1 expression: A potential link to accelerated arteriosclerosis. *Circulation* **100**(13): 1369–1373.

Dotsenko, O., Chackathayil, J., Patel, J.V., Gill, P.S., and Lip, G.Y. 2008. Candidate circulating biomarkers for the cardiovascular disease continuum. *Curr. Pharm. Des.* **14**(24): 2445–2461.

Dubey, L. and Hesong, Z. 2006. Role of leptin in atherogenesis. *Exp. Clin. Cardiol.* **11**(4): 269–275.

Du Clos, T.W. and Mold, C. 2004. C-reactive protein: An activator of innate immunity and a modulator of adaptive immunity. *Immunol. Res.* **30**(3): 261–277.

Duque-Guimaraes, D.E., de Castro, J., Martinez-Botas, J., Sardinha, F.L., Ramos, M.P., Herrera, E., and do Carmo, M.G. 2009. Early and prolonged intake of partially hydrogenated fat alters the expression of genes in rat adipose tissue. *Nutrition* **25**(7–8): 782–789.

Dzau, V.J., Braun-Dullaeus, R.C., and Sedding, D.G. 2002. Vascular proliferation and atherosclerosis: New perspectives and therapeutic strategies. *Nat. Med.* **8**(11): 1249–1256.

Edfeklt, K., Swedenborg, J., Hansson, J.K., and Yan, Z.Q. 2002. Expression of toll-like receptors in human atherosclerotic lesions: A possible pathway for plaque activation. *Circulation* **105**: 1158–1161.

Ehara, S., Ueda, M., Naruko, T., Haze, K., Itoh, A., Otsuka, M., Komatsu, R. et al. 2001. Elevated levels of oxidized low density lipoprotein show a positive relationship with the severity of acute coronary syndromes. *Circulation* **103**(15): 1955–1960.

Epstein, S.E., Zhou Y.F., and Zhu, J. 1999. Infection and atherosclerosis: Emerging mechanistic paradigms. *Circulation* **100**(4): e20–e28.

Erqou, S. et al. 2009. Lipoprotein(a) concentration and the risk of coronary heart disease, stroke, and nonvascular mortality. *JAMA* **302**(4): 412–423.

Fabricant, C.G., Fabricant, J., Litrenta, M.M., and Minick, C.R. 1978. *Virus*-induced atherosclerosis. *J. Exp. Med.* **148**(1): 335–340.

Fagot-Campagna, A., Balkau, B., Simon, D., Warnet, J.M., Claude, J.R., Ducimetiere, P., and Eschwege, E. 1998. High free fatty acid concentration: An independent risk factor for hypertension in the Paris Prospective Study. *Int. J. Epidemiol.* **27**(5): 808–813.

Flachs, P., Mohamed-Ali, V., Horakova, O., Rossmeisl, M., Hosseinzadeh-Attar, M.J., Hensler, M., Ruzickova, J., and Kopecky, J. 2006. Polyunsaturated fatty acids of marine origin induce adiponectin in mice fed a high-fat diet. *Diabetologia.* **49**(2): 394–397.

Galkina, E. and Ley, K. 2009. Immune and inflammatory mechanisms of atherosclerosis. *Annu. Rev. Immunol.* **27**: 165–197.

Gerrity, R.G., Naito, H.K., Richardson, M., and Schwartz, C.J. 1979. Dietary induced atherogenesis in swine. Morphology of the intima in prelesion stages. *Am. J. Pathol.* **95**(3): 775–792.

Gertow, K., Rosell, M., Sjogren, P., Eriksson, P., Vessby, B., de Faire, U., Hamsten, A., Hellenius, M.L., and Fisher, R.M. 2006. Fatty acid handling protein expression in adipose tissue, fatty acid composition of adipose tissue and serum, and markers of insulin resistance. *Eur. J. Clin. Nutr.* **60**(12): 1406–1413.

Gibson, W.T., Farooqui, I.S., Moreau, M., DePaoli, A.M., Lawrence, E., O'Rahilly, S. and Trussell, R.A. 2004. Congenital leptin deficiency due to homozygosity for the Delta133G mutation: Report of another case and evaluation of response to four years of leptin therapy. *J. Clin. Endocrinol. Metab.* **89**(10): 4821–4826.

Glass, C.K. and Witztum, J.L. 2001. Atherosclerosis. The road ahead. *Cell.* **104**(4): 503–516.

Gonzalez-Periz, A., Horrillo, R., Ferre, N., Gronert, K., Dong, B., Moran-Salvador, E., Titos, E. et al. 2009. Obesity-induced insulin resistance and hepatic steatosis are alleviated by omega-3 fatty acids: A role for resolvins and protectins. *FASEB J.* **23**(6): 1946–1957.

Goodnight, S.H. 1989. The vascular effects of omega-3 fatty acids. *J. Invest. Dermat.* **93**(2): 102S–106S.

Grayston, J.T., Kuo, C.C., Coulson, A.S., Campbell, L.A., Lawrence, R.D., Lee, M.J., Strandness, E.D., and Wang, S.P. 1995. *Chlamydia pneumoniae* (TWAR) in atherosclerosis of the carotid artery. *Circulation* **92**(12): 3397–3400.

Gu, L., Okada, Y., Clinton, S.K., Gerard, C., Sukhova, G.K., Libby, P., and Rollins, B.J. 1998. Absence of monocyte chemoattractant protein-1 reduces atherosclerosis in low density lipoprotein receptor-deficient mice. *Mol. Cell.* **2**(2): 275–281.

Gudbrandsen, O.A., Rodriguez, E., Wergedahl, H., Mork, S., Reseland, J.E., Skorve, J., Palou, A., and Berge, R.K. 2009. *Trans*-10, *cis*-12-conjugated linoleic acid reduces the hepatic triacylglycerol content and the leptin mRNA level in adipose tissue in obese Zucker fa/fa rats. *Br. J. Nutr.* **102**(6): 803–815.

Gyorkey, F., Melnick, J.L., Guinn, G.A., Gyorkey, P., DeBakey, M.E. 1984. Herpesviridae in the endothelial and smooth muscle cells of the proximal aorta in arteriosclerotic patients. *Exp. Mol. Pathol.* **40**(3): 328–339.

Hamwi, A., Vukovich, T., Wagner, O., Rumpold, H., Spies, R., Stich, M., and Langecker, C. 2001. Evaluation of turbidimetric high-sensitivity C-reactive protein assays for cardiovascular risk estimation. *Clin. Chem.* **47**(11): 2044–2046.

Hanke, H., Lenz, C., and Finking, G. 2001. The discovery of the pathophysiological aspects of atherosclerosis—A review. *Acta. Chir. Belg.* **101**(4): 162–169.

Hansson, G.K., Holm, J., and Jonasson, L. 1989. Detection of activated T lymphocytes in the human atherosclerotic plaque. *Am. J. Pathol.* **135**(1): 169–175.

Hattori, K., Heissig, B., Wu, Y., Dias, S., Tejada, R., Ferris, B., Hicklin, D.J. et al. 2002. Placental growth factor reconstitutes hematopoiesis by recruiting VEGFR1(+) stem cells from bone-marrow microenvironment. *Nat. Med.* **8**(8): 841–849.

Haugen, F., Zahid, N., Dalen, K.T., Hollung, K., Nebb, H.I., and Drevon, C.A. 2005. Resistin expression in 3T3-L1 adipocytes is reduced by arachidonic acid. *J. Lipid Res.* **46**(1): 143–153.

Heeschen, C., Dimmeler, S., Hamm, C.W., Fichtlscherer, S., Boersma, E., Simoons, M.L., and Zeiher, A.M. 2003. Serum level of the anti-inflammatory cytokine interleukin-10 is an important prognostic determinant in patients with acute coronary syndromes. *Circulation* **107**(16): 2109–2114.

Heeschen, C., Dimmeler, S., Fichtlscherer, S., Hamm, C.W., Berger, J., Simoons, M.L., and Zeiher, A.M. 2004. Prognostic value of placental growth factor in patients with acute chest pain. *JAMA* **291**(4): 435–441.

Heidenreich, P.A., Alloggiamento, T., Melsop, K., McDonald, K.M., Go, A.S., and Hlatky, M.A. 2001. The prognostic value of troponin in patients with non-ST elevation acute coronary syndromes: A meta-analysis. *J. Am. Coll. Cardiol.* **38**(2): 478–485.

Heikkila, H.M., Trosien, J., Metso, J., Jauhiainen, M., Pentikainen, M.O., Kovanen, P.T., and Lindstedt, K.A. 2010. Mast cells promote atherosclerosis by inducing both an atherogenic lipid profile and vascular inflammation. *J. Cell Biochem.* **109**(3): 615–623.

Hendricks, M.G., Salimans, M.M., van Boven, C.P., and Bruggeman, C.A. 1990. High prevalence of latently present cytomegalovirus in arterial walls of patients suffering from grade III atherosclerosis. *Am. J. Pathol.* **136**(1): 23–28.

Henrichot, E., Juge-Aubry, C.E., Pernin, A., Pache, J.C., Velebit, V., Dayer, J.M., Meda, P., Chizzolini, C., and Meier, C.A. 2005. Production of chemokines by perivascular adipose tissue: A role in the pathogenesis of atherosclerosis? *Arterioscler. Thromb. Vasc. Biol.* **25**(12): 2594–2599.

Hessler, J.R., Morel, D.W., Lewis, L.J., and Chisolm, G.M. 1983. Lipoprotein oxidation and lipoprotein-induced cytotoxicity. *Arteriosclerosis* **3**(3): 215–222.

Hirono, S., Dibrov, E., Hurtado, C., Kostenuk, A., Ducas, R., and Pierce, G.N. 2003. *Chlamydia pneumonia* proliferation of vascular smooth muscle cells through induction of endogenous heat shock protein 60. *Circ. Res.* **93**(8): 710–716.

Howie-Esquivel, J. and White, M. 2008. Biomarkers in acute cardiovascular disease. *J. Cardiovasc. Nurs.* **23**(2): 124–131.

Ibanez, B., Vilahur, G., and Badimon, J.J. 2007. Plaque progression and regression in atherothrombosis. *J. Thromb. Haemost.* **5**(Suppl. 1): 292–299.

Inoue, T., Uchida, T., Kamishirado, H., Takayanagi, K., Hayashi, T., and Marooka, S. 2001. Clinical significance of antibody against oxidized low density lipoprotein in patients with atherosclerotic coronary artery disease. *J. Am. Coll. Cardiol.* **37**(3): 775–779.

Jiang, S.J., Kuo, C.C., Berry, M.W., Lee, A.W., and Campbell, L.A. 2008. Identification and characterization of *Chlamydia pneumoniae*-specific proteins that activate tumor necrosis factor alpha production in RAW 264.7 murine macrophages. *Infect. Immun.* **76**(4): 1558–1564.

Johnson, B.D., Kip, K.E., Marroquin, O.C., Ridker, P.M., Kelsey, S.F., Shaw, L.J., Pepine, C.J. et al. 2004. Serum amyloid A as a predictor of coronary artery disease and cardiovascular outcome in women: The National Heart, Lung, and Blood Institute-Sponsored Women's Ischemia Syndrome Evaluation (WISE). *Circulation* **109**(6): 726–732.

Jongstra-Bilen, J., Haidari, M., Zhu, S.N., Chen, M., and Guha, M.I. 2006. Low-grade chronic inflammation in regions of the normal mouse arterial intima predisposed to atherosclerosis. *J. Ex. Med.* **203**: 2073–2083.

Jouven, X., Charles, M.A., Desnos, M., and Ducimetiere, P. 2001. Circulating nonesterified fatty acid level as a predictive risk factor for sudden death in the population. *Circulation* **104**(7): 756–761.

Jylhava, J., Haarala, A., Ecklund, C., Pertovaara, M., Kahonen, M., Hutri-Kahonen, N., Levula, M. et al. 2009. Serum amyloid A is independently associated with metabolic risk factors but not with early atherosclerosis: The Cardiovascular Risk in Young Finns Study. *J. Intern. Med.* **266**(3): 286–295.

Kannel, W.B., Wolf, R., Castelli, W.P., and D'Argostino, R.B. 1987. Fibrinogen and risk of cardiovascular disease. The Framingham Study. *JAMA* **258**(9): 1183–1186.

Karacalioglu, O., Arzian, Z., Kilic, S., Ozturk, E., and Ozguven, N. 2007. Baseline serum levels of cardiac biomarkers in patients with stable coronary artery disease. *Biomarkers* **12**(5): 533–540.

Kaski, J.C. and Holt, D.W. 2006. Pregnancy-associated plasma protein-A and cardiovascular risk. *Eur. Heart J.* **27**(14): 1637–1639.

Kaukoranta-Tolvanen, S.S., Ronni, T., Leinonen, M., Saikku, P., and Laitinen, K. 1996. Expression of adhesion molecules on endothelial cells stimulated by *Chlamydia pneumoniae*. *Microb. Pathog.* **21**(5): 407–411.

Kawachi, H., Yang, S.H., Hamano, A., Matsui, T., Smith, S.B., and Yano, H. 2007. Molecular cloning and expression of bovine (*Bos taurus*) leptin receptor isoform mRNAs. *Comp. Biochem. Physiol. B Biochem. Mol. Biol.* **148**(2): 167–173.

Khosravi, J., Diamandi, A., Krishna, R.G., Bodani, U., Mistry, J., and Khaja, N. 2002. Pregnancy associated plasma protein-A: Ultrasensitive immunoassay and determination in coronary heart disease. *Clin. Biochem.* **35**(7): 531–538.

Kinscherf, R., Kamencic, H., Deigner, H.P., and Metz, J. 2003. Hypercholesterolemia-induced long-term increase of macrophages in the myocardium of New Zealand White rabbits. *Cells Tissues Organs* **174**(4): 184–193.

Koba, S., Pakala, R., Watanabe, T., Katagiri, T., and Benedict, C.R. 1999. Vascular smooth muscle proliferation: Synergistic interaction between serotonin and low density lipoproteins. *J. Am. Coll. Cardiol.* **34**: 1644–1651.

Koutsari, C. and Jensen, M.D. 2006. Thematic review series: Patient-oriented research. Free fatty acid metabolism in human obesity. *J. Lipid Res.* **47**(8): 1643–1650.

Kuda, O., Jelenik, T., Jilkova, Z., Flachs, P., Rossmeisl, M., Hensler, M., Kazdova, L. et al. 2009. n-3 Fatty acids and rosiglitazone improve insulin sensitivity through additive stimulatory effects on muscle glycogen synthesis in mice fed a high-fat diet. *Diabetologia* **52**(5): 941–951.

Kutuk, O. and Basaga, H. 2003. Inflammation meets oxidation: NF-kappaB as a mediator of initial lesion development in atherosclerosis. *Trends Mol. Med.* **9**(12): 549–574.

Large, V., Peroni, O., Letexier, D., Ray, H., and Beylot, M. 2004. Metabolism of lipids in human white adipocyte. *Diabetes Metab.* **30**(4): 294–309.

Lee, J.H., Chan, J.L., Yiannakouris, N., Kontogianni, M., Estrada, E., Seip, R., Orlova, C., and Mantzoros, C.S. 2003. Circulating resistin levels are not associated with obesity or insulin resistance in humans and are not regulated by fasting or leptin administration: Cross-sectional and interventional studies in normal, insulin-resistant, and diabetic subjects. *J. Clin. Endocrinol. Metab.* **88**(10): 4848–4856.

Lee, M., Calasbresi, L., Chiesa, G., Franceschini, G., and Kovanen, P.T. 2002. Mast cell chymase degrades apoE and apoA-II in apoA-I-knockout mouse plasma and reduces its ability to promote cellular cholesterol efflux. *Arterioscler. Thromb. Vasc. Biol.* **22**: 1475–1481.

LeLeiko, R.M., Vacarri, C.S., Sola, S., Merchant, N., Nagamia, S.H., Thoenes, M., and Khan, B.V. 2009. Usefulness of elevations in serum choline and free F2)-isoprostane to predict 30-day cardiovascular outcomes in patients with acute coronary syndrome. *Am. J. Cardiol.* **104**(5): 638–643.

Lenderink, T., Heeschen, C., Fichtlscherer, S., Dimmeler, S., Hamm, C.W., Zeiher, A.M., Simoons, M.L., and Boersma, E. 2006. Elevated placental growth factor levels are associated with adverse outcomes at four-year follow-up in patients with acute coronary syndromes. *J. Am. Coll. Cardiol.* **47**(2): 307–311.

Libby, P., Ridker, P.M., and Maseri, A. 2002. Inflammation and atherosclerosis. *Circulation* **105**(9): 1135–1143.

Libby, P. 2002. Inflammation in atherosclerosis. *Nature* **420**(6917): 868–874.

Lihn, A.S., Bruun, J.M., He, G., Pedersen, S.B., Jensen, P.F., and Richelsen, B. 2004. Lower expression of adiponectin mRNA in visceral adipose tissue in lean and obese subjects. *Mol. Cell. Endocrinol.* **219**(1–2): 9–15.

Lindstedt, K., Mayranpaa, M.I., and Kovanen, P.T. 2007. Mast cells in vulnerable atherosclerotic plaques—A view to a kill. *J. Cell. Mol. Med.* **11**: 739–758.

Lo, J., Abbara, S., Shturman, L., Soni, A., Wei, J., Rocha-Filho, J.A., Nasir, K., and Grinspoon, S.K. 2010. Increased prevalence of subclinical coronary atherosclerosis detected by coronary computed tomography angiography in HIV-infected men. *AIDS* **24**(2): 243–253.

Lowe, G.D.O., Danesh, J., Lewington, S., Walker, M., Lennon, L., Thomson, A., Rumley, A., and Whincup, P.H. 2004. Tissue plasminogen activator antigen and coronary heart disease. Prospective study and meta-analysis. *Eur. Heart J.* **25**(3): 252–259.

Lopes, P.A., Martins, S.V., Pinho, M.S., Alfaia, C.M., Fontes, C.M., Rodrigues, P.O., Morais, G.S., Castro, M.F., Pinto, R., and Prates J.A. 2008. Diet supplementation with the *cis*-9, *trans*-11 conjugated linoleic acid isomer affects the size of adipocytes in Wistar rats. *Nutr. Res.* **28**(7): 480–486.

Luc, G., Arveiler, D., Evans, A., Amouyel, P., Ferrieres, J., Bard, J.M. Elkhalil, L., Fruchart, J.C., and Ducimetiere, P. 2003. Circulating soluble adhesion molecules ICAM-1 and VCAM-1 and incident coronary heart disease: The PRIME Study. *Atherosclerosis* **170**(1): 169–176.

Lund, J., Quin, Q-P., Ilva, T., Nikus, K., Eskola, M., Porela, P., Kokkala, S., Pulkki, K., Ptersson, K., and Voipio-Pulkki, L.M. 2006. Pregnancy-associated plasma protein A: A biomarker in acute ST-elevation myocardial infarction (STEMI). *Ann. Med.* **38**(3): 221–228.

Major, A.S., Fazio, S., and Linton, M.F. 2002. B-lymphocyte deficiency increases atherosclerosis in LDL receptor-null mice. *Arterioscler. Thromb. Vasc. Biol.* **22**(11): 1892–1898.

Mallat, Z., Gojova, A., Brun, V., Esposito, B., Fournier, N., Cottrez, F., Tedgui, A., and Groux, H. 2003. Induction of a regulatory T cell type 1 response reduces the development of atherosclerosis in apolipoprotein E-knockout mice. *Circulation* **108**(10): 1232–1237.

Malik, I., Danish, J., Whincup, P., Bhatia, V., Papacosta, O., Walker, M., Lennon, L., and Thomson, A. 2001. Soluble adhesion molecules and prediction of coronary heart disease: A prospective study and meta-analysis. *Lancet* **358**: 971–975.

Martin-Ventura, J.L., Blanco-Colio, L.M., Tunon, H., Munoz-Garcia, B., Madrigal-Matute, J., Moreno, J.A. Vega de Ceniga, M., and Egido, J. 2009. Biomarkers in cardiovascular medicine. *Rev. Esp. Cardiol.* **62**(6): 677–688.

McCullough, R.S., Edel, A.L., La Vallee, R.K., Dibrov, E., Blackwood, D.P., Ander, B.P., and Pierce, G.N. 2010. Diet-induced alterations in leptin expression can occur independently of caloric intake. Lipids, in press, 2011.

McKellar, G.E., McCarey, D.W., Sattar, N., and McInnes, I.B. 2009. Role for TNF in atherosclerosis? Lessons from autoimmune disease. *Nat. Rev. Cardiol.* **6**(6): 410–417.

Mehra, M.R., Lavie, C.J., Ventura, H.O., and Milani, R.V. 2006. Fish oils produce anti-inflammatory effects and improve body weight in severe heart failure. *J. Heart Lung. Transplant.* **25**(7): 834–838.

Meisinger, C., Baumert, J., Khuseyinova, N., Loewel, H., and Koenig, W. 2005. Plasma oxidized low-density lipoprotein, a strong predictor for acute coronary heart disease events in apparently healthy, middle-aged men from the general population. *Circulation* **112**(5): 651–657.

Mendall, M.A., Goggin, P.M., Molineaux, N., Levy, J., Toosy, T., Strachan, D., Camm, A.J., and Northfield, T.C. 1994. Relation of *Helicobacter pylori* infection and coronary heart disease. *Br. Heart J.* **71**(5): 437–439.

Mereno, P.R., Sans, J., and Fuster, V. 2009. Promoting mechanisms of vascular health: Circulating progenitor cells, angiogenesis, and reverse cholesterol transport. *J. Am. Coll. Cardiol.* **53**(25): 2315–2323.

Meuwese, M.C., Stroes, E.S.G., Hazen, S.L., van Miert, J.N., Kuivenhoven, J.A., Schaub, R.G., Wareham, M.J., Luben, R., Shaw, K-T., and Boekholdt, S.M. 2007. Serum myeloperoxidase levels are associated with the future risk of coronary artery disease in apparently healthy individuals: The EPIC-Norfolk Prospective Population Study. *J. Am. Coll. Cardiol.* **50**(2): 159–165.

Moncada, S. and Higgs, E.A. 2006. Nitric oxide and the vascular endothelium. *Handb. Exp. Pharmacol.* (**176** Pt 1): 213–254.

Mosorin, M., Surcel, H.M., Laurila, A., Lehtinen, M., Karttunen, R., Juvonen, J., Paavonen, J., Morrison, R.P., Saikku, P., and Juvonen, T. 2000. Detection of *Chlamydia pneumoniae*-reactive T lymphocytes in human atherosclerotic plaques of carotid artery. *Arterioscler. Thromb. Vasc. Biol.* **20**(4): 1061–1067.

Moutsopoulos, N.M. and Madianos, P.N. 2006. Low-grade inflammation in chronic infectious diseases: Paradigm of periodontal infections. *Ann. N. Y. Acad. Sci.* **1088**: 251–264.

Moynihan, A.T., Hehir, M.P., Glavey, S.V., Smith, T.J., and Morrison, J.J. 2006. Inhibitory effect of leptin on human uterine contractility *in vitro*. *Am. J. Obstet. Gynecol.* **195**(2): 504–509.

Mullick, A.E., Tobias, P.S., and Curtiss, L.K. 2005. Modulation of atherosclerosis in mice by Toll-like receptor 2. *J. Clin. Invest.* **115**(11): 3149–3156.

Myers, G.L., Rifai, N., Tracy, R.P., Roberts, W.L., Alexander, R.W., Biasucci, L.M., Catravas, J.D. et al. 2004. CDC/AHA workshop on markers of inflammation and cardiovascular disease: Application to clinical and public health practice. Report from the laboratory science discussion group. *Circulation* **110**(25): e545–e549.

Nagaev, I., Bokarewa, M., Tarkowski, A., and Smith, U. 2006. Human resistin is a systemic immune-derived proinflammatory cytokine targeting both leukocytes and adipocytes. *PLoS One* **1**: e31.

Nogueiras, R., Novelle, M.G., Vazquez, M.J., Lopez, M., and Dieguez, C. 2010. Resistin: Regulation of food intake, glucose homeostasis and lipid metabolism. *Endocr. Dev.* **17**: 175–184.

Packard, R.R. and Libby, P. 2008. Inflammation in atherosclerosis: From vascular biology to biomarker discovery and risk prediction. *Clin. Chem.* **54**(1): 24–38.

Pai, J.K., Pischon, T., Ma, J., Manson, J.E., Hankinson, S.E., Joshipura, K., Curhan, G.C. et al. 2004. Inflammatory makers and the risk of coronary heart disease in men and women. *N.J. Engl. J. Med.* **351**(25): 2599–2610.

Paulsson, G., Zhou, X., Tornquist, E., and Hansson, G.K. 2000. Oligoclonal T cell expansions in atherosclerotic lesions of apolipoprotein E-deficient mice. *Arterioscler. Thromb. Vasc. Biol.* **20**(1): 10–17.

Phillips, C.M., Goumidi, L., Bertrais, S., Field, M.R., Ordovas, J.M., Cupples, L.A., Defoort, C. et al. 2010. Leptin receptor polymorphisms interact with polyunsaturated fatty acids to augment risk of insulin resistance and metabolic syndrome in adults. *J. Nutr.* **140**(2): 238–244.

Pilz, S., Scharnagl, H., Tiran, B., Wellnitz, B., Seelhorst, U., Boehm, B.O., and Marz, W. 2007. Elevated plasma free fatty acids predict sudden cardiac death: A 6.85-year follow-up of 3315 patients after coronary angiography. *Eur. Heart J.* **28**(22): 2763–2769.

Pischon, T. 2009. Use of obesity biomarkers in cardiovascular epidemiology. *Dis Markers* **26**(5–6): 247–263.

Pischon, T., Hankinson, S.E., Hotamisligil, G.S., Rifai, N., Willett, W.C., and Rimm, E.B. 2003. Habitual dietary intake of n-3 and n-6 fatty acids in relation to inflammatory markers among US men and women. *Circulation* **108**(2): 155–160.

Procopio, C., Andreozzi, F., Laratta, E., Cassese, A., Beguinot, F., Arturi, F., Hribal, M.L., Perticone, F., and Sesti, G. 2009. Leptin-stimulated endothelial nitric-oxide synthase via an adenosine 5′-monophosphate-activated protein kinase/Akt signaling pathway is attenuated by interaction with C-reactive protein. *Endocrinology* **150**(8): 3584–3593.

Quinn, M.T., Parthasarathy, S., Fong, L.G., and Steinberg, D. 1987. Oxidatively modified low density lipoproteins: A potential role in recruitment and retention of monocyte/macrophages during atherogenesis. *Proc. Natl. Acad. Sci.* USA **84**(9): 2995–2998.

Raff, M., Tholstrup, T., Toubro, S., Bruun, J.M., Lund, P., Straarup, E.M., Christensen, R., Sandberg, M.B., and Mandrup, S. 2009. Conjugated linoleic acids reduce body fat in healthy postmenopausal women. *J. Nutr.* **139**(7): 1347–1352.

Rajappa, M. and Sharma, A. 2005. Biomarkers of cardiac injury: An update. *Angiology* **56**(6): 677–691.

Ramirez, J.A. 1996. Isolation of *Chlamydia pneumoniae* from the coronary artery of a patient with coronary atherosclerosis. The *Chlamydia pneumoniae*/Atherosclerosis Study Group. *Ann. Intern. Med.* **125**(12): 979–982.

Riccioni, C. 2009. Statins and carotid intimal-media thickness reduction: Up-to-date review. *Curr. Med. Chem.* **16**: 1799–1805.

Ridker, P.M., Hennekens, C.H., Buring, J.E., and Rifai, N. 2000. C-reactive protein and other markers of inflammation in the prediction of cardiovascular disease in women. *N. Engl. J. Med.* **342**(12): 836–843.

Ridker, P.M., Rafai, N., Pfeffer, M., Sacks, F., Lepage, S., and Braunwald, E. 2000. Elevation of tumor necrosis factor-alpha and increased risk of recurrent coronary events after myocardial infarction. *Circulation* **101**(18): 2149–2153.

Ridker, P.M., Buring, J.E., Cook, N.R., and Rifai, N. 2003. C-reactive protein, the metabolic syndrome, and risk of incident cardiovascular events: An 8-year follow-up of 14719 initially healthy American women. *Circulation* **107**(3): 391–397.

Rizvi, A.A. 2009. Cytokine biomarkers, endothelial inflammation, and atherosclerosis in the metabolic syndrome: Emerging concepts. *Am. J. Med. Sci.* **338**(4): 310–318.

Rizza, S., Tesauro, M., Cardillo, C., Galli, A., Iantorno, M., Gigli, F., Sbraccia, P., Federici, M., Quon, M.J., and Lauro, D. 2009. Fish oil supplementation improves endothelial function in normoglycemic offspring of patients with type 2 diabetes. *Atherosclerosis* **206**(2): 569–574.

Rodel, J., Prochnau, D., Prager, K., Pentcheva, E., Hartmann, M., and Straube, E. 2003. Increased production of matrix metalloproteinases 1 and 3 by smooth muscle cells upon infection with *Chlamydia pneumoniae*. *FEMS Immunol. Med. Microbiol.* **38**(2): 159–164.

Roden, M. 2004. How free fatty acids inhibit glucose utilization in human skeletal muscle. *News Physiol. Sci.* **19**: 92–96.

Romagnani, S. 2000. T-cell subsets (Th1 versus Th2). *Ann. Allergy Asthma Immunol.* **85**(1): 9–18; quiz 18, 21.

Rosamond, W., Flegal, K., Friday, G., Durie, K., Go, A., Greenlund, K., Haase, N. et al. 2007. Heart disease and stroke statistics 2007 update: A report from the American Heart Association Statistics Committee and Stroke Statistics Subcommittee. *Circulation* **115**(5): e69–e171.

Ross, R. 1993a. The pathogenesis of atherosclerosis: A perspective for the 1990s. *Nature* **362**(6423): 801–809.

Ross, R. 1993b. Atherosclerosis: Current understanding of mechanisms and future strategies in therapy. *Transplant. Proc.* **25**(2): 2041–2043.

Ross, R. 1999. Atherosclerosis—An inflammatory disease. *N. Engl. J. Med.* **340**(2): 115–126.

Rossmann, A., Henderson, B., Heidecker B., Seiler, R., Fraedrich, G., Singh, M., Parson, W., Keller, M., Grubeck-Loebenstein, B., and Wick, G. 2008. T-cells from advanced atherosclerotic lesions recognize hHSP60 and have a restricted T-cell receptor repertoire. *Exp. Gerontol.* **43**(3): 229–237.

Rudkowska, I., Marcotte, B., Pilon, G., Lavigne, C., Marette, A., and Vohl, M.C. 2010. Fish nutrients decrease expression levels of tumor necrosis factor alpha (TNF{alpha}) in cultured human macrophages. *Physiol. Genomics.* **40**(3): 189–194.

Sacks, H.S. and Fain, J.N. 2007. Human epicardial adipose tissue: A review. *Am. Heart J.* **153**(6): 907–917.

Saifullah, A., Watkins, B.A., Saha, C., Li, Y., Moe, S.M., and Friedman, A.N. 2007. Oral fish oil supplementation raises blood omega-3 levels and lowers C-reactive protein in haemodialysis patients—A pilot study. *Nephrol. Dial. Transplant.* **22**(12): 3561–3567.

Saikku, P., Leinonen, M., Mattila, K., Ekman, M.R., Nieminen, M.S., Makela, P.H., Huttunen, J.K., and Valtonen, V. 1988. Serologica evidence of an association of a novel *Chlamydia* TWAR with chronic heart disease and acute myocardial infarction. *Lancet* **2**(8618): 983–986.

Sakaguchi, S., Ono, M., Setoguchi, R., Yagi, H., Hori, S., Fehervari, Z., Shimizu, J., Takahashi, T., and Nomura, T. 2006. Foxp3+ CD25+ CD4+ natural regulatory T cells in dominant self-tolerance and autoimmune disease. *Immunol. Rev.* **212**: 8–27.

Sangiorgi, G., Mauriello, A., Bonanno, E., Oxvig, C., Conover, C.A., Christiansen, M., Trimarchi, S. et al. 2006. Pregnancy-associated plasma protein-a is markedly expressed by monocyte–macrophage cells in vulnerable and ruptured carotid atherosclerotic plaques: A link between inflammation and cerebrovascular events. *J. Am. Coll. Cardiol.* **47**(11): 2201–2211.

Sarafidis, P.A. and Bakris, G.L. 2007. Non-esterified fatty acids and blood pressure elevation: A mechanism for hypertension in subjects with obesity/insulin resistance? *J. Hum. Hypertens.* **21**(1): 12–19.

Sasu, S., LaVerda, D., Qureshi, N., Golenbock, D.T., and Beasley, D. 2001. *Chlamydia pneumoniae* and chlamydial heat shock protein 60 stimulate proliferation of human vascular smooth muscle cells via toll-like receptor 4 and p44/p42 mitogen-activated protein kinase activation. *Circ. Res.* **89**(3): 244–250.

Savory, D.J. and Pryce, J.D. 1980. Prognostic significance of LDH activity in ischaemic heart disease. *Lancet* **2**(8208–8209): 1375–1376.

Scherer, P.E., Williams, S., Fogliano, M., Baldini, G., and Lodish, H.F. 1995. A novel serum protein similar to C1q, produced exclusively in adipocytes. *J. Biol. Chem.* **270**(45): 26746–26749.

Schwenke, D.C. and Carew, T.E. 1988. Quantification *in vivo* of increased LDL content and rate of LDL degradation in normal rabbit aorta occurring at sites susceptible to early atherosclerotic lesions. *Circ. Res.* **62**(4): 699–710.

Scirica, B.M. and Morrow, D.A. 2004. Troponins in acute coronary syndromes. *Prog. Cardiovasc Dis.* **47**(3): 177–188.

Sharrett, A.R., Ballantyne, C.N., Coady, S.A., Heiss, G., Sorlie, P.D., Catellier, D., and Patsch, W. 2001. Coronary heart disease prediction from lipoprotein cholesterol levels, triglycerides, lipoprotein(a), apolipoproteins A-I and B, and HDL density subfractions: The Atherosclerosis Risk in Communities (ARIC) Study. *Circulation* **104**(10): 1108–1113.

Shibata, N. and Glass, C.K. 2009. Regulation of macrophage function in inflammation and atherosclerosis. *J. Lipid Res.* **50**: S277–S281.

Simopoulos, A.P. 2008. The importance of the omega-6/omega-3 fatty acid ratio in cardiovascular disease and other chronic diseases. *Exp. Biol. Med,* (Maywood). **233**(6): 674–688.

Slade, G.D., Offenbacher, S., Beck, J.D., Heiss, G., and Pankow, J.S. 2000. Acute-phase inflammatory response to periodontal disease in the US population. *J. Dent. Res.* **79**(1): 49–57.

Song, C., Shen, Y., Yamen, E., Hsu, K., Yan, W., Witting, P.K., Geczy, C.L., and Freedman, S.B. 2009. Serum amyloid A may potentiate prothrombotic and proinflammatory events in acute coronary syndromes. *Atherosclerosis* **202**(2): 596–604.

Sorlie, P.D., Adam, E., Melnick, S.L., Folsom, A., Skelton, T., Chambless, L.E., Barnes, R., and Melnick, J.L. 1994. Cytomegalovirus/herpesvirus and carotid atherosclerosis: The ARIC Study. *J. Med. Virol.* **42**(1): 33–37.

Sowers, J.R. 2008. *Endocrine* functions of adipose tissue: Focus on adiponectin. *Clin. Cornerstone.* **9**(1): 32–38.

Span, A.H., Mullers, W., Miltenburg, A.M., and Bruggeman, C.A. 1991. Cytomegalovirus induced PMN adherence in relation to an ELAM-1 antigen present on infected endothelial cell monolayers. *Immunology* **72**(3): 355–360.

Speir, E., Yu, Z.X., Ferrans, V.J., Huang, E.S., and Epstein, S.E. 1998. Aspirin attenuates cytomegalovirus infectivity and gene expression mediated by cyclooxygenase-2 in coronary artery smooth muscle cells. *Circ. Res.* **83**(2): 210–216.

Stein, E.A. and Myers, G.L. 1995. National cholesterol education program recommendations for triglyceride measurement: Executive summary. The National Cholesterol Education Program Working Group on Lipoprotein Measurement. *Clin. Chem.* **41**(10): 1421–1426.

Steppan, C.M., Bailey, S.T., Bhat, S., Brown, E.J., Banerjee, R.R., Wright, C.M., Patel, H.R., Ahima, R.S., and Lazar, M.A. 2001. The hormone resistin links obesity to diabetes. *Nature* **409**(6818): 307–312.

St-Onge, M.P., Zhang, S., Darnell, B., and Allison, D.B. 2009. Baseline serum C-reactive protein is associated with lipid responses to low-fat and high-polyunsaturated fat diets. *J. Nutr.* **139**(4): 680–683.

Sun, J., Sukhova, G.K., Wolters, P.J., Yang, M., Kitamoto, S., Libby, P., MacFarlane, L.A., Mallen-St Clair, J., and Shi, G.P. 2007. Mast cells promote atherosclerosis by releasing proinflammatory cytokines. *Nat. Med.* **13**(6): 719–724.

Sundstrom, J., Ingelsson, E., Berglund, L., Zethelius, B., Lind, L., Venge, P., and Arnlov, J. 2009. Cardiac troponin-I and risk of heart failure: A community-based cohort study. *Eur. Heart J.* **30**(7): 773–781.

Szymanski, F.M., Grabowski, M., Hrynkiewicz, A., Filipiak, K.J., Karpinski, G., and Opolski, G. 2008. Usefulness of myocardial necrosis triad markers for predicting 4-year mortality in patients with suspected acute coronary syndrome. *Acta Cardiol.* **63**(4): 473–477.

Taleb S., Herbin, O., Ait-Oufella, H., Verreth, W., Gourdy, P., Barateau, V., Merval, R. et al. 2007. Defective leptin/leptin receptor signaling improves regulatory T cell immune response and protects mice from atherosclerosis. *Arterioscler. Thromb. Vasc. Biol.* **27**(12): 2691–2698.

Tarnow, L., Astrup, A.S., and Parving, H.H. 2005. Elevated placental growth factor (PlGF) predicts cardiovascular morbidity and mortality in type 1 diabetic patients with diabetic nephropathy. *Scand. J. Clin. Lab. Invest. Suppl.* **240**: 73–79.

Thom, D.H., Grayston, J.T., Siscovick, D.S., Wang, S.P., Weiss, N.S., and Daling, J.R. 1992. Association of prior infection with *Chlamydia pneumoniae* and angiographically demonstrated coronary artery disease. *JAMA* **268**(1): 68–72.

Thompson, S.G., Kienast, J., Pyke, S.D.M., Haverkate, F., and van der Loo, J.C.W. 1995. Hemostatic factors and the risk of myocardial infarction or sudden death in patients with angina pectoris. European ConcAction on Thrombosis and Disabilities Angina Pectoris Study Group. *N. Engl. J. Med.* **332**(10): 635–641.

Toth, B., Fischl, A., Scholz, C., Kuhn, C., Friese, K., Karamouti, M., Makrigiannakis, A., and Jeschke, U. 2009. Insulin and leptin receptors as possible new candidates for endocrine control in normal and disturbed human pregnancy. *Mol. Hum. Reprod.* **15**(4): 231–239.

Trayhurn, P. and Wood, I.S. 2004. Adipokines: Inflammation and the pleiotropic role of white adipose tissue. *Br. J. Nutr.* **92**(3): 347–355.

Triantafilou, M., Gamper, F.G., Lepper, P.M., Mouratis, M.A., Schumann, C., Harokopakis, E., Schifferle, R.E., Hajishengallis, G., and Triantafilou, K. 2007. Lipopolysaccharides from atherosclerosis-associated bacteria antagonize TLR4, induce formation of TLR2/1/CD36 complexes in lipid rafts and trigger TLR2-induced inflammatory responses in human vascular endothelial cells. *Cell. Microbiol.* **9**(8): 2030–2039.

Tsimikas, S., Bergmark, C., Beyer, R.W., Patel, R., Pattison, J., Miller, E., Juliano, J., and Witztum, J.M. 2003. Temporal increases in plasma markers of oxidized low-density lipoprotein strongly reflect the presence of acute coronary syndromes. *J. Am. Coll. Cardiol.* **41**(3): 360–370.

Tzoulaki, I., Murray, G.D., Lee, A.J., Rumley, A., Lowe, G.D.O., and Fowkes, G.R. 2007. Relative value of inflammatory, hemostatic, and rheological factors for incident myocardial infarction and stroke: The Edinburgh Artery Study. *Circulation* **115**(16): 2119–2127.

Uhlar, C.M. and Whitehead, A.S. 1999. Serum amyloid A, the major vertebrate acute-phase reactant. *Eur. J. Biochem.* **265**(2): 501–523.

Varo, N., de Lemos, J.A., Libby, P., Morrow, D.A., Murphy, S.A., Nuzzo, R., Gibson, M., Cannon, C.P. Braunwald, E., and Shonbeck. U. 2003. Soluble CD40L: Risk prediction after acute coronary syndromes. *Circulation* **108**(9): 1049–1052.

Vasan, R.S. 2006. Biomarkers of cardiovascular disease: Molecular basis and practical considerations. *Circulation* **113**(19): 2335–2362.

Venkatesh, P.K., Caskey, D., and Reddy, P.C. 2008. Therapies to increase high-density lipoprotein cholesterol and their effect on cardiovascular outcomes and regression of atherosclerosis. *Am. J. Med. Sci.* **336**(1): 64–68.

Venugopal, S.K., Devaraj, S., and Jialal, I. 2005. Effect of C-reactive protein on vascular cells: Evidence for a proinflammatory, proatherogenic role. *Curr. Opin. Nephrol. Hypertens.* **14**(1): 33–37.

Verma, S., Li, S.H., Wang, C.H., Fedak, P.W., Li, R.K., Weisel, R.D., and Mickle, D.A. 2003. Resistin promotes endothelial cell activation: Further evidence of adipokine–endothelial interaction. *Circulation* **108**(6): 736–740.

Verma, S., Wang, C-H., Li, S-H., Dumont, A.S., Fedak, P.W.M., Badiwala, M.V., Dhillon, B. et al. 2002. A self-fulfilling prophecy: C-reactive protein attenuates nitric oxide production and inhibits angiogenesis. *Circulation* **106**(8): 913–919.

Virchow, R. 1856. Phlogose und Thrombose im Gefässystem. In: *Gesammelte Abhandlungen zur wissenschaftlichen Medizin*. Staatsdruckerei.

Wajchenberg, B.L. 2000. Subcutaneous and visceral adipose tissue: Their relation to the metabolic syndrome. *Endocr. Rev.* **21**(6): 697–738.

Wang, X., Collins, H.L., Ranaletta, M., Fuki, I.V., Billheimer, J.T., Rothblat, G.H., Tall, A.R., and Rader, D.J. 2007. Macrophage ABCA1 and ABCG1, but not SR-BI, promote macrophage reverse cholesterol transport *in vivo*. *J. Clin. Invest.* **117**: 2216–2224.

Wang, H., Chen, D.Y., Cao, J., He, Z.Y., Zhu, B.P., and Long, M. 2009. High serum resistin level may be an indicator of the severity of coronary disease in acute coronary syndrome. *Chin. Med. Sci. J.* **24**(3): 161–166.

Whincup, P.H., Danesh, J., Walker, M., Lennon, L., Thomson, A., Apleby, P., Rumley, A., and Lowe, G.D.A. 2002. Von Willebrand factor and coronary heart disease. Prospective study and meta-analysis. *Eur. Heart J.* **23**: 1764–1770.

Williams, K.J., Frig, J.E., and Fisher, E.A. 2008. Rapid regression of atherosclerosis: Insight from the clinical and experimental literature. *Nat. Clin. Pract. Cardiovasc. Med.* **5**: 91–102.

Won, J.C., Park, C.Y., Lee, W.Y., Lee, E.S., Oh, S.W., and Park, S.W. 2009. Association of plasma levels of resistin with subcutaneous fat mass and markers of inflammation but not with metabolic determinants or insulin resistance. *J. Korean Med. Sci.* **24**(4): 695–700.

Yan, J.C., Zhu, J., Gao, L., Wu, Z.G., Kong, X.T., Zong, R.Q., and Zhan, L.Z. 2004. The effect of elevated serum soluble CD40 ligand on the prognostic value in patients with acute coronary syndromes. *Clin. Chim. Acta* **343**(1–2): 155–159.

Young, R.A. and Elliott, T.J. 1989. Stress proteins, infection, and immune surveillance. *Cell* **59**(1): 5–8.

Yusuf, S., Hawken, S., Ounpuu, S., Dans, T., Avezum, A., Lanas, F., McQueen, M. et al. 2004. Effect of potentially modifiable risk factors associated with myocardial infarction in 52 countries (the INTERHEART study): Case–control study. *Lancet* **364**(9438): 937–952.

Zakynthinos, E. and Pappa, N. 2009. Inflammatory biomarkers in coronary artery disease. *J. Cardiol.* **53**(3): 317–333.

Zampelas, A., Paschos, G., Rallidis, L., and Yiannakouris, N. 2003. Linoleic acid to alpha-linolenic acid ratio. From clinical trials to inflammatory markers of coronary artery disease. *World Rev Nutr Diet.* **92**: 92–108.

Zeitlin, L., Segev, E., Fried, A., and Wientroub, S. 2003. Effects of long-term administration of N-3 polyunsaturated fatty acids (PUFA) and selective estrogen receptor modulator (SERM) derivatives in ovariectomized (OVX) mice. *J. Cell. Biochem.* **90**(2): 347–360.

Zhang, L., Geng, Y., Yin, M., Mao, L., Zhang, S., and Pan, J. 2009. Low omega-6/omega-3 polyunsaturated fatty acid ratios reduce hepatic C-reactive protein expression in apolipoprotein E-null mice. *Nutrition* **26**(7–8): 829–834.

Zhang, Y., Proenca, R., Maffei, M., Barone, M., Leopold, L., and Friedman, J.M. 1994. Positional cloning of the mouse obese gene and its human homologue. *Nature* **372**(6505): 425–432.

Zhao, T., Hou, M., Xia, M., Wang, Q., Zhu, H., Xiao, Y., Tang, Z., Ma, J., and Ling, W. 2005. Globular adiponectin decreases leptin-induced tumor necrosis factor-alpha expression by murine macrophages: Involvement of cAMP-PKA and MAPK pathways. *Cell. Immunol.* **238**(1): 19–30.

Zhao, W.S., Zhai, J.J., Wang, Y.H., Xie, P.S., Yin, X.J., Li, L.X., and Cheng, K.L. 2009. Conjugated linoleic acid supplementation enhances antihypertensive effect of ramipril in Chinese patients with obesity-related hypertension. *Am. J. Hypertens.* **22**(6): 680–686.

Zhu, J., Quyyumi, A.A., Rott, D., Csako, G., Wu, H., Halcox, J., and Epstein, S.E. 2001. Antibodies to human heat-shock protein 60 are associated with the presence and severity of coronary artery disease: Evidence for an autoimmune component of atherogenesis. *Circulation* **103**(8): 1071–1075.

Zwaka, T.P., Hombach, V., and Torzewski, J. 2001. C-reactive protein-mediated low density lipoprotein uptake by macrophages: Implications for atherosclerosis. *Circulation* **103**(9): 1194–1197.

2 Advances in Technology to Generate Cardiovascular-Friendly Functional Food Products

N. A. Michael Eskin, Curtis Rempel, and Michel Aliani
University of Manitoba

CONTENTS

2.1   INTRODUCTION

The rapidly expanding market for foods with defined health benefits has resulted in extensive research worldwide to find new functional foods to treat chronic diseases such as cardiovascular disease. The sustainable production and commercialization of functional foods and nutraceuticals is dependent on the availability and/or development of novel biofortification methods and processing technologies that will ensure the safe amplification or enhancement of bioactive components and their environmentally friendly yet cost-effective extraction from plants and other sources. A further challenge will be ensuring that bioactive components retain biological efficacy and still be bioavailable after processing, storage, and use (Day et al., 2009). This chapter will try to address the potential of new technologies to biofortify or amplify bioactives and extract them to provide reliable and stable functional foods and nutraceuticals for a changing planet. We will examine these in the context of cardiovascular health.

2.2 NEW TECHNOLOGIES

2.2.1 BIOFORTIFICATION VIA GENETIC MANIPULATION

The past decade has witnessed profound advances in both our understanding of genomes and in the functional analysis of key regulatory steps in many developmental and physiological processes in plants and animals. We are approaching the 15th anniversary of the commercialization of the first genetically modified crop (developed using recombinant DNA technology), and in these 15 years, the progress made with respect to understanding gene structure, function, expression, and manipulation or modification of genes is astounding. Genetic engineering, along with other developments in genomic science and marker-assisted breeding, will aid in producing plants with dramatically increased yields and concomitant elevated levels of desirable or necessary bioactives with less reliance on fossil fuel-based fertilizers, pesticides, and water. This is absolutely crucial to provide sufficient energy and nutrients to an expanding population with increasingly limited resources.

Genetic engineering traits for enhancing the nutritional value of plants for human and animal health is complex and technically challenging as it will involve the simultaneous manipulation of multiple steps in plant metabolic pathways. Traditional breeding approaches can only marginally enhance the nutritional value of our global staple food crops as many of these are deficient in some major nutrients (Bouis, 2005). Currently, genetic engineering programs in both private companies and public institutions are targeting elevated mineral content, improved fatty acid composition, improved carbohydrate/fiber profiles, increased amino acid and protein levels, and heightened antioxidant levels. Genetic engineering of plants targeting long-chain polyunsaturated fatty acid (LCPUFA) composition and increased antioxidant levels would have definite benefits, including impacting cardiovascular health.

2.2.1.1 Flavonoids

Anthocyanins, proanthocyanadins, flavones, isoflavones, flavanones, and flavonols (e.g. quercetin and kaemferol) (all collectively belong to a parent class called flavonoids) are naturally occurring polyphenols which impart vivid colors and flavors to flowers, fruits, vegetables, nuts, seeds, and vegetative tissue of higher plants (Schijlen et al., 2004). In plants, they perform various functions, including attracting insects for pollination and protecting the plant against fungal and insect pests (De Gara et al., 2003; Wink, 2003), and abiotic stress, including drought and UV light (Close and McArthur, 2002; Reddy et al., 2007). In addition to their role in plants, these compounds act as antioxidants offering protection against harmful free radicals in animals and humans. As such, they have been shown to offer protection against certain cancers (Lee et al., 2004b; Lee and Lee, 2006; Stuart et al., 2006; Ramos, 2008), cardiovascular disease (Wu et al., 2001a; Duffy and Vita, 2003; Vita, 2005) and age-related degenerative diseases (Lee et al., 2004a). There is also evidence that flavonoids have anti-inflammatory activity (Middleton et al., 2000; Sies et al., 2005). Beneficial effects for cardiovascular health appear to depend on relatively high levels of daily dietary intake, although daily dose remains to be defined (Parr and Bolwell, 2000).

Various health organizations have recognized the importance of naturally occurring antioxidants in the diet and recommend consumption of whole grains, nuts, fruits, and vegetables which are a source of flavonoids as are green tea and cocoa. However, diet surveys by health organizations indicate that adults and children in many parts of the world do not consume the recommended dietary servings of fruits, vegetables, and whole grains, and consequently, there is a growing interest in the development of widely available food crops with optimized levels of components of flavonoids. Additionally, several of these compounds have the ability to be natural food preservatives (Nijvelett et al., 2004).

Several of the enzymes involved in the biosynthesis of the different flavonoids, and their encoding and regulatory genes have already been isolated. Knowledge of these key genes allows for the upregulation or downregulation of these genes to result in increased overall flavonoid synthesis or to engineer pathways to new flavonoid compounds in targeted plants (Rice-Evans, 2001).

2.2.1.2 Tomato Plant

One targeted crop plant for transgenic enhancement of flavonoid content has been the tomato plant. It is an important food crop worldwide and grows in a variety of climates. Flavonoids are an important source of hydrophilic dietary antioxidants but in tomatoes, flavonoid levels are suboptimal to nonexistent (Butelli et al., 2008). The most abundant antioxidant in tomato fruit is the carotenoid lycopene, a lipophilic antioxidant (Le Gall et al., 2003). Generally, foods rich in both soluble and membrane-associated antioxidants are considered to offer the best protection against disease (Basu and Imrhan, 2007; Butelli et al., 2008; Singh and Goyal, 2008).

Initial experiments were conducted utilizing overexpression of a chalcone isomerase from petunia in the tomato fruit. This resulted in up to 78-fold increases in the levels of flavonoids in the fruit peel. However, the peel only accounts for about 5% of the fruit mass, so the total flavonoid levels were no more than 300 µg per g fresh weight (Muir et al. 2001).

Bovy et al. (2002) generated high-flavonoid tomatoes from the heterologous expression of transcription factor genes *Lc* and *C1* isolated from maize. The introduction and coordinated expression of these genes under the control of a combination of general and fruit-specific promoters was sufficient to upregulate the flavonoid pathway in the fruit flesh by 20-fold, this in tissue which does not normally produce flavonoids.

More recently, Butelli et al. (2008) reported enrichment of tomato fruit with anthocyanins by expression of two transcription factors (*Del* and *Ros1* genes) from snapdragon (*Antirrhinum majus*). They reported a significant increase in anthocyanins in both the peel and flesh, averaging 2.83 ± 0.46 mg per g fresh weight, without adversely affecting the liposoluble antioxidants. The level of anthocyanins in these transgenic tomatoes was on par with blackberries and blueberries suggesting that these tomatoes could play an important role in augmenting seasonal berries as a source of natural antioxidants for consumers. From a production perspective, these purple fruit transgenic tomatoes were stable and that the phenotype/genotype could be maintained after backcrossing into a number of commercial tomato varieties. In addition, the transgenes were not associated with any adverse effects on growth or yield.

2.2.1.3 Fatty Acids

Fatty acids are another target for biofortification as some of these are essential nutrients with diverse roles in the human body. There is now a considerable body of evidence from epidemiological and controlled dietary studies demonstrating the cardiovascular, metabolic, and neurological health benefits derived from the omega-3 LCPUFAs from marine fish. The main source of oils and fats in the human diet are from staple oilseed crops such as soybean, canola, flax, palm, peanut, and sunflower. Some of these crops (i.e., flax) are rich sources of the 18-carbon omega-3 fatty acid, α-linolenic acid (ALA), which is a dietary essential fatty acid as the human body cannot produce this. All these crops are rich in the 18-carbon omega-6 fatty acid, linoleic acid (LA), which is also a dietary essential fatty acid. It has been demonstrated that excess consumption of omega-6 fatty acids leads to the depletion of omega-3 fatty acids in human body tissues, with numerous negative health consequences (Lands, 2005; Simopoulous, 2008; Russo, 2009).

2.2.1.4 EPA and DHA

While plants are a source of essential ALA and LA, no higher plants produce the LCPUFAs (carbon-20 and greater) derived from fish which confer health benefits, specifically the omega-3 eicosapentaenoic acid (EPA) and the omega-3 docosahexaenoic acid (DHA). It is also important to remember that while fish are typically the dietary source of these LCPUFAs, they are not the primary producers of these key fatty acids. The primary producers are microbes such as algae which are then consumed by other aquatic organisms, with the fatty acids accumulating at the top of this aquatic food web in fish lipids (Bell et al., 2003; Williams and Burdge, 2006; Napier, 2007). It is also noteworthy that mammals have very limited ability to convert ALA in the body to EPA and

DHA and are therefore dependent upon fish sources in order to receive the cardiovascular and neurological health benefits (Simopoulous, 2008).

Many food products are now marketed or promoted on the basis of being rich in omega-3 fatty acids, though such claims frequently relate to the presence of plant oils which are completely lacking in LCPUFA. In fact, ALA-enriched meat and eggs now available, produced as a result of concentrating ALA-rich plant oils in the feed, contain little or no dietary omega-3 EPA/DHA (LCPUFAs).

While we know that the LCPUFAs from fish oils confer many health benefits, meeting the population needs for increased intake of these fats by eating fish raises several problems: (1) consumers do not eat enough fish or do not have ready access to marine fish; (2) if they did, the quantities needed could not be produced in an ecologically friendly or sustainable manner; and (3) oily fish at the top of the food chain accumulate many contaminants (heavy metals such as methylmercury, dioxins, and plasticizers) from the marine environment (Hites et al., 2004; Jacobs et al., 2004; Domergue et al., 2005). This latter reality has resulted in governments in the United States and Canada warning pregnant/lactating women and small children to limit marine fish servings, again ensuring that this segment of the population will not receive their dietary requirements.

The depletion of marine fish resources highlighted by Pauly et al. (2003) resulted in a UN resolution on restoring fisheries and marine ecosystems to sustainable levels (http://www.fao.org/fi/Prodn. asp). Since then, the marine fishery has not been replenished, but has suffered further decline [cite economist review on global state of fisheries (Pauley et al., 2002, 2003)]. Overfishing continues to manifest itself in declining global catches, the fishing down in marine food webs to lower trophic levels (i.e., replacing once staple fish species with fish species that they would have fed upon, further hindering recovery) and the extinction of whole fish populations (Opsahl-Ferstad et al., 2003; Graham et al., 2004; Domergue et al., 2005; De Alessi, 2008; Truska et al., 2009). None of this has resulted in any measurable counteraction by governments to halt the decline. In addition, aquaculture cannot compensate for the predicted shortfall in the fish supply and may even exacerbate the decline in wild populations. Fish farming disrupts coastal fish spawning habitat and also relies heavily on wild-caught fish which is processed into fish meal (Jackson et al., 2001; Dalton, 2004). As farmed fish still require dietary n-3 LCPUFA supplementation, aquaculture is currently the largest consumer of fish-derived oils, and this practice is also unsustainable. Many times, these processed fish species are not part of the natural trophic food chain for the species. As an example, most of the current farmed salmon is fed fish meal and the fish feed input: fish yield output is abysmal ranging from 2 to 3:1 (Naylor et al., 1998, 2000). Furthermore, there is overwhelming evidence that the levels of EPA/DHA in farmed fish species are much lower than equivalent wild fish species (Napier, 2007).

Many pundits suggest that fish EPA/DHA shortfalls can be made up by the production of single-cell algae or primitive fungi. However, these require bioreactors, fermentation, and/or other production facilities and their cost-effectiveness and sustainability to provide EPA/DHA for a growing population remain to be demonstrated (Lee, 2001; Griffiths and Morse, 2006). Production of EPA/DHA using single-cell fermentation will certainly not yield the protein content that much of the world also obtains from fish consumption. Therefore, the most promising solution appears to be the production of EPA/DHA using transgenic oilseed crops (Abbadi et al., 2000). Genetic engineering can produce these LCPUFAs in a sustainable fashion with oil free of environmental contaminants.

One key finding that makes the genetic engineering of an entire genetic or metabolic pathway present in one organism possible in another unrelated one is the relatively conserved nature of the LCPUFA biosynthetic pathway, extending from marine algae, bacteria, and fungi to invertebrates and mammals (Figure 2.1). This pathway has been tentatively called the "Δ6-pathway" (Napier, 2007). There are other variant forms which can also be exploited, but the Δ6-pathway appears to be the ancestral biosynthetic pathway from which LCPUFA biosynthesis evolved (Graham et al., 2007). Why higher plants have not evolved to include this pathway or retain this pathway is unclear. However, a few taxonomically unrelated phyla can synthesize Δ6-desaturated fatty acids (the initial step in the Δ6-pathway) such as the omega-6 Υ-linolenic acid and omega-3 stearidonic acid (Napier

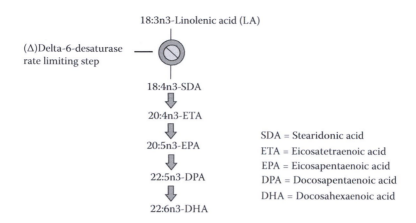

18:3n3-Linolenic acid (LA)

(Δ)Delta-6-desaturase
rate limiting step

18:4n3-SDA

20:4n3-ETA

20:5n3-EPA

22:5n3-DPA

22:6n3-DHA

SDA = Stearidonic acid
ETA = Eicosatetraenoic acid
EPA = Eicosapentaenoic acid
DPA = Docosapentaenoic acid
DHA = Docosahexaenoic acid

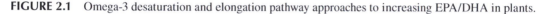

FIGURE 2.1   Omega-3 desaturation and elongation pathway approaches to increasing EPA/DHA in plants.

et al., 2006) and these are being utilized by some companies in a transgenic approach to synthesize LCPUFA but these will not be the focus of this chapter.

The production of LCPUFAs in transgenic oilseed crops has been the focus of several research groups in both the private and public sector for the past decade. Genetic engineering projects of this magnitude require reconstitution of the biochemical pathways existing in other organisms and involve the coordinated expression of multiple genes. Optimization frequently requires genes from several sources which are regulated by tissue-specific gene promoters.

One of the first "proof-of-concept" descriptions of expression of LCPUFA in plants was reported by Qi et al. (2004). This publication describes the reconstitution of a complete Δ9-elongase pathway expressed constitutively in *Arabidopsis*. Three individual pathway genes were each linked to Ca35S promoters and expressed in leaf tissue. EPA contents as high as 3.0% were reported and the overall omega-3-to-omega-6 ratio of fatty acids (2.2:1) was in the range of that found in fish oils. The drawback of this approach is that it is not economically feasible at this date to extract LCPUFA from leaf tissue.

Abbadi et al. (2004) engineered genes comprising the Δ6-pathway using seed-specific gene promoters in flax and tobacco. Flax was chosen as the production platform as its seeds naturally contain high levels of ALA, the omega-3 precursor of EPA. This approach resulted in a lower EPA content (<2%) than the approach taken by Qi et al. (2004). The rate-limiting step appeared to be elongation of 18-C PUFA attributed to a low pool of Δ6-acyl-CoA which is the required substrate for the Δ6-elongase enzyme.

A third approach described by Kinney et al. (2004) focused on expression of a Δ6-desaturase pathway expressed in soybean, under the control of efficient seed-specific gene promoters. This group used the Fad-3 gene from *Arabidopsis* (Yadav et al., 1993) and the *Saprolegnia diclina* Δ17-desaturase gene (Pereira et al., 2004a,b) in addition to the Δ6-pathway genes (Δ6-desaturase, Δ6-elongase, Δ5-desaturase). Utilization of this engineered metabolic pathway resulted in soybeans which accumulated up to 3.3% of total fatty acids as DHA. Additionally, seeds of plants derived from transgenic soy embryos transformed with the construct carrying the Δ6-desaturase, the Δ5-desaturase, and the Δ6-elongase produced up to 20% of the EPA.

Wu et al. (2005) transformed *Brassica juncea* with a series of binary vectors containing three, four, five, six, and nine genes, all controlled by the same seed-specific promoter. This stepwise process allowed for the reconstruction of the entire DHA synthesis pathway. This detailed study led the authors to conclude that, similar to Abbadi et al. (2004), the least efficient step was the elongation of desaturated intermediates. The addition of a second elongase in this model resulted in modest increases in elongation efficiency. Addition of an omega-3 desaturase from *Phytophthora* resulted in an average of 8% EPA production.

Robert et al. (2005) transformed *Arabidopsis thaliana* with Δ6/Δ5-desaturase enzymes from the fish *Danio rerio* and a Δ6-elongase from *Caenorhabditis elegans* with EPA production up to 3.2%. These seeds were further retransformed using two algal genes allowing levels of DHA to reach 0.5%.

Considering the levels of LCPUFA in the aforementioned studies, transgenic oilseed crops appear to be economically viable. Robert (2006) used the composition of the most common fish oil (18% EPA, 12% DHA) as a benchmark for evaluating EPA and DHA levels. Based upon this target, 18% EPA concentration is attainable as maximum values reported to date range from 15% to 20%. The main challenge is going to be further enhancing DHA levels in oilseeds, where the maximum values reported to date are 1.5% in *B. juncea* seeds and 3.3% in soybeans. There are a number of research programs which are focused on DHA improvement.

A group has also been generating cloned transgenic pigs which are rich in LCPUFAs. The researchers cloned pigs which expressed a humanized [i.e., codon usage more similar to that found in mammals (Duret and Mouchiroud, 1999)] *C. elegans* gene, fat-1, which encodes an omega-3 desaturase (Lai et al., 2006). The fat-1 transgenic pigs produced high levels of LCPUFA. The absolute level of omega-3 fatty acids in pig muscle was about 10–15% of that found in wild salmon (Prather, 2006). Additionally, the omega-6-to-omega-3 ratio was decreased in the surviving cloned pigs when compared to the age-matched control pigs. The ratio is 1:6 in the transgenic animals versus 8.5 in the control animals. This is the first report of a transgenic animal being utilized to produce LCPUFAs. The need for a transgenic pig with enhanced LCPUFA levels has been challenged emotively (Fiester, 2006, 2007) and defended (Kang and Leaf, 2007).

Genetic engineering has also been used to modify oils to achieve a reduction in the levels of saturated fats and *trans* fatty acids which are responsible for cholesterol production in the body (Uzogara, 2000). Examples of such modified oils include low- and zero-saturated fat canola, soybean and sunflower oils, canola oil containing medium-chain fatty acids, high-stearic-acid canola oil, and high-oleic-acid soybean and canola oil. Soybeans have been engineered to produce >80% oleic acid (23% is normal) (Hirschi, 2009).

Plant oils which are rich in monounsaturated fats provide improved oil stability, flavor, and nutrition qualities (Newell-McGloughin, 2008). High-oleic-acid soybean oil is more resistant to degradation by heat and oxidation and requires reduced postrefining processing, that is, less hydrogenation. Oils low in saturated or *trans* fatty acids but high in unsaturated fatty acids have important health benefits and better cooking performance characteristics, and consequently these genetically engineered plants offer better health for consumers and a higher economic value for the food industry (Shewry et al., 2008). Oils with lower levels of saturated and *trans* fatty acids can withstand higher temperatures used in frying and other processing methods, have improved temperature stability, and, in some instances, have improved shelf life. These enhanced-stability vegetable-based oils are excellent ingredients in cooking and frying, or in spray oils without the need for chemical hydrogenation (Damude and Kinney, 2008).

2.2.1.5 Lycopene, Resveratrol, and Other Nutraceuticals

Genetic engineering has also produced high-lycopene tomatoes (Pszczola, 1998) and increased resveratrol in white wines using transgenic wine yeast strains (Gonzales et al., 2000). Hugenholtz et al. (2002) showed how lactic acid bacteria can be manipulated to produce a wide range of nutraceuticals, including the B vitamins folate and riboflavin; the prebiotic tagatose; and a number of oligosaccharides. By altering the expression of homologous or heterologous genes, these lactic acid bacteria can be made to produce healthier food products and nutraceuticals. The complete genome of *Lactococcus lactis*, the most widely studied lactic acid bacterium, has been published (Bolotin et al., 2001). Once the complete genome sequences of other microorganisms are established, they will provide important information on the potential capacity of the organism to overexpress specific nutraceuticals. An earlier paper by Wall et al. (1997) showed the potential of transgenic dairy cattle for producing a wide range of pharmaceuticals for treating human diseases. While this technology is still in its infancy, and looked on with great caution by consumers, these researchers suggested that within the next 16 years the products of transgenic animal technology will be in the hands of consumers.

2.3 EXTRACTION OF NUTRACEUTICALS

Once a particular nutraceutical has been identified, a method must be developed for extracting it in large quantities. These methods have traditionally included the Soxhlet, distillation, and maceration with an alcohol–water mixture or hot fat. The Soxhlet method is not only time-consuming but uses large quantities of organic solvents (Luque de Castro and Garcia-Ayuso, 1998). Because of the environmental, health, and safety concerns associated with the use of hexane as the main extractant, alternative solvents have been examined. However, the use of isopropanol, ethanol, hydrocarbons, and even water generally result in lower recoveries due to the decreased affinity between the solvent and solute. As a result, considerable effort has been made to find more efficient and less time-consuming methods that are environmentally friendly and safe (Wang and Weller, 2006). Such methods include the use of sonication, microwaves, and high-pressure fluid extraction.

2.3.1 SONICATION

The application of high-powered ultrasound or ultrasonics for the extraction of bioactive or nutra-ceuticals from plant materials has been extensively reported (Salisova et al., 1997; Vinatoru et al., 1997, 1999; Vinatoru, 2001; Bruni et al., 2002, Melecchi et al., 2002, 2006; Albu et al., 2004; Schinor et al., 2004; Wang and Weller, 2006). Ultrasound is composed of sound waves with frequencies >20 kHz, which is above the upper limit of human hearing. It is a relatively simple and inexpensive alternative method that can be conducted at lower temperatures using any particular solvent. Ultrasonic sound waves are mechanical vibrations which disrupt the plant cell walls, resulting in the release of the cell contents. Microcavitations in the liquid surrounding the plant material are generated locally by the ultrasonic field. The overall effect is twofold: first, mechanical disruption releases the plant cell contents and second, the local heating of the liquid enhances the diffusion of the extract. This results in a greater penetration of solvent in the plant cell wall membranes and improved mass transfer (Keil, 2007).

Compared to conventional extraction methods, ultrasound-assisted extraction was shown by Wu et al. (2001a) to be far more effective and three times faster for extracting saponins from different types of ginseng. In addition, the sonication-assisted extraction could be conducted at lower temperatures and would be less detrimental to the more thermally labile bioactives. Using high-power ultrasound at a frequency of 30 kHz, Kadkhodaee and Hemmati-Kakhki (2007) extracted the three major constituents of saffron (picrocrocin, safranal, and crocin) from the flowers of *Crocus sativa* Linnaeus at 20°C. Compared to the water extraction procedure proposed by ISO, the ultrasonic method was far more efficient in extracting the active components from saffron in a much shorter time period. The extraction yield was found to increase over time as well as with the amplitude sonication. Sonication at short intervals proved to be far more effective than continuous sonication, indicating this method as a potent alternative to water extraction. Wang et al. (2008) showed that ultrasonification to extract phenolic compounds from wheat bran was not only as effective as Soxhlet extraction but was much quicker. Using response surface methodology, optimum extraction was achieved using 64% ethanol, a temperature of 60°C, and an extraction time of 25 min yielding 3.12 mg gallic acid.

Zhang et al. (2009) confirmed the ability of ultrasonic treatment to increase the extraction of epimedin C from *Epimedium*. Ultrasonic treatment disrupted the fresh leaf tissues and cell walls and enhanced the mass transfer of solvents. Compared to the Soxhlet method, ultrasonics reduced the extraction time and minimized the amount of solvent used while achieving a similar recovery.

2.3.2 Microwave

Microwaves are electronic radiations ranging in frequency from 0.3 to 300 GHz that can penetrate biomaterials and interact with polar molecules such as water to produce heat. Absorption of microwave energy by water in the plant cell matrix causes cell disruption by internal superheating which desorbs chemicals from the matrix, resulting in a much improved recovery of nutraceuticals (Kaufmann et al., 2001). The shorter extraction time and higher yields combined with the less use of solvent makes this technique a very attractive alternative for extracting nutraceuticals. Two different microwave-assisted extraction systems are available commercially, the closed extraction vessels under controlled pressure and temperature and the focused microwave ovens at atmospheric pressure (Kaufmann and Christen, 2002). A dynamic microwave-assisted extraction system was introduced by Ericsson and Colmsjo (2000) which produced a similar yield to that obtained using the Soxhlet but over a much shorter time period.

To be effective, microwave-assisted extractions require moist samples, as it depends on the dielectric properties of the solvent and matrix. Water, with a relatively high dielectric constant, allows the microwaves to facilitate the heating process which expands and ruptures the plant cell wall, releasing chemicals into the solvent (Spar Eskilsson and Borklund, 2000). The efficiency and selectivity of the microwave-assisted extraction of pigments from paprika using 30 different extracting solvents were shown by Csiktusnadi Kiss et al. (2000) to be highly dependent on the dielectric constant. The importance of the dielectric constant is to ensure the ability of the solvent to absorb microwave energy. Brachet et al. (2002) showed that, in addition to water, ethanol and methanol were sufficiently polar to be effective for microwave-assisted extraction. For essential oils, which are thermally labile, however, the use of solvents with a low dielectric constant would ensure that a cold environment was maintained during the microwave-assisted extraction (Brachet et al., 2002).

Martino et al. (2006) found that the microwave-assisted extraction of coumarin and related compounds from *Melilotus officinalis* (L) Pallas produced far better results compared to Soxhlet and ultrasound-assisted extraction. Using 50% v/v of aqueous ethanol as extractant and two heating cycles of 5 min at 50°C, they showed that on the basis of the ratio of extraction yield/extraction time, the microwave-assisted extraction procedure was far more efficient. A recent study by Gujar and et al. (2010) developed an efficient microwave-assisted extraction of thymol from the seeds of *Trachyspermum ammi* (ajwain) using methanol in a material-to-solvent ratio of 1:30 at a temperature of 45°C.

2.3.3 Pressurized Fluid Extraction

The use of pressurized fluid extraction systems have increased due to the versatility of pressurized solvents. Varying the temperature and pressure controls the physicochemical properties of the solvents, including density, diffusivity, viscosity, and dielectric constant. Controlling these properties effectively controls the solvating properties of these solvents (Pronyk and Mazza, 2009). High-pressure fluid extractors include supercritical fluid extraction (SFE), pressurized solvent extraction (SSE), and pressurized low-polarity water (PLPW) extraction.

2.3.3.1 Supercritical Fluid Extraction

In the late 1960s, Kurt Zosel at the Max Planck Institute for Coal Research in Mülheim recognized the potential of nontoxic and environmentally benign CO_2, used in a "supercritical" state, for natural product extraction (McHugh and Krukonis, 1986). Beyond a specific temperature and pressure, a gas such as CO_2 becomes a "supercritical" fluid, a state that is neither gas nor liquid, but has properties of both. An advantage of using CO_2 as a solvent is that the critical state is reached relatively readily—at a temperature of only 31°C and a pressure of 73.8 bar (Wang and Weller, 2006). No distinct gas or liquid phase can exist above the critical point, and the supercritical phase has a unique combination of properties from both states. In a supercritical state, CO_2 exhibits low viscosity and high diffusion rates, just like a gas, and has liquid-like densities (Eckert et al., 1996).

Because supercritical fluids such as carbon dioxide (SC-CO_2) have the characteristics of both liquids and gases, they have several major advantages over liquid solvents. First, the dissolving power of a supercritical solvent is dependent on density which can be adjusted by changing the pressure and temperature (De Simone, 2002). Second, supercritical fluids have a more favorable mass transfer due to their higher diffusion coefficient and lower viscosity. In addition, SFE is a more environmentally friendly method that leaves no undesirable residues. The solvent power and selectivity of supercritical CO_2 can be further controlled by fluid density and temperature. Even small changes in temperature or pressure result in dramatic changes in the density, viscosity, and dielectric properties of SC-CO_2 (License et al., 2003; Reverchon and De Marco, 2006; Khosravi-Darani, 2010). In addition to advantage of selective fractionation, the exclusion of oxygen from the SC-CO_2 system mitigates oxidation of compounds, the low operating temperatures minimize thermal degradation of sensitive materials, and the extracts are sterile as microorganisms and their spores are not soluble in SC-CO_2 (Rozzi and Singh, 2002; Dunford et al., 2003a).

Because of the selectivity and versatility of SC-CO_2, significant research is being conducted for use in drug/pharmaceutical synthesis and separation, polymer production and processing, biomedical engineering (controlled release devices and tissue scaffolding), garment cleaning, medical fabric sterilization, residual oil extraction from oil wells in the energy sector, microelectronics/processor chip manufacture, and food/nutraceutical separation and processing (Subramaniam et al., 1997; Leitner, 2000; Ginty et al., 2005; Pasquali and Bettini, 2008).

It is important to note that the use of SC-CO_2 for extraction/fractionation of lipids and bioactive molecules does not contribute directly to the greenhouse gas effect associated with global warming. The CO_2 which is utilized is isolated as a by-product from primary sources such as production of hydrogen or ammonia (De Simone, 2002). Furthermore, the SC-CO_2 system can be run as a "closed-loop" where the CO_2 is recycled. Finally, due to the low heat of vaporization of CO_2, energy costs may be significantly reduced relative to water-intensive processes, which often require large amounts of energy to heat water for extraction and then further energy to dry the final product.

For the food/nutraceutical sector, the primary factor determining the extraction efficacy of a supercritical fluid is the solubility of the bioactive of interest. Supercritical CO_2 is an excellent solvent for nonpolar compounds such as hydrocarbons (Vilegas et al., 1997; Sahena et al., 2009) but not for polar compounds (Temelli, 2009). The poor solubility of phenolics, alkaloids, and glycosides in supercritical CO_2 can be improved, however, by the addition of polar solvents such as ethanol, methanol, acetonitrile, acetone, water, ethyl ether, and dichloromethane. For use in food, however, ethanol is preferred due to its low toxicity compared to the other polar solvents (Lang and Wai, 2001; Hamburger et al., 2004).

If you are reading this chapter in the evening while drinking a cup of decaffeinated coffee or a pint of beer, chances are that the caffeine was removed from the coffee bean and the hops extracted for the beer using SC-CO_2. These were the first commercial-scale uses of SC-CO_2. Since its inception, use of a supercritical CO_2–cosolvent mixture has been found to be an effective way to produce nutraceutical ingredients or functional foods compared to organic solvent extraction (King, 2000).

Significant research has been conducted on extraction and fractionation of oils from plants using SC-CO_2 (Shi et al., 2006). Initially, research focused on oil extraction from staple oil crops—soy, canola, palm, sunflower, etc.—but the past decade has seen significant research on extraction of essential oils from vegetable (carrot, tomato), fruit/berry (apricot, cherry, grape, sea buckthorn, citrus zest), nut (hazelnut, walnut, almond, peanut, pecan), cereal (wheat germ, oat, rice bran), pseudocereal (amaranth), specialty oilseed (flax, chia, borage), and ethnobotanical plants (cloudberry, evening primrose, gardenia, chamomile, sage, veronica) as well as from dairy fat/whey.

The production of heart-healthy oils such as canola oil involves mechanical pressing and solvent extraction, typically *n*-hexane. This requires large amounts of solvent. Additional processing (desolventization/toasting) is required with an operating temperature of 100–110°C to evaporate the solvent from the meal. Some compounds with potential nutraceutical value may undergo thermal degradation from the heat or denaturation from the solvent and this economic value is lost in the processing. Additionally, the cost of evaporation of solvent from oil and meal is also significant and solvent is lost in the process, although process engineering has had a substantial impact on solvent recovery during the extraction process. Supercritical CO_2 promises shorter extraction times, no chemical residue, and a safer operating environment as a replacement for n-hexane extraction (Sahena et al., 2009). Several studies have shown that oil yields using SC-CO_2 are on par with solvent extraction and this is a crucial factor if SC-CO_2 is to be competitive economically with solvent extraction (Taylor et al., 1993; Bruhl and Matthaus, 1999; Perrut, 2000; Li et al., 2010).

Supercritical CO_2 may have an economic advantage over solvent extraction if one factors in the economic value of heart-healthy compounds such as phytosterols, tocopherols, tocotrienols, and other phenolic/aromatic compounds, as their recovery from the solvent "deodorizer distillate" fraction is questionable (Temelli, 2009; Sahena et al., 2009). Many studies have shown that fractionation of these compounds is effective when SC-CO_2 is utilized. Preserving bioactivity and unique flavor and aroma profiles of specialty oils during SC-CO_2 extraction is a major advantage since volatile aroma compounds are lost during hexane evaporation in traditional processing (Sun et al., 2008).

As noted earlier, many vegetable oils are traditionally extracted using hexane. For example, the processing of canola, sunflower, and soybean oil typically involves two main processes: mechanical pressing and extraction followed by further processing to remove impurities. Due to the high residual oil content, the press cake which is generated as a result of the mechanical pressing is further extracted using n-hexane to recover the residual oil. The remaining press cake is then used as a feed meal for animal and aquaculture production.

Several research studies have focused on oil yield (Dunford and Temelli, 1997; Bruhl and Matthias, 1999; Fattori et al., 1988), fatty acid composition (Stahl et al., 1980), and oxidative stability of extracted oils (Przybylski et al., 1998; Jenab et al., 2006) using SC-CO_2 when compared to solvent extraction. Only two studies have examined the extraction of phenolic compounds such as sinapines using SC-CO_2 (Vuorela et al., 2004; Li et al., 2010). The extraction of sinapine, sinapic acid, and vinyl syringol from rapeseed meal was investigated using 70% methanol, 70% ethanol, hot water, enzymes, and SC-CO_2 (Vuorela et al., 2004). SC-CO_2 resulted in the lowest yields of these compounds while 70% methanol resulted in the highest yield of phenolic compounds. A limitation of this study was the fact that the SC-CO_2 operating parameters such as temperature and CO_2 flow rate were not necessarily optimal for efficient extraction of phenol compounds.

Li et al., (2010) investigated the effects of SC-CO_2 operating parameters on extraction yield of oil and recovery of phenolic compounds from canola meal when compared to traditional solvent extraction. These investigators found that canola meal samples were extracted using SC-CO_2 at a comparable oil level to that obtained when extracting with n-hexane. The study also showed that the lowest residual oil levels remaining in the canola meal were achieved with SC-CO_2 operating parameters that are attainable in most SC-CO_2 extraction systems.

The yield of phenolic compounds such as sinapine and sinapic acid were significantly lower with SC-CO_2 than yields obtained from n-hexane extraction. Retention of phenolic compounds is influenced by using a cosolvent such as ethanol and operating parameters for the ethanol cosolvent requires further investigation.

The use of SC-CO_2 for extraction of essential oils has also been extensively investigated. Recently, He et al. (2010) utilized SC-CO_2 for the extraction of gardenia (*Gardenia jasminoides*) fruit. Gardenia has been utilized for centuries in Chinese herbal medicine and the extracts are used for their anti-inflammatory and cholagogue properties (Wang et al., 2004). The major constituents of gardenia fruits are irridoid glycosides. In this study, the total oil yield, yields of particular fatty acids such as stearic, linoleic, linolenic, and eicosaenoic acids as well as tocopherols were all on par with n-hexane extraction.

Although cereals are a modest source of lipids, they are a rich source of antioxidants. These include tocochromanols (tocopherols and tocotrienols) as well as phytosterols. The hulls of wheat, rice, and oats, by-products of milling or processing, are major sources of these bioactive molecules but are considered to be of low value and are typically not consumed by humans despite their health benefits.

Supercritical CO_2, however, has been used to extract oil and tocopherols from wheat germ in several research studies (Ge et al., 2002; Panfili et al., 2003; Eisenmenger et al., 2006; Piras et al., 2009; Kwon et al., 2010). These have focused on the effects of extraction parameters (i.e., temperature, pressure, CO_2 flow rate, cosolvent flow rate, extraction time) on oil and tocopherol yield and sterol and phospholipid content of the extracted oil. A recent study (Gelmez et al., 2009) optimized SC-CO_2 extraction for antioxidant concentration and antioxidant activity of the SC-CO_2 extracts rather than simply oil yield. The effects of pressure (148–602 bar), temperature (40–60°C), and extraction time were modeled. The optimum extraction conditions were 336 bar, 58°C, and 10 min, resulting in 5.3% tocopherol yield, 6 mg gallic acid equivalent (GAE) phenolics/g extract, 6.7 mg tocopherol/g extract, and 57.3 mg scavenged 2,2-diphenyl-1-picrylhydrazyl (DPPH) extract. The tocopherol yield under these conditions corresponded to almost complete recovery.

An example of recovering bioactives with demonstrated cardiovascular benefits from a waste product is the use of SC-CO_2 to extract and fractionate rice bran oil (Shen et al., 1997; Dunford et al., 2003a). Rice bran oil is extremely rich in bioactive phytochemicals such as Υ-oryzanol (10,000–20,000 ppm), phytosterols (15,000–20,000 ppm), and tocopherol/tocotrienols (tocols) (1500–2000 ppm) with proven health benefits (Kaimal, 1999). Υ-Oryzanols are unique to rice bran oil and are potent hypocholesteremic agents (Ramsay et al., 1991). The tocotrienols that comprise 70% of the tocols in rice bran oil have been shown to be powerful antioxidants with antithrombotic properties as well (Yoshino et al., 1989). The conventional method of chemical refining destroys the entire oryzanol complement and substantial amounts of tocols in addition to heavy neutral oil loss. Therefore, chemical refining is not suitable for refining rice bran oil (Gopala Krishna, 1992). Kuk and Dowd (1988) found that the quality of rice extracted by SC-CO2 was superior to that of oil obtained by hexane extraction.

Several studies have demonstrated the suitability of SC-CO_2 for enrichment of rice bran oil with oryzols, tocols, and phytosterols (Dunford et al., 2003a). Recently, Balachandran et al. (2008) showed that rice bran oil extracted with SC-CO_2 had negligible phosphatides and prooxidant metals (Fe and Cu), and the oil was superior in color quality when compared to rice bran oil extracted with hexane. The total rice bran oil yield using optimal SC-CO_2 parameters was comparable to that of hexane extraction (22.5%) and the tocols, sterol, and oryzol yields ranged from 1500 to 1800 ppm, 15,350 to 19,120 ppm, and 5800 to 11,100 ppm, respectively. In addition to high recovery of these bioactives, significant cost savings could be realized using SC-CO_2 as there was no need for a "degumming" process to remove phosphatides nor was bleaching of the oil required (typical with hexane extraction) when extracted with SC-CO_2.

In addition to rice, oats have also been shown to be a source of plant sterols (phytosterols). Plant sterols have been demonstrated to reduce the risk of cardiovascular disease due to their ability to lower serum cholesterol levels in humans (John et al., 2007). Yield of the major sterols found in oats (stigmasterol, campesterol, β-sitosterol, and stigmastanol) were all shown to be significantly greater when extracted with SC-CO_2 than with hexane (Lu et al., 2007). Total plant sterol yield for oats extracted with SC-CO_2 was 105.7 mg/100 g while the yield for hexane-extracted oats was 86.4 mg/100 g.

Choi et al. (2007) showed that the amount of squalene extracted from *Spirodela polyrhiza* was much greater than stigmasterol at 10 MPa and 50–60°C. Using a continuous supercritical CO_2 extraction, Lau et al. (2008) selectively extracted carotene and vitamin E from fresh palm-pressed mesocarp fiber (*Elaeis guineenis*).

In summary, the potential of SC-CO_2 to replace solvent extraction as an environmentally friendly option appears promising. Economics likely favor extraction of specialty oils and bioactives but the use of SC-CO_2 for commodity oil extraction/processing appears attainable as well.

2.3.3.2 Subcritical Water Extraction

Subcritical water extraction (SWE) is a technique using water as an extractant between 100°C and 374°C with the pressure high enough (around 10–60 bar) to maintain water in the liquid state. It is an environmentally friendly technique that results in much higher extraction yields from solid samples (Li-Hsun et al., 2004; Luque de Castro et al., 1998). The principle of this technique is based on the variability in the dielectric properties of water. At room temperature, water is very polar with a dielectric constant of around 80. As water is heated under pressure to maintain its liquid state, the dielectric constant decreases so that at 250°C the dielectric constant is around 27 (Figure 2.2) (Herrero et al., 2006). This value is very similar to that for ethanol (Miller and Hawthorne, 2000). The basic process involved is relatively simple with a water reservoir coupled to a high-pressure pump which introduces the solvent into the system, an oven, in which the extraction cell is placed with a restrictor or valve to maintain pressure. Extracts are collected in a vial at the end of the extraction system which can be cooled rapidly to stabilize the bioactive removed (Herrero et al., 2006). Extraction with subcritical water has proved to be a very effective alternative method for concentrating bioactives, such as antioxidants, lignans, and anthocyanins, from natural materials (Ibanez et al., 2003; Ya-Chuang and Chieh-Ming, 2004; Ju and Howard, 2005; Cacace and Mazza, 2006).

Cacace and Mazza (2006) used subcritical water to extract lignans from whole flaxseed. While the maximum amount of lignans and other protein bioactives were extracted at 160°C and 5.2 MPa, the most concentrated extracts of lignans and phenolic compounds (on a dry weight basis) were obtained at the lower temperature of 140°C and 5.2 MPa. Other factors affecting the rate of extraction were higher flow rates and bed depth. Later work by Guclu-Ustundag and Mazza (2008) examined the effects of flow rate, flow direction, and sample size on the SWE of saponins and cyclopeptides from cow cockle seed.

Using subcritical water at 20–260°C for 5 min, Wiboonsirikul et al. (2007) obtained extracts from black rice bran that exhibited strong antioxidant properties. Their results, shown in Figure 2.3, indicate greater radical scavenging activity at the higher temperature. Analysis of the protein and carbohydrate content also showed the protein and carbohydrate contents to be significantly higher at higher temperatures. However, above 200°C, there was a precipitous decline in the carbohydrate content. The higher protein content at the higher temperatures was attributed to hydrolysis of disulfide or peptide bonds while the drop in the carbohydrate content was ascribed to the hydrolysis of poly- and oligosaccharides as well as monosaccharide degradation at the high ion product of water and temperature (Sasaki et al., 1998; Haghighat et al., 2005). They also found that a short heating period (within 5 min) was preferable as prolonged heating destroyed the beneficial antioxidant effects of the functional ingredients extracted from black rice bran.

Hassas-Roudsari et al. (2009) reported that the highest yield of total phenolics was obtained from canola meal using SWE at 160°C compared to water extraction at 80°C and ethanolic (95% v/v)

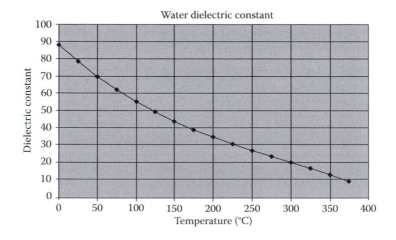

FIGURE 2.2 Graphical representation of dielectric constant of water versus temperature. (From Herrero, M., Cifuentes, A. and Ibanez, E. 2006. *Food chem.* **98**: 136–148. With permission.)

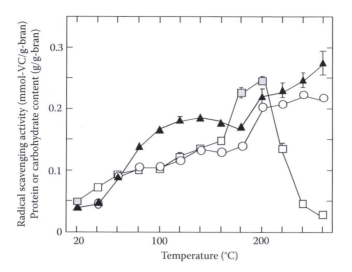

FIGURE 2.3 Effect of temperature treatment on the radical scavenging activity and protein and carbohydrate contents of wheat bran extract. The radical activity was expressed as L-ascorbic acid (VC) equivalent antioxidative capacity. The error bars indicate the standard deviation of the three replicates. ▲, DPPH radical scavenging activity; ○, protein content; □, carbohydrate content. (From Wiboonsirikul, J. et al. 2007. *LWT* **40**: 1732–1740. With permission.)

extraction. The highest antioxidant activity was also reported in the subcritical water extract as measured by DPPH scavenging assay, the Trolox equivalent antioxidant capacity (TEAC) method, and the β-carotene–linoleic acid model system.

Because of the poor solvent power of supercritical CO_2 for polar compounds, Kim et al. (2009) used subcritical water to extract bioactive components, astatic acid, and astaticoside, from *Centella asiatica*. Under optimal extraction of 40 MPa and 250°C, supercritical extraction yielded 7.8 mg/g and 10.0 mg/g asiatic acid and astaticoside, respectively. This was higher compared to yields obtained using conventional liquid solvents such as methanol and ethanol.

Mangiferin, 1,3,6,7-tetrahydroxyxanthone-C2-β-d-glucoside, a bioactive compound found in higher plants, has been reported to have a number of beneficial pharmacological effects, including treating inflammatory diseases, atherosclerosis, and septic shock (Eskin and Tamir, 2006). Using subcritical water, Kim et al. (2010) extracted mangiferin from *Mahkota Dewa*, a popular herbal plant grown in South Asia, in comparison to water, ethanol, and methanol extraction at room temperature, heat of reflux, and using the Soxhlet. They found that the extraction yield with subcritical water was influenced more strongly by temperature than by pressure. Their results in Table 2.1 showed that nothing was extracted using supercritical CO_2 due to the polar nature of mangiferin and its low solubility in supercritical CO_2. In comparison, irrespective of the method used, methanol produced a fairly consistent extract ranging from 23.4 to 25.0 mg/g. Lower extracts were obtained with water ranging from 15.1 to 18.7 mg/g, while the lowest extracts were evident with ethanol ranging from 7.4 to 13.2 mg/g. In comparison, a maximum yield of 21.7 mg/g was obtained using SWE at 373 K and 4.0 MPa over a 5-h period. The latter value was relatively close to the yields obtained using methanol but had the distinct advantage of being environmentally benign.

2.3.4 PULSED ELECTRIC FIELD EXTRACTION

Pulsed electric field (PEF) is a nonthermal method of food preservation and bioactive extraction from natural materials that utilizes short bursts of electricity (Yeom et al., 2002). Where the technology has been used for food processing, it has resulted in microbial inactivation with minimal

TABLE 2.1

Comparison of Mangiferin Extraction Yields Obtained from
Mahkota Dewa **Using Various Extraction Solvents and Extraction**
Methods

Extraction Method	Solvent	Extraction Yield (mg/g)
Supercritical CO_2	CO_2	0
Subcritical water	Water	21.7
Room temperature extraction	Methanol	23.4
	Ethanol	7.4
	Water	15.1
Heat of reflux extraction	Methanol	25.0
	Ethanol	13.2
	Water	18.6
Soxhlet extraction	Methanol	24.6
	Ethanol	12.1
	Water	18.7

Source: Kim, W-j. et al. 2010. *J. Ind. Eng. Chem.* **16**: 425–430. With permission.

or no detrimental effect on food quality attributes (Mosqueda-Melgar et al., 2008). Foods processed with PEF retain their aroma, flavor, and appearance which are not always the case when thermal processing such as pasteurization is used (Knorr et al., 2002). In addition to retention of hedonic characteristics, PEF is attractive as a technology as it is designated as gentle and waste-free, and has short treatment time, low energy requirements, and instant distribution throughout an electrically conductive food (Knorr et al., 2008).

PEF involves treatment of material, which is placed between electrodes, with very short electric pulses (μs or ms) at high electric field strengths (kV/cm) and moderate temperatures. This sudden capacitor discharge is transmitted to the food or plant material via the electrodes. The configuration and geometry of the electrodes determine the course of the field lines and therefore the homogeneity of the electric field. If the electrodes are positioned to be in direct contact with the material being treated, the selection of the electrode material and coating is significant (Barbosa-Canovas et al., 2000; Wouters et al., 2001). Additional parameters which can affect the process and can thus be optimized include electric field strength, pulse shape, pulse duration, number of pulses, and the repetition rate of the specific energy input as well as heating of the product and temperature distribution within the treatment cell. Finally, the electrical conductivity of the product to be treated will also impact the process. Typically, PEF is used for processing liquid or semiliquid material, but wetted milled material has also been investigated. Currently, the technology is restricted to food products with no air bubbles and with low electrical conductivity (Knorr et al., 2002).

The PEF technique is similar to that of electroporation, which has had successful application in biomedicine, cell biology, and biotechnology (Chang et al., 1992). The principle is straightforward—a cell membrane exposed to high-intensity electric field can be temporarily destabilized or irreversibly ruptured. Since the application of PEF is based on the permeabilization of biological membranes, the electrical damage may involve one to several mechanisms such as alteration of transmembrane potential, visco-elastic properties, exploitation or induction of structural defects, compression of the membrane, and colloidal osmotic swelling (Bouzrara and Vorobiev, 2000). The membranes of PEF-treated cells become permeable to small molecules, and the permeation causes swelling and eventual rupture of cell membranes.

While a substantive body of research exists on the use of PEF for destruction of microorganisms and impact on enzymes, effectively demonstrating efficacy as a preservation technology (Barsotti et al., 2002), there are relatively few articles pertaining to the use of PEF in the permeabilization of plant or animal material in order to increase the extraction yield, the potential to induce stress response reactions for concentration of foods with functional constituents, or the impact of PEF on the nutritional quality of health-related compounds of foods or plant materials. The few studies that have been conducted have looked at fruit and vegetable juices (Min et al., 2003a, 2003b, Elez-Martinez et al., 2006, Torregrosa et al., 2005, 2006, Elez-Martinez and Martin-Belloso, 2007), egg (Barsotti et al., 2002), milk (Bendicho et al., 2002, Sepulveda et al., 2005, Kelly and Zeece, 2009), and wine (Puertolas et al., 2009) and have focused on the impact of PEF on preservation of vitamin, carotenoid, phenolic compounds and antioxidant activity, proteins and amino acids, and fatty acids in material versus degradation, presumably to demonstrate to regulatory bodies that no health-promoting constituents of foods are lost when processing with PEF (i.e., demonstration of substantial equivalence with heat treatment).

Conventional heat treatment of products such as juices ensure safety and acceptable shelf life, but the undesirable brown color development is a result of the Maillard reaction between amino and carbonyl compounds and the subsequent formation of 5-hydroxymethylfurfural (HMF). Among the harmful Maillard reaction compounds, acrylamide has received considerable attention this past decade. Acrylamide is spontaneously formed during heat treatment such as frying of foods rich in reducing sugars and amino acids. PEF treatment of raw foods such as potato could be applied as a new method for cell disintegration. The occurring increase in membrane permeability by an exposure of cells to an external electric field positively affects the mass transfer rate. Subsequently, the diffusion of intercellular components in extracellular liquid is increased, while leaving the product matrix relatively unchanged. PEF treatment can be considered a method to assist in removing sugars or amino acids that represent the necessary substrates for the Maillard reaction (Jaeger et al., 2010).

The studies that have been conducted using PEF to investigate extraction yield or concentration of bioactives include grapes (Puertolas et al., 2009), ginseng (Hou et al., 2010), green tea (Zhao et al., 2009), frog (*Rana temporaria chensinensis*) (Yongguang), maize, olives, and soybean (Guderjan et al., 2005) as well as anthocyanins from red cabbage (Gachovska et al., 2010).

Rana temporaria chensinensis is a species of frog which has a long history of use in Chinese medicine. The component which imparts benefit to cardiovascular health and other pharmacological activity has been shown to be a polysaccharide. Yongguang et al. (2006) compared PEF extraction with various factorials of electric field intensity, pulse duration, and inclusion of solvent and then compared this to conventional extraction methods, including alkali and enzyme extraction. In this study, the optimized PEF extraction resulted in higher extraction ratio and polysaccharide content than the other methods. A PEF extraction time of 6 μs gave higher extraction yield of polysaccharide than the other traditional extractions running from 2 to 6 h in length.

Grape skins contain large amounts of different phenolic compounds with cardiovascular benefits, including resveratrol, which are partially extracted during wine making. The cell wall and associated membranes are limiting barriers that prevent the release of phenols into the must during fermentation. Various techniques have been employed to enhance the extraction of these compounds during vinification, with the utilization of macerating enzymes such as pectinases, cellulases, etc. being the most popular. The effect of two enzymatic preparations and the application of PEF on phenolic content and color of Cabernet Sauvignon wine was compared (Puertolas et al., 2009). The researchers demonstrated that PEF treatment was more effective than the enzymatic preparations. After 3 months of storage, anthocyanin content, total polyphenol index, and color intensity were all significantly higher than control and enzyme-treated wines. The color index, anthocyanin content, and total polyphenol index were 28%, 26%, and 11% higher, respectively, than the control wine.

Researchers have also investigated the use of PEF to produce a sterol-enriched maize oil. Plant sterols have been demonstrated to competitively inhibit cholesterol intestinal uptake; a major metabolic effect of dietary plant sterols is the inhibition of absorption and subsequent compensatory stimulation of the synthesis of cholesterol. Higher dietary consumption of plant sterols results in lower cholesterol absorption with a concomitant lowering of serum cholesterol levels, which are associated with atherosclerosis. Guderjan et al. (2005) used a PEF process to produce a maize germ oil which had up to 32.4% higher plant sterol content while achieving a higher oil yield (up to 88.4%). This was done by using hull fractions in addition to the germ. The PEF was efficient at altering cell membrane permeability of the hull fractions in order to release the bound sterol components.

Microbial inactivation coupled with hedonic quality retention makes PEF processing important in order to fulfill consumers' demands for high-quality, minimally processed but safe foods with acceptable shelf life. In addition to these benefits, PEF should be considered by consumers and industry as an environmentally friendly method for the extraction of bioactive compounds from plant and animal material, resulting in food products with increased health potential via improvement of bioavailability of compounds.

REFERENCES

Abbadi, A., Domergue, F., Bauer, J., Napier, J.A., Welti, R., Zahringer, U., Cirpus, P. and Heinz, E. 2004. Biosynthesis of long-chain polyunsaturated fatty acids in transgenic oilseeds: Constraints on their accumulation. *Plant Cell* **16**: 2734–2748.

Abbadi, A., Domergue, F., Meyer, A., Riedel, K., Sperling, P., Zank, T. and Heinz, E. 2001. Transgenic oilseeds as sustainable source of nutritionally relevant C_{20} and C_{22} polyunsaturated fatty acids? *Eur. J. Lipid Sci. Technol.* **103**: 106–113.

Albu, S., Joyce, E., Paniwnyk, L., Lorimer, J.P. and Mason, T.J. 2004. Potential for the use of ultrasound in the extraction of antioxidants from *Rosmarinus officinalis* for the food and pharmaceutical industry. *Ultrason. Sonochem.* **11**: 261–265.

Balachandran, C., Mayamol, P.N., Thomas, S., Sukumar, D., Sundaresan, A. and Arumughan, S. 2008. An ecofriendly approach to process rice bran for high quality rice bran oil using supercritical carbon dioxide for nutraceutical applications. *Bioresour. Technol.* **99**: 2905–2912.

Barbosa-Canovas, G., Pierson, M.D., Zhang, Q.H., and Schaffner, D. 2000. Pulsed electric fields. *J. Food Safety* **65**: 65–79.

Barsotti, L., Dumay, E. Mu, T.H., Diaz, M.D.F. and Cheftel, J.C. 2002. Effects of high voltage electric pulses on protein-based food constituents and structures. *Trends Food Sci. Tech.* **12**: 136–144.

Basu, A. and Imrhan, V. 2007. Tomatoes versus lycopene in oxidative stress and carcinogenesis: Conclusions from clinical trials. *Eur. J. Clin. Nutr.* **61**: 295–503.

Bell, J.G., McGhee, F., Campbell, P.J. and Sargent, J.R. 2003. Rapeseed oil as an alternative to marine fish oil in diets of post-smolt salmon (*Salmo salari*) changes in flesh fatty acid composition and effectiveness of subsequent fish oil "wash out". *Aquaculture* **281**: 515–528.

Bendicho, S., Barbosa-Canovas, G.V. and Martin, O. 2002. Milk processed by high intensity pulsed electric fields. *Trends Food Sci. Technol.* **13**: 195–204.

Bolotin, A., Wincker, P., Mauger, S., Jaillon, O., Melarme, K., Weissenbach, J., Ehrlich, S.D. and Sorokin, A. 2001. The complete genome sequence of lactic acid bacterium *Lactococcus lactis* ssp. *lactis* IL 1403. *Genome Res.* **11**: 731–753.

Bouis, H.E. 2005. Micronutrient fortification of plants through plant breeding: Can it improve nutrition in man at low cost? *Proc. Natl. Acad. Sci. USA* **62**: 403–411.

Bouzrara, H. and Vorobiev, V. 2000. Beet juice extraction by pressing and pulsed electric fields. *Int. Sugar J.* **102**: 194–200.

Bovy, A., De Vos, R., Kemper, M., Schijlen, E., Almenar Pertejo, M., Muir, S. et al. 2002. High-flavonol tomatoes resulting from heterologous expression of the maize transcription factor gene LC and C1. *Plant Cell* **14**: 2509–2526.

Brachet, A., Christen, P. and Veuthey, J.L. 2002. Focussed microwave-assisted extraction of cocaine and benzoylecgonine from coca leaves. *Phytochem. Anal.* **13**: 162–169.

Bruhl, L. and Matthaus, B. 1999. Extraction of oilseeds by SFE—A comparison with other methods for the determination of oil content. *Fresenius J. Anal. Chem.* **364**: 631–634.

Bruni, R., Guerrini, A., Scalla, S., Romagnoli, C. and Sacchetti, G. 2002. Rapid techniques for the extraction of vitamin E isomers from *Amaranthus candatus* seeds: Ultrasonic and supercritical fluid extraction. *Phytochem. Anal.* **13**: 257–261.

Butelli, E., Titta, L., Giorgio, M., Mock, H-P., Schijlen, E.G.W.M., Hall, R.D., Bovy, A.G., Luo, J. and Martin, C. 2008. Enrichment of tomato fruit with health-promoting anthocyanins by expression of select transcription factors. *Nat. Biotechnol.* **26**: 1301–1308.

Cacace, J.E. and Mazza, G. 2006. Pressurized low polarity water extraction of lignans from whole flaxseed. *J. Food Eng.* **77**: 1087–1095.

Chang, D.C., Chassy, B.M. and Saunders, J.A. 1992. *Guide to Electroporation and Electrofusion.* Academic Press Inc., San Diego, CA.

Choi, Y.H., Kim, J., Noh, M.J., Choi, E.S. and Yoo, K.P. 2007. Comparison of supercritical carbon dioxide with solvent of nonacosan-10-ol, α-amyrin acetate, squalene and stigmasterol from medicinal plants. *Phytochem. Anal.* **8**: 233–237.

Close, D.C. and McArthur, C. 2002. Rethinking the role of many plant phenolics-protection from photodamage and herbivores? *Oikos* **99**: 166–172.

Csiktusnadi Kiss, G.A., Forgais, E., Cserhati, T., Mora, T., Morais, H. and Ramos, A. 2000. Optimisation of microwave-assisted extraction of pigments from paprika (*Capsicum annum* L.) powders. *J. Chromatogr. A* **889**: 41–49.

Dalton, R. 2004. Aquaculture: Fishing for trouble. *Nature* **431**: 502–504.

Damude, H.G. and Kinney, A.J. 2008. Enhancing plant seed oils for human nutrition. *Plant Physiol.* **147**: 962–968.

Day, L., Seymour, R.B., Pitts, K.F., Konczak, I. and Lundin, L. 2009. Incorporation of functional ingredients into foods. *Trends Food Sci. Technol.* **20**: 388–395.

De Alessi, M. 2008. Measuring the biological sustainability of marine fisheries: Property rights, politics, science. *Electronic J. Sust. Dev.* **1**: 1–11.

De Gara, L., De Pinto, M.C. and Tommasi, F. 2003. The antioxidant systems vis-a-vis reactive oxygen species during plant-pathogen interaction. *Plant Physiol. Biochem.* **41**: 863–870.

De Simone, J.M. 2002. Practical approaches to green solvents. *Science* **297**: 799–803.

Domergue, F., Abbadi, A. and Heinz, E. 2005. Relief for fish stocks: Oceanic fatty acid acids in transgenic oilseeds. *Trends Plant Sci.* **10**: 112–116.

Duffy, S.J. and Vita, L.A. 2003. Effects of phenolics on vascular endothelial function. *Curr. Opin. Lipodol.* **14**: 21–27.

Dunford, N.T., Teel, J.A. and King, J.W. 2003a. A continuous counter current supercritical fluid deacidification process for phytosterol ester fortification in rice bran oil. *Food Res. Int.* **36**: 175–181.

Dunford, N.T. and Temelli, F. 1997. Extraction conditions and moisture content of canola flakes as related to lipid composition of supercritical CO_2 extracts. *J. Food Sci.* **62**: 155–159.

Dunford, N.T., King, J.W. and List, G.R. 2003b. Supercritical fluid extraction in food engineering. In *Extract Optimization in Food Engineering*, C. Tzia and G. Liadakis, eds. Marcel Dekker, New York.

Duret, L.C. and Mouchiroud, D. 1999. Expression pattern and, surprisingly, gene length, shape codon usage in *Caenorhabditis*, *Drosophila*, and *Arabidopsis*. *Proc. Natl. Acad. Sci. USA* **98**: 4482–4487.

Eckert, C.A., Knutson, B.L. and Debenedetti, P.G. 1996. Supercritical fluids as solvents for chemical and materials processing. *Nature* **383**: 313–318.

Eisenmenger, M., Dunford, N.T., Eller, F., Taylor, S. and Martinez, J. 2006. Pilot-scale supercritical carbon dioxide extraction and fractionation of wheat germ oil. *J. Am. Oil Chem. Soc.* **83**: 863–868.

Elez-Martinez, P., Soliva-Fortuny, R.C. and Martin-Belloso, O. 2006. Comparative study on shelf-life of orange juice processed by high intensity pulsed electric fields or heat treatment. *Eur. Food Res. Technol.* **222**: 321–329.

Elez-Martinez, P. and Martin-Belloso, O. 2007. Effects of high intensity pulsed electric field processing conditions on vitamin C and antioxidant capacity of orange juice and "gazpacho" a cold vegetable soup. *Food Chem.* **102**: 201–209.

Ericsson, M. and Colmsjo, A. 2000. Dynamic microwave-assisted extraction. *J. Chromatogr. A* **877**: 141–151.

Eskin, N.A.M. and Tamir, S. 2006. *Dictionary of Nutraceuticals and Functional Foods.* CRC/Taylor & Francis, Boca Raton, FL.

Fattori, M., Bulley, N.R. and Meisen, A. 1988. Carbon dioxide extraction of canola seed: Oil solubility and effect of seed treatment. *J. Am. Oil Chem. Soc.* **65**: 968–974.

Fiester, A. 2006. Why the omega-3 piggy should not go to market. *Nat. Biotechnol.* **24**: 1472–1473.

Fiester, A. 2007. Response to "why the omega-3 piggy should go to market". *Nat. Biotechnol.* **25**: 506.

Gachovska, T., Cassada, D., Subbiah, J., Hanna, M., Thippareddi, H. and Snow, D. 2010. Enhanced anthocyanin extraction from red cabbage using pulsed electric field processing. *J. Food Sci.* **75**: E323–E329.

Ge, Y., Ni, Y., Yan, H., Chen, Y. and Cai, T. 2002. Optimization of the supercritical fluid extraction of natural vitamin E from wheat germ using response surface methodology. *J. Food Sci.* **67**: 239–243.

Gelmez, N., Kincal, N.S. and Yener, M.E. 2008. Optimization of supercritical carbon dioxide extraction of antioxidants from roasted wheat germ based on yield, total phenolic and tocopherol contents, and antioxidant activities of extracts. *J. Supercrit. Fluids* **48**: 217–224.

Ginty, P.J., Whitaker, M.J., Shakesheff, K.M. and Howdle, S.M. 2005. Drug delivery goes supercritical. *Nanotoday* **8**: 42–48.

Gonzales, C.L., Gil, J.V., Lamuela Raventos, R.M. and Ramn, D. 2000. The use of transgenic yeasts expressing a gene encoding a glycosyl-hydrolase as a tool to increase resveratrol content in wine. *Int. J. Food Microbiol.* **86**: 231–236.

Gopala Krishna, A.G. 1992. A method for bleaching rice bran oil with silica gel. *J. Am. Oil Chem. Soc.* **69**: 1257–1259.

Graham, I.A., Cirpus, P., Rein, D. and Napier, J.A. 2004. The use of very long chain polyunsaturated fatty acids to ameliorate metabolic syndrome: Transgenic plants as an alternative sustainable source of fish oils. *Nutr. Bull.* **29**: 228–233.

Graham, I.A., Larson, T. and Napier, J.A. 2007. Rational metabolic engineering of transgenic plants for biosynthesis of omega-3 polyunsaturates. *Curr. Opin. Biotechnol.* **18**: 142–147.

Griffiths, G. and Morse, N. 2006. Clinical applications of C18 and C20 chain length polyunsaturated fatty acids and their biotechnological production in plants. *J. Am. Oil Chem. Soc.* **83**: 171–185.

Guclu-Ustundag, O. and Mazza, G. 2008. Extraction of saponins and cyclopeptides from cow cockle seed with pressurized low polarity water. *LWT. Food Sci. Technol.* **41**: 1600–1606.

Guderjan, M., Topfl, S., Angersbach, A. and Knorr, D. 2005. Impact of pulsed electric field treatment on the recovery and quality of plant oils. *J. Food Eng.* **67**: 281–287.

Gujar, J.G., Wagh, S.J. and Gaikar, V.G. 2010. Experimental and modeling studies on microwave-assisted extraction of thymol from seeds of *Trachyspermum ammi* (TA). *Separation Purification Technol.* **70**: 257–264.

Haghighat Khajavi, S., Kimura, Y., Oomori, T., Matsuno, R. and Adachi, S. 2005. Degradation kinetics of monosaccharides in subcritical water. *J. Food Eng.* **68**: 309–313.

Hamburger, M., Baumann, D. and Adler, S. 2004. Supercritical carbon dioxide extraction of selected medicinal plants—Effects of high pressure and added ethanol on yield of extracted substances. *Phytochem. Anal.* **15**: 46–54.

Hassas-Roudsari, M., Chang, P.R., Pegg, R.B. and Tyler, R.T. 2009. Antioxidant capacity of bioactives extracted from canola meal by subcritical water, ethanolic and hot water extraction. *Food Chem.* **114**: 717–726.

He, W., Gao, Y., Yuan, F., Bao, Y., Liu, F. and Dong, J. 2010. Optimization of supercritical carbon dioxide extraction of *Gardenia* fruit oil and the analysis of functional components. *J. Am. Oil Chem. Soc.* **87**: 1071–1079.

Herrero, M., Cifuentes, A. and Ibanez, E. 2006. Sub- and supercritical fluid extraction of functional ingredients from different natural sources. Plants, food-by-products, algae and microalgae. A review. *Food Chem.* **98**: 136–148.

Hirschi, K.D. 2009. Nutrient biofortification of food crops. *Annu. Rev. Nutr.* **29**: 401–421.

Hites, R.A., Foran, J.A., Carpenter, D.O., Hamilton, M.C., Knuth, B.A. and Schwage, S.J. 2004. Global assessment of organic contaminants in farmed salmon. *Science* **303**: 2707–2713.

Hou, J., He, S., Ling, M., Li, W., Dong, R., Pan, Y. and Zheng, Y. 2010. A method of extracting Kauginsenoosides from *Panax ginseng* by pulsed electric field. *J. Sep. Sci.* **33**: 2707–2713.

Hugenholtz, J., Sybesma, W., Groot, M.N., Wisselink, W., Ladero, V., Burgess, K., et al. 2002. Metabolic engineering of lactic acid bacteria for the production of nutraceuticals. *Antonie van Leeuwenhoek* **82**: 217–235.

Ibanez, E., Kubatova, A., Senorans, F.J., Cavero, S., Reglero, G. and Hawthorne, S.B. 2003. Subcritical water extraction of antioxidant compounds from rosemary plants. *J. Agric. Food Chem.* **51**: 375–382.

Jackson, J.B.C., Kirby, M.X., Berger, W.H. et al. 2001. Historical overfishing and the recent collapse of coastal ecosystems. *Science* **293**: 629–637.

Jacobs, M.N., Covaci, A., Gheorghe, A. and Schephens, P. 2004. Time trend investigations of PCBs, PBDEs, and organochlorine pesticides in selected *n*-3 polyunsaturated fatty acid rich dietary fish oil and vegetable oil supplements; nutritional relevance for human essential n-3 fatty acid requirements. *J. Agric. Food Chem.* **52**: 1780–1788.

Jaeger, H., Janositz, A. and Knorr, D. 2010. The Maillard reaction and its control during food processing. The potential of emerging technologies. *Pathol. Biol.* **58**: 207–213.

Jenab, E., Razael, K. and Emam-Djomeh, Z. 2006. Canola oil extracted by supercritical carbon dioxide and a commercial organic solvent. *Eur. J. Lipid Sci. Technol.* **108**: 488–492.

John, S., Sorokin, A.V. and Thompson, P.D. 2007. Phytosterols and vascular disease. *Curr. Opin. Lipidol.* **18**: 35–40.

Ju, Z.Y. and Howard, L.R. 2005. Effects of solvent and temperature on pressurized liquid extraction of antioxidant compounds from dried red grapes. *J. Agric. Food Chem.* **51**: 5207–5213.

Kadkhodaee, R. and Hemmati-Kakhki, A. 2007. Ultrasonic extraction of active compounds from saffron. *Acta Horticulturae* **739**: 417–426.

Kaimal, T.N.B. 1999. Rice bran as a food supplement. *J. Oil Technol. Assoc. India* **31**: 25–37.

Kang, J.X. and Leaf, A. 2007. Why the omega-3 piggy should go to market. *Nat. Biotechnol.* **25**: 505–506.

Kaufmann, B. and Christen, Ph. 2002. Recent extraction techniques for natural products: Microwave-assisted extraction and pressurized solvent extraction. *Phytochem. Anal.* **13**: 105–113.

Kaufmann, B., Christen, P., and Veuthey, J.L. 2001. Parameters affecting microwave-assisted extraction of withanolides. *Phytochem. Anal.* **12**: 327–331.

Keil, F.J. 2007. *Modeling Process Intensification.* Wiley-VCH Verlag GmbH & Co., KGaA, Weinheim.

Kelly, A.L. and Zeece, M. 2009. Applications of novel technologies in processing of functional foods. *Aus. J. Dairy Technol.* **64**: 12–16.

Khosravi-Darani, K. 2010. Research activities on supercritical fluid science in food biotechnology. *Crit. Rev. Food Sci. Nutr.* **50**: 479–488.

Kim, W-J., Kim, J., Veriansyah, B., Kim, J-D., Lee, Y-W., Oh, S-G. and Tjandrawinata, R.R. 2009. Extraction of bioactive components from *Centella asiatica* using subcritical water. *J. Supercrit. Fluids.* **48**: 211–216.

Kim, W-j., Veriansyah, B., Lee, Y-W., Kim, J. and Kim, J-D. 2010. Extraction of mangiferin from Mahkota Dewa (*Phaleria macrocarpa*) using subcritical water. *J. Ind. Eng. Chem.* **16**: 425–430.

King, J.W. 2000. Advances in critical fluid technology for food processing. *Food Sci. Technol. Today* **14**: 186–191.

Kinney, A.J., Cahoon, E.B., Damude, H.G., Hitz, W.D., Kolar, C.W. and Liu, Z-B. 2004. Production of very long chain polyunsaturated fatty acids in oilseed plants. El Du Pont de Nemours WO 2004/2007/071 1467 A2.

Knorr, D., Ade-Omowaye, B.I.O. and Heinz, V. 2002. Nutritional improvement of plant foods by non-thermal processing. *Proc. Nutr. Soc.* **61**: 311–318.

Knorr, D., Engel, K-H., Vogel, R., Kochte-Clemens, B. and Eisenbrand, G. 2008. Statement on the treatment of food using a pulsed electric field. *Mol. Nutr. Food Res.* **52**: 1539–1542.

Kuk, M.S. and Dowd, M.K. 1998. Supercritical fluid extraction of rice bran. *J. Am. Oil Chem. Soc.* **75**: 623–628.

Kwon, K-T., Uddin, Md.S., Jung, G-W., Sim, J-E. and Chun, B-S. 2010. Supercritical carbon dioxide extraction of phenolics and tocopherols enriched oil from wheat bran. *World Acad. Sci. Eng. Technol.* **64**: 255–260.

Lai, L., Kang, J.X., Li, R., Wang, J., Witt, W.T., Yong, H.Y., et al. 2006. Generation of cloned transgenic pigs rich in omega-3 fatty acids. *Nat. Biotechnol.* **24**: 435–436.

Lands, W.E.M. 2005. Dietary fat and health: The evidence and politics of prevention: Careful use of dietary fats can improve life and prevent disease. *Ann. N.Y. Acad. Sci.* **1055**: 179–192.

Lang, Q. and Wai, C.M. 2001. Supercritical fluid extraction in herbal and natural product studies. *Talanta.* **53**: 771–782.

Lau, H.L.N., Choo, Y.M., Ma, A.N. and Chuah, C.H. 2008. Selective extraction of palm carotene and vitamin E from fresh palm-pressed mesocarp fibre (*Elaeis guineenis*) using supercritical CO_2. *J. Food Eng.* **84**: 289–296.

Le Gall, G., Dupont, M.S., Melton, F.A., Davies, A.L., Collins, G.J., Verhoeyen, M.E. and Colquhoun, I.J. 2003. Characterization and content of flavonoid glycosides in genetically modified tomato (*Lycopersicon esculentum*) fruits. *J. Agric. Food Chem.* **51**: 2438–2446.

Lee, J., Koo, N. and Min, D.B., 2004a. Reactive oxygen species, ageing, and antioxidative nutraceuticals. *Comp. Rev. Food Sci.* **3**: 21–33.

Lee, K.W. and Lee, H.J. 2006. Biphase effects of dietary antioxidants on oxidative stress-mediated carcinogenesis. *Mech. Aging Develop.* **127**: 424–431.

Lee, K.W., Lee, H.J. and Lee, C.Y. 2004b. Vitamins, phytochemicals, diets and their implications in cancer chemoprevention. *Crit. Rev. Food Sci. Nutr.* **44**: 437–452.

Lee, Y.K. 2001. Microalgal mass culture systems and methods: Their limitation and potential. *J. Appl. Phycol.* **13**: 307–315.

Leitner, W. 2000. Designed to dissolve. *Nature* **405**: 129–130.

Li, H., Wu, J., Rempek, C.B. and Thiyam, U. 2010. Effect of operating parameters on oil and phenolic extraction using supercritical CO_2. *J. Am. Oil Chem. Soc.* **87**: 1081–1089.

License, P., Ke, J., Sokolova, M., Ross, S.K. and Poliakoff, M. 2003. Chemical reactions in supercritical carbon dioxide: From laboratory to commercial plant. *Green Chem.* **5**: 99–104.

Li-Hsun, C., Ya-Chuan, C. and Chieh-Ming, C. 2004. Extracting and purifying isoflavones from defatted soybean flakes using superheated water at elevated pressures. *Food Chem.* **84**: 279–284.

Lu, B., Zhang, Y., Wu, X. and Shi, J. 2007. Separation and determination of diversiform phytosterols in food materials using supercritical carbon dioxide extraction and ultraperformance liquid chromatography-atmospheric pressure chemical ionization-mass spectrometry. *Anal. Chim. Acta* **588**: 50–63.

Luque de Castro, M.D. and Garcia-Ayuso, L.E. 1998. Soxhlet extraction of solid materials: A outdated technique with promising innovative future. *Anal. Chim. Acta* **369**: 1–10.

Martino, E., Ramaiola, I., Urbano, M., Bracco, F. and Collins, S. 2006. Microwave-assisted extraction of coumarin and related compounds from *Melilotus officinalis* (L) Pallas as an alternative to Soxhlet and ultrasound-assisted extraction. *J. Chromatogr. A* **1125**(2): 147–151.

McHugh, M.A. and Krukonis, V.J. 1986. *Supercritical Fluid Extraction: Principles and Practice*, Butterworth, Stoneham, MA.

Melecchi, M.I.S., Martinez, M.M., Abad, F.C., Zini, P.P., Filho, I. and Caramao, E.B. 2002. Chemical composition of *Hibiscus tillaceus* L. flowers: A study of extraction methods. *J. Sep. Sci.* **25**: 86–90.

Melecchi, M.I.S., Peres, V.F., Dariva, C., Zini, C.A., Abad, F.C., Martinez, M.M. and Caramao, E.B. 2006. Optimization of the sonication extraction method of *Hibiscus tiliaceus* L. flower. *Ultrason. Sonochem.* **13**: 242–250.

Middleton, E., Kandaswami, C. and Theoharides, T.C. 2000. The effects of plant flavonoids on mammalian cells: Implications for inflammation, heart disease, and cancer. *Pharmacol. Rev.* **52**: 673–751.

Miller, D.J. and Hawthorne, S.B. 2000. Solubility of liquid organic flavour and fragrance compounds in supercritical (hot/liquid) water from 298 to 473 K. *J. Chem. Eng. Data* **45**: 315–318.

Min, S., Jin, Z.T. and Zhang, Q.H. 2003b. Commercial scale pulsed electric field processing of tomato juice. *J. Agric. Food Chem.* **51**: 3338–3344.

Min, S., Jin, Z.T., Min, S.K., Yeom, H. and Zhang, Q.H. 2003a. Commercial-scale pulsed electric field processing of orange juice. *J. Food Sci.* **68**: 1265–1271.

Mosqueda-Melgar, J., Elez-Martinez, P., Raybaudi-Massilia, R.M. and Martin-Belloso, O. 2008. Effects of pulsed electric fields on pathogenic microorganisms of major concern in fluid foods: A review. *Crit. Rev. Food Sci. Nutr.* **48**: 747–759.

Muir, S.R., Collins, G.J., Robinson, S., Hughes, S., Bovy, A., Ric de Vos, C.H., Van Tunen, A.J. and Verhoeyen, M.E. 2001. Overexpression of petunia chalcone isomerise in tomato results in fruit containing increasing levels of flavonols. *Nat. Biotechnol.* **19**: 470–474.

Napier, J.A. 2007. Transgenic plants as a source of fish oils: Healthy, sustainable and GM. *J. Sci. Food Agric.* **87**: 8–12.

Napier, J.A., Haslan, R., Caleron, M.V., Michaelson, L.V., Beaudoin, F. and Sayanova, O. 2006. Progress towards the production of very long chain polyunsaturated fatty acid in transgenic plants: Plant metabolic engineering comes of age. *Physiologia Plantarum* **126**: 398–406.

Naylor, R.L., Goldburg, R.J., Mooney, H., Beveridge, M.C.M., Clay, J., Folke, C., Kautsky, N., Lubchenco, J., Primavera, J.H. and Williams, M. 1998. Nature's subsidies to shrimp and salmon farming. *Science* **282**: 883–884.

Naylor, R.L., Goldburg, R.J., Primavera, J.H., Kautsky, N., Beveridge, M.C.M., Clay, J., Folke, C., Luchenco, J., Mooney, H. and Troell, M. 2000. Effect of aquaculture on world fish supplies. *Nature* **405**: 1017–1024.

Newell-McGloughin, M. 2008. Nutritionally improved agricultural crops. *Plant Physiol.* **147**: 939–953.

Nijveldt, R.J., Nood, V.E., van Hoorn, D.E.C., Boelends, P.G., van Norren, K. and van Leeuwen, P.A.M. 2001. Flavonoids: A review of probable mechanisms of action and potential applications. *Am. J. Clin. Nutr.* **74**: 418–425.

Opsahl-Ferstad, H-G., Rudi, H., Ruyter, B. and Refstie, S. 2003. Biotechnological approaches to modifying rapeseed oil composition for application in aquaculture. *Plant Sci.* **165**: 349–357.

Panfili, G., Cinquanta, L., Fratianni, A. and Cubadda, R. 2003. Extraction of wheat germ oil by supercritical CO2: Oil and defatted cake characterization. *J. Am. Oil Chem. Soc.* **80**: 157–161.

Parr, A.J. and Bolwell, G.P. 2000. Phenols in the plant and in man. The potential for possible nutritional enhancement of the diet by modifying the phenols content or profile. *J. Sci. Food Agric.* **80**: 985–1012.

Pasquali, I. and Bettini, R. 2008. Are pharmaceutics really going supercritical? *Int. J. Pharm.* **364**: 176–187.

Pauly, D., Christensen, V., Guenette, S., Pitcher, T.J., Sumaila, U.R., Walters, C.J., Watson, R. and Zeller, D. 2002. Towards sustainability in world fisheries. *Nature* **418**: 689–695.

Pauly, D., Alder, J., Bennett, E., Christensen, V., Tyedmere, P. and Watson, R. 2003. The future of fisheries. *Science* **302**: 1359–1361.

Pauly, D., Watson, R. and Alder, J. 2005. Global trends in world fisheries: Impacts on marine ecosystems and food security. *Philos. Trans. R. Soc. Lond. B. Biol. Sci.* **360**: 5–12.

Pereira, S.L., Huang, Y.S., Bobik, E.G., Kinney, A.J., Stecca, K.L., Packer, J.C. and Mukerji, P. 2004. A novel omega-3 fatty acid desaturase involved in the biosynthesis of eicopentaenoic acid. *Biochem. J.* **378**: 665–671.

Pereira, S.L., Leonard, A.E., Huang, Y.S., Chuang, L.T. and Mukerji, P. 2004. Identification of two novel micro-algal enzymes involved in the conversion of omega-3 fatty acid, eicosapentaenoic acid (EPA) to docosa-hexaenoic acid (DHA). *Biochem. J.* **384**: 357–366.

Perrut, M. 2000. Supercritical fluid applications: Industrial developments and economic issues. *Ind. Eng. Chem. Res.* **39**: 4531–4535.

Piras, A., Rosa, A., Falconieri, D., Porcedda, S., Dessi, M.A. and Marongiu, B. 2009. Extraction of oil from wheat germ by supercritical CO_2. *Molecules* **14**: 2573–2581.

Prather, R.S. 2006. Cloned transgenic heart-healthy pork? *Transgenic Res.* **15**: 405–407.

Pronyk, C. and Mazza, G. 2009. Design and scale-up of pressurized fluid extractors for food and bioproducts. *J. Food Eng.* **95**: 215–226.

Przybylski, R., Lee, Y.C. and Kim, I.H. 1998. Oxidative stability of canola oils extracted with supercritical carbon dioxide. *Lebensmittel-Wissenschaft und-Technologie* **31**: 687–693.

Pszczola, D.E. 1998. The ABCs of nutraceutical ingredients. *Food Technol.* **52**: 30–37.

Puertolas, E., Saldana, G., Condon, S., Alvarez, I. and Raso, J. 2009. A comparison of the effect of macerating enzymes and pulsed electric fields technology on phenolic content and color of red wine. *J. Food Sci.* **74**: 647–652.

Qi, B., Fraser, T., Mugford, S., Diobson, G., Sayanova, O., Butler, J., Napier, J.A. and Lazarus, C.M. 2004. Production of very long chain polyunsaturated omega-3 and omega-6 fatty acids in plants. *Nat. Biotechnol.* **22**: 739–745.

Ramos, S. 2008. Cancer chemoprevention and chemotherapy: Dietary polyphenols and signalling pathways. *Mol. Nutr. Food Res.* **52**: 507–526.

Ramsay, M.E., Novak, R.A. and Reightler, W.J. 1991. Processing rice bran oil by supercritical fluid extraction. *Food Technol.* **45**: 98–104.

Reddy, A.M., Reddy, V.S., Scheffler, B.E., Wienand, U. and Reddy, A.R. 2007. Novel transgenic rice over-expressing anthocyanidin synthase accumulates a mixture of flavonoids leading to an increased antioxi-dant potential. *Metab. Eng.* **9**: 95–111.

Reverchon, E. and De Marco, I. 2006. Supercritical fluid extraction and fractionation of natural matter. *J. Supercrit. Fluids* **38**: 146–166.

Rice-Evans, C. 2001. Flavonoid antioxidants. *Curr. Med. Chem.* **8**: 797–807.

Robert, S.S., Singh, S., Zhou, X-R., Petrie, J.R., Blackburn, S.L., Mansour, P.M., Nichols, P.D., Liu, Q. and Green, A.G. 2005. Metabolic engineering of *Arabidopsis* to produce nutritionally important DHA in seed oil. *Funct. Plant Biol.* **32**: 473–479.

Robert, S.S. 2006. Production of eicosapentaenoic and docosahexaenoic acid-containing oils in transgenic land plants for human and aquaculture nutrition. *Mar. Biotechnol.* **8**: 103–109.

Rozzi, N.L. and Singh, R.K. 2002. Supercritical fluids in the food industry. *Com. Rev. Food Sci. Food Safety* **1**: 33–44.

Russo, G.L. 2009. Dietary n-6 and n-3 polyunsaturated fatty acids: From biochemistry to clinical implications in cardiovascular prevention. *Biochem. Pharmacol.* **77**: 937–946.

Sahena, F., Zaidul, I.S.M., Jinap, S., Karim, A.A., Norulaini, N.A.N. and Omar, A.K.M. 2009. Application of supercritical CO_2 in lipid extraction-A review. *J. Food Eng.* **95**: 240–253.

Salisova, M.M., Toma, M. and Mason, T.J. 1997. Comparison of conventional and ultrasonically assisted extractions of pharmaceutically active compounds from *Salvia officinalis*. *Ultrason. Sonochem.* **4**: 131–134.

Sasaki, M., Kabyemela, B., Malaluan, R., Hirose, S., Takeda, N., Adschiri, T. and Arai, K. 1998. Cellulose hydrolysis in subcritical and supercritical water. *J. Supercrit. Fluids* **13**(1–3): 261–268.

Schijlen, E.G.W.M., de Vos, C.H.R., van Tunen, A.J. and Bovy, A.G. 2004. Modification of flavonoid biosyn-thesis in crop plants. *Phytochemistry* **65**: 2631–2648.

Schinor, E.C., Salvador, M.J. and Turatti, I.C.C. 2004. Comparison of classical and ultrasound-assisted extrac-tions of steroids and terpenoids from three Chresta spp. *Ultrason. Sonochem.* **11**: 415–421.

Sepulveda, D.D., Gongora-Nieto, M.M., Guerrero, J.A. and Barbosa-Canovas G.V. 2005. Production of extended shelf-life milk by processing pasteurized milk with pulsed electric fields. *J. Food Eng.* **67**: 81–86.

Shen, Z., Palmer, M.V., Ting, S.S.T. and Fairclough, R.J. 1997. Pilot scale extraction and fractionation of rice bran oil using supercritical carbon dioxide. *J. Agric. Food Chem.* **45**: 4540–4544.

Shewry, P.R., Jones, H.D. and Halford, N.G. 2008. Plant biotechnology: Transgenic crops. *Adv. Biochem. Eng. Biotechnol.* **111**: 149–186.

Shi, J., Kassama, S. and Kakuda, Y. 2006. Supercritical fluid extraction for bioactive components. In *Functional Food Ingredients and Nutraceuticals*: *Processing Technologies,* Shi, J. ed., CRC Press, Boca Raton, FL.

Sies, H., Schewe, T., Heiss, C. and Kelm, M. 2005. Cocoa polyphenols and inflammatory mediators. *Am. J. Clin. Nutr.* **81**: 3045–3125.

Simopoulous, A.P. 2008. The importance of the omega-6/omega-3 fatty acid ratio in cardiovascular disease and other chronic diseases. *Exp. Biol. Med.* (Maywood) **223**: 674–688.

Singh, P. and Goyal, G.K. 2008. Dietary lycopene: Its properties and anticarcinogenic effects. *Comp. Rev. Food Sci. Food Safety* **7**: 255–270.

Spar Eskilsson, C. and Borklund, E. 2000. Analytical-scale microwave-assisted extraction. *J. Chromatogr. A* **902**: 227–250.

Stahl, E., Schultz, E. and Mangold, H.K. 1980. Extraction of oil seeds with liquor and supercritical carbon dioxide. *J. Agric. Food Chem.* **28**: 1153–1157.

Stuart, E.C., Scandlyn, M.J. and Rosengreen, R.J. 2006. The role of epigallocatechin gallate (EGCG) in the treatment of breast and prostate cancer. *Life Sci.* **79**: 2329–2336.

Subramaniam, B., Rajewski, R.A. and Snavely, K. 1997. Pharmaceutical processing with supercritical carbon dioxide. *J. Pharm. Sci.* **86**: 885–890.

Sun, M., Xu, L., Saldana, M.D.A. and Temelli, F. 2008. Comparison of canola meals obtained by conventional methods and supercritical CO_2 with and without ethanol. *J. Am. Oil Chem. Soc.* **85**: 667–675.

Taylor, S.L., King, J.W. and List, G.R. 1993. Determination of oil content in oilseeds by analytical supercritical fluid extraction. *J. Am. Oil Chem. Soc.* **70**: 437–439.

Temelli, F. 2009. Perspectives on supercritical fluid processing of fats and oils. *J. Supercrit. Fluids* **47**: 583–590.

Torregrosa, F., Cortes, C., Esteve, M.J. and Frigola, A. 2005. Effect of high-intensity pulsed electric fields processing and conventional heat treatment on orange-carrot juice carotenoids. *J. Agric. Food Chem.* **53**: 9519–9525.

Torregrosa, F., Esteve, M.J., Frigola, A. and Cortes, C. 2006. Ascorbic acid stability during refrigerated storage of orange-carrot juice treated by high pulsed electric field and comparison with pasteurized juice. *J. Food Eng.* **73**: 339–345.

Truska, M., Vrinten, P. and Qui, X. 2009. Metabolic engineering of plants for polyunsaturated fatty acid production. *Mol. Breeding* **23**: 1–11.

Uzogara, S.G. 2000. The impact of genetic modification of human foods in the 21st century: A review. *Biotech. Adv.* **18**: 179–206.

Vilegas, J.H.Y., de Marchi, E. and Lancas, F.M. 1997. Extraction of low-polarity compounds (with emphasis on coumarin and kaurenoic acid) from *Mikania glomerata* ('Guaco') leaves. *Phytochem. Anal.* **8**: 266–270.

Vinatoru, M., Toma, M., Radu, O., Filip, P., Lazurca, D. and Mason, T.J. 1997. The use of ultrasound for the extraction of bioactive principles from plant materials. *Ultrason. Sonochem.* **4**: 125–139.

Vinatoru, M., Toma, M. and Mason, T.J. 1999. Ultrasonic assisted extraction of bioactive principles from plants and its constituents. *Adv. Sonochem.* **5**: 209–249.

Vinatoru, M. 2001. An overview of the ultrasonically assisted extraction of bioactive from herbs. *Ultrason. Biochem.* **8**: 303–313.

Vita, J.A. 2005. Polyphenols and cardiovascular disease: Effects on endothelial and platelet function. *Am. J. Clin. Nutr.* **81**: 2925–2975.

Vuorela, S., Meyer, A.S. and Heinonen, M. 2004. Impact of isolation method on the antioxidant activity of rapeseed meal phenolics. *J. Agric. Food Chem.* **52**: 8202–8207.

Wall, R.J., Kerr, D.E. and Bondioli, K.R. 1997. Transgenic dairy cattle: Genetic engineering on a large scale. *J. Dairy Sci.* **80**: 2213–2224.

Wang, J., Sun, B., Cao, Y., Tian, Y. and Li, X. 2008. Optimisation of ultrasound-assisted extraction of phenolic compounds from wheat bran. *Food Chem.* **106**: 804–810.

Wang, L. and Weller, C.L. 2006. Recent advances in extraction of nutraceuticals from plants. *Trends Food Sci. Technol.* **117**: 300–312.

Wang, S.C., Tseng, T.Y., Huang, C.M. and Tsai, H. 2004. Gardenia herbal active constituents: Applicable separation procedures. *J. Chromatogr. B* **812**: 193–202.

Wiboonsirikul, J., Hata, S., Tsuno, T., Kimira, Y. and Adachi, S. 2007. Production of functional substances from black rice bran by its treatment in subcritical water. *LWT* **40**: 1732–1740.

Williams, C.M. and Burdge, G. 2006. Long chain *n*-3 PUFA: Plant v. marine sources. *Proc. Nutr. Soc.* **65**: 1–9.

Wink, M. 2003. Evolution of secondary metabolites from an ecological and molecular phylogenetic perspective. *Phytochemistry* **64**: 3–19.

Wouters, P.C., Alvarez, I. and Raso, J. 2001. Critical factors determining inactivation kinetics by pulsed electric field food processing. *Trends Food Sci. Technol.* **12**: 112–121.

Wu, G., Truska, M., Datla, N., Vrinten, P., Bauer, J., Zank, T., Cirpus, P., Heinz, E. and Qiu, X. 2005. Stepwise engineering to produce high yields of very long-chain polyunsaturated fatty acids in plants. *Nat. Biotechnol.* **23**: 1013–1017.

Wu, J., Lin, L. and Chau, F-t. 2001a. Ultrasound-assisted extraction of ginseng saponins from ginseng roots and cultured ginseng cells. *Utrason. Sonochem.* **6**(4): 347–352.

Wu, L.M., Wang, Z.R., Hsieh, T.C., Bruder, J.L., Zhou, J.G. and Huang, Y.Z. 2001b. Mechanisms of cardioprotection by resveratrol, a phenolic antioxidant in red wine (review). *Int. J. Mol. Med.* **8**: 3–17.

Yadav, N.S., Wierzbicki, A., Aergerter, M., Caster, C.S., Perez-Grau, L., Kinney, A.J., Hitz, W.D., Booth, J.R., Schweiger, B.J., Stecka, K.L. et al. 1993. Cloning of higher plant w-3 fatty acid desaturases. *Plant Physiol.* **103**: 487–476.

Yeom, H.W., McCann, K.T., Streaker, C.B. and Zhang, Q.H. 2002. Pulsed electric field processing of high acid liquid foods: A review. *Adv. Food Nutr. Res.* **44**: 2–8.

Yongguang, Y., Yuzhu, H. and Yong, H. 2006. Pulsed electric field extraction of polysaccharide from *Rana temporaria chensinensis* David. *Int. J. Pharmaceutics* **312**: 33–36.

Yoshino, G., Kazumi, T., Amano, M., Tateiwa, M., Yamasaki, T., Takashima, S., Iwai, M., Hatanaka, H. and Baba, S. 1989. Effects of gamma oryzanol on hyperlipidemic subjects. *Curr. Theor. Res. Clin. Exp.* (USA). **45**: 543–552.

Zhang, H-F., Yang, X-H, Zhao, L-D. and Wang, Y. 2009. Ultrasonic-assisted extraction of epimedin C from fresh leaves of *Epimedium* an extraction mechanism. *Innov. Food Sci. Emerg. Sci.* **10**(1): 54–60.

Zhao, W., Yang, R., Wang, M. and Lu, R. 2009. Effects of pulsed electric fields on bioactive components, colour, and flavour of green tea infusions. *Int. J. Food Sci. Tech.* **44**: 312–321.

3 Clinical and Experimental Evidence on Cardiovascular Benefits of Fish Oil

Mohammed H. Moghadasian and Natalie D. Riediger
University of Manitoba

CONTENTS

3.1   INTRODUCTION

The beneficial role of fish oil in health has been investigated since the early 1950s (Brusch and Johnson, 1959; Spoor, 1960; Wood and Biely, 1960). Specifically, the connection between fish intake and reduced cardiovascular risk has been known for some time. Early ecological studies indicated Canadian Inuit had a low rate of cardiovascular disease, despite high total fat intake; this phenomenon was attributed to the high fish intake of this northern population (Kromann and Green, 1980; Kromhout et al., 1985). Marine or cold-water fish, as compared to fresh-water fish, are generally high in long-chain n-3 polyunsaturated fatty acids (PUFA) (Bistrian, 2004). This could be explained by the fact that PUFA remain in liquid form, while saturated and shorter fatty acids (FA) are solid at low temperatures. The particular n-3 FA from fish oil to which the beneficial cardiovascular effects are attributed are eicosapentaenoic acid (EPA) and docosahexaenoic acid (DHA). The contents of EPA and DHA of common fish and shellfish are listed in Table 3.1. It is important to note that n-3 FA content of fish is significantly influenced by seasonal variation, type of fish (i.e., Atlantic

TABLE 3.1

Dietary Sources of Docosahexaenoic and Eicosapentaenoic Acid

Dietary Source (100 g edible portion)	DHA and EPA (g)[a]	Reference
Salmon, Atlantic	2.3	Soltan and Gibson (2008)[b]
Mackerel	1.8	Mahaffey et al. (2008)
Herring, Atlantic	1.2	Copeman and Parrish (2004)[b]
Anchovy	1.2	Soriguer et al. (1997)[b]
Sardines	1.0	Mahaffey et al. (2007)
Bass, farmed	1.0	Cahu et al. (2004)
Squid	0.6	Soltan and Gibson (2008)[b]
Trout	0.6	Mahaffey et al. (2007)
Perch, wild	0.5	Cahu et al. (2004)
Shrimp	0.4	Mahaffey et al. (2007)
Lobster	0.4	Mahaffey et al. (2007)
Pollock	0.3	Mahaffey et al. (2007)
Tuna	0.2	Soriguer et al. (1997)[b]
Mahimahi, wild, Hawaii	0.2	Ako et al. (1994)
Bass, wild	0.2	Cahu et al. (2004)
Cod, wild	0.1	Cahu et al. (2004)
Nori	0.1	Ako et al. (1994)

Note: DHA, docosahexaenoic acid; EPA, eicosapentaenoic acid.

[a] Important note: Values vary throughout season and dietary changes (Cahu et al., 2004; Soriguer et al., 1997).

[b] Values noted are for total n-3 fatty acids.

versus Pacific or "farmed" salmon), type of meat (i.e., organ vs. muscle meat), and preparation method (Ackman, 1989). The content of EPA and DHA of fish oil also varies for similar reasons.

Nutrition recommendations for the public now include n-3 FA and fish intake, not only to prevent deficiency because n-3 FA are essential, but also to obtain the cardiovascular and other health-related benefits (Riediger et al., 2009). In this regard, the Dietary Reference Intakes (DRIs), used in both Canada and the United States, indicate a Recommended Dietary Allowance (RDA) for n-3 FA of 1.6 g/day for males and 1.1 g/day for females; the type of n-3 FA is not distinguished (National Academy of Sciences, 2005). Furthermore, Canada's Food Guide, released in 2007, and the American Heart Association Nutrition Committee recommends consuming at least two meals containing fish per week, especially oily fish (Lichtenstein et al., 2006). Efforts are now being made to establish separate DRI recommendations for EPA and DHA; available literature supports a DRI of 500 mg/day for EPA and DHA (Harris et al., 2009).

The pathogenesis of cardiovascular (CV) disease is multifactorial and although we have just begun to understand its etiology, it still remains as the leading cause of death in developed countries. Plasma lipid profile, inflammatory state, hypertension, atherosclerosis, body weight, glucose metabolism, and arrhythmia all influence the development and outcomes of CV disease and have also all been shown to be influenced by fish oil intake. Evidence from epidemiological studies, experimental animal studies, and randomized controlled trials has been reported and mechanisms have been postulated in this chapter.

3.2   EPIDEMIOLOGICAL EVIDENCE

Epidemiological evidence of associations between fish/fish oil and reduced cardiovascular risk has provided the rationale for the many experimental studies conducted in this area. The Chicago

Western Electric Study reported an inverse association between fish intake and both myocardial infarction and all coronary heart disease, but not sudden cardiac death (Daviglus et al., 1997). Conversely, another prospective cohort study, the Physicians' Health Study revealed that fish intake (fish oil supplement use was not included) was associated with reduced risk of sudden cardiac death, but not myocardial infarction, after adjusting for other risk factors (Albert et al., 1998). These studies in addition to many other major epidemiological and clinical studies on fish oil were conducted in male populations; therefore studies in a female population were required. As part of the Nurses' Follow-up Study, Hu et al. (2002) was the first to report this inverse association between fish and coronary heart disease death independent of age and other cardiovascular risk factors among women. Major observational studies have been summarized in Table 3.2.

3.3 PLASMA LIPIDS

3.3.1 TRIGLYCERIDES

Early work indicated that cardiovascular benefits from n-3 FA may be mediated through beneficial modifications in lipoprotein profile. In this regard, reductions in plasma triglyceride (TG) are the most consistent finding among all plasma lipids as a result of long-chain n-3 FA intake (Harris, 1989; Kudo and Kawashima, 1997; Maki, 2003; Harris and Bulchandani, 2006). Importantly, plasma TG is a significant and independent risk factor for cardiovascular disease (Austin et al., 1998). This reduction has been observed in several animal models, including mouse (Qi et al., 2008), rat (Ukropec et al., 2003), and swine (Larson et al., 2003); and most relevantly, humans. For example, supplementation with 4 g/day of EPA decreased plasma concentrations of TG by 23% in mildly hyperlipidemic subjects (Mori et al., 2000), and by 12% in healthy subjects (Grimsgaard et al., 1997). Similarly, supplementation with as little as 1 g/day of DHA alone or in combination with EPA (1252 mg total) in hypertriglyceridemic subjects resulted in similar reductions in plasma TG levels (21.8%) (Schwellenbach, 2006). There may be a threshold effect of EPA and DHA on plasma TG levels. In this regard, Kris-Etherton and colleagues (Kris-Etherton et al., 2003) reported that supplementation with 2–4 g/day of EPA + DHA can lower plasma TG levels by approximately 25–30% in hypertriglyceridemic patients. It should be noted that other clinical trials (Yamamoto et al., 1995; Sanders et al., 2006) did not report significant TG-lowering effects.

There are several possible mechanisms for the TG-lowering effects of fish oil: (1) n-3 FA are more susceptible to β-oxidation compared to shorter length FA (Guo et al., 2005) and decrease the uptake of nonesterified FA by the liver, which reduces the availability of the FA necessary for TG synthesis; (2) n-3 FA may reduce the activity of enzymes essential for TG synthesis (diacylglycerol acyltransferase and phosphatidic acid phosphohydrolase); (3) phospholipid synthesis is increased, which reduces the diglycerides required for TG synthesis (Harris and Bulchandani, 2006; Schwalfenberg, 2006); and/or (4) increased activity of lipoprotein lipase and clearance of TG from blood (Qi et al., 2008). Possible mechanisms by which EPA/DHA may reduce plasma TG concentrations have been reviewed in more detail by Davidson (2006).

3.3.2 HDL CHOLESTEROL

The influence of fish oil on plasma HDL cholesterol (HDL-C) is inconsistent. One should be reminded that HDL cholesterol is significantly and inversely associated with cardiovascular risk because of its role in reverse cholesterol transport (Assmann et al., 1997). We have shown a significant increase in HDL cholesterol as a result of fish oil feeding as compared to safflower oil feeding in C57BL/6 mice after 16 weeks (Riediger et al., 2008). Others have also reported increases, although small, in HDL-C as a result of long-chain n-3 FA intake in humans (Ferrier et al., 1995; Calabresi et al., 2004; Engler et al., 2004; Breslow, 2006). The influence of EPA and DHA on HDL

TABLE 3.2
Epidemiological Evidence from Observational Studies Investigating Relationship between Fish Oil and Cardiovascular Risk

Reference	Population	Sample Size and Follow-Up Period[a]	Measurements	Main Findings
Yamagishi et al. (2008) (JACC Study)	Japanese men and women aged 40–79	57,972 participants followed for 12.7 years	Mortality rates, type of mortality, fish consumption, gender, and age	• Intakes of fish and n-3 FA were associated with 18% to 19% lower risk of mortality from total cardiovascular disease, IHD, myocardial infarction, and heart failure
Chrysohoou et al. (2007) (ATTICA Study)	Greek men and women	3042 participants (cross-sectional study)	Fish consumption, QTc (heart rate corrected-QT) duration	• Those who consumed >300 g fish/week had a mean 13.6% lower QTc ($P < 0.01$) and also had a 29.2% lower likelihood of having QTc intervals >0.45 s ($P = 0.03$)
Mozaffarian et al. (2008)	American men and women aged 65 years and older	4465 participants (cross-sectional study)	Heart rate variability (HRV), fish consumption	• Consumption of fish improved HRV indices: increased vagal predominance and moderated baroreceptor responses, higher normalized high-frequency power ($P = 0.008$) • Lower low-frequency/high-frequency ratio ($P = 0.03$) • Less erratic sinoatrial node firing ($P = 0.02$) • Higher short-term fractal scaling exponent ($P = 0.005$)
Virtanen et al. (2008) (The Health Professionals Follow-Up Study)	American male health professionals aged 40–75 years	40,230 healthy participants followed for 18 years	Whole fish and fish oil intake, lifestyle, physical and environmental risk factors for chronic diseases	• Fish consumption is inversely related to risk for chronic disease ($P = 0.02$) • Fish consumption of 1 serving/wk (RR: 0.86; 95% CI: 0.75, 0.98), and 2–4 servings/wk (RR: 0.85; 95% CI: 0.73, 0.99) was associated with a lower risk of CVD

Study	Subjects	Number	Methods	Findings
Murakami et al. (2008)	Japanese young women aged 18–22 years	443 participants (cross-sectional study)	Self-administered diet history questionnaires and CRP detection using nephelometry	• A significant relationship was reported between n-3 FA intake and lower levels of circulating C-reactive protein ($P = 0.02$)
Hu et al. (2002)	American female nurses involved in the Nurses' Health Study aged 34–59 years without existing CHD	84,688 women followed for 16 years	Food frequency questionnaires and incidence of CHD or MI (including non fatal types)	• Significant inverse relationship between fish or n-3 FA intake and risk of CHD (P for trend <0.001)
Albert et al. (1998)	US Physicians' Health Study; 40–84 years of age without baseline CHD or cancer	20551 US male physicians followed for 11 years	Food frequency questionnaire and health status follow-up	• Consumption of at least 1 fish meal per week significantly reduced risk for sudden cardiac death (P for trend $= 0.03$)
Daviglus et al. (1997)	Chicago Western Electric Study; men aged 40–55 free of CVD at baseline	1822 men followed for 30 years	Dietary history, food frequency questionnaire, CVD mortality data from death certificates	• Significant inverse relationship between fish intake (35 g fish or higher) and death from coronary heart disease (P for trend $= 0.04$)

[a] For studies which are not longitudinal studies, the type of study is indicated in parentheses.

cholesterol may be mediated by dose, duration of supplementation, and animal model. Therefore, studies with no observed benefits of fish oil on HDL may vary in these properties, sample size, or both.

3.3.3 TOTAL AND LDL CHOLESTEROL

Effects of fish oil on plasma total cholesterol, LDL cholesterol (LDL-C), and apolipoprotein B (apoB) concentrations have also been inconsistent. Although elevated LDL-C and apoB levels have been observed with DHA supplementation (Maki et al., 2003; Goyens and Mensink, 2006), long-chain n-3 FA have been shown to reduce LDL particle size (Contacos et al., 1993; Mori et al., 2000). Kelley and associates (2007) observed a significant 21% reduction in the number of small, dense LDL particles and a 0.6 nm increase in LDL particle size in hypertriglyceridemic men receiving 3 g/day DHA. Contacos et al. (1993) also observed a 1 nm increase in the diameter of LDL particles after consumption of 3 g/day fish oil for 6 weeks. The change in particle size may partially explain the increased LDL-C levels observed in other clinical trials (Sanders et al., 2006). Therefore, apoB levels should also be measured when LDL particle size is assessed. In this regard, an increase in apoB concentrations following n-3 FA supplementation has been observed in healthy elderly subjects (Goyens and Mensink, 2006). Others have observed no significant changes in plasma total cholesterol (Ågren et al., 2006). Overall, influences of fish oil on total or LDL cholesterol metabolism appear inconsistent, while influences of particle size seem to be important.

3.4 BLOOD PRESSURE

n-3 FA from fish oil may also play a role in the regulation of blood pressure (Mozaffarian, 2007). This effect may be mediated through an alteration in the balance between vasoconstrictive prostaglandins and increasing production of vasodilatory prostacyclin, response to angiotensin II (Kenny et al., 1992), and/or nitric oxide production (Omura et al., 2001). A meta-analysis of 36 trials with fish oil supplementation by Geleijnse et al. (2002) showed a weighted reduction of 2.09 and 1.63 mmHg for systolic and diastolic blood pressure, respectively. However, the effect of fish oil on blood pressure is significantly mediated by both age and baseline blood pressure (Geleijnse et al., 2002). Several factors including the dose of fish oil, concurrent use of medications, an inadequate sample size, population type, the choice of placebo oil, and inadequate statistical power may be the reasons for the lack of antihypertensive effects of these oils observed in other studies (Wing et al., 1990; Woodman et al., 2002; Kelley et al., 2007).

3.5 INFLAMMATION AND THROMBOTIC FACTORS

Perhaps the greatest effect of long-chain n-3 FA, with respect to a multitude of adverse health conditions including cardiovascular disease, is their anti-inflammatory activities (Ross, 1999; Lusis, 2000; Mori and Beilin, 2004; Willerson and Ridker, 2004). This effect may be mediated by the change in eicosanoid balance previously mentioned to occur following long-chain n-3 FA consumption (Gallai et al., 1995). Another possible mechanism by which n-3 FA may reduce inflammation is via an interaction with peroxisome proliferator-activated receptor-alpha, a transcription factor that breaks down leukotrienes (but again involved with the eicosanoid pathway) (Ergas et al., 2002). Improvements in production or gene expression (by either an increase or decrease) of specific cytokines, including IL-1β, IL-6, TNF-α, IL-12, adiponectin, and interferon-δ have been reported in either animals and/or humans (Endres et al., 1989; Caughey et al., 1996; Fritsche et al., 1999; James et al., 2000; Duda et al., 2009). Philips et al. (2003) have found that dietary DHA supplementation decreased exercise-induced inflammation by reducing CRP and IL-6 in healthy subjects. Conversely, Mori et al. (2003) showed that neither purified EPA nor DHA given at 4 g/day for 6 weeks to type 2 diabetic subjects significantly decreased IL-6 or CRP levels. However, both FA remarkably reduced the levels of TNF-α by 25%. The effect of n-3 FA on many other cytokines is yet to be investigated.

3.6 ARRHYTHMIA

It is postulated that many of the beneficial effects of fish oil on cardiovascular outcomes are related to the incorporation of DHA and EPA into cell membranes and their consequent antiarrhythmic effects (Kang and Leaf, 1994, 1995; Wang et al., 2005). Arrhythmias occur as a result of poor electrical signaling in the heart muscle to other chambers (atria or ventricles) for a fully coordinated beat and often occur following myocardial infarction. The antiarrhythmic effect may be due to the improvement in membrane fluidity with the incorporation of EPA and DHA into cardiac cell membrane, thereby preventing atrial fibrillation (rapid twitching of cardiac muscle fiber) by altering the sodium and calcium ion channels (Schwalfenberg, 2006). Improved membrane fluidity may also influence the binding of cytokines to the membrane (Ergas et al., 2002). Both EPA and DHA are readily incorporated into cell membranes following supplementation (Gallai et al., 1995; Wilkinson et al., 2005).

Mozaffarian et al. (2006) has observed slower heart rates, reduced atrioventricular conduction, and lower risk of prolonged ventricular repolarization among participants with higher fish consumption compared to those with the lowest intake. Moreover, habitual consumption of fish and marine n-3 FA is linked with particular heart rate variability constituents, including indices of vagal activity, baroreceptor responses, and sinoatrial node function among American adults (Mozaffarian et al., 2008). Such enhancement of vagal control by tuna and other fish consumption could explain, in part, improved endothelial function and reduced resting heart rate after fish oil supplements in a randomized study with healthy men and women (Shah et al., 2007). Consuming 3 g/day of encapsulated fish oil for 6 weeks reduced inducible ventricular tachycardia and risk of sudden cardiac death among patients with coronary artery disease (Metcalf et al., 2008). These findings indicate that fish oil may exert an overall improvement in heart rhythm. Generally, observational studies support the theory of reduced risk of arrhythmias as a result of fish/fish oil intake, because of the inverse association between fish intake and sudden cardiac death (which are mostly accounted for by arrhythmia), but not myocardial infarction (Albert et al., 1998; Streppel et al., 2008). However, there is also evidence against an antiarrhythmic effect of fish oil from the Rotterdam Study (Brouwer et al., 2006).

Animal studies also support the antiarrhythmic effects of fish oil. In this regard, McLennan et al. (1993) has reported beneficial effects of fish oil on ventricular fibrillation in marmoset monkeys and tuna oil in rats, respectively (McLennan et al., 1988). Not only is dietary DHA beneficial, but pericardial delivery has also shown to be effective; in this regard pericardial delivery of DHA reduced heart rate and ventricular arrythmias in pigs with induced myocardial infarctions (Xiao et al., 2008). However, McLennan (1993) also reported in a separate study that dietary n-6 FA also reduced incidence and severity of arrythmias in rats, which is contrary to majority of scientific opinion.

3.7 ATHEROSCLEROSIS

A reduction in atherosclerosis may be secondary to the other influences of the aforementioned fish oil. Hino et al. (2004) reported an inverse association between long-chain n-3 FA intake and carotid intima-media thickness, a marker of atherosclerosis, using ultrasonography, in an epidemiological study. Furthermore, Thies et al. (2003) have shown that long-chain n-3 FA intake enhances plaque stability. Despite these positive results from epidemiological studies, three large randomized controlled clinical trials failed to show that n-3 FA prevent restenosis (reoccurrence of an obstructed artery) after angioplasty (Leaf et al., 1994; Cairns et al., 1996; Johansen et al., 1999).

Some of the antiatherosclerotic associations of dietary n-3 FA reported (Hino et al., 2004; Erkikilä et al., 2006) may be due to their beneficial impacts on platelet activities. In this regard, a 35% decline in platelet–monocyte aggregates was reported after supplementation of 14 healthy participants with 500 g/week of fish oil for 4 weeks (Din et al., 2008). Other studies have also reported a reduction in platelet aggregation and platelet count following long-chain n-3 fatty acid intake (Mori et al., 1997; Yamada et al., 1998).

3.8 GLUCOSE AND INSULIN METABOLISM

Although blood glucose and insulin are not thought of as classic cardiovascular risk factors, subsequent development of impaired glucose tolerance and diabetes do increase cardiovascular risk. For this reason, the effects of fish oil on glucose metabolism are discussed. Results from animal studies have been promising. In this regard, the Storlien group conducted several studies demonstrating the beneficial effects of fish oil on insulin resistance in rats by replacing other dietary fats with fish oil (Storlien et al., 1987, 1991). Others have also reported benefits of fish oil on preventing sucrose-induced insulin resistance in rats, that is, hyperinsulinemia (Luo et al., 1996; Podolin et al., 1998; Peyron-Caso et al., 2002). However, plasma glucose in particular was not significantly changed (Luo et al., 1996; Peyron-Caso et al., 2002).

Clinical trials have not been as promising. A systematic review of 18 clinical trials (prior to 1998) by Montori et al. (2000) revealed that fish oil did not reduce plasma glucose in patients with type 2 diabetes; plasma insulin was not reported. It should be noted that although fish oil did not reduce plasma glucose in those with type 2 diabetes in the majority of trials, plasma TG were often significantly decreased.

3.9 BODY WEIGHT MANAGEMENT

Maintenance of body weight and/or weight loss is not considered main effects of fish oil supplementation as little evidence exists. However, this possible effect of n-3 FA is discussed to be comprehensive and because of high body mass index, a marker for obesity, is known to be an independent risk factor for cardiovascular disease (Hubert et al., 1983). In this regard, Cunnane et al. (1986) have demonstrated that cod liver oil given to ob/ob mice reduced weight gain compared to mice given evening primrose oil. Similarly, Ruzickova et al. (2004) reported reduced weight gain in C57BL/6J mice fed fish oil as part of a high-fat diet compared to control groups. Purported mechanisms for this EPA/DHA-associated reduction in weight gain in mice are limited hypertrophy and hyperplasia of adipose cells (Ruzickova et al, 2004). On the other hand, we and others have shown no change in body weight in animals fed fish oil compared to control (Murphy et al., 1997; Riediger et al., 2008, 2009; Duda et al., 2009). No clinical trials were found to report weight loss as a result of fish oil consumption.

3.10 TRANSPLANTATION

It must be noted that cardiovascular disease may lead to the requirement for a heart transplant. Although a transplant may prolong life of a patient, they also further negatively influence health via tissue rejection and the use of antirejection drugs. In this regard, fish oil may also have beneficial effects by reducing the negative effects of rejection and immune-suppressing agents, such as cyclosporine (Gibson et al., 2000; Othman et al., 2008; Yin et al., 2008).

3.11 RANDOMIZED CONTROLLED TRIALS

Many randomized controlled trials of fish oil have been discussed throughout this chapter as they pertain to a respective cardiovascular risk factor. Overall, many of these trials of fish oil supplements may be regarded as successful. The success of a trial by reducing cardiovascular risk is dependent on many factors, including dose, type of n-3 FA (EPA vs. DHA), duration of treatment, inclusion criteria of participants, and variability of participants. A lack of success compared to other studies may be attributed to one of these trial features. A summary of major clinical trials is summarized in Table 3.3.

TABLE 3.3

Summary of Major Clinical Randomized Controlled Trials on Fish Oil and Cardiovascular Risk

Study	Subjects (n)[a]	Dose (g)	Duration	Outcomes
Kelley et al. (2007)	Hypertriglyceridemic men aged 39–66 years (34)	3 g DHA/day	90 days	• Decrease in plasma TG ($P = 0.03$), large VLDL particles ($P < 0.05$), and small HDL particles ($P = 0.0003$) • Increase in plasma small VLDL particles ($P = 0.02$), large HDL particles ($P = 0.0002$) • No significant change in heart rate, systolic, and diastolic blood pressures.
Schwellenbach et al. (2006)	Hypertriglyceridemic (200–750 mg/dL) men and women (57–59)	Either 1000 mg/day DHA or 1252 mg/day DHA + EPA	8 weeks	• 21.8% and 18.3% decrease in plasma TG in DHA alone ($P < 0.001$) and DHA + EPA group ($P = 0.001$), respectively • No change in TG-lowering between DHA only and DHA + EPA combined • DHA alone showed greater ($P < 0.05$) increase in HDL-C
Goyens and Mensink (2006)	Mildly hyper-cholesterolemic elderly men and women (14)	1.05 g/day EPA + 0.55 g/day DHA	6 weeks	• No change in plasma lipids between groups or compared to baseline • EPA/DHA-induced subjects had an increase in apoB ($P = 0.0031$)
Sanders et al. (2006)	Healthy men and women (40)	1.5 g DHA/day + 0.6 g DPA/day	4 weeks	• Total, LDL, and HDL cholesterol increased ($P = 0.001$) • Factor VII (FVII) coagulant activity increased ($P = 0.006$) • No changes in blood pressure, serum C-reactive protein, plasma FVII antigen, or fibrinogen
Wilkinson et al. (2005)	Healthy men (17–21)	3 g EPA + DHA/day	12 weeks	• EPA and DHA increased in erythrocyte membranes ($P < 0.001$) • Plasma total cholesterol, HDL, TG, and small dense LDL decreased ($P < 0.05$)
Engler et al. (2004)	Children (9–19 y old) with familial hypercholeserolemia or familial combined hyperlipidemia (20)	1.2 g DHA/day	6 months	• Endothelium-dependent flow-mediated dilation of brachial artery increased with DHA supplementation ($P < 0.012$) compared to placebo • Total cholesterol ($P < 0.01$), LDL and HDL increased ($P < 0.001$)

continued

TABLE 3.3 (continued)
Summary of Major Clinical Randomized Controlled Trials on Fish Oil and Cardiovascular Risk

Study	Subjects (n)[a]	Dose (g)	Duration	Outcomes
Nodari et al. (2009)	Adult patients with idiopathic dilated cardiomyopathy (IDC) (44)	1.0 g EPA + DHA/day	6 months	• Fish oil supplementation was associated with a reduced risk of sudden cardiac death • Fish oil supplementation reduced arrhythmic risk in 58% of patients with IDC • Signal averaged ECG was normalized ($P = 0.001$) and decreases in both nonsustained ventricular tachycardia episodes and heart rate ($P = 0.0002$ and 0.0003 respectively) was shown
Yusof et al. (2008)	Healthy men (35–60)	2.1 g of EPA + DHA/day	8 weeks	• Fish oil did not produce significant changes in blood pressure, plasma LDL-C, HDL-C, or TG • Plasma inflammatory marker sIACM-1 was significantly lowered by 10% in fish oil group ($P = 0.05$)
Wang, S et al. (2007)	Overweight adult hypertensive patients (52)	3 g of EPA + DHA/day	8 weeks	• Fish oil supplementation showed significant increases in arterial elasticity 15.5 ± 1.5 mL mmHg^{-1} ×10 compared to placebo group • No alterations found in small arterial elasticity, blood pressure and pulse pressure

[a] The number of subjects are indicated per study group; where the number of subjects per group differ, a range of subjects has been given.

3.12   CURRENT N-3 FATTY ACID CONSUMPTION

Currently, the n-6:n-3 FA ratio of the typical Western diet is 20–30:1; a far cry from a 2:1 ratio reported during the Paleolithic era (Eaton and Konner, 1985). Some researchers hypothesize that the ratio of dietary n-6:n-3 FA may be equally important as total n-3 FA because of the metabolic competition between n-6 and n-3 FA. According to the Multiple Risk Factor Intervention Trial, a longitudinal trial with over 12,000 male participants, the average intake of long-chain n-3 FA was approximately 175 mg/day, with 20% reporting no intake (Dolecek and Granditis, 1991). This intake is well-below the DRI mentioned previously of 1.6 g/day for males. This increase in the n-6 fatty acid intake and reduction in n-3 fatty acid intake is due to both a reduction in fish intake and the emphasis on mass agricultural production, which has reduced the n-3 fatty acid contents in many foods and increased the n-6 fatty acid contents (Simopoulos et al., 1995; Simopoulos, 1999). Furthermore, sources of n-6 fatty acid are much more available than sources of n-3 fatty acid and there are many limitations to fish intake, a major source of n-3 fatty acid. Even populations with typically high n-3 fatty acid intake, for example Japan, are decreasing their n-3 fatty acid intake while also increasing their n-6 FA, as they are influenced by the Western culture (Sugano and Hirahara, 2000). In addition, populations with increased needs for n-3 fatty acid intake, pregnant women, are also reported to have low consumption (Innis and Elias, 2003; Denomme, 2005; Innis and Friesen, 2008).

3.13   LIMITATIONS OF FISH OIL

Some limitations of regular fish oil supplement consumption are poor patient acceptability because of fishy taste, belching, nausea, and diarrhea. Fish are also known to be high in methyl mercury due to bioaccumulation. This, combined with high absorption, makes mercury poisoning a reasonable danger with regular fish consumption (Mozaffarian and Rimm, 2006; Innis et al., 2006). Fish particularly high in mercury include shark, swordfish, king mackerel, and tilefish (Food and Drug Administration, 2004). Therefore, eating fish species known to contain high quantities of mercury should be cautioned, particularly in high-risk populations such as young children and pregnant/breastfeeding women (Helland et al., 2001). It should be noted that less mercury is found in fish oil alone compared to fish (Foran et al., 2003). However, dioxin concentration and other sources of contamination can also be a safety issue in fish oil supplements (Bays, 2007). There is no defined upper limit for fish oil, although the United States Food and Drug Administration do specify that 3 g of n-3 FA from fish oil per day is Generally Recognized as Safe (GRAS). Lastly, there may be increased risk of bleeding/hemorrhage with high n-3 FA intake. Therefore, caution should be taken with high intake, especially for those taking blood thinners or who suffer from bleeding disorders (Lichtenstein, 2005).

3.14   SUMMARY AND CONCLUSIONS

In summary, fish oil appears to be beneficial in regards to cardiovascular health by improving plasma lipid profile, reducing inflammation, reducing hypertension, preventing arrhythmia, and consequently slowing atherosclerosis. The mechanisms of these effects are thought to be regulated by the change in balance of eicosanoid production. The cardiovascular benefits of fish oil may be particularly magnified among populations with low fish consumption and it appears n-3 fatty acid intake is low among Western populations. However, caution for excessive fish oil intake should be advised.

REFERENCES

Ackman, R.G. 1989. Nutritional composition of fats in seafoods. *Progr. Food and Nutr. Sci.* **13**:161–241.
Ågren, J.J., Hanninen, O., Julkunen, A., Fogelholm, L., Vidgren., H., Schwab, U., Pynnönen, O., and Uusitupa, M. 1996. Fish diet, fish oil and docosahexaenoic acid rich oil lower fasting and postprandial plasma lipid levels. *Eur. J. Clin. Nutr.* **50**:765–771.

Ako, H., Ota, E., and Ogasawara, A. 1994. Omega-3 fatty acids in Hawaii seafood. *Hawaii Med. J.* **53**:142–145.

Albert, C.M., Hennekens, C.H., O'Donnell, C.J., Ajani, U.A., Carey, V.J., Willett, W.C., Ruskin, J.N., and Manson, J.E. 1998. Fish consumption and risk of sudden cardiac death. *JAMA* **279**:23–28.

Assmann, G., Schulte, H., and Cullen, P. 1997. New and classical risk factors—the Münster Heart Study (PROCAM). *Eur. J. Med. Res.* **2**:237–242.

Austin, M.A., Hokanson, J.E., and Edwards, K.L. 1998. Hypertriglyceridemia as a cardiovascular risk factor. *Am. J. Cardiol.* **81**(4A):7B–12B.

Bays, H.E. 2007. Safety considerations with omega-3 fatty acid therapy. *Am J. Cardiol.* **99**:35C–43C.

Bistrian, B.R. 2004. Practical recommendations for immune-enhancing diets. *J. Nutr.* **134**(Suppl):2868S–2872S.

Breslow, J.L. 2006. n-3 Fatty acids and cardiovascular disease. *Am. J. Clin. Nutr.* **83**(Suppl):1477S–1482S.

Brouwer, I.A., Heeringa, J., Geleijnse, J.M., Zock, P.L. and Witteman, J.C. 2006. Intake of very long-chain n-3 fatty acids from fish and incidence of atrial fibrillation. The Rotterdam Study. *Am. Heart J.* **151**:857–862.

Brusch, C.A. and Johnson, E.T. 1959. A new dietary regimen for arthritis: Value of cod liver oil on a fasting stomach. *J. Natl. Med. Assoc.* **51**:266–270.

Calabresi, L., Villa, N., Canavesi, M., Sirtori, C.R., James, R.W., Bernini, F., and Franceschini, G. 2004. An omega-3 polyunsaturated fatty acid concentrate increases plasma high-density lipoprotein 2 cholesterol and paraoxonase levels in patients with familial combined hyperlipidemia. *Metabolism* **53**:153–158.

Cahu, C., Salen, P., and de Lorgeril, M. 2004. Farmed and wild fish in the prevention of cardiovascular disease: Assessing possible differences in lipid nutritional values. *Nutr. Metab. Cardiovasc. Dis.* **14**:34–41.

Caughey, G.E., Mantzioris, E., Gibson, R.A., Cleland, L.G., and James, M.J. 1996. The effect on human tumor necrosis factor α and interleukin1 β production of diets enriched in n-3 fatty acids from vegetable oil or fish oil. *Am. J. Clin. Nutr.* **63**:116–22.

Chrysohoou, C., Panagiotakos, D.B., Pitsavos, C., Skoumas, J., Krinos, X., Chloptsios, Y., Nikolaou, V., and Stefanadis, C. 2007. Long-term fish consumption is associated with protection against arrhythmia in healthy persons in a Mediterranean region—The ATTICA Study. *Am. J. Clin. Nutr.* **85**:1385–1391.

Contacos, C., Barter, P.J., and Sullivan, D.R. 1993. Effect of pravastatin and omega-3 fatty acids on plasma lipids and lipoproteins in patients with combined hyperlipidemia. *Arterioscler. Thromb.* **13**:1755–1762.

Copeman, L.A. and Parrish, C.C. 2004. Lipid [corrected] classes, fatty acids, and sterols in seafood from Gilbert Bay, southern Labrador. *J. Agric. Food. Chem.* **52**:4872–4881.

Cunnane, S.C., McAdoo, K.R., and Horrobin, D.F. 1986. n-3 essential fatty acids decrease weight gain in genetically obese mice. *Br. J Nutr.* **56**:87–95.

Davidson, M.H. 2006. Mechanisms for the hypotriglyceridemic effect of marine omega-3 fatty acids. *Am. J. Cardiol.* **98**:27i–33i.

Daviglus, M.L., Stamler, J., Orencia, A.J., Dyer, A.R., Liu, K., Greenland, P., Walsh, M.K., Morris, D., and Shekelle, R.B. 1997. Fish consumption and the 30-year risk of fatal myocardial infarction. *N. Eng. J. Med.* **336**:1046–1053.

Denomme, J., Stark, K.D., and Holub, B.J. 2005. Directly quantitated dietary (n-3) fatty acid intakes of pregnant Canadian women are lower than current dietary recommendations. *J. Nutr.* **135**:206–211.

Din, J.N., Harding, S.A., Valerio, C.J., Sarma, J., Lyall, K., Riemersma, R.A., Newby, D.E., and Flapan, A.D. 2008. Dietary intervention with oil rich fish reduces platelet–monocyte aggregation in man. *Atherosclerosis* **197**:290–296.

Dolecek, T.A. and Granditis, G. 1991. Dietary polyunsaturated fatty acids and mortality in the multiple risk factor intervention trial (MRFIT). *World Rev. Nutr. Diet.* **66**:205–216.

Duda, M.K., O'Shea, K.M., Tintinu, A., Xu, W., Khairallah, R.J., Barrows, B.R., Chess, D.J., et al. 2009. Fish oil, but not flaxseed oil, decreases inflammation and prevents pressure overload-induced cardiac dysfunction. *Cardiovasc. Res.* **81**:319–327.

Eaton, S.B., and Konner, M. 1985. Paleolithic nutrition. A consideration of its nature and current implications. *N. Eng. J. Med.* **312**:283–289.

Endres, S., Ghorbani, R., Kelley, V.E., Georgilis, K., Lonnemann, G., van der Meer, J.W., Cannon, J.G., et al. 1989. The effect of dietary supplementation with n-3 polyunsaturated fatty acids on the synthesis of interleukin-1 and tumor necrosis factor by mononuclear cells. *N. Engl. J. Med.* **320**:265–271.

Engler, M.M., Engler, M.B., Malloy, M., Chiu, E., Besio, D., Paul, S., Stuehlinger, M., et al. 2004. Docosahexaenoic acid restores endothelial function in children with hyperlipidemia: Results from the EARLY study. *Int. J. Clin. Pharmacol. Ther.* **42**(12):672–679.

Ergas, D., Eilat, E., Mednlovic, S., and Sthoeger, Z.M. 2002. n-3 fatty acids and the immune system in autoimmunity. *Isr. Med. Assoc. J.* **4**:34–38.

Erkikilä, A.T., Matthan, N.R., Herrington, D.M., and Lichtenstein, A.H. 2006. Higher plasma docosahexaenoic acid is associated with reduced progression of coronary atherosclerosis in women with CAD. *J. Lipid. Res.* **47**:2814–2819.

Ferrier, L.K., Caston, L.J., Leeson, S., Squires, J., Weaver, B.J., and Holub, B.J. 1995. alpha-Linolenic acid- and docosahexaenoic acid-enriched eggs from hens fed flaxseed: Influence on blood lipids and platelet phospholipid fatty acids in humans. *Am. J. Clin. Nutr.* **62**:81–86.

Foran, S.E., Flood, J.G., and Lewandrowski, K.B. 2003. Measurement of mercury levels in concentrated over-the-counter fish oil preparations: Is fish oil healthier than fish? *Arch. Pathol. Lab. Med.* **127**:1603–1605.

Fritsche, K.L., Byrge, M., and Feng, C. 1999. Dietary omega-3 polyunsaturated fatty acids from fish oil reduce interleukin-12 and interferon-gamma production in mice. *Immunol. Lett.* **65**:167–173.

Gallai, V., Sarchielli, P., Trequattrini, A., Franceschini, M., Floridi, A., Firenzi, C., Alberti, A., Di Benedetto, D., and Stragliotto, E. 1995. Cytokine secretion and eicosanoid production in the peripheral blood mononuclear cells of MS patients undergoing dietary supplementation with n-3 polyunsaturated fatty acids. *J. Neuroimmunol.* **56**:143–153.

Geleijnse, J.M., Giltay, E.J., Grobbee, D.E., Donders, A.R., and Kok, F.J. 2002. Blood pressure response to fish oil supplementation: Meta-regression analysis of randomized trial. *J. Hypertens.* **20**:1493–1499.

Gibson, S.W., Valente, J.F., Alexander, J.W., Custer, D.A., Li, B.G., Frede, S., Babcock, G.F., and Ogle, C.K. 2000. Nutritional immunomodulation leads to enhanced allograft survival in combination with cyclosporine A and rapamycin, but not FK506. *Transplantation* **69**:2034–2038.

Goyens, P.L. and Mensink, R.P. 2006. Effects of alpha-linolenic acid versus those of EPA/DHA on cardiovascular risk markers in healthy elderly subjects. *Eur. J. Clin. Nutr.* **60**:978–984.

Grimsgaard, S., Bonaa, K.H., Hansen, J.B., and Norday, A. 1997. Highly purified eicosapentaenoic acid and docosahexaenoic acid in humans have similar triacylglycerol-lowering effects but divergent effects on serum fatty acids. *Am. J. Clin. Nutr.* **66**:649–659.

Guo, W., Xie, W., Lei, T., and Hamilton, J.A. 2005. Eicosapentaenoic acid, but not oleic acid stimulates beta-oxidation in adipocytes. *Lipids* **40**:815–821.

Harris, W.S. 1989. Fish oils and plasma lipid and lipoprotein metabolism in humans: A critical review. *J. Lipid. Res.* **30**:785–807.

Harris, W.S., and Bulchandani, D. 2006. Why do omega-3 fatty acids lower serum triglycerides?. *Curr. Opin. Lipidol.* **17**:387–393.

Harris, W.S., Mozaffarian, D., Lefevre, M., Toner, C.D., Colombo, J., Cunnane, S.C., Holden, J.M., Klurfeld, D.M., Morris, M.C., and Whelan, J. 2009. Towards establishing dietary reference intakes for eicosapentaenoic and docosahexaenoic acids. *J. Nutr.* **139**:804S–819S.

Helland, I.B., Saugsted, O.D., Smith, L., Saarem, K., Solvoll, K., Ganes, T., and Drevon, C.A. 2001. Similar effects on infants of n-3 and n-6 fatty acids supplementation to pregnant and lactating women. *Pediatrics* **108**:E82.

Hino, A., Adachi, H., Toyomasu, K., Yoshida, N., Enomoto, M., Hiratsuka, A., Hirai, Y., Satoh, A., and Imaizumi, T. 2004. Very long chain n-3 fatty acids intake and carotid atherosclerosis: An epidemiological study evaluated by ultrasonography. *Atherosclerosis* **176**:145–149.

Hu, F.B., Bronner, L., Willett, W.C., Stampfer, M.J., Rexrode, K.M., Albert, C.M., Hunter, D., and Manson, J.E. 2002. Fish and omega-3 fatty aicd intake and risk of coronary heart disease in women. *JAMA* **287**:1815–1821.

Hubert, H.B., Feinleib, M., McNamara, P.M., and Castelli, W.P. 1983. Obesity as an independent risk factor for cardiovascular disease: A 26-year follow-up of participants in the Framingham Heart Study. *Circulation* **67**:968–77.

Innis, S.M. and Elias, S.L. 2003. Intakes of essential n-6 and n-3 polyunsaturated fatty acids among pregnant Canadian women. *Am. J. Clin. Nutr.* **77**:473–478.

Innis, S.M., Palaty, J., Vaghri, Z., and Lockitch, G. 2006. Increased levels of mercury associated with high fish intakes among children from Vancouver, Canada. *J. Pediatr.* **148**:759–763.

Innis, S.M. and Friesen, R.W. 2008. Essential n-3 fatty acids in pregnant women and early visual acuity maturation in term infants. *Am. J. Clin. Nutr.* **87**:548–557.

James, M.J., Gibson, R.A., and Cleland, L.G. 2000. Dietary polyunsaturated fatty acids and inflammatory mediator production. *Am. J. Clin. Nutr.* **71**(Suppl):343S–348S.

Johansen, O., Brekke, M., Sejeflot, L., Abdelnoor, M., and Arnesen, H. 1999. n-3 fatty acids do not prevent restenosis after coronary angioplasty: Results from the CART study. Coronary Angioplasty Restenosis Trial. *J. Am. Coll. Cardiol.* **33**:1619–1626.

Kang, J.X., and Leaf, A. 1994. Effects of long-chain polyunsaturated fatty acids on the contraction of neonatal rat cardiac myocytes. *Proc. Natl. Acad. Sci. USA* **91**:9886–9890.

Kang, J.X. and Leaf, A. 1995. Prevention and termination of the β-adrenergic agonist-induced arrhythmias by free polyunsaturated fatty acids in neonatal rat cardiac myocytes. *Biochem. Biophys. Res. Commun.* **208**:629–636.

Kelley, D.S., Siegel, D., Vemuri, M., and Mackey, B.E. 2007. Docosahexaenoic acid supplementation improves fasting and postprandial lipid profiles in hypertriglyceridemic men. *Am. J. Clin. Nutr.* **86**:324–333.

Kenny, D., Warltier, D.C., Pleuss, J.A., Hoffmann, R.G., Goodfriend, T.L. and Egan, B.M. 1992. Effect of omega-3 fatty acids on the vascular response to angiotensin in normotensive men. *Am. J. Cardiol.* **70**:1347–1352.

Kris-Etherton, P.M., Harris, W.S., and Appel, L.J. 2003. Fish consumption, fish oil, omega-3 fatty acids, and cardiovascular disease. *Arterioscler. Thromb. Vasc. Biol.* **23**:20–30.

Kromann, N. and Green, A. 1980. Epidemiological studies in the Upernavik district, Greenland. Incidence of some chronic diseases 1950–1974. *Acta. Med. Scand.* **208**:401–406.

Kromhout, D., Bosschieter, E.B., and de Lezenne Coulander, C. 1985. The inverse relation between fish consumption and 20-year mortality from coronary heart disease. *N. Engl. J. Med.* **312**:1205–1209.

Kudo, N. and Kawashima, Y. 1997. Fish oil-feeding prevents perfluorooctanoic acid-induced fatty liver in mice. *Toxicol. Appl. Pharmacol.* **145**:285–293.

Larson, L.F., Olsen, A.K., Hansen, A.K., Bukhave, K., and Marckmann, P. 2003. Feeding minipigs fish oil for four weeks lowers postprandial triacylglycerolemia. *J. Nutr.* **133**:2273–2276.

Leaf, A., Jorgensen, M.B., Jacobs, A.K., Cote, G., Schoenfeld, D.A., Scheer, J., Weiner, B.H., Slack, J.D., Kellett, M.A., and Raizner, A.E. 1994. Do fish oils prevent restenosis after coronary angioplasty? *Circulation* **90**:2248–2257.

Lichtenstein, A.H. 2005. Remarks on clinical data concerning dietary supplements that affect antithrombotic therapy. *Thromb. Res.* **117**:71–73.

Lichtenstein, A.H., Appel, L.J., Brands, M., Carnethon, M., Daniels, S., Franch, H.A., Franklin, B. et al. 2006. Diet and lifestyle recommendations Revision 2006: A scientific statement from the American Heart Association Nutrition Committee. *Circulation* **114**:82–96.

Luo, J., Rizkalla, S.W., Boillot, J., Alamowitch, C., Chaib, H., Bruzzo, F., Desplanque, N., Dalix, A.M., Durand, G., and Slama, G. 1996. Dietary (n-3) polyunsaturated fatty acids improve adipocyte insulin action and glucose metabolism in insulin-resistant rats: Relation to membrane fatty acids. *J. Nutr.* **126**:1951–1958.

Lusis, A.J. 2000. Atherosclerosis. *Nature* **407**:233–241.

Mahaffey, K.R., Clickner, R.P., and Jeffries, R.A. 2008. Methylmercury and omega-3 fatty acids: Co-occurrence of dietary sources with emphasis on fish and shellfish. *Environ. Res.* **107**:20–29.

Maki, K.C., Van Elswyk, M.E., McCarthy, D., Seeley, M.A., Veith, P.E., Hess, S.P., Ingram, K.A., Halvorson, J.J., Calaguas, E.M., and Davidson, M.H. 2003. Lipid responses in mildly hypertriglyceridemic men and women to consumption of docosahexaenoic acid-enriched eggs. *Int. J. Vitam. Nutr. Res.* **73**:357–368.

McLennan, P.L., Bridle, T.M., Abeywardena, M.Y., and Charnock, J.S. 1993. Comparative efficacy of n-3 and n-6 polyunsaturated fatty acids in modulating ventricular fibrillation threshold in marmoset monkeys. *Am. J. Clin. Nutr.* **58**:666–669.

McLennan, P.L. 1993. Relative effects of dietary saturated, monounsaturated, and polyunsaturated fatty acids on cardiac arrhythmias in rats. *Am. J. Clin. Nutr.* **57**:207–212.

McLennan, P.L., Abeywardena, M.Y., and Charnock, J.S. 1988. Dietary fish oil prevents ventricular fibrillation following coronary artery occlusion and reperfusion. *Am. Heart. J.* **116**:709–717.

Metcalf, R.G., Sanders, P., James, M.J., Cleland, L.G., and Young, G.D. 2008. Effect of dietary n-3 polyunsaturated fatty acids on the inducibility of ventricular tachycardia in patients with ischemic cardiomyopathy. *Am. J. Cardiol.* **101**:758–761.

Montori, V.M., Farmer, A., Wollan, P.C., and Dinneen, S.F. 2000. Fish oil supplementation in type 2 diabetes: A quantitative systematic review. *Diabetes Care* **23**:1407–1415.

Mori, T.A., Beilin, L.J., Burke, V., Morris, J., and Ritchie, J. 1997. Interactions between dietary fat, fish, and fish oils and their effects on platelet function in men at risk of cardiovascular disease. *Arterioscler. Thromb. Vasc. Biol.* **17**:279–286.

Mori, T.A., Woodman, R.J., Burke, V., Puddey, I.B., Croftt, K.D., and Beilin, L.J. 2003. Effect of eicosapentaenoic acid and docosahexaenoic acid on oxidative stress and inflammatory markers, in treated-hypertensive Type 2 diabetic subjects. *Free. Rad. Biol. Med.* **35**:772–781.

Mori, T.A. and Beilin, L.J. 2004. Omega-3 fatty acids and inflammation. *Curr. Atheroscler. Rep.* **6**:461–467.

Mori, T.A., Burke, V., Puddey, I.B., Watts, G.F., O'Neal, D.N., Best, J.D., and Beilin, L.J. 2000. Purified eicosapentaenoic and docosahexaenoic acids have differential effects on serum lipids and lipoproteins, LDL particle size, glucose, and insulin in mildly hyperlipidemic men. *Am. J. Clin. Nutr.* **71**:1085–1094.

Mozaffarian, D. and Rimm, E.B. 2006. Fish intake, contaminants, and human health: Evaluating the risks and the benefits. *JAMA* **296**:1885–1899.

Mozaffarian, D., Prineas, R.J., Stein, P.K., and Siscovick, D.S. 2006. Dietary fish and n-3 fatty acid intake and electrocardiographic parameters in humans. *J. Am. Coll. Cardiol.* **48**:478–484.

Mozaffarian, D., Stein, P.K., Prineas, R.J., and Siscovick, D.S. 2008. Dietary fish and omega-3 fatty acid consumption and heart rate variability in US adults. *Circulation* **117**:1130–1137.

Mozaffarian, D. 2007. Fish, n-3 fatty acids, and cardiovascular haemodynamics. *J. Cardiovasc. Med. (Hagerstown).* **8**:S23-S26.

Murakami, K., Sasaki, S., Takahashi, Y., Uenishi, K., Yamasaki, M., Hayabuchi, H., Goda, T., et al. 2008. Total n-3 polyunsaturated fatty acid intake is inversely associated with serum C-reactive protein in young Japanese women. *Nutr. Res.* **28**:309–314.

Murphy, M.G., Wright, V., Ackman, R.G., and Horackova, M. 1997. Diets enriched in menhaden fish oil, seal oil, or shark liver oil have distinct effects on the lipid and fatty-acid composition of guinea pig heart. *Mol. Cell. Biochem.* **177**:257–269.

National Academy of Sciences. Institute of Medicine. Food and Nutrition Board. Dietary Reference Intakes for energy, carbohydrate, fiber, fat, fatty acids, cholesterol, protein, and amino acids (2002/2005). Accessed March 27, 2009 from http://www.iom.edu/Object.File/Master/7/300/Webtablemacro.pdf

Nodari, S., Metra, M., Milesi, G., Manerba, A., Cesana, B.M., Gheorghiade, M., and Dei Cas, L. 2009. The role of n-3 PUFAs in preventing the arrhythmic risk in patients with idiopathic dilated cardiomyopathy. *Cardiovasc. Drugs. Ther.* **23**:5–15.

Omura, M., Kobayashi, S., Mizukami, Y., Mogami, K., Todoroki-Ikeda, N., Miyake, T., and Matsuzaki, M. 2001. Eicosapentaenoic acid (EPA) induces Ca(2+)-independent activation and translocation of endothelial nitric oxide synthase and endothelium-dependent vasorelaxation. *FEBS Lett.* **487**:361–366.

Othman, R.A., Suh, M., Fischer, G., Azordegan, N., Riediger, N., Le, K., Jassal, D.S., and Moghadasian, M.H. 2008. A comparison of the effects of fish oil and flaxseed oil on cardiac allograft chronic rejection in rats. *Am. J. Physiol. Heart. Circ. Physiol.* **294**:H1452–H1458.

Peyron-Caso, E., Fluteau-Nadler, S., Kabir, M., Guerre-Millo, M., Quignard-Boulangé, A., Slama, G., and Rizkalla, S.W. 2002. Regulation of glucose transport and transporter 4 (GLUT-4) in muscle and adipocytes of sucrose-fed rats: Effects of n-3 poly- and monounsaturated fatty acids. *Horm. Metab. Res.* **34**:360–366.

Philips, T., Childs, A.C., Dreon, D.M., Phinney, S., and Leeuwenburgh, C. 2003. A dietary supplement attenuates IL-6 and CRP after eccentric exercise in untrained males. *Med. Sports Exerc.* **35**:2032–2037.

Podolin, D.A., Gayles, E.C., Wei, Y., Thresher, J.S., and Pagliassotti, M.J. 1998. Menhaden oil prevents but does not reverse sucrose-induced insulin resistance in rats. *Am. J. Physiol.* **274**:R840–R848.

Qi, K., Fan, C., Jiang, J., Zhu, H., Jiao, H., Meng, Q., and Deckelbaum, R.J. 2008. Omega-3 fatty acid containing diets decrease plasma triglyceride concentrations in mice by reducing endogenous triglyceride synthesis and enhancing the blood clearance of triglyceride-rich particles. *Clin. Nutr.* **27**:424–430.

Riediger, N.D., Othman, R., Suh, M., and Moghadasian, M.H. 2009. A systemic review of n-3 fatty acids in health and disease. *J. Am. Diet. Assoc.* **109**:668–679.

Riediger, N.D., Othman, R., Fitz, E., Pierce, G.N., Suh, M., and Moghadasian, M.H. 2008. Low n-6:n-3 fatty acid ratio, with fish- or flaxseed oil, in a high fat diet improves plasma lipids and beneficially alters tissue fatty acid composition in mice. *Eur. J. Nutr.* **47**:153–160.

Riediger, N.D., Azordegan, N., Harris-Janz, S., Ma, D.W., Suh, M., and Moghadasian, M.H. 2009. 'Designer oils' low in n-6:n-3 fatty acid ratio beneficially modifies cardiovascular risks in mice. *Eur. J. Nutr.* **48**:307–314.

Ross, R. 1999. Atherosclerosis—An inflammatory disease. *N. Eng. J. Med.* **340**:115–126.

Ruzickova, J., Rossmeisl, M., Prazak, T., Flachs, P., Sponarova, J., Veck, M., Tvrzicka, E., Bryhn, M., and Kopecky, J. 2004. Omega-3 PUFA of marine origin limit diet-induced obesity in mice by reducing cellularity of adipose tissue. *Lipids* **39**:1177–85.

Sanders, T.A., Gleason, K., Griffin, B., and Miller, G.J. 2006. Influence of an algal triacylglycerol containing docosahexaenoic acid (22:6n-3) and docosapentaenoic acid (22:5n-6) on cardiovascular risk factors in healthy men and women. *Br. J. Nutr.* **95**:525–531.

Sanders, T.A.B., Lewis, F., Slaughter, S., Griffin, B.A., Griffen, M., Davies, I., Millward, D.J., Cooper, J.A., and Miller, G.J. 2006. Effect of varying ratio of n-6 to n-3 fatty acids by increasing the dietary intake of α-linolenic acid, eicosapentaenoic and docosahexaenoic acid, or both on fibrinogen and clotting factors VII and XII in persons aged 45–70 y: The OPTILIP Study. *Am. J. Clin. Nutr.* **84**:513–522.

Schwalfenberg, G. 2006. Omega-3 fatty acids: Their beneficial role in cardiovascular health. *Can. Fam. Phys.* **52**:734–740.

Schwellenbach, L.J., Olson, K.L., McConnell, K.J., Stolcpart, R.S., Nash, J.D., and Merenich, J.A. 2006. Clinical pharmacy cardiac risk service study group. The triglyceride-lowering effects of a modest dose of docosahexaenoic acid alone versus in combination with low dose eicosapentaenoic acid alone versus in combination with low dose eicosapentaenoic acid in patients with coronary artery disease and elevated triglycerides. *J. Am. Coll. Nutr.* **25**:480–485.

Shah, A.P., Ichiuji, A.M., Han, J.K., Traina, M., El-Bialy, A., Meymandi, S.K., and Wachsner, R.Y. 2007. Cardiovascular and endothelial effects of fish oil supplementation in healthy volunteers. *J. Cardiovasc. Pharmacol. Ther.* **12**:213–219.

Simopoulos, A.P., Norman, H.A., and Gillapsy, J.E. 1995. Purslane in human nutrition and its potential for world agriculture. *World. Rev. Nutr. Diet* **77**:47–74.

Simopoulos, A.P. 1999. Essential fatty acids in health and chronic disease. *Am. J. Clin. Nutr.* **70**(Suppl):560S–569S.

Soltan, S.S., and Gibson, R.A. 2008. Levels of Omega 3 fatty acids in Australian seafood. *Asia. Pac. J. Clin. Nutr.* **17**:385–390.

Soriguer, F., Serna, S., Valverde, E., Hernando, J., Martin-Reyes, A., Soriquer, M., Pareja, A., Tinahones, F., and Esteva, I. 1997. Lipid, protein, and calorie content of different Atlantic and Mediterranean fish, shell-fish, and mollusks commonly eaten in the south of Spain. *Eur. J. Epidemiol.* **13**:451–463.

Spoor, H.J. 1960. External cod liver oil therapy in infantile and atopic eczema. *N. Y. State. J. Med.* **60**:2863–2868.

Storlien, L.H., Jenkins, A.B., Chisholm, D.J., Pascoe, W.S., Khouri, S., and Kraegen, E.W. 1991. Influence of dietary fat composition on development of insulin resistance in rats. Relationship to muscle triglyceride and omega-3 fatty acids in muscle phospholipid. *Diabetes* **40**:280–289.

Storlien, L.H., Kraegen, E.W., Chisholm, D.J., Ford, G.L., Bruce, D.G., and Pascoe, W.S. 1987. Fish oil prevents insulin resistance induced by high-fat feeding in rats. *Science* **237**:885–888.

Streppel, M.T., Ocké, M.C., Boshuizen, H.C., Kok, F.J., and Krohout, D. 2008. Long-term fish consumption and n-3 fatty acid intake in relation to (sudden) coronary heart disease death: The Zutphen Study. *Eur. Heart. J.* **29**:2024–2030.

Sugano, M. and Hirahara, F. 2000. Polyunsaturated fatty acids in the food chain in Japan. *Am. J. Clin. Nutr.* **71**(Suppl):189S–196S.

Thies, F., Garry, J.M., Yaqoob, P., Rerkasem, K., Williams, J., Shearman, C.P., Gallagher, P.J., Calder, P.C., and Grimble, R.F. 2003. Association of n-3 polyunsaturated fatty acids with stability of atherosclerotic plaques: A randomised controlled trial. *Lancet* **361**:477–485.

Ukropec, J., Reseland, J.E., Gasperikova, D.., Demcakova, E., Madsen, L., Berge, R.K., Rustan, A.C., Klimes, I., Drevon, C.A., and Sebökova, E. 2003. The hypotriglyceridemic effect of dietary n-3 FA is associated with increased beta-oxidation and reduced leptin expression. *Lipids* **38**:1023–1029.

Virtanen, J.K., Mozaffarian, D., Chiuve, S.E., and Rimm, E.B. 2008. Fish consumption and risk of major chronic disease in men. *Am. J. Clin. Nutr.* **88**:1618–1625.

Wang, Y., Botolin, D., Christian, B., Busik, J., Xu, J., and Jump, D.B. 2005. Tissue-specific, nutritional, and developmental regulation of rat fatty acid elongases. *J. Lipid. Res.* **46**:706–715.

Wilkinson, P., Leach, C., Ah-Sing, E.E., Hussain, N., Miller, G.J., Millward, D.J., and Griffin, B.A. 2005. Influence of alpha-linolenic acid and fish-oil on markers of cardiovascular risk in subjects with an athero-genic lipoprotein phenotype. *Atherosclerosis* **181**:115–124.

Willerson, J.T. and Ridker, P.M. 2004. Inflammation as a cardiovascular risk factor. *Circulation* **109**(Suppl 1): II2–II10.

Wing, L.M., Nestel, P.J., Chalmers, J.P., Rouse, I., West, M.J., Bune, A.J., Tonkin, A.L., and Russell, A.E. 1990. Lack of effect of fish oil supplementation on blood pressure in treated hypertensives. *J. Hypertens.* **34**:943–949.

Wood, J.D. and Biely, J. 1960. The effect of dietary marine fish oils on the serum cholesterol levels in hyper-cholesterolemic chickens. *Can. J. Biochem. Physiol.* **38**:19–24.

Woodman, R.J., Mori, T.A., Burke, V., Puddey, I.B., Watts, G.F., and Beilin, L.J. 2002. Effects of purified eicosapentaenoic and docosahexaenoic acids on glycemic control, blood pressure, and serum lipids in type 2 diabetic patients with treated hypertension. *Am. J. Clin. Nutr.* **76**:1007–1015.

Xiao, Y.F., Sigg, D.C., Ujhelyi, M.R., Wilhelm, J.J., Richardson, E.S., and Iaizzo, P.A. 2008. Pericardial delivery of omega-3 fatty acid: A novel approach to reducing myocardial infarct sizes and arrhythmias. *Am. J. Physiol. Heart. Circ. Physiol.* **294**:H2212–H2218.

Yamada, N., Shimizu, J., Wada, M., Takita, T., and Innami, S. 1998. Changes in platelet aggregation and lipid metabolism in rats given dietary lipids containing different n-3 polyunsaturated fatty acids. *J. Nutr. Sci. Vitaminol. (Tokyo).* **44**:279–289.

Yamagishi, K., Iso, H., Date, C., Fukui, M., Wakai, K., Kikuchi, S., Inaba, Y., Tanabe, N., and Tamakoshi, A. Japan Collaborative Cohort Study for Evaluation of Cancer Risk Study Group. 2008. Fish, omega-3 polyunsaturated fatty acids, and mortality from cardiovascular diseases in a nationwide community-based cohort of Japanese men and women the JACC (Japan Collaborative Cohort Study for Evaluation of Cancer Risk) study. *J. Am. Coll. Cardiol.* **52**:988–996.

Yamamoto, H., Yoshimura, H., Noma, M., Suzuki, S., Kai, H., Tajimi, T., Sugihara, M., and Kikuchi, Y. 1995. Improvement of coronary vasomotion with eicosapentaenoic acid does not inhibit acetylcholine-induced coronary vasospasm in patients with variant angina. *Jap. Circ. J.* **59**:608–616.

Yin, R., Huang, H., Zhang, J., Zhu, J., Jing, H., and Li, Z. 2008. Dietary n-3 fatty acids attenuate cardiac allograft vasculopathy via activating peroxisome proliferators-activated receptor-gamma. *Pediatr. Transplant.* **12**:550–556.

Yusof, H.M., Miles, E.A., and Calder, P. 2008. Influence of very long-chain n-3 fatty acids on plasma markers of inflammation in middle-aged men. *Prostaglandins Leukot. Essent. Fatty. Acids* **78**:219–228.

4 Alpha-Linolenic Acid and Cardiovascular Disease
Flaxseed Oil

Kelley C. Fitzpatrick
Flax Canada

CONTENTS

4.1 INTRODUCTION

Oils rich in the omega-3 fatty acid, alpha(α)-linolenic acid (ALA) are gaining increased attention because of anticipated health benefits related to the cardioprotective effects of this fatty acid. Flax and perilla seed oils are the richest sources of ALA, followed by the seed oils of camelina, hempseed, canola, soy, red and black currants, sea buckthorn, lingonberry, blueberry, cranberry, cloud berry, raspberry, and walnut. Flaxseed or linseed (*Linum usitatissimum*, L., subspecies *usitatissimum*, Linaceae) has been used for food and industrial fiber since ancient times (Vaisey-Genser and Morris, 2003). Flaxseed cultivation was reported to date back to around 9000–8000 BC in the Middle East; Turkey (van Zeiste, 1972), Iran (Hopf, 1983), Jordan (Rollefson et al., 1985), and Syria (Hillman, 1975; Hillman et al., 1989). Domestication of flaxseed is dated back to 7000–4500 BC (Zohary and Hopf, 2000; Vaisey-Genser and Morris, 2003). About 2 million metric tons of flaxseed are produced annually with Canada being the main producer (ca. 33%), followed by China (20%), the United States (16%), and India (11%) (Vaisey-Genser and Morris, 2003).

Flaxseed contains lipid (40%), protein (21%), dietary fiber (28%), ash (4%), and other soluble components such as sugars, phenolic acids, and lignans (ca. 6%). The oil content in flaxseed represents between 29% and 45% of the seed depending on the cultivar, location, and agroclimatic conditions (Oomah and Mazza, 1997; Daun et al., 2003; Wakjira et al., 2004). The main nutritional advantage of flaxseed oil is related to the high level of ALA in the oil (50–60%). About 20% of the flaxseed is a mucilagenous hull. Flaxseed mucilage is comprised of gum-like polysaccharides containing acidic (54.5% rhamnose and 23.4% galactose) and neutral arabinoxylan (62.8% xylose) (Cui et al., 1994a; Warrand et al., 2005). Flaxseed contains about 1–2% total phenolic compounds (Oomah et al., 1995; Hall and Shultz, 2001), of which the lignan secoisolariciresinol diglucoside (SDG) is a major component. SDG is present in the seed as a mixture of oligomers with hydroxymethylglutaric acid having an average molecular weight of 4000 Da (Kamal-Eldin et al., 2001). A number of bioactivities are claimed for SDG including antioxidant and estrogenic/oestrogenic effects (Adlercreutz et al., 1992; Hutchins and Slavin, 2003) leading to health benefits with respect to cardiovascular diseases and diabetes.

Perilla (*Perilla frutescens* (L.) Britton, Lamiaceae), also known as beefsteak plant, Chinese basil, or purple mint, is a perennial herb that belongs to the mint family and grows mainly in India and South East Asia. The plant is well known for an essential oil extracted from its leaves that contains perillaldehyde (*p*-mentha-1,8(9)-dien-7-al), limonene, linalool, β-caryophyllene, l-menthol, limonene, α-pinene, perillene (2-methyl-5-(3-oxolanyl)-2-pentene), and elemicin as main components (Yuba et al., 1995). The leaves also contain rosmarinic acid that might be responsible for an antiallergic effect (Makino et al., 2003). Perilla seeds contain 35–45% oil that is comprised of approximately 55–60% ALA (Lee et al., 1993).

Camelina (*Camelina sativa*, L. Crantz, Brassicaceae), known also as false flax or gold of pleasure, is an oilseed with cultivation history extending back to the Bronze Age (Schultze-Motel, 1979). The seeds contain 30–40% oil that is comprised of approximately 35–40% of ALA (Plessers et al., 1962; Seehuber, 1984; Marquard and Kuhlmann, 1986; Budin et al., 1995; Zubr, 1997), enabling its utilization as a drying oil in painting and coating applications. The camelina seed contains much lower levels of glucosinolates compared to other Brassicaceae species (Lange et al., 1995), which encourages the utilization of meals in feed applications.

The most widely studied source of ALA for health outcomes is flaxseed oil which is the focus of this chapter.

4.2 METABOLISM OF ALA

ALA is found in plants, animals, plankton, and marine species but flax and perilla seed oils are the richest sources (Morris, 2007). ALA is an essential fatty acid (EFA) that plays an important role in: growth and development, reproduction, vision; maintaining healthy skin, maintaining cell structure, the metabolism of cholesterol, and gene regulation. ALA, which is the most commonly consumed omega-3 fatty acid in the typical Western diet (Lanzmann-Petithory, 2001), has also been linked to the prevention and/or amelioration of several chronic conditions including cardiovascular disease, certain cancers, rheumatoid arthritis, and autoimmune disorders.

EFAs are required in the diet as they cannot be synthesized by humans. The two established EFAs are the omega-6 fatty acid linoleic acid (C18:2n-6, LA) and the omega-3 fatty acid ALA. LA and ALA are components of cellular membranes and act to increase membrane fluidity. These fatty acids are necessary for cell membrane function, as well as for the proper functioning of the brain and nervous system (Davis and Kris-Etherton, 2003; Harper and Jacobson, 2001). ALA is converted into the long-chain omega-3 fatty acids, eicosapentaenoic acid (EPA) and docosapentaenoic acid (DPA), and to some extent to docosahexaenoic acid (DHA), which are commonly found in fish and fish oil. The conversion of ALA into EPA, DPA, and DHA occurs primarily in the liver in the endoplasmic reticulum and involves a series of elongation enzymes that sequentially add

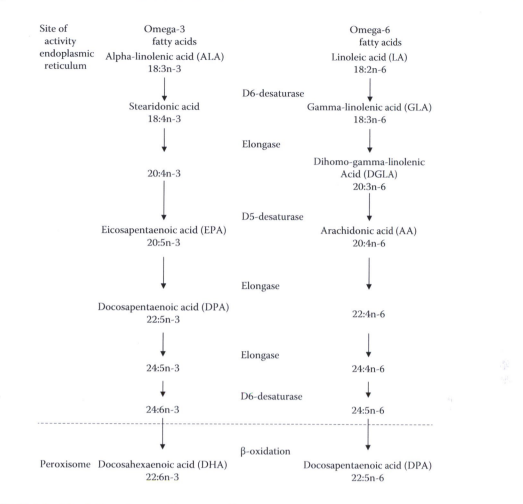

FIGURE 4.1 Metabolic pathways of the omega-3 and omega-6 fatty acids. *Note:* The conversion pathway shown is the "Sprecher pathway," which is believed to be the major route (Burdge, 2006).

2-carbon units to the fatty acid backbone and desaturation enzymes that insert double bonds into the molecules (Figure 4.1). The final conversion of ALA into DHA requires a translocation to the peroxisome for a β-oxidation reaction. Similarly, LA is converted into long-chain omega-6 fatty acids, in particular arachidonic acid (AA), also by the same series of desaturations and elongations that metabolize ALA.

The desaturation and elongation of LA and ALA, as well as the subsequent production of eicosanoids occur competitively using the same group of enzymes. Thus, an excess of one family of fatty acids can interfere with the metabolism of the other, reducing its incorporation into tissue lipids and altering their biological effects (Harper and Jacobson, 2001). Although the rate-limiting enzyme D6-desaturase shows greater substrate specificity for ALA, the overabundance of dietary LA gives this fatty acid a quantitative advantage that is believed to limit the conversion of ALA into EPA *in vivo* (Burdge and Calder, 2005). The intake of LA in the American diet, which is about 15 g/day, is approximately an order of magnitude greater than the intake of ALA (Arterburn et al., 2006).

About 96% of dietary ALA appears to be absorbed in the gut (Burdge, 2006). After absorption, ALA has several metabolic fates, including desaturation and elongation to the longer chain omega-3 polyunsaturated fatty acids (PUFA) (Figure 4.1) or shortening by β-oxidation which is considered the major catabolic route. In men, 24–33% of an ingested dose of ALA undergoes β-oxidation

(Bretillon et al., 2001; DeLany et al., 2000) compared to 19–22% in women (Burdge and Wootton, 2002; McCloy et al., 2004). The greater β-oxidation of ALA in men probably reflects a larger mass of active tissues such as muscles, heart, liver, and kidney compared with women. Furthermore, the figures may underestimate by about 30% the actual amount of dietary ALA that undergoes β-oxidation due to the trapping of labeled CO_2 in bicarbonate pools (Burdge, 2006). The amount of ingested ALA shunted into the β-oxidation pathway appears to be stable and is not affected by dietary intake. In a study of 14 healthy men aged 40–64 years, the proportion of ALA undergoing β-oxidation did not differ between the men who consumed a diet rich in ALA (10 g/day) versus those who consumed a diet rich in EPA + DHA (1.5 g/day) for 8 weeks (Burdge et al., 2003).

Like other fatty acids, ALA can be stored in adipose tissue. In a typical 75-kg man with a fat mass of 15%, adipose tissue is calculated to contain 79 g of ALA. In a typical 65-kg woman with a fat mass of 23%, adipose tissue is calculated to contain 105 g of ALA (Burdge and Calder, 2005). The greater capacity for ALA storage by women probably reflects their greater fat mass compared with men.

4.3   ALA CONVERSION INTO LONGER CHAIN POLYUNSATURATED FATTY ACIDS

Estimates of the amount of ALA converted into EPA range from 0.2% to over 10% (Burdge and Calder, 2005; Burdge et al., 2002; Cao et al., 2006), with young women showing a conversion rate of as high as 21% (Burdge and Wootton, 2002). Conversion of ALA into DPA is estimated to range from 0.13% to 6% (Burdge, 2006; Cao et al., 2006). The conversion rate for young women is on the higher end (6%) (Burdge and Wootton, 2002).

Conversion of ALA into DHA appears to be limited in humans, with most studies showing a conversion rate of about 0.05% (Burdge, 2006; Pawlosky et al., 2001), although one study reported a value of 4% (Emken et al., 1994). A conversion rate of 9% was found in young women (Burdge and Wootton, 2002) and upregulation of the conversion of EPA into DHA which may be the result of the actions of estrogen on D6-desaturase, and may be of particular importance in maintaining adequate provision of DHA in pregnancy (Williams and Burdge, 2006).

However, stable isotope tracer studies have shown that healthy adults have the ability to synthesize DHA from ALA (Emken et al., 1990; Salem Jr, et al., 1999; Vermunt et al., 2000). The large differences in the rates of ALA conversion may be due to major differences in study methodologies. In addition, some have argued that a failure of ALA to elevate DHA levels in blood compartments does not necessarily mean that DHA concentrations do not increase in tissues (Barceló-Coblijn and Murphy, 2009; Brenna, 2002).

Conversion and conservation of ALA may be efficient in developing neural tissue and in very active tissues such as retina which actively recycles DHA (Barceló-Coblijn et al., 2005). Further, the conversion of ALA into EPA and DHA appears to be dependent on the tissue and phospholipid class, with significant accumulation of ALA, DPA, and EPA, but not DHA, in the heart and liver phospholipids of rats fed flax oil. Additionally, diets enriched in either flax or fish oil diets increased phospholipid DHA mass in the brains of rats. In all tissues, both oils decreased the AA mass, although the effect was more marked in the fish oil than in the flax oil group. This study was not able to identify the origin of the DHA in the rats fed the flax oil diet, that is, whether it was imported from the blood as preformed DHA or synthesized in the brain from plasma-derived ALA. However, several studies demonstrate minimal elongation and desaturation of ALA in the plasma, with conversion limited to EPA and DPA (Burdge et al., 2002; Zhao et al., 2004; de Groot, et al., 2004) and thus suggesting that ALA, DPA, and EPA are taken up by the brain and converted into DHA.

In 20 humans who received supplementation with either fish oil (1296 mg EPA and 864 mg DHA/day) or flaxseed oil (3510 mg ALA; 900 mg LA/day) for 8 weeks, erythrocyte membrane EPA and DHA increased 300% and 42%, respectively following fish oil supplementation (Cao et al., 2006). Flaxseed oil supplementation increased erythrocyte membrane EPA to 133% and DPA to 120% of baseline. The rapid conversion between EPA and DPA indicates the possibility that DPA can be a potential storage form for EPA. ALA supplementation enriches EPA and DPA composition in erythrocyte membranes which may act to sustain a constant supply of EPA to body tissues.

Similarly, flaxseed oil (17 g/day ALA) increased phospholipid ALA (>3-fold); EPA (>2-fold); and DPA (50%), but did not change DHA, in 21 moderately hyperlipidemic men supplemented for 12 weeks (Hussein et al., 2005).

The relationship between the dietary intake of ALA and changes in membrane EPA is positive and linear over intakes of ALA between 2 and 10 g but strongly influenced by several factors most significantly being dietary intakes of LA. An early demonstration of the competitive nature of LA and ALA showed that an increase in dietary concentrations of LA causes a decrease in products of omega-3 long-chain PUFA, and vice versa (Mohrhauer and Holman, 1963). Further, a diet rich in LA can reduce ALA conversion by as much as 40%, with a net reduction in long-chain omega-3 fatty acid accumulation of 70%. It is important to note that considerable variability in the conversion rates among individuals has been reported, even when the subjects have similar background diets (Emken, 1995).

In a study of 22 healthy men, an LA-rich diet (10.5% energy) reduced the EPA content of plasma phospholipids significantly after 4 weeks compared with a low LA diet (3.8% energy), even though both diets contained the same amount of ALA (1.1% energy) (Liou et al., 2007). Optimal conversion of ALA to n-3 long-chain PUFA is expected when the diet is low in both n-6 fatty acids, particularly LA and in omega-3 long-chain PUFA. Additionally, a high intake of LA by pregnant women has been reported to lower EPA and DHA levels in umbilical plasma, suggesting reduced ALA conversion and availability of omega-3 long-chain PUFA for the developing fetus (Al et al., 1996).

Maximum conversion of ALA was observed in human hepatoma cells (HepG2) incubated with a mixture of [13C]LA/[13C]ALA at a ratio of 1:1, where 0.7% and 17% of the recovered [13C]ALA was converted into DHA and EPA, respectively (Harnack et al., 2009). Regulative cellular signal transduction pathways involved in conversion were studied through the determination of transcript levels of the genes encoding delta-5 desaturase and delta-6 desaturase, peroxisome proliferator-activated receptor alpha (PPARα) and sterol regulatory element binding protein 1c (SREBP-1c). Gene expression of PPARα, SREBP-1c, and D5D were higher in the presence of ALA solely. When comparing the percentage rates of conversion of [13C]LA and [13C]ALA into AA and EPA/DHA, respectively, the conversion of [13C]ALA into EPA/DHA was higher than the conversion of [13C] LA into AA. This effect might be attributed to differential effects of omega-6 and omega-3 fatty acids on desaturase activity and/or gene expression.

Using stable isotope tracers, the absolute amounts of linoleic acid and ALA were shown to be of greater importance in influencing the conversion of ALA into EPA and DHA than the relative proportions of these fatty acids (Goyens et al., 2006). This study which employed a randomly controlled intervention design of 258 subjects, examined the optimal ratio of omega-6/omega-3 fatty acids in the United Kingdom diet, using a six-month, food-based intervention in older men and women. Four dietary treatments with omega-6/omega-3 ratios of 3:1 and 5:1, consisting of either ALA or EPA/DHA or combinations of both, versus a control (omega-6/omega-3 ratio of 10:1) were assessed. The results showed that lowering LA was more effective in promoting the conversion of ALA to EPA, while increasing ALA facilitated the conversion of EPA to DHA. The authors argued that a reduction in dietary LA together with an increase in ALA intake would be the most appropriate way to enhance EPA and DHA synthesis from ALA. However, the study also noted no differences between the ALA and EPA plasma phospholipid contents between the two low-ratio groups which support the hypothesis that incorporation and bioconversion of ALA are rather influenced by the ratio of dietary LA/ALA. In additional work by the same group, 29 healthy subjects consumed for 28 days a diet which provided 7% of energy from LA and 0.4% from ALA (Goyens et al., 2005). On day 19, subjects received a single bolus of 30 mg of uniformly labeled [13 C]ALA and for the next 8 days 10 mg twice daily. Nearly 7% of dietary ALA was incorporated into plasma phospholipids. From this pool, 99.8% was converted into EPA and 1% was converted into DPA and subsequently into DHA. The quantification of the separate conversion reactions remains complex.

Most of the investigations of ALA metabolism in human subjects have focused on groups of relatively young, healthy or slightly hypercholesterolemic individuals. Research suggests that age does not seem to be a major determining factor in the metabolism of ALA to EPA. Replacing soybean oil (SO) with perilla oil (PO) was used to increase ALA intake to 3 g/day in 20 Japanese subjects over the age of 60 years (Ezaki et al., 1999). As a result, the omega-6/omega-3 ratio in the diet changed from 4:1 to 1:1. Following 10 months and in comparison to the SO diet, the higher ALA diet resulted in significant increases in serum EPA and DHA from 2.5% to 3.6% and 5.3% to 6.4%, respectively. These data indicate that in elderly subjects, a 3 g/day increase of dietary ALA could increase serum EPA and DHA.

Subjects aged 18–29 or 45–69 years consuming 6 g/day of ALA in the form of ground flaxseed (30 g) or flaxseed oil showed significant increases in plasma ALA and EPA concentrations over a period of 4 weeks (Patenaude et al., 2009). The diets induced no major changes in platelet aggregation, plasma total cholesterol, low-density lipoprotein or high-density lipoprotein cholesterol levels in any of the groups. However, younger subjects showed a decrease in triacylglycerols (TAG) values compared with older subjects. In contrast, studies of a longer duration that administered larger ALA doses to older populations resulted in lower plasma TG concentrations (Djoussé et al., 2003b; Zhao et al., 2004).

High intakes of EPA and DHA can also block ALA conversion, possibly by signaling that tissue levels of omega-3 fats are adequate. A diet containing more than 12 g of ALA per day can reduce ALA conversion (Cunnane et al., 1993). Other factors that influence the rates of ALA conversion include the intake of high levels of dietary cholesterol (Garg et al., 1988; Leiken and Brenner, 1987), saturated fat, oleic acid (Berger et al., 1992; Li et al., 1999), *trans* fatty acids (Houwelingen and Hornstra, 1994), and the ratio of polyunsaturated to saturated fats in the diet (Layne et al., 1996).

Individuals who do not eat fish or fish oils (vegans and non-fish-eating vegetarians and meat-eaters) could be at risk of low or inadequate omega-3 status as plasma concentrations are lower in vegetarians and in vegans than in fish-eaters (Sanders et al., 1978). Although non-fish-eating meat-eaters and vegetarians have much lower intakes of EPA and DHA than do fish-eaters, their omega-3 status is higher than would be expected. Using data from a cross-sectional study of 196 meat eating, 231 vegetarian, and 232 vegan men in the United Kingdom, the proportions of plasma EPA and DHA were found to be lower in the vegetarians and in the vegans than in the meat-eaters (Rosell et al., 2005). Only small differences were seen for DPA. Plasma EPA, DPA, and DHA proportions were not significantly associated with the duration of time since the subjects became vegetarian or vegan, which ranged from <1 year to >20 years. In the vegetarians and the vegans, plasma DHA was inversely correlated with plasma LA. When animal foods are excluded from the diet, these data show that the endogenous production of EPA and DHA results in low but stable plasma concentrations of these fatty acids.

Using data from the EPIC (European Prospective Investigation into Cancer and Nutrition)-Norfolk cohort, Welch et al. assessed intakes of omega-3 fatty acids in 14,422 men and women aged 39–78 with 7-day diary data (Welch et al., 2010). Plasma phospholipid fatty acid measures were conducted in a subgroup of 4902 individuals. ALA intake was highest in fish-eaters and lowest in vegans, women, and meat-eaters. ALA contributed 82% of total dietary omega-3 fatty acids in the whole population, including 80% in fish-eaters, 98% in vegetarian men, 99% in vegetarian women, and 97% in meat-eaters. EPA intakes in meat-eaters were only 15% (men) and 18% (women) of those in fish-eaters and in vegetarians were 9% (women) and 15% (men) of those in fish-eaters. The ratio of EPA/DHA:ALA in plasma phospholipids was 209% higher in vegan men and 184% higher in vegan women than in fish-eaters; 14% higher in vegetarian men and 6% higher in vegetarian women than in fish-eaters; and 17% and 18% higher in male and female meat-eaters, respectively, than in fish-eaters, suggesting that statistically estimated conversion may be higher in non-fish-eaters than in fish-eaters. This is the first large population study to investigate intakes, status, and the precursor–product ratio by using statistical models as, surrogate estimates of conversion of ALA to EPA and DHA in different dietary groups.

As summarized here, a number of studies have reported the effects of consuming increased amounts of dietary ALA on the fatty acid composition of plasma or cell lipids and consistently demonstrate that intakes ranging from <5 to >18 g/day result in enhancement of EPA and increased proportions of DPA. Many studies also demonstrate that increased consumption of ALA does not result in increased proportions of DHA in plasma or cell lipids but some do report a tendency for DHA to increase. What is important to note is the variation in the response between studies, which might reflect differences in the age and gender mix of the subjects studied and variations in background diet (e.g., habitual omega-3 long-chain PUFA and LA intakes), as well as differences in the way in which ALA was provided (capsules, oils, margarines, prepared foods), the duration of studies, and differences in the analytical procedures used.

Preliminary data suggest that there are important differences between men and women in their capacity for synthesis of EPA and DHA from ALA, and that this capacity may be affected by physiological state (e.g., pregnancy). The ability to upregulate this pathway during pregnancy may be one of the adaptational mechanisms by which circulating maternal DHA levels are increased and provision of fetal DHA needs are met. This capacity for adaptation may be of particular importance in vegan pregnancies and in multiple and sequential pregnancies, where demand for DHA will be much greater than normal. Clearly, more research in this area is required.

The conversion of ALA into EPA in the body may be physiologically and clinically important. As described in subsequent sections, dietary supplementation with ALA does result in cardiovascular benefits similar to that seen with EPA, but whether these effects are due to its conversion into EPA or another mechanism unrelated to EPA (i.e., improvements in endothelial function, inflammation, lipid changes, or antiarrhythmic effect) require further assessment. The consumption of ALA-containing products has important clinical and public health implications because many people do not consume fish or do not have access to fish rich in EPA. Additionally, ALA intake is feasible and realistic through a number of different sources, supplements, and foods.

4.4 ALA AND CARDIOVASCULAR DISEASE

Cardiovascular disease (CVD) includes all diseases of the blood vessels and circulatory system such as coronary heart disease (CHD), ischemic heart disease (IHD), myocardial infarction (MI), and stroke. CVD is the leading cause of death in the United States and Canada (Rosamond et al., 2007; Heart and Stroke Foundation of Canada, 2003). ALA affects cardiovascular health through its effects on blood lipid levels, blood pressure, endothelial function, and inflammation.

Four case–control studies (Lemaitre et al., 2003; Baylin et al., 2003, 2007; Guallar et al., 1999; Rastogi et al., 2004), one cross-sectional study (Manav et al., 2004), three prevention trials (Pietinen et al., 1997; de Lorgeril et al., 1994, 1999; Dolecek, 1992), and three cohort studies (Djoussé et al., 2001, 2003a,b, 2005a; Ascherio et al., 1996; Mozaffarian et al., 2005; Hu et al., 1999; Albert et al., 2005) found a benefit of ALA-rich diets in lowering the risk of CHD, IHD, nonfatal MI, and stroke. One prevention trial found no change in the estimated 10-year IHD risk but reported a significant decrease in the levels of the prothrombotic protein, fibrinogen and the proinflammatory C-reactive protein (CRP) following ALA-rich diets (Bemelmans et al., 2002, 2004). The number of participants in these studies ranged from 233 to 76,283.

Modest intakes of ALA appear to have a significant effect on reducing nonfatal MI (Campos et al., 2008). A nonlinear inverse relationship between 0.7% adipose tissue ALA and dietary ALA intake of about 1.8 g/day (1/2 teaspoon of flax oil) and risk of nonfatal MI has been observed in a study of 1819 patients who survived an MI and 1817 matching controls. The relationship between ALA and MI was nonlinear; risk did not decrease with intakes above 0.65% energy (1.8 g/day). These observations are significant in that ALA as assessed both by questionnaire and in adipose tissue was associated with reduced risk of MI in a large population. The maximum benefit of ALA was obtained within a realistic and achievable range of intake, and the association between ALA and MI was independent of fish intake.

These results confirm earlier studies in which the ALA content of adipose tissue was reported to be inversely related to risk of MI in one case–control study conducted in Europe and Israel (Guallar et al., 1999) and inversely related to nonfatal acute MI in another study in Costa Rica (Baylin et al., 2003). In the Nurse's Health Study, which involved a 10-year follow-up of 76,283 women with no previously diagnosed CVD, a higher intake of ALA was associated with a lower relative risk of fatal and nonfatal MI (Hu et al., 1999; Albert et al., 2005). A recent evaluation of food balance sheets and CHD outcomes for 11 Eastern European countries revealed that populations which experienced the greatest increase in ALA consumption since 1990 also experienced a substantial decline in CHD mortality. These results were consistent in men and women (Zantonski, 2008). It was noted that in the countries that achieved an ALA increase of more than 0.6 g/day between 1990 and 2002 had substantial reductions in CHD risk. It is possible that the partial replacement of oils that do not have ALA, such as sunflower oil, with oils that are rich in ALA could lead to considerable health benefits.

ALA appears to have an important role among populations with low fish intake in part because EPA can inhibit the action of delta-5 and delta-6 desaturase activity. Consistent with this hypothesis, 1 g/day ALA intake has been associated with a 50% lower risk of nonfatal MI among men consuming very low (<100 mg/day) omega-3 long-chain PUFA from fish, but no association was found among those with a higher intake (Mozaffarian et al., 2005). The data assessed was from the Health Professional Follow-up Study, which began in 1986 with a cohort of 45,772 health professionals. These data strongly support a direct role of ALA consumption in decreasing CHD risk and further indicate that ALA may be of particular importance in sectors of the population that do not eat fatty fish.

The Lyon Diet Heart Study included participants who had previously survived a myocardial infarction compared to an experimental group who consumed a typical Mediterranean-style diet rich in ALA. The control group consumed a typical Western-type diet low in ALA. The results were impressive with a 75% reduction in nonfatal myocardial infarctions, and a 70% reduction in total death noted amongst the ALA group in comparison to the control group (de Lorgeril et al., 1994, 1999).

Using the National Health and Nutrition Examination Survey (NHANES), a higher intake of ALA was associated with lower prevalence of peripheral arterial disease (PAD) (Lane et al., 2008). Data from the period 1999 to 2004 from 7203 lower extremity examinations, of which 422 individuals had prevalent PAD (5.9%), were included in the analysis.

The beneficial effects of ALA seen in these studies is most likely not due to changes in serum lipids as most clinical observations show no effect of flax oil consumption (2–20 g/day) consumed for 4–20 weeks, on blood total cholesterol (TC) and LDL-cholesterol (LDL-C) levels in normal and hypercholesterolemic subjects (Sanders and Roshanai, 1983; Mantzioris et al., 1994; Kestin et al., 1990; Nestel et al., 1997; Clandinin et al., 1997; Goh et al., 1997; Paschos et al., 2005; Rallidis et al., 2004; Schwab et al., 2006; Singer et al., 1986, 1990).

In a recent study, 86 healthy male and female volunteers completed a 12-week double-blinded, placebo-controlled trial supplemented with two 1-g capsules of placebo, fish oil, flaxseed oil, or hempseed oil per day for 12 weeks (Kaul et al., 2008). The lipid parameters (TC, high-density HDL-C, LDL-C, and TG) did not show any significant differences nor was the oxidative modification of LDL affected. None of the dietary interventions induced any significant change in collagen or thrombin-stimulated platelet aggregation or the level of inflammatory markers.

A significant decrease in TC was however, noted among men who consumed 2 tbsp of flax oil daily for 12 weeks (Wilkinson et al., 2005). HDL-C decreased significantly between 4% and 10% in four of the 13 studies (Nestel et al., 1997; Paschos et al., 2005; Rallidis et al., 2004; Wilkinson et al., 2005). TG decreased significantly between 9% and 25% in three studies (Schwab et al., 2006; Singer et al., 1986, 1990).

Elderly subjects appear to react favorably to ALA. Goyens and Mensink studied an ALA-rich diet (6.8 g/day) compared to EPA/DHA-rich diet (1.05 g EPA/day + 0.55 g DHA/day) in 37 mildly hypercholesterolemic subjects, aged between 60 and 78 years (Goyens and Mensink, 2006). Both EPA/DHA and ALA induced increases in tissue factor pathway inhibitor (TFPI) of 14.6% and 18.3%, respectively. TFPI is a critical inhibitor of tissue factor-induced coagulation and low levels are involved in the development of deep-vein thrombosis. Additionally, ALA affected concentrations of LDL-C and apoB more favorably than EPA and DHA. Results from well-controlled and larger clinical trials are needed to provide a more conclusive answer regarding the effects of ALA on blood lipids.

Two population studies reported a benefit of ALA in reducing stroke risk. In the Edinburgh Artery Study, significantly lower levels of ALA were found in the red blood cell phospholipids of men and women who had had a stroke compared with participants who had no evidence of the disease (Leng et al., 1999). In the Multiple Risk Factor Intervention Trial (MRFIT), 96 men who had had a stroke were compared with 96 men without stroke who were matched for age. In the multivariate model, each increase of 0.13% in serum ALA level was associated with a 37% decrease in risk of stroke (Simon et al., 1995). After controlling for risk factors of stroke such as smoking and blood pressure, ALA emerged as an independent predictor of stroke risk. In one clinical trial, supplementing the diet with flax oil (1 tbsp providing 8 g ALA/day) for 12 weeks lowered systolic and diastolic blood pressure significantly in middle-aged hypercholesterolemic men compared with a safflower oil group. The magnitude of the effect (5 mmHg) was clinically relevant (Paschos et al., 2007).

Endothelial dysfunction is the earliest detectable stage in the development of atherosclerosis. An increase in systemic arterial compliance (SAC) denoting an improvement in endothelial function, combined with a reduction in mean arterial pressure, was reported among 15 obese adults who ate daily a diet enriched with flax oil (providing 20 g of ALA) for 4 weeks (Sanders and Roshanai, 1983). The increase in SAC with flax oil was similar to that achieved through exercise training. West et al. (2005) measured endothelial function by the method of flow-mediated vasodilation (FMD) in 18 healthy adults with type 2 diabetes. FMD was measured before and 4 h after three test meals, each providing 50 g of a specific type of fat—monounsaturated fat (MUFA) obtained from high-oleic safflower and canola oils; the MUFA diet plus EPA and DHA from sardine oil; or the MUFA diet plus ALA from canola oil. In volunteers with high fasting triacylglycerols, meals containing omega-3 fatty acids increased FMD by 50–80%. Sardine and plant omega-3 fats were equally effective in improving endothelial function as measured by FMD.

Endothelial dysfunction is also characterized by a tendency for leukocytes to adhere to the endothelium in a process controlled by cell adhesion molecules, including E-selectin, vascular cell adhesion molecule type 1 (VCAM-1), and intercellular adhesion molecule type 1 (ICAM-1) (Hwang et al., 1997). A diet rich in ALA significantly decreased VCAM-1, ICAM-1, and E-selectin compared to an average American diet in 23 hypercholesterolemics (Zhao et al., 2004). Consuming 1 tbsp of flax oil daily for 12 weeks reduced VCAM-1 levels by 18.7% in a group of male hypercholesterolemic subjects (Rallidis et al., 2004). These findings suggest that an ALA-rich diet containing flax oil has a beneficial effect on the endothelium.

4.4.1 Anti-Inflammatory Effects

In recent years, medical research has moved toward almost a unifying theory—of chronic disease as a consequence of low-grade, chronic inflammation. Inflammation is a controlled, ordered process whereby the body responds to infection or injury. Symptoms of inflammation include redness, swelling, heat, and pain. Chronic inflammation is linked with age-related diseases such as CHD, obesity, diabetes, and cancer. Agents that exert anti-inflammatory actions are likely to be important in both prevention and therapy of a wide range of human diseases and conditions. An increasing amount of research suggests that the consumption of ALA may provide protection against inflammatory diseases by reducing inflammatory eicosanoids and cytokines (Figure 4.2). Proinflammatory eicosanoids such as thromboxane A_2 (TXA_2) and leukotriene B_4 (LTB_4) are derived from AA. TXA_2 is one of the most potent promoters of platelet aggregation known (Reiss and Edelman, 2006;

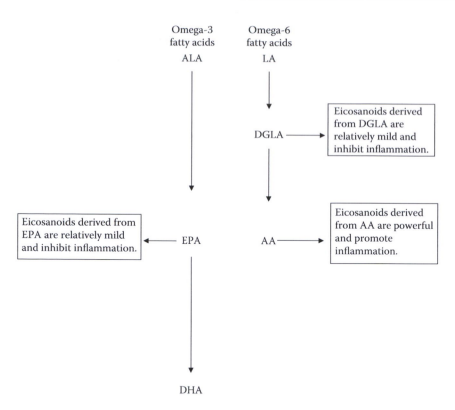

FIGURE 4.2   Sources and actions of eicosanoids. (Adapted from Stark, A.H., Crawford, M., and Reifen, R. 2008. Update on alpha-linolenic acid. *Nutr. Rev.* **66**: 326–332.)

Ross, 1999). LTB_4 increases the release of reactive oxygen species and cytokines like tumor necrosis factor α (TNF-α), interleukin 1β (IL-1β), IL-6, and IL-8 (Calder, 2006).

The potential anti-inflammatory effects of ALA could be mediated in part through its conversion to EPA or through direct protective effects. In cell membranes, omega-3 PUFA replace the omega-6 long-chain AA, thereby reducing the potential release of AA under basal conditions and during pathophysiological insults which precipitate inflammation. Mechanistically, this would effectively reduce the basal levels of proinflammatory eicosanoids.

In a clinical study of healthy men, consumption of 13/4tbsp of flax oil daily for 4 weeks led to a 30% reduction in the immune cells concentration of TXB_2, which is an inactive metabolite of TXA_2 (Caughey et al., 1996). Concentrations of the proinflammatory cytokines TNF-α and IL-1β in immune cells decreased 26% and 28%, respectively. In 64 patients with chronic obstructive pulmonary disease (COPD), serum and sputum LTB_4 levels decreased 32% and 41%, respectively, in those patients who received an ALA-rich nutritional support (1.4% ALA) daily for 24 months compared to those who received a low-ALA nutritional support (0.18% ALA) (Matsuyama et al., 2005). Serum levels of IL-6 decreased 25% in men who consumed 1 tbsp of flax oil daily for 12 weeks (Paschos et al., 2005). The serum levels of TNF-α decreased by 43% and the production by immune cells of TNF-α, IL-6, and IL-1β, decreased between 18% and 22% in hypercholesterolemics who consumed a diet rich in ALA compared with the average American diet (Zhao et al., 2007).

During inflammation, the liver releases acute-phase proteins such as CRP and serum amyloid A (SAA) in response to acute injury, infection, malignancy, hypersensitivity reactions, and trauma. CRP and SAA are markers of systemic inflammation, and are present in the lesions of atherosclerosis. CRP is an independent risk factor for CVD (Getz, 2005). Consuming flax oil reduced CRP by

48% and serum SAA by 32% in 50 hypercholesterolemic men who consumed 1 tbsp of flax oil daily for 12 weeks (Paschos et al., 2005). In a U.S. study of 23 adults with high blood cholesterol levels, consuming a high-ALA diet based on walnuts, walnut oil, and flax oil resulted in a 75% decrease in CRP levels after 6 weeks (Zhao et al., 2004).

In a recent assessment, inverse relationships were reported between dietary intake of both omega-3 and omega-6 PUFA and serum CRP concentrations in 300 Japanese men aged 21–67 years (Poudel-Tandukara et al., 2009). Self-administered diet history questionnaire were used to assess the dietary intake of the preceding month in all subjects. In men, the mean serum CRP concentrations in the highest ALA intake group were 47% lower than that with the lowest intake. Although not statistically significant, serum CRP concentrations tended to decrease with increasing intakes of EPA and DHA in women.

4.4.2 Other Mechanisms of ALA

ALA may lower the risk of fatal or nonfatal MI appears to involve an effect on cardiac rhythm. In the Family Heart Study, Djoussé et al. (2005b) found that the higher the dietary ALA intake, the lower the risk of abnormally prolonged repolarization of the heart muscle, an indicator of cardiac arrhythmia. In a clinical study among women referred for elective coronary angiography, ALA content of adipose tissue was positively correlated with 24-h heart rate variability (HRV), a strong predictor of arrhythmic events and sudden cardiac death (Christensen et al., 2005). Decreased HRV is a strong predictor of SCD and arrhythmic events and thus this association supports an antiarrhythmic effect of ALA. ALA may reduce ventricular fibrillation (Ander et al., 2004) and its cardio-protective effects have also been attributed to improvements in arrhythmia (Vos and Cunnane, 2003).

ALA may also have antithrombotic activities. An increase in activated protein C resistance (APC™ resistance) which demonstrates increased anticoagulant activity was noted in 15 healthy male subjects who consumed an ALA-rich diet with 31.5% energy fat diet and approximately 7% energy from PUFA. The high ALA diet had an ALA:LA ratio of either 1:1.2 and was compared to a diet with an ALA:LA ratio of 1:21 (LA-rich) (Allman-Farinelli et al., 1999).

The effects of doubling the ALA intake from canola-type rapeseed oil (RSO) was assessed in 42 volunteers for 6 weeks in a parallel design (Seppanen-Laakso et al., 2010). Efficient competitive inhibition by ALA was deemed to be responsible for a decrease in long-chain omega-6 PUFA at 3 weeks. Initial elevated levels of fibrinogen (2.6–3.9 g/L) decreased by 30% (0.95 g/L) at 6 weeks. Fibrinogen, a protein involved in coagulation processes, is found in elevated levels in prothrombotic and proinflammatory states, associated with higher risk of CHD, stroke, diabetes, Alzheimer's disease, and dementia. In addition, DHA in plasma phospholipids increased when fibrinogen levels were reduced following the enhancement in ALA intakes.

It has been shown that ALA decreases the nuclear transcription factor $\kappa\beta$, a major transcription factor involved in the regulation of inflammatory genes (Perez-Martinez et al., 2007; Ren and Chung, 2007). Furthermore, ALA inhibits the production of nitric oxide and downregulates inducible nitric oxide synthase, cyclooxygenase-2, and tumor necrosis factor-R gene expression in murine macrophages (Ren and Chung, 2007).

Overall, ALA appears to protect against cardiovascular diseases by altering the omega-3 fat content of cell membranes (Harper et al., 2006), by improving blood lipids and endothelial function and by exerting significant anti-inflammatory and antithrombotic effects (Bloedon and Szapary, 2004). These beneficial effects have been reported with ranges of about 3–20 g of ALA per day (equivalent to 1/2 tsp to 2½ tbsp of flax oil). In epidemiological studies, ALA intakes associated with reduced CVD risk averaged about 2 g/day (range = 0.7–6.3 g). A meta-analysis of prospective studies suggested that increasing the intake of ALA by 1.2 g/day decreases the risk of fatal CHD by at least 20% (Brouwer et al., 2004). The Institute of Medicine has set an Adequate Intake for ALA, based on the median daily intake of healthy Americans who are not likely to be deficient in this

TABLE 4.1

Estimated Dietary Intakes of Major Omega-6 and Omega-3 Fatty Acids in Canada and the United States (g/day)[a]

Country	Omega-6 Fatty Acid Intake (Linoleic Acid)	Omega-3 Fatty Acid Intake	
		ALA	Long-Chain Fatty Acids (EPA, DHA, and/or DPA)
Europe[b]	15	1–2	0.1–0.5
Canada[c]	8–11	1.3–1.6	0.14–0.24
United States[d]			
Men	18	1.7	0.13
Women	14	1.3	0.10

[a] Abbreviations: ALA, alpha-linolenic acid; DPA, docosapentaenoic acid; DHA, docosahexaenoic acid; EPA, eicosapentaenoic acid.

[b] Values for the general European population (Sanders, 2000).

[c] Values are for pregnant women living in British Columbia and Ontario (Innis and Elias, 2003; Denomme et al., 2005).

[d] Values are for men and women aged 20–39 years (Gebauer et al., 2006).

nutrient as shown in Table 4.1 (Institute of Medicine, 2002). The Adequate Intake is 1.6 g ALA per day for men and 1.1 g ALA per day for women. Up to 10% of the Adequate Intake for ALA can be provided by EPA and DHA.

More studies are needed to clarify the role of ALA in reducing CVD risk. In particular, there is an urgent need for randomized, controlled clinical trials with good study designs, clearly defined outcomes, appropriate control groups, realistic dietary interventions, and thorough statistical analyses (Stark et al., 2008).

4.5   THE DIETARY OMEGA-6 TO OMEGA-3 FATTY ACID RATIO

The dietary omega-6/omega-3 ratio affects inflammation and gene expression, thus influencing the development of chronic disease. This ratio may be as high as 17:1 in some Western diets (Simpouolos, 2006) and is estimated to be 10:1 in the U.S. diet (Kris-Etherton et al., 2002). In the Women's Health Study, participants had an average dietary ratio of about 8:1, although some women ate diets with a low ratio of about 1:1 while others ate diets with a ratio as high as 33:1 (Miljanović et al., 2005). The omega-6/omega-3 ratio recommended by international agencies and some European countries ranges from 4:1 to 10:1 (Gebauer et al., 2006). The Institute of Medicine supports a ratio of 5:1 for the U.S. and Canadian populations (Institute of Medicine, 2002). ALA comprises about 57% of the total fatty acids in flax, whereas the omega-6 fatty acids comprise about 16%. Thus, flax contains more than three times as much omega-3 as omega-6 fatty acids, giving an omega-6/omega-3 ratio of 0.3:1 (Morris, 2007) compared to the omega-6/omega-3 ratio of 58:1 in corn oil, 7:1 in soybean oil, and 2:1 in canola/rapeseed oil.

A dietary imbalance of omega-6 and omega-3 fats leads to a high ratio of omega-6 to omega-3 fatty acids in cell membranes (Harris et al, 2006) which can result in the overproduction of proinflammatory eicosanoids, many of which are derived from AA. These eicosanoids in turn stimulate the release of inflammatory cytokines and acute-phase proteins. The end result is low-grade chronic inflammation that contributes to health problems such as atherosclerosis, Alzheimer's disease, cancer, cardiovascular disease, metabolic syndrome, obesity, osteoporosis, type 2 diabetes, and periodontitis (Cordain et al., 2005; Calder, 2006; Hotamisligil, 2006; Kornman, 2006). Table 4.2

TABLE 4.2

Comparison of Health Consequences of Diets Rich in Omega-6 versus Omega-3 Fats

Consequences of Eating a Diet Rich in Omega-6 Fats	Benefits of Eating a Diet Rich in Omega-3 Fats
↑ n-6/n-3 in cell membrane phospholipids	↓ n-6 fatty acids in cell membranes
↑ production of arachidonic acid	↓ n-6/n-3 in cell membrane phospholipids
↑ release of proinflammatory eicosanoids derived from arachidonic acid	↓ levels of pro-inflammatory compounds like eicosanoids and cytokines
↑ production of proinflammatory cytokines	↓ clumping (aggregation) of blood platelets
↑ expression (activation) of proinflammatory genes	↓ expression (activation) of proinflammatory genes
↑ biomarkers of inflammation such as C-reactive protein	↓ biomarkers of inflammation such as C-reactive protein
↑ blood viscosity	↓ production of interleukin-10, an anti-inflammatory cytokine
↑ constriction of blood vessels	Decreased risk of chronic diseases
↑ oxidative modification of low-density-lipoprotein (LDL) cholesterol	
Increased risk of chronic diseases	

Sources: Adapted from Gebauer, S.K. et al., 2006. *Am. J. Clin. Nutr.* **83**: 1526S-1535S; Simopoulos, A.P. 2006. *Biomed. Pharmacother.* **60**: 502–507.

outlines some consequences of eating a diet rich in omega-6 fats versus the benefits of eating a diet rich in omega-3 fats.

A recent report suggested that omega-3 deficiency is the sixth highest cause of death among Americans (Danaei et al., 2009). It was estimated that 72,000–96,000 preventable deaths occurred each year due to omega-3 deficiency, compared to 63,000–97,000 for high *trans* fat intake. Tobacco smoking ranked as the highest risk factor with 436,000–500,000 attributed preventable deaths, followed by high blood pressure (372,000 to 414,000), obesity (188,000–237,000), physical inactivity (164,000–222,000), high blood glucose (163,000–217,000), high LDL-C (94,000–124,000), and high salt intake (97,000–107,000).

4.6 THE MARKET PRODUCTS CONTAINING ALA

Because of limitations in increasing the public's consumption of fish, the use of ALA may be an important alternative for providing optimal EPA and DHA concentrations in the plasma and cell membranes. Unlike its longer chain metabolites, ALA can be obtained from several types of nuts, seeds, and seed oils, including flaxseed oil, English walnuts, canola oil, and soybean oil. Flaxseed meal or flaxseed oil can easily be incorporated into common dietary items such as breads, rolls, cereals, muffins, margarines, and salad dressings.

4.6.1 NORTH AMERICA

The market is responding to increases in demand for omega-3 oils. Estimates for fish- and plant-based omega-3 oils in the United States were US$291.7 million in 2004. By 2007, this had risen to US$514.9 million at a CAGR of 20.9%. The market has experienced a major shift since 2004 as what was described as an immature marketplace for omega-3 has grown driven by consumer and end-product manufacturer enthusiasm. Although smaller than the market for fish and algae oils, plant oils are expected to see the highest value growth in the market, rising at a CAGR of 22.0% between 2007 and 2011 to US$63.9 million (Datamonitor, 2009; Mintel International, 2008; Frost and Sullivan, 2008; Packaged Facts, 2009). The major advantage that plant oils hold in the market is less resistance from both manufacturers and consumers as to the addition of plant oils versus fish oils to functional foods.

Market analyst Packaged Facts has estimated that the overall omega-3 market will be valued at US$7 billion by 2011 (Packaged Facts, 2009). Using sales data, new product roll out information, and product availability, grain-based foods (bars, breads, cereals, etc.) represented 86% of the omega-3-enhanced food and beverage market in 2008. Eggs were second with 6% share, and dairy third with 4% share. Spreads and dressings represent 2% share, while all other products have 2% share. Packaged Facts projects that by 2011, percent share will shift with dairy (cheese, ice cream, milk, yogurt, etc.) gaining a larger piece of the market.

In volume terms, at 4.0 million kg, bakery is the leading additive category, up at a CAGR of 18.7% since 2004. It is expected that although growth in these (and other additive categories) will slow in 2011, value-generation opportunities will increase as demand shifts away from "basic" omega-3 additives such as oils towards concentrates (Frost and Sullivan, 2008). Microencapsulation and similar technologies will increase the use of oils in various food products.

Omega-3 oil sales to the supplements industry are healthy but not as dynamic as those to the food industry. The average consumer views the concept of omega-3 fortified food as much more convenient and inexpensive than a supplement regime. Within the category, the trend is towards capsule forms as more palatable omega-3 formats in comparison to "traditional" liquid oil products.

Like the United States, Canada has witnessed significant development in the market for omega-3 for food, beverage, and other markets such as personal care. Increasingly, supplements sales are lagging, although the outlook for that sector is reasonably solid through 2011, recording a CAGR of 22.1% by value, 10.3% by volume. In 2007 in Canada, omega-3 in the food and beverages market had sales of US$34.2 million and US$19.0 million for supplements.

In North America, new food and beverage products containing flaxseed oil grew from less than 100 in the year 2000 to over 400 by 2008 and the trend is continuing (Datamonitor, 2009). Baked products including snack foods, cereals and breads, as well as nutritional bars are leading categories for introduction of new flax ingredients in the functional food area. Flax oil is often blended with other oils to provide EFA combinations including borage and evening primrose (sources of omega 6 PUFA, in particular gamma linolenic acid), fish oil, and canola or high oleic sunflower oils as a source of omega-9 monounsaturated fatty acids. Flax oil is often sold in combination with flax lignans.

Spreads are another popular medium for delivering omega-3 fatty acids which are added to margarines and butter to improve the nutritional characteristics of the products. In addition, omega-3-fortified milk was introduced in the United States and Canada in June 2004 and continues to expand in sales and availability of products.

4.6.2 European Union

Europe has been a more stable omega-3 market than North America since 2004. Omega-3 additives in foods and supplements account for the majority of the market both in value and volume terms, US$222.8 million in 2007 at a volume of 11.5 million kg, up at CAGRs of 23.2% and 14.7%, respectively since 2004 (Frost and Sullivan, 2008). Notably, growth in value terms is expected to be fairly consistent over the forecast period of up to 2011, for a number of categories. Oil-based foods, and particularly snack foods, confectionery, and beverages are all likely to register CAGRs similar to those for 2007 as they benefit from the concept of incorporating functional attributes into products that may not have been traditionally associated with "better for you" formulations.

Dairy is the dominant category for omega-3 additive sales in Europe. Sales to the bakery sector have also gained importance. Supplements are also a leading product category for marketing new products with omega-3 health claims.

4.7 REGULATIONS FOR ALA

In this section, the most relevant claims for ALA in the United States, Canada, and the European Union are summarized.

4.7.1 United States

4.7.1.1 Nutrient Content Claims

On May 16, 2004, the U.S. Food and Drug Administration approved a petition to establish Daily Values (DV) and Nutrient Content Claims for ALA, EPA, and DHA. There was no upper-limit established for omega-3 consumption in the form of ALA as there was for EPA and DHA (U.S. Food and Drug Administration, Food and Nutrition, 2010). The FDA action established a minimum recommended Daily Value for ALA at 1300 mg per day. Recommended Daily Values for EPA and DHA were provided at 130 mg per day. Only "high" claims can be made for EPA and DHA while ALA declarations can include "high," "good," and "more."

When making a claim, the omega-3 fatty acid in the product must be identified as ALA omega-3.

The packaging label claims that can be made for foods and in dietary supplements are as follows:

"contains — mg of ALA per serving, which is —% of the Daily value for ALA (1.3g)"
"contains — mg of ALA per serving. The Daily Value for ALA is 1.3g."

For "*more*" claims: "*—% more of the Daily Value of ALA per serving than [reference food]. This product contains —mg ALA omega-3 per serving, which is —% of the Daily Value for ALA omega-3 (1.3g). [Reference Food] contains —mg ALA omega-3 per serving.*"

Nutrient Content Claim	Amount of ALA-Omega-3 (per serving) (mg)
"high," "rich," or "excellent" source of ALA omega-3	260
"good" source of ALA omega-3	130
"more" ALA omega-3 (than reference food)	130

4.7.1.2 Structure/Function (S/F) Claims

S/F claims for food and dietary supplement products describe the effect that the product has on the normal structure or function of the body (U.S. Food and Drug Administration, 2010a). These need not be preapproved by the FDA, but they must be true and not misleading to the consumer. Products containing flax oil qualify for S/F claims such as "*Now with Omega-3 ALA To Help Support A Healthy Heart.*"

4.7.1.3 Health Claims

Health claims allow a statement on a food label which describes the relationship between a substance and a reduction in risk of a disease (U.S. Food and Drug Administration, 2010a). In 2003, the FDA launched the Consumer Health Information for Better Nutrition Initiative for foods and supplements. The result of the initiative saw the FDA allow the use of *qualified health claims* (U.S. Food and Drug Administration, 2010b). These claims do not have sufficient scientific agreement in support of them and would be required to have a qualifying statement detailing the limitations of the evidence in support of the claim. Since 2004, producers of foods containing omega-3 from fish and algal oils are able to make a qualified health claim on the benefits of their products:

"Supportive but not conclusive research shows that consumption of EPA and DHA Omega3 fatty acids may reduce the risk of coronary heart disease."

The claim does not include ALA because this omega-3 was not included in the petition reviewed by the FDA as it was submitted by fish oil companies.

4.7.2 CANADA

4.7.2.1 Nutrient Content Claims

Similar to the United States, nutrient content claims in Canada are statements or expressions which describe, directly or indirectly, the level of a nutrient in a food or a group of foods. Food manufacturers may claim the nutrient content of specific nutrients if the food meets criteria described by regulations of the Canadian Food Inspection Agency (CFIA). The label can state the food is "low," "high," "a good source," or other descriptor of a particular nutrient. In order to make these claims, the food must meet the specifications set out in the table in Section B.01.513 of the Food and Drug Regulations (Department of Justice Canada, 2010).

Health Canada requires the following guidelines to be met ("Guide" refers to the CFIA "Nutrition Labeling Guide") for foods claiming omega-3 fatty acids. The claims in quotation marks in Column 1 are those which are permitted by the *Food and Drug Regulations*. The reference amounts are found in Part D, Schedule M of the *Food and Drug Regulations* (Canadian Food Inspection Agency, 2010).

Omega-3 and Omega-6 Polyunsaturated Fatty Acid Claims

Column 1 Claim	Column 2 Conditions—Food	Column 3 Conditions—Label or Advertisement	FDR Reference
a. Source of omega-3 polyunsaturated fatty acids "source of omega-3 polyunsaturated fatty acids" "contains omega-3 polyunsaturated fatty acids" "provides omega-3 polyunsaturated fatty acids" Note: "polyunsaturated fatty acids" may be substituted with "polyunsaturated fat" or "polyunsaturates" in the above claims	The food contains: a. 0.3 g or more of omega-3 polyunsaturated fatty acids per reference amount and serving of stated size; or b. 0.3 g or more of omega-3 polyunsaturated fatty acids per 100 g, if the food is a prepackaged meal.	Must comply with the general requirements for nutrient content claims—see 7.5 of the *Guide* Nutrition Facts table must include a declaration of omega-3 polyunsaturated fatty acids, omega-6 polyunsaturated fatty acids, and monounsaturated fatty acids Nutrition Facts table required on products otherwise exempted by B.01.401(2) (a) and (b) When used in an advertisement, must comply with the requirements for advertisements—see 7.11 of the *Guide*	[B.01.402 (3) and (4)] [B.01.401(3)(*e*)(ii)] Table following B.01.513, item 25
b. Source of omega-6 polyunsaturated fatty acids "source of omega-6 polyunsaturated fatty acids" "contains omega-6 polyunsaturated fatty acids" "provides omega-6 polyunsaturated fatty acids" Note: "polyunsaturated fatty acids" may be substituted with "polyunsaturated fat" or "polyunsaturates" in the above claims	The food contains: a. 2 g or more of omega-6 polyunsaturated fatty acids per reference amount and serving of stated size; or b. 2 g or more of omega-6 polyunsaturated fatty acids per 100 g, if the food is a prepackaged meal.	See conditions set out for item (a) of this table.	Table following B.01.513, item 26

4.7.2.2 Health Claims

A health claim is a statement or representation that states, suggests, or implies that a relation exists between a food or component of that food and health, and of disease reduction. There are no health claims allowed in Canada for any edible oil or seed containing omega-3 fatty acids.

4.7.3 European Union

The European Food Safety Authority (EFSA) was established in January 2002, following a series of food crises in the late 1990s, as an independent source of scientific advice and communication on risks associated with the food chain. EFSA's responsibility includes food and feed safety, nutrition and health claim guidance, animal health and welfare, plant protection, and plant health. In all these fields, EFSA provides objective and independent science-based advice and clear communication grounded in the most up-to-date scientific information and knowledge.

Under Article 13 of Regulation (EC) No 1924/20063, a general health claim is permissible on products containing ALA (EFSA, 2009) related to blood cholesterol. The target population is defined as the general population. In order to bear the claim, a food should contain at least 15% of the proposed labeling reference intake value of 2 g ALA per day. The allowable claim is *"contributes to healthy blood cholesterol level/helps to maintain normal cholesterol level/maintenance of normal blood cholesterol level"* or *"Alpha-linolenic acid contributes to maintenance of normal blood cholesterol concentrations."*

A second claim is permissible under Article 14 of Regulation (EC) No 1924/20061 and is specific to either ALA or LA and a relationship to the normal growth and development of children (EFSA, 2008). The target population for the health claim is children from 1 to 12 years of age.

REFERENCES

Adlercreutz, H., Mousavi, Y., Clark, J., Hockerstedt, K., Hämäläinen, E., Wähälä, K., Mäkelä, T., and Hase, T. 1992. Dietary phytoestrogens and cancer: *In vitro* and *in vivo* studies. *J. Steroid Biochem. Mol. Biol.* **41**: 331–337.

Al, M.D.M., Badart-Smook, A., Houwelingen, A., Hasaart, T., and Hornstra. G. 1996. Fat intake of women during normal pregnancy: Relationship with maternal and neonatal essential fatty acid status. *J. Am. Coll. Nutr.* **15**: 49–55.

Albert, C.M., Oh, K., Whang, W., Manson, J.E., Chau, C.E., Stampfer, M., Willett, W., and Hu, F.B. 2005. Dietary Alpha-linolenic acid intake & risk of sudden cardiac death & coronary heart disease. *Circulation* **112**: 3232–3238.

Allman-Farinelli, M.A., Hall, D., Kingham, K., Pang, D., Petocz, P., and Favaloro, E.J. 1999. Comparison of the effects of two low fat diets with different alpha-linolenic:linoleic acid ratios on coagulation and fibrinolysis *Atherosclerosis* **142**(1): 159–168.

Ander, B.P., Weber, A.R., Rampersad, P.P., Gilchrist, J., Pierce, G., and Lukas. A. 2004. Dietary flaxseed protects against ventricular fibrillation induced by ischemia-reperfusion in normal and hypercholesterolemic rabbits. *J. Nutr.* **134**: 3250–3256.

Arterburn, L.M., Hall, E.B., and Oken, H. 2006. Distribution, interconversion, and dose response of n-3 fatty acids in humans. *Am. J. Clin. Nutr.* **83**(Suppl), 1467S–1476S.

Ascherio, A., Rimm, E.B., Giovannucci, E.L., Spiegelman, D., Stampfer, M., and Willett, W.C. 1996. Dietary fat and risk of coronary heart disease in men: Cohort follow up study in the United States. *Br. Med. J.* **313**: 84–90.

Barceló-Coblijn, G. and Murphy, E.J. 2009. Alpha-linolenic acid and its conversion to longer chain n-3 fatty acids: Benefits for human health and a role in maintaining tissue n-3 fatty acid levels. *Prog. Lipid Res.* **48**: 355–374.

Barceló-Coblijn, G., Collison, L.W., Jolly, C.A., and Murphy, E.J. 2005. Dietary α-linolenic acid increases brain but not heart and liver docosahexaenoic acid levels. *Lipids* **40**:787–798.

Baylin, A., Kabagambe, E.K., Ascherio, A., Spiegelman, D., and Campos, H. 2003. Adipose tissue α-linolenic acid and nonfatal acute myocardial infarction in Costa Rica. *Circulation* **107**: 1586–1591.

Baylin, A., Ruiz-Narvaez, E., Kraft, P., and Campos, H. 2007. α-Linoleic acid, Δ6-desaturase gene polymorphism, and the risk of nonfatal myocardial infarction. *Am. J. Clin. Nutr.* **85**: 554–560.

Bemelmans, W.J.E., Broer, J., Feskens, E.J.M., Smit, A., Muskiet, F., Lefrandt, J., Bom, V., May, J., and Meyboom-de Jong, B. 2002. Effect of an increased intake of α-linolenic acid and group nutritional education on cardiovascular risk factors: The Mediterranean Alpha-linolenic Enriched Groningen Dietary Intervention (MARGARIN) study. *Am. J. Clin. Nutr.* **75**: 221–227.

Bemelmans, W.J.E., Lefrandt, J.D., Feskens, E.M.J., van Haelst, P.L., Broer, J., Meyboom-de Jong, B., May, J.F., Cohen, T., and Smit, A. 2004. Increased alpha-linolenic acid intake lowers C-reactive protein, but has no effect on markers of atherosclerosis. *Eur. J. Clin. Nutr.* **58**: 1083–1089.

Berger, A., Gershwin, M.E., and German. J.B. 1992. Effects of various dietary fats on cardiolipin acyl composition during ontogeny of mice. *Lipids* **27**: 605–612.

Bloedon, L.T. and Szapary, P.O. 2004. Flaxseed and cardiovascular risk. *Nutr. Rev.* **62**: 18–27.

Brenna, J.T. 2002. Efficiency of conversion of alpha-linolenic acid to long chain n-3 fatty acids in man. *Curr. Opin. Clin. Nutr. Metab. Care.* **5** :127–132.

Bretillon, L., Chardigny, J.M., Sébédio, J.L., Noel, J.P., Scrimgeour, C.M., Fernie, C.E., Loreau, O., Gachon, P., and Beaufrere, B. 2001. Isomerization increases the postprandial oxidation of linoleic acid but not α-linolenic acid in men. *J. Lipid Res.* **42**: 995–997.

Brouwer I.A., Katan, M.B., and Zock, P.L. 2004. Dietary α-linolenic acid is associated with reduced risk of fatal coronary heart disease, but increased prostate cancer risk: A meta-analysis. *J. Nutr.* **134**: 919–922.

Budin, J.T., Breene, W.M., and Putnam D.H. 1995. Some compositional properties of camelina (*Camelina sativa* L. Crantz) seeds and oils. *J. Am. Oil Chem. Soc.* **72**: 309–315.

Burdge, G.C. 2006. Metabolism of α-linolenic acid in humans. *Prostaglandins Leukot. Essent. Fatty Acids.* **75**: 161–168.

Burdge, G.C. and Calder, P.C. 2005. Conversion of α-linolenic acid to longer-chain polyunsaturated fatty acids in human adults. *Reprod. Nutr. Dev.* **45**: 581–597.

Burdge, G.C. and Wootton, S.A. 2002. Conversion of α-linolenic to eicosapentaenoic, docosapentaenoic and docosahexaenoic acids in young women. *Br. J. Nutr.* **88**: 411–420.

Burdge, G.C., Finnegan, Y.E., Minihane, A.M., Williams, C.M., and Wootton, S.A. 2003. Effect of altered dietary n-3 fatty acid intake upon plasma lipid fatty acid composition, conversion of [^{13}C]α-linolenic acid to longer-chain fatty acids and partitioning towards β-oxidation in older men. *Br. J. Nutr.* **90**: 311–321.

Burdge, G.C., Jones, A.E., and Wootton, S.A. 2002. Eicosapentaenoic and docosapentaenoic acids are the principal products of α-linolenic acid metabolism in young men. *Br. J. Nutr.* **88**: 355–363.

Calder, P.C. 2006. n-3 Polyunsaturated fatty acids, inflammation, and inflammatory diseases. *Am. J. Clin. Nutr.* **83**(Suppl): 1505S–1519S.

Campos, H., Baylin, A., and Willett, W.C. 2008. α-Linolenic acid and risk of nonfatal acute myocardial infarction, *Circulation* **118**: 339–345.

Canadian Food Inspection Agency, 2010. *Guide to Food Labelling and Advertising Chapter 7—Nutrient Content Claims.* http://www.inspection.gc.ca/english/fssa/labeti/guide/ch7be.shtml.).

Cao, J., Schwichtenberg, K.A., Hanson, N.Q., and Tsai, M.Y. 2006. Incorporation and clearance of omega-3 fatty acids in erythrocyte membranes and plasma phospholipids. *Clin. Chem.* **52**(12): 2265–2272.

Caughey, G.E., Mantzioris, E., Gibson, R.A., Cleland, L.G., and James, M.J. 1996. The effect on human tumor necrosis factor α and interleukin 1β production of diets enriched in n-3 fatty acids from vegetable oil or fish oil. *Am. J. Clin. Nutr.* **63**: 116–122.

Christensen, J.H., Schmidt, E.B., Mølenberg, D., and Toft, E. 2005. Alpha-linolenic acid and heart rate variability in women examined for coronary artery disease. *Nutr. Metab. Cardiovasc. Dis.* **15**: 345–351.

Clandinin, M.T., Foxwell, A., Goh, Y.K., Layne, K., and Jumpsen, J. 1997. Omega-3 fatty acid intake results in a relationship between the fatty acid composition of LDL cholesterol ester and LDL cholesterol content in humans. *Biochim. Biophys. Acta* **1346**: 247–252.

Cordain, L., S.B. Eaton, S.B. Sebastian, A., Mann, N., Lindeberg, S., Watkins, B., O'Keefe, J., and Brand-Miller, J. 2005. Origins and evolution of the Western diet: Health implications for the 21st century. *Am. J. Clin. Nutr.* **81**: 341–354.

Cui, W., Mazza, G., and Biliaderis, C.G. 1994a. Chemical structure, molecular size distributions and rheological properties of flaxseed gum. *J. Agric. Food Chem.* **42**: 1891–1895.

Cunnane, S.C., Ganguli, S., Menard, C., Liede, A. C., Hamadeh, M.J., Chen, Z-Y., Wolever, T.M.S., and Jenkins, D.J.A. 1993. High α-linolenic acid flaxseed (*Linum usitatissimum*): Some nutritional properties in humans. *Br. J. Nutr.* **69**: 443–453.

Danaei, G., Ding, E.L., Mozaffarian, D., Taylor, B., Rehm, J., Murray, C.J., and Ezzati, M. 2009. The preventable causes of death in the United States: Comparative risk assessment of dietary, lifestyle, and metabolic risk factors. *PLoS Med.* **6**(4): E1000058.

Datamonitor. Omega 3 Oils Market Analysis. 2009.

Daun, J.K., Barthet, V.J., Chornick, T.L., and Duguid, S. 2003. Structure, composition and variety development of flaxseed. In: *Flaxseed in Human Nutrition*, 2nd ed. L.U. Thompson and S.C. Cunnane (eds.), Champaign: AOCS Press, Champaign, IL, USA, pp. 1–40.

Davis, B.C. and Kris-Etherton, P.M. 2003. Achieving optimal essential fatty acid status in vegetarians: Current knowledge and practical implications. *Am. J. Clin. Nutr.* **78**(Suppl): 640S–660S.

de Groot, R.H.M., Hornstra, G., van Houwelingen, A.C., and Roumen, F. 2004. Effect of a-linolenic acid supplementation during pregnancy on maternal and neonatal polyunsaturated fatty acid status and pregnancy outcome. *Am .J. Clin. Nutr.* **79**: 251–260.

DeLany, J.P., Windhauser, M.M., Champagne, C.M., and Bray, G.A. 2000. Differential oxidation of individual dietary fatty acids in humans. *Am. J. Clin. Nutr.* **72**: 905–911.

De Lorgeril, M., Salen, P., Martin, J-L., Monjaud, I., Delaye, J., and Mamelle, N. 1999. Mediterranean diet, traditional risk factors, and the rate of cardiovascular complications after myocardial infarction: Final report of the Lyon Diet Heart Study. *Circulation* **99**: 779–785.

De Lorgeril, M., Renaud, S., Mamelle, N., Salen, P., Martin, J., Monjaud, I., Guidollet, J., Touboul, P., and Delaye, J. 1994. Mediterranean alpha-linolenic acid-rich diet in secondary prevention of coronary heart disease. *Lancet* **343**: 1454–1459.

Denomme, J., Stark, K.D., and Holub, B.J. 2005. Directly quantitated dietary (n-3) fatty acid intakes of pregnant Canadian women are lower than current dietary recommendations. *J. Nutr.* **135**: 206–211.

Department of Justice Canada, 2010. *Food and Drug Regulations*. (http://laws.justice.gc.ca/eng/F-27/index.html) Accessed November 23, 2010.

Djoussé, L., Arnett, D.K., Carr J., Eckfeldt, J.H., Hopkins, P, N., Province, M.A., and Ellison, R.C. 2005a. Dietary linolenic acid is inversely associated with calcified atherosclerotic plaque in the coronary arteries: The National Heart, Lung, and Blood Institute Family Heart Study. *Circulation* **111**: 2921–2926.

Djoussé, L., Folsom, A.R., Province, M.A., Hunt, S.C., and Ellison, R.C. 2003a. Dietary linolenic acid and carotid artherosclerosis: The National Heart, Lung, and Blood Institute Family Heart Study. *Am. J. Clin. Nutr.* **77**: 819–825.

Djoussé, L., Hunt, S.C., Arnett, D.K., Province, M.A., Eckfeldt, J.H., and Ellison, R.C. 2003b. Dietary linolenic acid is inversely associated with plasma triacylglycerol: The National Heart, Lung, and Blood Institute Family Heart Study. *Am. J. Clin. Nutr.* **78**: 1098–1102.

Djoussé, L., Pankow, J.S., Eckfeldt, J.H., Folsom, A.R., Hopkins, P.N., Province, M.A., Hong, Y., and Ellison, R.C. 2001. Relationship between dietary linolenic acid and coronary artery disease in the national Heart, Lung, and Blood Institute Family Heart Study. *Am. J. Clin. Nutr.* **74**: 612–619.

Djoussé, L., Rautaharju, P.M., Hopkins,P.N., Whitsel, E.A., Arnett, D.K., Eckfeldt, J.H., Province, M.A., and Ellison, R.C. 2005b. Dietary linolenic acid and adjusted QT and JT intervals in the National Heart, Lung, and Blood Institute Family Heart Study. *J. Am. Coll. Cardiol.* **45**: 1716–1722.

Dolecek, T.A. 1992. Epidemiological evidence of relationships between dietary polyunsaturated fatty acids and mortality in the multiple risk factor intervention trial. *Pro. Soc. Exp. Biol. Med.* **200**: 177–182.

EFSA, 2008. Scientific Opinion of the panel on dietetic products, nutrition and allergies on a request from unilever PLC/NV on α-linolenic acid and linoleic acid and growth and development of children. *EFSA J.* **783**: 1–9.

EFSA, 2009. Panel on Dietetic Products, Nutrition and Allergies (NDA); Scientific opinion on the substantiation of health claims related to alpha-linolenic acid and maintenance of normal blood cholesterol concentrations (ID 493) and maintenance of normal blood pressure (ID 625). *EFSA J.* **7**(9): 1252.

Emken, E.A. 1995. Influence of linoleic acid on conversion of linolenic acid to omega-3 fatty acids in humans. In: *Proceedings from the Scientific Conference on Omega-3 Fatty Acids in Nutrition, Vascular Biology, and Medicine*, American Heart Association, Dallas, TX, pp. 9–18.

Emken, E.A., Adlof, R.O., and Gulley, R.M. 1994. Dietary linoleic acid influences desaturation and acylation of deuterium-labeled linoleic and linolenic acids in young adult males. *Biochim. Biophys. Acta* **1213**: 277–288.

Emken E.A., Adlof, R.O., Rakoff, H., Rohwedder, W.K., and Gulley, R.M. 1990. Metabolism *in vivo* of deuterium labelled linolenic and linoleic acids in humans. *Biochem. Soc. Trans.* **18**: 766–769.

Ezaki, O., M. Takahashi, M., Shigematsu, T., Shimamura, K., Kimura, J., Ezaki, H. and Gotoh, T. 1999. Long-term effects of dietary alpha-linolenic acid from perilla oil on serum fatty acids composition and on the risk factors of coronary heart disease in Japanese elderly subjects, *J. Nutr. Sci. Vitaminol. (Tokyo)*. **45**: 759–772.

Frost and Sullivan. Opportunities in the Omega 3 Market. 2008.

Garg, M.L., Wierzbicki, A.A., Thomson, A.B.R., and Clandinin, M.T. 1988. Dietary cholesterol and/or n-3 fatty acid modulate delta 9—desaturase activity in rat liver microsomes. *Biochim. Biophys. Acta* **962**: 330–336.

Gebauer, S.K., Psota, T.L., Harris, W.S., and Kris-Etherton, P.M. 2006. n-3 Fatty acid dietary recommenda-
    tions and food sources to achieve essentiality and cardiovascular benefits. *Am. J. Clin. Nutr.* **83**:
    1526S–1535S.
Getz, G.S. 2005. Immune function in atherogenesis. *J. Lipid Res.* **46**: 1–10.
Goh, Y.K., Jumpsen, J.A., Ryan, E.A., and Clandinin, M.T. 1997. Effect of ω3 fatty acid on plasma lipids,
    cholesterol and lipoprotein fatty acid content in NIDDM patients. *Diabetologia* **40**: 45–52.
Goyens, P.L.L., Spilker, M.., Zock, P.L., Katan, M.B., and Mensink, R.P. 2005. Compartmental modeling to
    quantify alpha-linolenic acid conversion after longer term intake of multiple tracer boluses. *J. Lipid Res.*
    46: 1474–1483.
Goyens, P.P.L. and Mensink, R.P. 2006. Effects of alpha-linolenic acid versus those of EPA/DHA on cardiovas-
    cular risk markers in healthy elderly subjects. *Eur. J. Clin. Nutr.* **60**: 978–984.
Goyens, P.L.L., Spilker, M.E., Zock, P.L., Katan, M., and Mensink, R. 2006. Conversion of α-linolenic acid in
    humans is influenced by the absolute amounts of α-linolenic acid and linoleic acid in the diet and not by
    their ratio. *Am. J. Clin. Nutr.* **84**: 44–53.
Guallar, E., Aro A., Jiménez, F.J., Martin-Moreno, J.M., Salminen, I., vant Veer, P., Kardinaal, A.F.M. et al.
    1999. Omega-3 fatty acids in adipose tissue and risk of myocardial infarction. The EURAMIC study.
    Arterioscler. Thromb. Vasc. Biol. **19**: 1111–1118.
Hall III, C. and Shultz, K. 2001. Phenolic antioxidant interactions. In: *Abstracts of the 92nd American Oil
    Chemists Society Annual Meeting and Expo.* p. S88.
Harnack, K., Andersen, G., and Somoza,V. 2009. Quantitation of alpha-linolenic acid elongation to eicosapen-
    taenoic and docosahexaenoic acid as affected by the ratio of n6/n3 fatty acids. *Nutr. Metab.* **6**: 8.
Harper, C.R. and Jacobson, T.A. 2001. The fats of life. *Arch. Intern. Med.* **161**: 2185–2192.
Harper, C.R., Edwards, M.J., DeFilipis, A.P., and Jacobson, A.T. 2006. Flaxseed oil increases the plasma con-
    centrations of cardioprotective (n-3) fatty acids in humans. *J. Nutr.* **136**: 83–87.
Harris W.S., Assaad, B., and Poston, W.C. 2006. Tissue omega-6/omega-3 fatty acid ratio and risk for coronary
    artery disease. *Am. J. Cardiol.* **98**(Suppl.): 19i–26i.
Heart and Stroke Foundation of Canada. 2003. The growing burden of heart disease and stroke in Canada 2003.
    http://www.heartandstroke.ca. Accessed July 17, 2008.
Hillman, G. 1975. The plant remains from Tell Abu Hureyra: A preliminary report. *Proc. Prehist. Soc.* **41**: 70–73.
Hillman, G.C., Colledge, S.M., and Harris, D.R. 1989. Plant-food economy during the Epipalaeolithic period
    at Tell Abu Hureyra, Syria: Dietary diversity, seasonality, and modes of exploitation. In: *Foraging and
    Farming: the Evolution of Plant Exploitation* (D.R. Harris and G.H. Hillman, eds.), Unwin & Hyman,
    London. pp. 240–268.
Hopf, M. 1983. Jericho plant remains. In:*Excavations at Jericho*, Vol. 5.Kenyon, K.M. and Holland, T.A. (eds.),
    British School of Archaeology in Jerusalem, London, pp. 576–621.
Hotamisligil, G.S. 2006. Inflammation and metabolic disorders. *Nature* **444**: 860–867.
Houwelingen, A.C. and Hornstra, G. 1994. Trans fatty acids in early human development. *World Rev. Nutr. Diet*
    75: 175–178.
Hu, F.B., Stampfer, M.J., Manson, J.E., Rimm, E.B., Wolk, A., Colditz, G.A., Hennekens, C.H., and Willett,
    W.A. 1999. Dietary intake of α-linolenic acid and risk of fatal ischemic heart disease among women. *Am.
    J. Clin. Nutr.* **69**: 890–897.
Hussein, N., Ah-Sing, E., Wilkinson, P., Leach, C., Griffin, B.A., and Millward, D.J. 2005. Long-chain conver-
    sion of [13C]linoleic acid and alpha-linolenic acid in response to marked changes in their dietary intake
    in men. *J. Lipid Res.* **46**: 269–280.
Hutchins, A.M. and Slavin, J.L. 2003. Effects of flaxseed on sex hormone metabolism. In: *Flaxseed in Human
    Nutrition*, 2nd ed. L.U. Thompson and S.C. Cunnane (eds.), AOCS Press, Champaign, IL, pp. 126–149.
Hwang, S.J., Ballantyn, C.M., Sharrett, A.R., Smith, J., Davis, C., Gotto Jr., A., and Boerwinkle, E. 1997.
    Circulating adhesion molecules VCAM-1, ICAM-1, and E-selectin in carotid atherosclerosis and inci-
    dent coronary heart disease cases: The Atherosclerosis Risk in Communities (ARIC) study. *Circulation*
    96: 4219–4225.
Innis, S.M. and Elias, S.L. 2003. Intakes of essential n-6 and n-3 polyunsaturated fatty acids among pregnant
    Canadian women. *Am. J. Clin. Nutr.* **77**: 473–478.
Institute of Medicine. 2002. Dietary reference intakes for energy, carbohydrate, fiber, fat, fatty acids, choles-
    terol, protein, and amino acids. *National Academies Press*, Washington, DC, pp. 7-1–7-69 (dietary fiber),
    8-1–8-97 (fat and fatty acids).
Kamal-Eldin, A., Peerlkamp, N., Johnsson, P., Andersson, R., Andersson, R.E., Lundgren, L., and Åman, P.
    2001. An oligomer from flaxseed composed of secoisolariciresinoldiglucoside and 3-Hydroxy-3-Methyl
    glutaric acid residues. *Phytochemistry* **58**: 587–590.

Kaul, N., Kreml, R., Austria, J.A., Richard, M.N., Edel, A.L., Dibrov, E., Hirono, S., Zettler, M.E., and Pierce, G.N. 2008. A comparison of fish oil, flaxseed oil and hempseed oil supplementation on selected parameters of cardiovascular health in healthy volunteers. *J. Am. Coll. Nutr.* **27**(1): 51–58.

Kestin, M., Clifton, P., Belling, G.B., and Nestel, P.J. 1990. n-3 Fatty acids of marine origin lower systolic blood pressure and triglycerides but raise LDL cholesterol compared with n-3 and n-6 fatty acids from plants. *Am. J. Clin. Nutr.* **51**: 1028–1034.

Kornman, K.S. 2006. Interleukin 1 genetics, inflammatory mechanisms, and nutrigenetic opportunities to modulate diseases of aging. *Am. J. Clin. Nutr.* **83**: 475S–483S.

Kris-Etherton, P.M., Harris, W.S., and Appel, L.J. 2002. AHA scientific statement—Fish consumption, fish oil, omega-3 fatty acids, and cardiovascular disease. *Circulation* **106**: 2747–2757.

Lane, J.S., Magno, C.P., Lane, K.T., Chan, T. Hoyt, D.B., and Greenfield, S. 2008. Nutrition impacts the prevalence of peripheral arterial disease in the United States. *J. Vasc. Surg.* **48**: 897–904.

Lange, R., Schumann, W., Petrzika, M., Busch, H., and Marquard, R. 1995. Glucosinolates in linseed dodder. *Fat Sci. Technol.* **97**: 146–152.

Lanzmann-Petithory, D. 2001. Alpha-linolenic acid and cardiovascular diseases. *J. Nutr. Health Aging* **5**: 79–183.

Layne, K.S., Goh, Y.K., Jumpsen, J.A., Ryan, E.A., Chow, P., and Clandinin, M.T. 1996. Normal subjects consuming physiological levels of 18:3(n-3) and 20:5(n-3) from flaxseed or fish oils have characteristic differences in plasma lipid and lipoprotein fatty acid levels. *J. Nutr.* **126**: 2130–2140.

Lee, B.H., Lee, J.I., Park, C.B., Lee, S.W., and Kim, Y.H. 1993. Fatty acid composition and improvement of seed oil in perilla. *Crop Prod. Improvement Technol. in Asia* 471–479.

Leiken, A.I. and Brenner, R.R. 1987. Cholesterol-induced microsomal changes modulate desaturase activities. *Biochim. Biophys. Acta.* **922**: 294–303.

Lemaitre, R., King, I., Mozaffarian, D., Kuller, L., Tracy, R., and Siscovick, D. 2003. N-3 polyunsaturated fatty acids, fatal ischemic heart disease, and nonfatal myocardial infarction in older adults: The cardiovascular study. *Am. J. Clin. Nutr.* **77**: 319–325.

Leng, G.C., Taylor, G.S., Lee, A.L., Fowkes, F.G., and Horrobin, D. 1999. Essential fatty acids and cardiovascular disease: The Edinburgh Artery Study. *Vasc. Med.* **4**: 219–226.

Li, D., Mann. N.J., and Sinclair, A.J. 1999. Comparison of n-3 polyunsaturated fatty acids from vegetable oils, meat and fish in raising platelet eicosapentaenoic acid levels in humans. *Lipids* **34**: S309.

Liou, Y.A., King, D.J., Zibrik, D., and Innis, S.M. 2007. Decreasing linoleic acid with constant α-linolenic acid in dietary fats increases (n-3) eicosapentaenoic acid in plasma phospholipids in healthy men. *J. Nutr.* **137**: 945–952.

Makino, T., Furuta, Y., Wakushima, H., Fujii, H., Saito, K., and Kano, Y. 2003. Anti-allergic effect of *Perilla frutescens* and its active constituents. *Phytotherapy Res.* **17**: 240–243.

Manav, M., Su, J., Hughes, K., Lee, H.P., and Ong, C.N. 2004. ω-3 Fatty acids and selenium as coronary heart disease risk modifying factors in Asian Indian and Chinese males. *Nutr.* **20**: 967–973.

Mantzioris, E., James, M.J., Gibson, R.A., and Cleland, L.G. 1994. Dietary substitution with an α-linolenic acid rich vegetable oil increases eicosapentaenoic acid concentrations in tissues. *Am. J. Clin. Nutr.* **59**, 1304–1309.

Marquard, R. and Kuhlmann, H. 1986. Investigations of productive capacity and seed quality of linseed dodder (*Camelina sativa* Crtz.). *Fette Seifen Anstrichmittel.* **88**: 245–249.

Matsuyama, W., Mitsuyama, H., Watanabe, M., Oonakahara, K., Higashimoto, I., Osame, M., and Arimura, K. 2005. Effects of omega-3 polyunsaturated fatty acids on inflammatory markers in COPD. *Chest* **128**: 3817–3827.

McCloy, U., Ryan, M.A., Pencharz, P.B., Ross, R., and Cunnane, S. 2004. A comparison of the metabolism of eighteen-carbon ^{13}C-unsaturated fatty acids in healthy women. *J. Lipid Res.* 2004, **45**, 474–485.

Miljanović, B., Trivedi, K.A., Dana, M.R., Gilbard, J., Buring, J., and Schaumberg, D. 2005. Relation between dietary n-3 and n-6 fatty acids and clinically diagnosed dry eye syndrome in women. *Am. J. Clin. Nutr.* **82**: 887–893.

Mintel International. United States Omega 3 Market. 2008.

Mohrhauer, H. and Holman, R.T. 1963. The effect of dose level of essential fatty acids upon fatty acid composition of the rat liver. *J. Lipid Res.* **6**:494–497.

Morris, D. 2007. Flax Nutrition Primer. Flax Council of Canada. www.flaxcouncil.ca.

Mozaffarian, D., Ascherio, A., Hu, F.B., Stampfer, M.J., Willett, W.C., Siscovick, D.S., and Rimm, E.B. 2005. Interplay between different polyunsaturated fatty acids and risk of coronary heart disease in men. *Circulation* **111**: 157–164.

Nestel, P.J., Pomeroy, S.E., Sasahara, T., Yamashita, T., Liang, Y., Dart, A., Jennings, G., Abbey, M., and Cameron, J. 1997. Arterial compliance in obese subjects is improved with dietary plant n-3 fatty acid from flaxseed oil despite increased LDL oxidizability. *Arterioscler. Thromb. Vasc. Biol.* **117**: 1163–1170.

Oomah, B.D. and Mazza, G. 1997. Effect of dehulling on chemical composition and physical properties of flaxseed. *Lebensm. Wiss. U. Technol.* **30**: 135–140.

Oomah, B.D., Kenaschuk, E., Cui, W., and Mazza, G. 1995. Variation in the composition of water-soluble polysaccharides in flaxseed. *J. Agric. Food Chem.* **43**: 1484–1488

Packaged Facts. Omega 3 foods and the U.S. Food and Beverage market. 2009.

Paschos, G.K., Magkos, F., Panagiotakos, D.B., Votteas, V., and Zampelas, A. 2007. Dietary supplementation with flaxseed oil lowers blood pressure in dyslipidaemic patients. *Eur. J. Clin. Nutr.* **31**: 1–6.

Paschos, G.K., Yiannakouris, N., Rallidis, L.S., Davies, I., Griffin, B.A., and Panagiotakos, D. 2005. Apolipoprotein E genotype in dyslipidemic patients and response of blood lipids and inflammatory markers to alpha-linolenic acid. *Angiology* **56**: 56–59.

Patenaude, A., Rodriguez-Leyva, D., Edel, A.L., Dibrov, E., Dupasquier, C.M., Austria, J.A., Richard, M.N., Chahine, M.N., Malcolmson, L.J., and Pierce, G.N. 2009. Bioavailability of alpha-linolenic acid from flaxseed diets as a function of the age of the subject. *Eur. J. Clin. Nutr.* **63**: 1123–1129.

Pawlosky, R.J., Hibbeln, J.R., Novotny, J.A., and Salem Jr., N. 2001. Physiological compartmental analysis of α-linolenic acid metabolism in adult humans. *J. Lipid Res.* **42**: 1257–1265.

Perez-Martinez, P., Lopez-Miranda, J., Blanco-Colio, L., Bellido, C., Jimenez, Y., Moreno, J.A., Delgado-Lista, J., Egido, J., and Perez-Jimenez, F. 2007. The chronic intake of a Mediterranean diet enriched in virgin olive oil, decreases nuclear transcription factor kappaB activation in peripheral blood mononuclear cells from healthy men. *Atherosclerosis* **194**: e141–e146.

Pietinen, P., Ascherio, A., Korhonen, P., Hartman, A., Willett, W., Albanes, D., and Virtamo, J. 1997. Intake of fatty acids and risk of coronary heart disease in a cohort of Finnish men: The Alpha-Tocopherol, Beta-Carotene Cancer Prevention Study. *Am. J. Epidemiol.* **145**: 876–887.

Plessers, A.G., McGregor, W.G., Carson, R.B., and Nadoneshny, W. 1962. Species trials with oilseed crops, *Camelina. Can. J. Plant Sci.* **42**: 452–459.

Poudel-Tandukar, K., Nanri, A., Matsushita, Y., Sasaki, S., Ohta, M., Sato, M., and Mizoue, T. 2009. Dietary intakes of α-linolenic and linoleic acids are inversely associated with serum C-reactive protein levels among Japanese men. *Nutr. Res.* **29**: 363–337.

Rallidis, L.S., Paschos, G., Papaioannou, M.L., Liakos, G., Panagiotakos, D., Anastasiadis, G., and Zampelas, A. 2004. The effect of diet enriched with α-linolenic acid on soluble cellular adhesion molecules in dyslipidaemic patients. *Atherosclerosis* **174**: 127–132.

Rastogi, T., Reddy, K.S.,Vaz, M., Spiegelman,D., Prabhakaran, D.,Willett, W., Stampfer, M., and Ascherio, A. 2004. Diet and risk of ischemic heart disease in India. *Am. J. Clin. Nutr.* **79**: 582–592.

Reiss, A.B. and Edelman, S.D. 2006. Recent insights into the role of prostanoids in atherosclerotic vascular disease. *Curr. Vasc. Pharmacol.* **4**: 395–408.

Ren, J. and Chung, S.H. 2007. Anti-inflammatory effect of α-linolenic acid and its mode of action through the inhibition of nitric oxide production and inducible nitric oxide synthase gene expression via NF-κβ and nitrogen-activated protein kinase pathways. *J. Agric. Food Chem.* **55**: 5073–5080.

Rollefson, G.O., Simmons, A.H., Donaldson, M.L., Gillespie, W., Kafafi, Z., Kohler-Rollefson, I.U., McAdam, E., Ralston, S., and Tubb, M. 1985. Excavation at the pre-pottery neolithic B village of 'Ain Ghazal (Jordan). *Mitteilungen der Deuschen Orient-Gesellschaft zu Berlin.* **117**: 69–116.

Rosamond, W., Flegal, K., Friday, G., Furie, K., Go, A., Greenlund, K., Haase, N. et al. 2007. Heart Disease and Stroke Sttistics-2007 Update. A report from the American Heart Association Statistics Committee and Stroke Statistics Subcommittee. *Circulation.* **115**: e69–e171.

Rosell, M.S., Lloyd-Wright, Z., Appleby, P.N., Sanders, T.A., Allen, N.E., and Key, T.J. 2005. Long-chain n-3 polyunsaturated fatty acids in plasma in British meat-eating, vegetarian, and vegan men. *Am. J. Clin. Nutr.* **82**: 327–334.

Ross, R. 1999. Atherosclerosis—An inflammatory disease. *N. Engl. J. Med.* **340**: 115–126.

Salem Jr., N., Pawlosky, R., Wegher, B., and Hibbeln, J. 1999. *In vivo* conversion of linoleic acid to arachidonic acid in human adults. *Prostaglandins Leukot. Essent. Fatty Acids* **6**: 407–410.

Sanders, T.A.B. 2000. Polyunsaturated fatty acids in the food chain in Europe. *Am. J. Clin. Nutr.* **71**: 176S–178S.

Sanders, T.A.B. and Roshanai, F. 1983. The influence of different types of ω3 polyunsaturated fatty acids on blood lipids and platelet function in healthy volunteers. *Clin. Sci.* **64**: 91–99.

Sanders, T.A., Ellis, F.R., and Dickerson, J.W. 1978. Studies of vegans: The fatty acid composition of plasma choline phosphoglycerides, erythrocytes, adipose tissue, and breast milk, and some indicators of susceptibility to ischemic heart disease in vegans and omnivore controls. *Am. J. Clin. Nutr.* **31**: 805–813.

Schultze-Motel, J. 1979. Die Anbaugeschichte des Leindotters, *Camelina sativa* (L.) Crantz. *Archaeo-Physika* **8**: 267–281.

Schwab, U.S., Callaway, J.C., Erkkilä, A.T., Gynther, J., Uusitupa, M., and Jarvinen, T. 2006. Effects of hemp-seed and flaxseed oils on the profile of serum lipids, serum total and lipoprotein lipid concentrations and haemostatic factors. *Eur. J. Nutr.* **45**: 470–477.

Seehuber, R. 1984. Genotypic variation for yield- and quality-traits in poppy and false flax. *Fette-Seifen-Anstrichmittel.* **86**: 177–180.

Seppanen-Laakso, T., Laakso, I., Lehtimaki, T., Rontu, R., Moilanen, E., Solakivi, T., Seppo, L., Vanhanen, H., Kiviranta, K., and Hiltunen, R.2010. Elevated plasma fibrinogen caused by inadequate a-linolenic acid intake can be reduced by replacing fat with canola-type rapeseed oil. *Prostaglandins Leukot. Essent. Fatty Acids* **83**: 45–54.

Simon, J.A., Fong, J., Bernert, J.T., and Browner, W.S. 1995. Serum fatty acids and the risk of stroke. *Stroke* **26**: 778–782.

Simopoulos, A.P. 2006. Evolutionary aspects of diet, the omega-6/omega-3 ratio and genetic variation: Nutritional implications for chronic diseases. *Biomed. Pharmacother.* **60**: 502–507.

Singer, P., Berge, I., Wirth, M., Goedicke, W., Jaeger, W., and Voigt, S. 1986. Slow desaturation and elongation of linoleic and α-linolenic acids as a rationale of eicosapentaenoic acid-rich diet to lower blood pressure and serum lipids in normal, hypertensive and hyperlipemic subjects. *Prostaglandins Leuko. Med.* **24**: 173–193.

Singer, P., Wirth, M., and Berger, I. 1990. A possible contribution of decrease in free fatty acids to low serum triglyceride levels after diets supplemented with n-6 and n-3 polyunsaturated fatty acids. *Atherosclerosis* **83**: 167–175.

Stark, A.H., Crawford, M., and Reifen, R. 2008. Update on alpha-linolenic acid. *Nutr. Rev.* **66**: 326–332.

U.S. Food and Drug Administration. 2010a. Food and Nutrition. (http://www.fda.gov/Food/GuidanceComplianceRegulatoryInformation/GuidanceDocuments/FoodLabelingNutrition/FoodLabelingGuide/ucm064908.htm) Accessed November 28, 2010.

U.S. Food and Drug Administration. 2010b. Food Labeling and Nutrition. http://www.fda.gov/Food/GuidanceComplianceRegulatoryInformation/GuidanceDocuments/ FoodLabelingNutrition/ucm073332.htm) Accessed November 28, 2010.

Vaisey-Genser, M. and Morris, D. 2003. Introduction: History of the cultivation and uses of flaxseed. In: *Flax: The Genus Linum*, A. Muir and N. Westcott (eds.), Taylor & Francis, Ltd. London, England, pp. 1–21.

Van Zeiste, W. 1972. Palaeobotanical results in the 1970 seasons at Cayonu, Turkey. *Helinium.* **12**: 3–19 (Cited by Zohary and Hopf, 1993).

Vermunt, S.H., Mensink, R.P., Simonis, M.M., and Hornstra, G. 2000. Effects of dietary alpha linolenic acid on the conversion and oxidation of 13C-alpha-linolenic acid. *Lipids* **35**: 137–142.

Vos, E. and Cunnane, S.C. 2003. α-Linolenic acid, linoleic acid, coronary artery disease, and overall mortality (letter). *Am. J. Clin. Nutr.* **77**: 521–522.

Wakjira, A., Labuschagne, M.T., and Hugo, A. 2004. Variability in oil content and fatty acid composition of Ethiopian and introduced cultivars of linseed. *J. Sci. Food Agric.* **84**: 601–607.

Warrand, J., Michaud, P., Picton, L., Muller, G., Courtois, B., Ralainirina, R., and Courtois, J. 2005. Structural investigations of the neutral polysaccharide of *Linum usitatissimum* L. Seeds mucilage. *Int. J. Biol. Macromol.* **35**: 121–125.

Welch, A.A., Shakya-Shrestha, S., Lentjes, M.A.H., Wareham, M.J., and Khaw, K-T. 2010. Dietary intake and status of n-3 polyunsaturated fatty acids in a population of fish-eating and non-fish-eating meat-eaters, vegetarians, and vegans and the precursor–product ratio of alpha-linolenic acid to long-chain n23 poly-unsaturated fatty acids: results from the EPIC-Norfolk. *Am. J. Clin. Nutr.* **92**: 1040–1051.

West, S.G., Hecke, K.D., Mustad, V.A., Nicholson, S., Schoemer, S., Wagner, P., Hinderliter, A., Ulbrech, J., Ruey, P., and Kris-Etherton, P. 2005. Acute effects of monounsaturated fatty acids with and without omega-3 fatty acids on vascular reactivity in individuals with type 2 diabetes. *Diabetologia* **48**: 113–122.

Wilkinson, P., Leach, C., Ah-Sing, E.E., Eric, E., Hussain,N., Miller, G., Millward, D., and Griffin, B. 2005. Influence of α-linolenic acid and fish-oil on markers of cardiovascular risk in subjects with an athero-genic lipoprotein phenotype. *Atherosclerosis* **181**: 115–124.

Williams, C.M and Burdge, G. 2006. Long-chain n-3 PUFA: plant v. marine sources. *Proceedings of the Nutrition Society* **65**: 42–50.

Yuba, A., Honda, G., Koezuka, Y., and Tabata, M.1995. Genetic analysis of essential oil variants in *Perilla frutescens. Biochem. Genet.* **33**: 341–348.

Zatonski, W., Campos, H., and Willett, W.C. 2008. Rapid declines in coronary heart disease mortality in Eastern Europe are associated with increased consumption of oils rich in alphalinolenic acid. *Eur J. Epidemiol.* **23**(1): 3–10.

Zhao, G., Etherton, T.D., Martin, K.R., Gillies, P., West, S., and Kris-Etherton, P. 2007. Dietary alpha-linolenic acid inhibits proinflammatory cytokine production by peripheral blood mononuclear cells in hypercholesterolemic subjects. *Am. J. Clin. Nutr.* **85**: 385–391.

Zhao, G., Etherton, T.D., Martin, K.R., Vanden Heuvel, J., Gillies, P., West, S., and Kris-Etherton, P. 2004. Dietary α-linolenic acid reduces inflammatory and lipid cardiovascular risk factors in hypercholesterolemic men and women. *J. Nutr.* **134**: 2991–2997.

Zohary, D. and Hopf, M. 2000. Oil and fibre crops. In: *Domestication of Plants in the Old World*, 3rd ed. D. Zohary and M. Hopf (eds.), Oxford University Press, Oxford, pp. 125–132.

Zubr, J. 1997. Oil-seed crop: *Camelina sativa. Industrial Crops Products* **6**: 113–119.

5 Folic Acid and Pathogenesis of Cardiovascular Disease

James D. House, Mingyan Jing, Sun-Young Hwang, and Karmin O
University of Manitoba

CONTENTS

5.1 INTRODUCTION

Folate is the generic term for the water-soluble B-complex vitamin that includes various chemical structures with similar biological activity. Folic acid, the common synthetic form of the vitamin, consists of three subunits: (1) a pteridine linked to, (2) para-aminobenzoic acid (PABA) which forms pteroic acid, and (3) glutamic acid (Combs, 2008). When one or more glutamic acid residues bond together, pteroylpolyglutamates are formed, and these represent the main cellular forms of folates in plants and animals (Combs, 2008). The oxidation state of the pteridine structure varies from the fully oxidized form (folic acid) to various levels of reduction (e.g., dihydrofolate, tetrahydrofolate, 5,10-methylene tetrahydrofolate; 5-methyltetrahydro-folate). While animal cells contain the necessary-enzymatic capacity to interconvert most folate species, they cannot synthesize the pteroic acid moiety, and are, therefore, dependent on an exogenous source of the pteroylglutamate (irrespective of oxidation state) in order to replace obligatory losses. Folate inadequacy limits one-carbon transfer reactions, thus limiting the ability of folate to serve as a substrate for the transfer of single carbon atoms in the metabolism of pyrimidines and purines (Fox and Stover, 2008), formate (Sokoro et al., 2008), and amino acids, including glycine, serine, and the sulfur amino acids methionine and homocysteine (Hcy) (House et al., 1999). The current review will focus on the recent advances in our understanding of folate nutrition, with specific emphasis on the potential for folate to mitigate risk related to vascular disease.

5.2 FOLATE NUTRITION AND METABOLISM

The intestine is exposed to two sources of folate: a dietary source and a bacterial source, where the vitamin is synthesized by the normal microflora in the distal part of the small intestine and the colon. The folate content of selected foods is illustrated in Table 5.1. Folate in the diet consists of either natural folates or synthetic oxidized folic acid, principally added as a fortificant. Natural dietary folates are generally present in a polyglutamated form. A notable exception to this rule is the egg in which all of the folate is found in the monoglutamate form (Seyoum and Selhub, 1998). When in the poly-glutamated form, the polyglutamate tail must be hydrolyzed prior to absorption (Mason et al., 1990; Combs, 2008). In humans, hydrolysis of the glutamate residues is thought to occur primarily through the action of the enzyme glutamate carboxypeptidase II (GCPII), an enzyme expressed on the brush border membrane of enterocytes within the proximal colon (Lievers et al., 2002). A second enzyme, gamma-glutamyl hydrolase is active within cells, and functions to mobilize intracellular folates.

It is now well-established that the duodenum and upper jejunum are the preferred sites of absorption of dietary folate and that the process involves specialized, carrier-mediated systems (Said and Strum, 1983; Said et al., 1987; Said, 2004). Another folate source is derived from microbial synthesis. The normal microflora can synthesize considerable amounts of folate, and a significant portion of this folate exists in the lumen in the absorbable monoglutamate form (Crittenden et al., 2003; Kim et al., 2004). Studies in rats (Rong et al., 1991) provided some of the first direct evidence *in vivo* that bacteri-ally synthesized folates could be absorbed across the intact large intestine and incorporated in tissues.

TABLE 5.1
Folate Content of Selected Foods

Food	Representative Serving Size	Natural Folate (μg/100 g)	Folic Acid[a] (μg/100 g)	Total Folate[b] (μg/100 g)	Total Dietary Folate Equivalents (DFE)[c] (μg/100 g)	Total DFE per Representative Serving (μg)
		Un-Enriched Foods				
Navy beans (cooked)	1 cup = 182 g	140	0	140	140	255
Orange juice, condensed	1 cup = 249 g	44	0	44	44	110
Broccoli, raw	1 stalk = 148 g	63	0	63	63	93
Spinach, raw	1 cup = 30 g	194	0	194	194	58
Egg, whole, hard-boiled	1 large egg = 50 g	44	0	44	44	22
Milk, 2% fat	1 cup = 244 g	5	0	5	5	12
Beef, top sirloin, broiled	4 oz = 113 g	9	0	9	9	10
Cheese, cheddar	1 slice = 28 g	18	0	18	18	5
Chicken breast, broiled	1 half breast = 86 g	4	0	4	4	3
		Enriched Foods				
Formulated energy bar	1 bar = 68 g	0	615	615	1046	711
Raisin bran (RTE cereal)[d]	1 cup = 59 g	19	236	255	421	248
Spaghetti, cooked	1 cup = 140 g	7	66	73	119	167
White bread	2 slice = 50 g	25	86	111	171	86
Water plus vitamins	1 serving = 237 g	0	8	8	14	33

Source: Adapted from USDA Agricultural Research Services. *USDA Nutrient Database, Standard Reference, Release 22,* 2010. Accessed: http://www.nal.usda.gov/fnic/foodcomp/search/.

[a] Represents added synthetic folic acid (monoglutamate, oxidized form).

[b] Represents summation of natural food folate and added folic acid.

[c] Calculated according to the DRI formula ascribing a bioavailability equivalency of 0.6 μg folic acid = 1 μg DFE.

[d] RTE = ready-to-eat cereals; fortification rates of RTE cereals differ by jurisdiction.

Similarly, recent studies (Asrar and O'Connor, 2005) showed that supplemental folic acid and bacterially synthesized folate could be absorbed across the large intestine of piglets and incorporated into their tissues. They predicted that approximate 18% of the dietary folate requirement for the piglet could be met by folate absorption across the large intestine. More recently, the same group showed that $^{13-}$C 5-formyltetrahydrofolate was absorbed from the large intestine during cecal infusion studies performed during colonoscopies in human (Aufreiter et al., 2009). Several studies have shown that the colon is indeed capable of absorbing some luminal folate via an efficient, specialized, carrier-mediated system (Kumar et al., 1997; Sirotnak and Tolner, 1999; Dudeja et al., 2001), which is very similar (or identical) to that found in the small intestine (Said et al., 1987; Schron et al., 1985). Taken together, the data provide evidence that folate produced from commensal microorganisms may make a significant contribution to endogenous folate pools, and that this source of folate may be influenced by factors affecting microbial populations (i.e., dietary fiber sources, prebiotics, probiotics, etc.).

With respect to intestinal folate uptake, two carrier-mediated transport processes have been proposed for intestinal uptake: (1) the reduced folate carrier (RFC), and (2) the proton-coupled folate transporter (PCFT). The RFC is an efficient, pH-dependent, transport protein that is ubiquitously expressed (Schron et al., 1985; Dudeja et al., 2001). Within the intestine, RFC is expressed in the apical brush border membrane of the small intestine and colon (Dudeja et al., 2001; Wang et al., 2005; Hayashi et al., 2007). Expression of both the mRNA and protein are modified by dietary factors, including upregulation during folate deficiency (Said et al., 2000), and downregulation during folate oversupplementation (Ashokkumar et al., 2007). Studies with a rat intestinal epithelial cell culture system documented that, through specific silencing of the RFC via lentivirus-mediated short hairpin RNA, transport of labeled folic acid was effectively abolished (Balamurugan and Said, 2006). These data were used by the authors to support the position of the RFC as the major, if not only, transport carrier for intestinal folate uptake. However, recent lines of evidence have been established to contest this. When RFC expression was inhibited by chemical mutagenesis, folate transport at low pH (5.5), as would be expected in the intestinal lumen, was not affected (Wang et al., 2005). These data supported the presence of an RFC-independent folate transport process as low pH operational in the intestinal tract. Subsequent research identified another protein, previously recognized as heme carrier protein 1 (HCP1), with folate transport activity at low pH (Qiu et al., 2006). The PCFT was shown to have a high affinity for folic acid at low pH. Furthermore, examination of patients with familial folate malabsorption syndrome, characterized by extremely low serum folate concentrations, had a mutation in the gene encoding this protein (SLC46A1) (Qiu et al., 2006), yet the RFC gene did not possess any mutations. The latter results argue against a major role of the RFC for intestinal folate transport. Similar to the case with the RFC, expression of PCFT mRNA is upregulated by folate restriction (Ashokkumar et al., 2007). Therefore, in mammalian systems, in particular, two folate transporters, the RFC and PCFT, have been identified as major folate transporters; however, the relative contribution of each to folate uptake remains contested.

Following intestinal absorption, folates are delivered via the hepatic portal system to the liver where they undergo intracellular polyglutamylation for storage and metabolic functions (Combs, 2008). Following release of the folate monoglutamate (almost exclusively, 5-methyltetrahydro-folate (5-MTHF) from the liver, folates are then transported to, and taken up by, specific transporters in peripheral tissues (Shane and Stokstad, 1983). Folates delivered to the kidney are largely filtered at the glomerulus then reabsorbed by the renal tubular epithelial cells (Damaraju et al., 2008). Folates are especially critical to the one-carbon needs of rapidly proliferating cells of the bone marrow and intestinal mucosa (Damaraju et al., 2008; Fox and Stover, 2008). The latter plays a significant role in influencing dietary folate requirements.

5.3 FOLATE REQUIREMENTS

A joint review of nutrient requirement estimates led to the publication of harmonized estimate values for American and Canadian populations, as published in the Dietary Reference Intake (DRI) reports (Institute of Medicine, 1998). With respect to folate, the DRI process introduced a new term, the dietary folate equivalent (DFE), an expression of food folate values that corrects for the bioavailability of folate from natural sources. The DFE, in essence, assigns a bioavailability value of 50% to all food folates relative to crystalline folic acid, irrespective of the nature of the food. This approach is likely oversimplified, given that foods will differ in their bioavailability values for folate. As an example, we have shown that, using a rat bioassay, the folate contained in folate-enriched eggs had a relative bioavailability greater than 100%, in comparison with crystalline folic acid (House et al., 2003).

The estimated Recommended Daily Allowance (RDA) requirements for dietary folate equivalents vary by life stage, with those over the age of 14 requiring 400 µg DFE per day (Institute of Medicine, 1998). The DRI process made no allowances for differences due to gender, as was done with other nutrients (i.e., thiamin, niacin, riboflavin, pyridoxine), with the exception of those women who are pregnant or lactating. In the latter cases, requirements are increased to 600 µg DFE per day, to account for the increased metabolic demands arising from fetal development and milk production. During the process of establishing the RDA for folate, additional factors were considered beyond the classic criteria used for establishing adequacy, namely the alleviation of deficiency symptoms. For folate, attention was turned to a growing evidence base that linked folate to the reduction of developmental disorders and chronic degenerative diseases. Of the disorders related to development, the potential for folate to reduce the risk of both occurrence and recurrence of neural tube defects (NTDs) is now well-established (House et al., 2006). NTDs, including spina bifida, have been linked to maternal folate supply for over 40 years (Hibbard and Smithells, 1965). While the DRI process stopped short of increasing the RDA to account for the NTDs risk reduction, a special recommendation was put forth for all women capable of becoming pregnant, which read:

> To reduce the risk of neural tube defects for women capable of becoming pregnant, the recommendation is to take 400 µg of folic acid daily from fortified foods, supplements, or both in addition to consuming food folate from a varied diet (Institute of Medicine, 1998).

With respect to disease states, the one chronic disease for which a potential link exists with folate supply is cardiovascular disease. This is the topic of the next section.

5.4   FOLATE AND CARDIOVASCULAR DISEASE

5.4.1   FOLATE, HOMOCYSTEINE, AND RISK OF CARDIOVASCULAR DISEASE

Cardiovascular disease due to atherosclerosis is the leading cause of death worldwide. Atherosclerosis is an inflammatory process characterized by thickening, hardening, and plaque formation in the arteries. Plaque rupture and the consequent thrombosis may lead to sudden blockage of the arteries, causing stroke and heart attack. More than 250 factors associated with the development of coronary artery disease have been identified. The traditional risk factors include hypercholesterolemia, hypertension, smoking, gender, diabetes mellitus, and family history. Hyperhomocysteinemia, or elevated plasma concentrations of the sulfur amino acid Hcy, has emerged as an independent risk factor for cardiovascular and cerebral vascular disease (Clarke et al., 1991; Duell and Malinow, 1997a; Refsum et al., 1998; Welch and Loscalzo, 1998).

Hcy is a sulfhydryl-containing amino acid formed during the metabolism of methionine to cysteine. Homocysteine metabolism serves as an important methyl donor in cell function (Refsum et al., 1998). The cellular homeostasis of Hcy is tightly regulated under normal conditions. Hcy can be metabolized by two major pathways, namely the *transsulfuration pathway* to form cysteine which requires vitamin B_6 as a cofactor and the *remethylation pathway* to form methionine (Figure 5.1). As depicted in Figure 5.1, folate serves as an important co-substrate for Hcy metabolism in cells, specifically through the remethylation pathway. Hcy can be remethylated to methionine

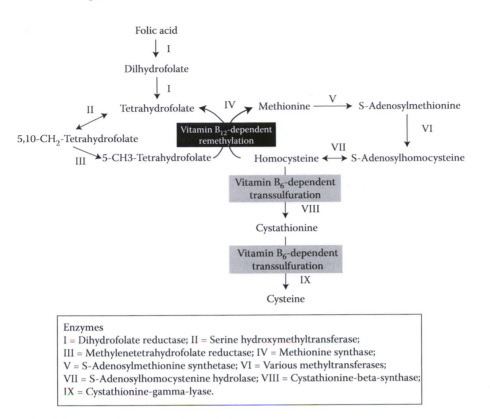

FIGURE 5.1 Folate and sulfur amino acid metabolism.

using either 5-MTHF as a substrate catalyzed by methionine synthase or using betaine as a substrate catalyzed by betaine Hcy methyltransferase. Previous studies have documented a strong inverse relationship between dietary folate supply and plasma Hcy levels, particularly at folate intakes below the RDA (400 μg DFE/day) (Kang et al., 1992; Refsum et al., 1998). The form of folate that directly serves as a co-substrate for the remethylation of Hcy is 5-MTHF formed via the action of the enzyme 5,10-methylenetetrahydrofolate reductase (Figure 5.1). Factors that perturb steps in Hcy metabolic pathways can cause an increase in its cellular levels and lead to hyperhomocysteinemia (plasma Hcy level above 16 μmol/L) (Kang et al., 1992; Refsum et al., 1998). Moderate increases in plasma Hcy levels often occur in patients with deficiencies of folate, vitamin B_6 or vitamin B_{12}, heterozygous enzyme deficiency, impaired renal function, as well as in elderly people (Di Minno et al., 2010). Severe hyperhomocysteinemia seen in children is usually the result of a rare homozygous deficiency of enzymes necessary for Hcy catabolism (Zavadakova et al., 2002).

Many studies have shown that Hcy, at pathological concentrations, elicits inflammatory responses and impairs endothelial function (Wang et al., 2002; Weiss et al., 2002; Au-Yeung et al., 2004; Edirimanne et al., 2007). Although the precise molecular mechanisms responsible for the pathogenesis of hyperhomocysteinemia remain uncertain, several potential mechanisms have been proposed. These include endothelial dysfunction (Edirimanne et al., 2007), increased proliferation of smooth muscle cells (Wang et al., 2000, 2002), enhanced coagulability (Duell and Malinow, 1997), and increased cholesterol biosynthesis in hepatocytes (Woo et al., 2005). Endothelial injury and dysfunction are considered to be one of the leading mechanisms contributing to atherogenesis. Upon injury, endothelial cells are capable of producing various cytokines and growth factors that in turn participate in the development of atherosclerotic lesions.

5.5 FOLIC ACID SUPPLEMENTATION

Folic acid supplementation is regarded as a promising approach in reducing blood Hcy levels. The current treatment for patients with hyperhomocysteinemia is supplementation of folic acid alone or in combination with vitamin B_6 or vitamin B_{12} (Bazzano et al., 2006; Antoniades et al., 2009). It has been postulated that the beneficial effect of folic acid on cardiovascular disease is mediated by its Hcy-lowering effect. However, more evidence has suggested that some benefits of folic acid supplementation are independent of the Hcy-lowering effect.

5.5.1 Homocysteine-Lowering Effect

Folic acid supplementation alone can reduce plasma Hcy levels, which is thought to be one of the key mechanisms underlying the beneficial effects of folic acid. The Hcy-lowering effect of folic acid is attributed to its ability to enhance the remethylation of Hcy in cells and hence reduce the intracellular level of Hcy. This, in turn, lowers the efflux of Hcy into the blood compartment (Marinou et al., 2005). Oral folic acid supplementation (0.4–5 mg daily) for 6 weeks has been shown to improve the endothelium-dependent vascular function of the brachial artery in individuals with mild hyperhomocysteinemia (Bellamy et al., 1999). In another study, administration of folic acid (5 mg daily) and vitamin B_{12} for 8 weeks to patients with coronary heart disease and hyperhomocysteinemia is shown to improve vascular endothelial function as assessed by brachial artery flow-mediated dilatation (Chambers et al., 2000). In animal studies, supplementation of folic acid has been shown to prevent dietary-induced hyperhomocysteinemia in rats (Wang et al., 2002; Woo et al., 2006). Consequently, the Hcy-stimulated chemokine expression in the aortic endothelium can be abolished (Wang et al., 2002).

5.5.2 Homocysteine-Independent Effect

Although lowering plasma Hcy levels may contribute to the improved vascular function, folic acid has been shown to possess some independent effects (Stroes et al., 1998; Doshi et al., 2001). One of the mechanisms underlying the acute beneficial effect of folic acid on endothelial function may be mediated by a reduction of intracellular superoxide levels (Doshi et al., 2001). Many risk factors causing atherosclerosis share a common feature of generating intracellular oxidative stress (Upchurch et al., 1997; Kanani et al., 1999; Dayal et al., 2002). Superoxide anion is one of the potent reactive oxygen species (ROS) and its overproduction can lead to cell injury. Nicotinamide adenine dinucleotide phosphate (NADPH)-dependent oxidase is the major source of superoxide anions generated in macrophages (Van Heerebeek et al., 2002; Bey et al., 2004). NADPH oxidase is composed of membrane-bound components (p22[phox] and gp91[phox] subunits) and cytosolic components (p40[phox], p47[phox], p67[phox], and Rac 1/2). It is generally believed that phosphorylation and subsequent translocation of p47[phox] subunit to the membrane are essential steps for NADPH oxidase activation (Babior, 1999; Groemping et al., 2003; Robinson et al., 2004). It has been shown that NADPH oxidase activity is significantly elevated in atherosclerotic lesions leading to increased superoxide anion production (Kalinina et al., 2002; Sorescu et al., 2002). Increased superoxide anion generation via NADPH oxidase not only impairs endothelial function but also stimulates the expression of inflammatory factors in vascular cells (Au-Yeung et al., 2004; Edirimanne et al., 2007). For example, increased superoxide generation is shown to be responsible for Hcy-induced nuclear factor-κB (NF-κB) activation and subsequently monocyte chemoattractant protein-1 (MCP-1) expression in vascular smooth muscle cells and monocyte-derived macrophages (Au-Yeung et al., 2004, 2006). In our recent study, concomitant supplementation of folic acid to rats fed a high-methionine diet significantly reduced plasma Hcy levels as well as inhibited the expression of MCP-1 and adhesion molecules in the aortic endothelium (Wang et al., 2002). Further investigation has revealed that folic acid can directly antagonize Hcy-induced

NADPH oxidase activation by inhibiting the phosphorylation of NADPH oxidase subunits, P47^{phox} and p67^{phox} (Au-Yeung et al., 2004).

In addition to putative antioxidant effects, the vascular protective effect of folic acid may derive from its effect in restoration of endothelial nitric oxide synthase (eNOS)-mediated nitric oxide (NO) production (Verhaar et al., 1998; Wilmink et al., 2000). It is generally believed that eNOS-mediated NO production plays an important role in regulating vessel tone (Verhaar et al., 1998; Wilmink et al., 2000). Under physiological conditions, eNOS catalyzes the formation of NO by incorporating molecular oxygen into the substrate L-arginine, a reaction that requires NADPH, the allosteric activator calmodulin, and several cofactors such as tetrahydrobiopterin (BH$_4$) (Beckman and Koppenol, 1996). However, under pathophysiological conditions, eNOS can switch from mainly NO synthesis to superoxide production, a process called NOS uncoupling (Stroes et al., 1998). Reduced NO synthesis and increased ROS generation due to uncoupling of NOS contributes to cardiovascular diseases such as hypertension, atherosclerosis, and cardiac hypertrophy (Ohara et al., 1993, 1995; Seiler et al., 1993; Egashira et al., 1995; Harrison and Ohara, 1995; Williams et al., 1996). Under oxidative stress, BH$_4$ is oxidized to its inactive form BH$_2$, leading to eNOS uncoupling with decreased NO synthesis and increased superoxide production (Pritchard et al., 1995; Stroes et al., 1998). Folic acid or 5-MTHF can restore BH$_4$ bioavailability by enhancing the binding affinity of BH$_4$ to eNOS and the regeneration of BH$_4$ from BH$_2$ or by direct interaction with eNOS (Verhaar et al., 1998; Wilmink et al., 2000). A recent study (Moens et al., 2008) demonstrated the protective effect of high-dose folic acid pretreatment against myocardial dysfunction during ischemia and postreperfusion injury in Wistar rats. It is hypothesized that such a beneficial effect is due to (1) preservation of high-energy phosphate (ATP) levels in the heart by increasing purine synthesis; (2) reduced superoxide production; and (3) increased NO synthesis (Moens et al., 2008).

5.5.3 Effect of Folic Acid on Other Organs

Besides endothelial function, the effect of folic acid has also been examined in other organs such as in the liver that is the largest internal organ in our body and the kidney that removes and metabolizes about 70% of Hcy in plasma (Refsum, 1998). It has been reported that depletion of folic acid in the diet-increased plasma Hcy levels and eventually promoted oxidative stress in rat liver (Huang et al., 2001; Woo et al., 2008). Another study has demonstrated that supplementation of folic acid for 4 weeks improves liver morphology in aged rats (Roncales et al., 2004). In our recent study, hepatic protective effect of folic acid supplementation is observed in hyperhomocysteinemic rats (Woo et al., 2006). It has been found that diet-induced hyperhomocysteinemia causes liver injury due to oxidative stress (Woo et al., 2006, 2008). Increased superoxide anion generation may serve as one of the important mechanisms for Hcy-induced oxidative stress and subsequently liver injury. Folic acid supplementation can effectively inhibit NADPH oxidase-mediated superoxide anion production leading to reduced lipid peroxidation in the liver, which in turn, alleviates liver injury (Woo et al., 2006).

Impaired kidney function is one of the common factors causing hyperhomocysteinemia. However, recent studies suggest that hyperhomocysteinemia may cause renal injury. Studies have demonstrated that hyperhomocysteinemia causes activation of NF-κB, induction of inducible NOS (iNOS) and chemokine expression in rat kidneys (Zhang et al., 2004; Hwang et al., 2008). NF-κB is a transcriptional factor that plays an important role in regulating gene expression of various inflammatory factors in the kidney and is a redox-sensitive transcription factor. It has been also demonstrated that hyperhomocysteinemia stimulates monocyte chemoattractant protein-1 (MCP-1) expression in rat kidneys as well as human proximal tubular cells via NF-κB activation indicating that an inflammatory response may contribute to renal injury associated with hyperhomocysteinemia (Hwang et al., 2008). Moreover, it has been also observed that Hcy induces MCP-1 expression in rat mesangial cells mediated by oxidative stress and NF-κB activation (Cheung et al., 2008).

It is increasingly recognized that oxidative stress is an important factor in the development and progression of kidney disease. It has been suggested that increased NADPH oxidase-mediated superoxide generation contributes to the development of diabetic nephropathy (Etoh et al., 2003; Inoguchi et al., 2003). Hcy treatment was shown to increase collagen production and cell proliferation in rat mesangial cells (Yang and Zou, 2003). Such a stimulatory effect by Hcy could be blocked by inhibition of NADPH oxidase activation. In a rat model of hyperhomocysteinemia induced by folate-free diet, glomerulosclerosis was characterized by enhanced oxidative stress, mesangial expansion, podocyte dysfunction, and fibrosis. When these rats with hyperhomocysteinemia were treated with apocynin, an inhibitor of NADPH oxidase, the glomerular injury was significantly attenuated (Yi et al., 2006, 2009). Therefore, it is suggested that the role of folic acid in maintaining good health may extend beyond the cardiovascular system.

5.5.4 FOLIC ACID AND VASCULAR DISEASE RISK

Although observational data have clearly demonstrated an inverse association between folate status and the risk of cardiovascular disease, interventional data give equivocal results. A recent study analyzing the data from 16,958 participants in 12 randomized controlled trials shows no reduction of cardiovascular risk by folic acid supplementation in patients with a history of end-stage renal disease or vascular diseases including stroke, myocardial infarction, coronary heart disease, and/or intermittent claudication (Bazzano et al., 2006). The controversy regarding the outcome of folate supplementation may be due to (1) the severity of the preexisting cardiovascular diseases or renal disease that may contribute to the negative result of folic acid; (2) the physiological and health effects exerted by folate may not necessarily operate on a linear continuum: (3) folate supplementation may not necessarily impact all individuals in the population surveyed in an equal manner due to genotypic differences; and (4) differences in the absorption and metabolism of naturally occurring folate and oxidized folic acid that is used in supplements or fortification may have different impacts on health and disease.

With respect to cerebrovascular disease, the linkage between Hcy and disease progression appears to be stronger than with cardiovascular disease (Lonn et al., 2006; Saposnik et al., 2009). Results from the Heart Outcomes Prevention Evaluation (HOPE) 2 Trial, examining the effect of daily supplementation with 2.5 mg of folic acid, 50 mg of B_6, and 1 mg of B_{12} to older adults with history of vascular disease, over the course of 5 years provided evidence of a 25% reduction in stroke risk with the Hcy-lowering therapy (Lonn et al., 2006). Follow-up analysis on the HOPE 2 data set (Saposnik et al., 2009) provided evidence that those benefitting from the Hcy-lowering intervention, from the perspective of overall stroke risk, were those under the age of 70 not receiving lipid-lowering drugs, and with existing hyperhomocysteinemia. Additionally, those patients who lived in a country without a folic acid fortification policy also tended to benefit more from vitamin intervention (see below). It does appear that Hcy-lowering therapy, principally using folic acid as a mainstay of the regimen, may have more of an impact in those individuals with the highest Hcy concentrations. A recent study by Hodis and colleagues (2009), in which a randomized controlled trial design was employed, examined the impact of high-dose B vitamin supplementation, including 5 mg of folic acid/day, on measures of carotid intima media thickness. This study found that when subjects presented with Hcy concentrations greater than 9.1 μM at study onset, high-dose B vitamin therapy led to significantly lower carotid intimal thicknesses as compared to placebo. These data provide support for a role of B vitamin supplementation, including folic acid, earlier on in the disease cycle to reduce the risk for later progression toward vascular disease. The lack of beneficial effects of folic acid supplementation in previous intervention studies may be due to the fact that, in subjects with established vascular disease, the damage induced by elevated Hcy concentrations has already been done. For those that may be at risk for hyperhomocysteinemia, including those individuals with genetic mutations in one or more of enzymes of the folate cycle, such as the thermolabile 5, 10-methylenetetrahydrofolate reductase variant (Sazci et al., 2006), earlier interventions designed to increase the intake of folate may be warranted.

5.6 STRATEGIES TO INCREASE FOLATE INTAKE: THE ROLE OF FUNCTIONAL FOODS

Strategies to increase folate intake include

1. Encouraging the consumption of foods naturally rich in folates, including green, leafy vegetables
2. Encouraging the consumption of supplements containing folic acid
3. Folic acid fortification policies—mandatory or discretionary

With respect to the first two approaches, their effectiveness in contributing to overall folate intake will depend on (a) the eating habits of the specific population concurrent with the availability of foods naturally rich in folate and (b) the prevalence of supplement usage within a given population. In a recent study of the folate intake in a sample population of young college women in Manitoba, Canada, major contributors to total folate intake included vegetables (17.6%), juices (13.0%), and dairy and eggs (7.5%) (Shuaibi et al., 2008). The largest contributors to total dietary folate equivalent intakes were bakery products (27.7%), rice and pasta (15.0%), and ready-to-eat cereals (5.1%), with the bulk of the folate coming from synthetic folic acid due to the fortification of these food groups in North America (see below). In the absence of folic acid fortification, the median intake of natural folate would have been 295 µg/day of folate, well below the RDA value of 400 µg/day. Supplement usage in this population was 26% (Shuaibi et al., 2008), a value consistent with national trends in Canada (De Wals et al., 2007). These data highlight challenges with respect to relying on supplement usage or the consumption of foods naturally rich in folate as a means of increasing the intake of this important vitamin for the potential mitigation of vascular disease risk. Fortification strategies, on the other hand, are proving effective in increasing folate intake in the North American population (Ray et al., 2002).

Implemented in the late 1990s, the policy of mandatory fortification of cereal grain products, including enriched white flour, has contributed to an increase in the folic acid intake of approximately 100–150 µg/day (Ray et al., 2002). Folic acid fortification strategies are widely recognized as a public health success story with respect to the reduction in NTDs. For example, the province of Newfoundland saw its rate of NTDs drop from 4 per 1000 births to approximately 1 per 1000 births in the immediate period postfortification (House et al., 2006). Whether existing folic acid fortification strategies will lead to reductions in the rates of vascular disease is another matter entirely, as it may prove impossible to conclusively establish cause and effect given the time required to develop the disease and the presence of confounding factors. However, one of the challenges of the current fortification strategy remains the choice of vehicle. Enriched white flour, along with other cereal products, was chosen as the delivery vehicle for the mandatory folic acid fortification policy based on population exposure modeling exercises. Given recent interest in certain circles to reduce carbohydrate intakes, these vehicles may be actively avoided by segments of the population. As such, the opportunity exists to position other foods as potential vehicles for the delivery of folate into the human diet.

While numerous food products are available with added vitamins and minerals, the addition of vitamins to foods of animal origin, especially whole, unprocessed foods, is challenging. The enrichment of meat, milk, or eggs is governed by the biological processes regulating the assimilation and transfer of the respective nutrient into the final product. Previous work in our laboratory has documented that eggs can be fortified with folate by increasing the level of folic acid in the laying hen diet. The inclusion of 4 mg of folic acid per kg of laying hen diet led to a 2.5 fold increase in egg folate levels (from 20 to 50 µg/egg) (House et al., 2002). Further enrichment was not possible given the saturable nature of the process, regulated principally by plasma folate concentrations (Hebert et al., 2005). With respect to the folate content, the egg is somewhat unique in that the majority (>90%) of the folate is in the form of 5-MTHF and in the monoglutamate form (Seyoum and Selhub, 1998). This form, coupled with the absence of fibrous antinutritive factors in eggs, may confer advantages to this

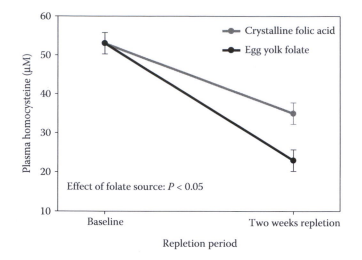

FIGURE 5.2 Slope-ratio assay comparing Hcy-lowering effects of equimolar amounts of folic acid or egg folate (5-MTHF) in a rat model of folate depletion–repletion. (Adapted from House, J. D., O'Connor, C. P., and Guenter, W. 2003. *J. Agric. Food Chem.* 51(15): 4461–4467.)

dietary source of folate, from the perspective of bioavailability. In a rodent model of folate depletion–repletion, egg folate was superior to an equimolar amount of folic acid in reducing plasma Hcy concentrations (Figure 5.2) (House et al., 2003). Therefore, the potential exists to position folate-enriched eggs as a protein-rich vehicle for the delivery of the folate into the human diet (Sahlin and House, 2006). Given emerging evidence to distance egg consumption specifically from cardiovascular disease risk (Hu et al., 1999), this vehicle may prove to be an attractive one for certain segments of the population.

5.7 SUMMARY

With respect to vascular disease, folate, along with other B vitamins, may play an important role in mitigating disease risk. While the precise mechanisms continue to be elucidated, a primary focus continues to be the Hcy-lowering effects of folate. Ensuring that plasma Hcy concentrations remain lower, particularly early in life before the initiation of damage to the walls of blood vessels, may require a focus on the folate status. Mandatory folic acid fortification of the food supply has worked to increase the folate intake of the North American population, however, additional opportunities exist to position alternative foods enriched in folate, including eggs.

REFERENCES

Antoniades, C., Antonopoulos, A. S., Tousoulis, D., Marinou, K., and Stefanadis, C. 2009. Homocysteine and coronary atherosclerosis: From folate fortification to the recent clinical trials. *Eur. Heart J.* 30(1): 6–15.

Ashokkumar, B., Mohammed, Z. M., Vaziri, N. D., and Said, H. M. 2007. Effect of folate oversupplementation on folate uptake by human intestinal and renal epithelial cells. *Am. J. Clin. Nutr.* 86(1): 159–166.

Asrar, F. M. and O'Connor, D. L. 2005. Bacterially synthesized folate and supplemental folic acid are absorbed across the large intestine of piglets. *J. Nutr. Biochem.* 16(10): 587–593.

Aufreiter, S., Gregory III, J. F., Pfeiffer, C. M., Fazili, Z., Kim, Y., Marcon, N., Kamalaporn, P., Pencharz, P. B., and O'Connor, D. L. 2009. Folate is absorbed across the colon of adults: Evidence from cecal infusion of 13C-labeled [6S]-5-formyltetrahydrofolic acid. *Am. J. Clin. Nutr.* 90(1): 116–123.

Au-Yeung, K. K., Woo, C. W., Sung, F. L., Yip, J. C., Siow, Y. L., and Karmin, O. 2004. Hyperhomocysteinemia activates nuclear factor-kappa B in endothelial cells via oxidative stress. *Circ. Res.* 94(1): 28–36.

Au-Yeung, K. K., Yip, J. C., Siow, Y. L., and Karmin, O. 2006. Folic acid inhibits homocysteine-induced superoxide anion production and nuclear factor kappa B activation in macrophages. *Can. J. Physiol Pharmacol.* 84(1): 141–147.

Babior, B. M. 1999. NADPH oxidase: An update. *Blood* 93(5): 1464–1476.

Balamurugan, K. and Said, H. M. 2006. Role of reduced folate carrier in intestinal folate uptake. *Am. J. Physiol. Cell Physiol.* 291(1): C189–C193.

Bazzano, L. A., Reynolds, K., Holder, K. N., and He, J. 2006. Effect of folic acid supplementation on risk of cardiovascular diseases: A meta-analysis of randomized controlled trials. *JAMA* 296(22): 2720–2726.

Beckman, J. S. and Koppenol, W. H. 1996. Nitric oxide, superoxide, and peroxynitrite: The good, the bad, and ugly. *Am. J. Physiol.* 271(5 Pt 1): C1424–C1437.

Bellamy, M. F., McDowell, I. F., Ramsey, M. W., Brownlee, M., Newcombe, R. G., and Lewis, M. J. 1999. Oral folate enhances endothelial function in hyperhomocysteinaemic subjects. *Eur. J. Clin. Invest.* 29(8): 659–662.

Bey, E. A., Xu, B., Bhattacharjee, A., Oldfield, C. M., Zhao, X., Li, Q., Subbulakshmi, V., Feldman, G. M., Wientjes, F. B., and Cathcart, M. K. 2004. Protein kinase C delta is required for p47phox phosphorylation and translocation in activated human monocytes. *J. Immunol.* 173(9): 5730–5738.

Chambers, J. C., Ueland, P. M., Obeid, O. A., Wrigley, J., Refsum, H., and Kooner, J. S. 2000. Improved vascular endothelial function after oral B vitamins: An effect mediated through reduced concentrations of free plasma homocysteine. *Circulation* 102(20): 2479–2483.

Cheung, G. T., Siow, Y. L., and Karmin, O. 2008. Homocysteine stimulates monocyte chemoattractant protein-1 expression in mesangial cells via NF-kappaB activation. *Can. J. Physiol. Pharmacol.* 86(3): 88–96.

Clarke, R., Daly, L., Robinson, K., Naughten, E., Cahalane, S., Fowler, B., and Graham, I. 1991. Hyperhomocysteinemia: An independent risk factor for vascular disease. *N. Engl. J. Med.* 324(17): 1149–1155.

Combs, G. F. 2008. Folate. *The Vitamins: Fundamental Aspects in Nutrition and Health* (3rd edition). Burlington, MA: Elsevier. pp. 355–380.

Crittenden, R. G., Martinez, N. R., and Playne, M. J. 2003. Synthesis and utilisation of folate by yoghurt starter cultures and probiotic bacteria. *Int. J. Food Microbiol.* 80(3): 217–222.

Damaraju, V. L., Cass, C. E., and Sawyer, M. B. 2008. Renal conservation of folates. Role of folate transport proteins. *Vitam. Hor.* 79: 185–202.

Dayal, S., Brown, K. L., Weydert, C. J., Oberley, L. W., Arning, E., Bottiglieri, T., Faraci, F. M., and Lentz, S. R. 2002. Deficiency of glutathione peroxidase-1 sensitizes hyperhomocysteinemic mice to endothelial dysfunction. *Arterioscler. Thromb. Vasc. Biol.* 22(12): 1996–2002.

De Wals, P., Tairou, F., Van Allen, M. I., Uh, S., Lowry, R. B., Sibbald, B., Evans, J. A. et al. 2007. Reduction in neural-tube defects after folic acid fortification in Canada. *New Eng. J. Med.* 357(2): 135–142.

Di Minno, M. N., Tremoli, E., Coppola, A., Lupoli, R., and Di Minno, G. 2010. Homocysteine and arterial thrombosis: Challenge and opportunity. *Thromb. Haemost.* 103(5): 942–961.

Doshi, S. N., McDowell, I. F., Moat, S. J., Lang, D., Newcombe, R. G., Kredan, M. B., Lewis, M. J., and Goodfellow, J. 2001. Folate improves endothelial function in coronary artery disease: An effect mediated by reduction of intracellular superoxide? *Arterioscler. Thromb. Vasc. Bio.* 21(7): 1196–1202.

Dudeja, P. K., Kode, A., Alnounou, M., Tyagi, S., Torania, S., Subramanian, V. S., and Said, H. M. 2001. Mechanism of folate transport across the human colonic basolateral membrane. *Am. J. Physiol.— Gastrointestinal and Liver Physiology.* 281(1, 44-1): G54–G60.

Duell, P. B. and Malinow, M. R. 1997. Homocyst(e)ine: An important risk factor for atherosclerotic vascular disease. *Curr. Opin. Lipidol.* 8(1): 28–34.

Edirimanne, V. E., Woo, C. W., Siow, Y. L., Pierce, G. N., Xie, J. Y., and Karmin, O. 2007. Homocysteine stimulates NADPH oxidase-mediated superoxide production leading to endothelial dysfunction in rats. *Can. J. Physiol. Pharmacol.* 85(12):1236–1247.

Egashira, K., Suzuki, S., Hirooka, Y., Kai, H., Sugimachi, M., Imaizumi, T., and Takeshita, A. 1995. Impaired endothelium-dependent vasodilation of large epicardial and resistance coronary arteries in patients with essential hypertension. Different responses to acetylcholine and substance P. *Hypertension* 25(2): 201–6.

Etoh, T., Inoguchi, T., Kakimoto, M., Sonoda, N., Kobayashi, K., Kuroda, J., Sumimoto, H., and Nawata, H. 2003. Increased expression of NAD(P)H oxidase subunits, NOX4 and p22phox, in the kidney of streptozotocin-induced diabetic rats and its reversibility by interventive insulin treatment. *Diabetologia* 46(10): 1428–1437.

Fox, J. T. and Stover, P. J. 2008. Folate-mediated one-carbon metabolism. *Vitam. Hor.* 79: 1–44.

Groemping, Y., Lapouge, K., Smerdon, S. J., and Rittinger, K. 2003. Molecular basis of phosphorylation-induced activation of the NADPH oxidase. *Cell* 113(3): 343–355.

Harrison, D. G. and Ohara, Y. 1995. Physiologic consequences of increased vascular oxidant stresses in hypercho-lesterolemia and atherosclerosis: Implications for impaired vasomotion. *Am. J. Cardiol.* 75(6): 75B–81B.

Hayashi, I., Sohn, K., Stempak, J. M., Croxford, R., and Kim, Y. 2007. Folate deficiency induces cell-specific changes in the steady-state transcript levels of genes involved in folate metabolism and 1-carbon transfer reactions in human colonic epithelial cells. *J. Nutr.* 137(3): 607–613.

Hebert, K., House, J. D., and Guenter, W. 2005. Effect of dietary folic acid supplementation on egg folate content and the performance and folate status of two strains of laying hens. *Poult. Sci.* 84(10): 1533–1538.

Hibbard, E. and Smithells, R. W. 1965. Folic acid metabolism and human embryopathy. *The Lancet* 285(7398): 1254.

Hodis, H. N., Mack, W. J., Dustin, L., Mahrer, P. R., Azen, S. P., Detrano, R., Selhub, J. et al. 2009. High-dose B vitamin supplementation and progression of subclinical atherosclerosis: A randomized controlled trial. *Stroke* 40(3): 730–736.

House, J. D., Braun, K., Ballance, D. M., O'Connor, C. P., and Guenter, W. 2002. The enrichment of eggs with folic acid through supplementation of the laying hen diet. *Poult. Sci.* 81(9): 1332–1337.

House, J. D., Jacobs, R. L., Stead, L. M., Brosnan, M. E., and Brosnan, J. T. 1999. Regulation of homocysteine metabolism. *Adv. Enz. Reg.* 39: 69–91.

House, J. D., March, S. B., Ratnam, S., Crowley, M., and Friel, J. K. 2006. Improvements in the status of folate and cobalamin in pregnant Newfoundland women are consistent with observed reductions in the incidence of neural tube defects. *Can. J. Pub. Health* 97(2): 132–135.

House, J. D., O'Connor, C. P., and Guenter, W. 2003. Plasma homocysteine and glycine are sensitive indices of folate status in a rodent model of folate depletion and repletion. *J. Agric. Food Chem.* 51(15): 4461–4467.

Hu, F. B., Stampfer, M. J., Rimm, E. B., Manson, J. E., Ascherio, A., Colditz, G. A., Rosner, B. A. et al. 1999. A prospective study of egg consumption and risk of cardiovascular disease in men and women. *J. Am. Med. Assoc.* 281(15): 1387–1394.

Huang, R. F., Hsu, Y. C., Lin, H. L., and Yang, F. L. 2001. Folate depletion and elevated plasma homocysteine promote oxidative stress in rat livers. *J. Nutr.* 131(1): 33–38.

Hwang, S. Y., Woo, C. W., Au-Yeung, K. K., Siow, Y. L., Zhu, T. Y., and Karmin, O. 2008. Homocysteine stimulates monocyte chemoattractant protein-1 expression in the kidney via nuclear factor-kappaB activation. *Am. J. Physiol. Renal Physiol.* 294(1): F236–F244.

Inoguchi, T., Tsubouchi, H., Etoh, T., Kakimoto, M., Sonta, T., Utsumi, H., Sumimoto, H. et al. 2003. A possible target of antioxidative therapy for diabetic vascular complications—Vascular NAD(P)H oxidase. *Curr. Med. Chem.* 10(17): 1759–1764.

Institute of Medicine. 1998. Folate. *DRI Dietary Reference Intakes for Thiamin, Riboflavin, Niacin, Vitamin B_6, Folate, Vitamin B_{12}, Pantothenic Acid, Biotin, and Choline.* National Academy Press, Washington, DC.

Kalinina, N., Agrotis, A., Tararak, E., Antropova, Y., Kanellakis, P., Ilyinskaya, O., Quinn, M. T., Smirnov, V., and Bobik, A. 2002. Cytochrome b558-dependent NAD(P)H oxidase-phox units in smooth muscle and macrophages of atherosclerotic lesions. *Arterioscler. Thromb. Vasc. Biol.* 22(12): 2037–2043.

Kanani, P. M., Sinkey, C. A., Browning, R. L., Allaman, M., Knapp, H. R., and Haynes, W. G. 1999. Role of oxidant stress in endothelial dysfunction produced by experimental hyperhomocyst(e)inemia in humans. *Circulation* 100(11):1161–1168.

Kang, S. S., Wong, P. W., and Malinow, M. R. 1992. Hyperhomocyst(e)inemia as a risk factor for occlusive vascular disease. *Annu. Rev. Nutr.* 12: 279–298.

Kim, T. H., Yang, J., Darling, P. B., and O'Connor, D. L. 2004. A large pool of available folate exists in the large intestine of human infants and piglets. *J. Nutr.* 134(6): 1389–1394.

Kumar, C. K., Moyer, M. P., Dudeja, P. K., and Said, H. M. 1997. A protein-tyrosine kinase-regulated, pH-dependent, carrier-mediated uptake system for folate in human normal colonic epithelial cell line NCM460. *J. Biol. Chem.* 272(10): 6226–6231.

Lievers, K. J. A., Kluijtmans, L. A. J., Boers, G. H. J., Verhoef, P., Den Heijer, M., Trijbels, F. J. M., and Blom, H. J. 2002. Influence of a glutamate carboxypeptidase II (GCPII) polymorphism (1561C → T) on plasma homocysteine, folate and vitamin B12 levels and its relationship to cardiovascular disease risk. *Atherosclerosis* 164(2): 269–273.

Lonn, E., Yusuf, S., Arnold, M. J., Sheridan, P., Pogue, J., Micks, M., McQueen, M. J. et al. 2006. Homocysteine lowering with folic acid and B vitamins in vascular disease. *N. Engl. J. Med.* 354(15): 1567–1577.

Marinou, K., Antoniades, C., Tousoulis, D., Pitsavos, C., Goumas, G., and Stefanadis, C. 2005. Homocysteine: A risk factor for coronary artery disease? *Hellenic J. Cardiol.* 46(1): 59–67.

Mason, J. B., Shoda, R., Haskell, M., Selhub, J., and Rosenberg, I. H. 1990. Carrier affinity as a mechanism for the pH-dependence of folate transport in the small intestine. *Biochim. Biophys. Acta–Biomembranes* 1024(2): 331–335.

Moens, A. L., Champion, H. C., Claeys, M. J., Tavazzi, B., Kaminski, P. M., Wolin, M. S., Borgonjon, D. J. et al. 2008. High-dose folic acid pretreatment blunts cardiac dysfunction during ischemia coupled to maintenance of high-energy phosphates and reduces postreperfusion injury. *Circulation* 117(14): 1810–1819.

Ohara, Y., Peterson, T. E., and Harrison, D. G. 1993. Hypercholesterolemia increases endothelial superoxide anion production. *J. Clin. Invest.* 91(6): 2546–2551.

Ohara, Y., Peterson, T. E., Sayegh, H. S., Subramanian, R. R., Wilcox, J. N., and Harrison, D. G. 1995. Dietary correction of hypercholesterolemia in the rabbit normalizes endothelial superoxide anion production. *Circulation* 92(4): 898–903.

Qiu, A., Jansen, M., Sakaris, A., Min, S. H., Chattopadhyay, S., Tsai, E., Sandoval, C., Zhao, R., Akabas, M. H., and Goldman, I. D. 2006. Identification of an intestinal folate transporter and the molecular basis for hereditary folate malabsorption. *Cell* 127(5): 917–928.

Pritchard, K. A., Jr, Groszek, L., Smalley, D. M., Sessa, W. C., Wu, M., Villalon, P., Wolin, M. S., and Stemerman, M. B. 1995. Native low-density lipoprotein increases endothelial cell nitric oxide synthase generation of superoxide anion. *Circ. Res.* 77(3): 510–518.

Ray, J. G., Vermeulen, M. J., Boss, S. C., and Cole, D. E. C. 2002. Declining rate of folate insufficiency among adults following increased folic acid food fortification in Canada. *Can. J. Public Health* 93(4): 249–253.

Refsum, H. 1998. Hyperhomocysteinemia in terms of steady-state kinetics. *Eur. J. Pediatr. Suppl.* 157(2): S45–S49.

Refsum, H., Ueland, P. M., Nygard, O., and Vollset, S. E. 1998. Homocysteine and cardiovascular disease. *Ann. Rev. Med.* 49: 31–62.

Robinson, J. M., Ohira, T., and Badwey, J. A. 2004. Regulation of the NADPH-oxidase complex of phagocytic leukocytes. Recent insights from structural biology, molecular genetics, and microscopy. *Histochem. Cell Biol.* 122(4): 293–304.

Roncales, M., Achon, M., Manzarbeitia, F., Maestro de las Casas, C., Ramirez, C., Varela-Moreiras, G., and Perez-Miguelsanz, J. 2004. Folic acid supplementation for 4 weeks affects liver morphology in aged rats. *J. Nutr.* 134(5): 1130–1133.

Rong, N., Selhub, J., Goldin, B. R., and Rosenberg, I. H. 1991. Bacterially synthesized folate in rat large intestine is incorporated into host tissue folyl polyglutamates. *J. Nutr.* 121(12): 1955–1959.

Sahlin, A. and House, J. D. 2006. Enhancing the vitamin content of meat and eggs: Implications for the human diet. *Can. J. Animal Sci.* 86(2): 181–195.

Said, H. M. 2004. Recent advances in carrier-mediated intestinal absorption of water-soluble vitamins. *Ann. Rev. Physiol.* 66: 419–446.

Said, H. M., Chatterjee, N., Ul Haq, R., Subramanian, V. S., Ortiz, A., Matherly, L. H., Sirotnak, F. M., Halsted, C., and Rubin, S. A. 2000. Adaptive regulation of intestinal folate uptake: Effect of dietary folate deficiency. *Am. J. Physiol.—Cell Physiol.* 279: C1889–C1895.

Said, H. M., Ghishan, F. K., and Redha, R. 1987. Folate transport by human intestinal brush-border membrane vesicles. *Am. J. Physiol.—Gastrointest. Liver Physiol.* 252(2): G229–G236.

Said, H. M. and Strum, W. B. 1983. A pH-dependent, carrier-mediated system for transport of 5-methyltetrahydrofolate in rat jejunum. *J. Pharmacol. Exp. Ther.* 226(1): 95–99.

Saposnik, G., Ray, J. G., Sheridan, P., McQueen, M., and Lonn, E. 2009. Homocysteine-lowering therapy and stroke risk, severity, and disability: Additional findings from the HOPE 2 trial. *Stroke* 40(4): 1365–1372.

Sazci, A., Ergul, E., Tuncer, N., Akpinar, G., and Kara, I. 2006. Methylenetetrahydrofolate reductase gene polymorphisms are associated with ischemic and hemorrhagic stroke: Dual effect of MTHFR polymorphisms C677T and A1298C. *Brain Res. Bull.* 71(1–3): 45–50.

Schron, C. M., Washington Jr., C., and Blitzer, B. L. 1985. The transmembrane pH gradient drives uphill folate transport in rabbit jejunum. Direct evidence for folate/hydroxyl exchange in brush border membrane vesicles. *J. Clin. Invest.* 76(5): 2030–2033.

Seiler, C., Hess, O. M., Buechi, M., Suter, T. M., and Krayenbuehl, H. P. 1993. Influence of serum cholesterol and other coronary risk factors on vasomotion of angiographically normal coronary arteries. *Circulation* 88(5 Pt 1): 2139–2148.

Seyoum, E. and Selhub, J. 1998. Properties of food folates determined by stability and susceptibility to intestinal pteroylpolyglutamate hydrolase action. *J. Nutr.* 128(11): 1956–1960.

Shane, B. and Stokstad, E. L. 1983. The interrelationships among folate, vitamin B12, and methionine metabolism. *Adv. Nutr. Res.* 5: 133–170.

Shuaibi, A. M., House, J. D., and Sevenhuysen, G. P. 2008. Folate status of young Canadian women after folic acid fortification of grain products. *J. Am. Diet. Assoc.* 108(12): 2090–2094.

Sirotnak, F. M. and Tolner, B. 1999. Carrier-mediated membrane transport of folates in mammalian cells. *Annu. Rev. Nutr.* 19: 91–122.

Sokoro, A. A. H., Zhang, Z., Eichhorst, J. C., Zello, G. A., House, J. D., Alcorn, J., and Lehotay, D. C. 2008. Formate pharmacokinetics during formate administration in folate-deficient young swine. *Metabolism: Clinical and Experimental* 57(7): 920–926.

Sorescu, D., Weiss, D., Lassegue, B., Clempus, R. E., Szocs, K., Sorescu, G. P., Valppu, L. et al. 2002. Superoxide production and expression of nox family proteins in human atherosclerosis. *Circulation* 105(12): 1429–1435.

Stroes, E., Hijmering, M., van Zandvoort, M., Wever, R., Rabelink, T. J., and van Faassen, E. E. 1998. Origin of superoxide production by endothelial nitric oxide synthase. *FEBS Lett.* 438(3):161–164.

Upchurch, G.R., Jr, Welch, G. N., Fabian, A. J., Freedman, J. E., Johnson, J. L., Keaney, J. F. Jr., and Loscalzo, J. 1997. Homocyst(e)ine decreases bioavailable nitric oxide by a mechanism involving glutathione peroxidase. *J. Biol. Chem.* 272(27): 17012–17017.

USDA Agricultural Research Services. *USDA Nutrient Database, Standard Reference, Release 22*, 2010. Accessed: http://www.nal.usda.gov/fnic/foodcomp/search/.

Van Heerebeek, L., Meischl, C., Stooker, W., Meijer, C. J., Niessen, H. W., and Roos, D. 2002. NADPH oxidase(s): New source(s) of reactive oxygen species in the vascular system? *J. Clin. Pathol.* 55(8): 561–568.

Verhaar, M. C., Wever, R. M., Kastelein, J. J., van Dam, T., Koomans, H. A., and Rabelink, T. J. 1998. 5-Methyltetrahydrofolate, the active form of folic acid, restores endothelial function in familial hypercholesterolemia. *Circulation* 97(3): 237–241.

Wang, G., Siow, Y. L., and Karmin, O. 2000. Homocysteine stimulates nuclear factor kappaB activity and monocyte chemoattractant protein-1 expression in vascular smooth-muscle cells: A possible role for protein kinase C. *Biochem. J.* 352(Pt 3): 817–826.

Wang, G., Woo, C. W., Sung, F. L., Siow, Y. L., and Karmin, O. 2002. Increased monocyte adhesion to aortic endothelium in rats with hyperhomocysteinemia: Role of chemokine and adhesion molecules. *Arterioscler. Thromb. Vasc. Biol.* 22(11): 1777–1783.

Wang, Y., Rajgopal, A., Goldman, I. D., and Zhao, R. 2005. Preservation of folate transport activity with a low-pH optimum in rat IEC-6 intestinal epithelial cell lines that lack reduced folate carrier function. *Am. J. Physiol.—Cell Physiol.* 288(1, 57-1): C65–C71.

Weiss, N., Heydrick, S., Zhang, Y. Y., Bierl, C., Cap, A., and Loscalzo, J. 2002. Cellular redox state and endothelial dysfunction in mildly hyperhomocysteinemic cystathionine beta-synthase-deficient mice. *Arterioscler. Thromb. Vasc. Biol.* 22(1): 34–41.

Welch, G. N. and Loscalzo, J. 1998. Homocysteine and atherothrombosis. *N. Engl. J. Med.* 338(15): 1042–1050.

Williams, S. B., Cusco, J. A., Roddy, M. A., Johnstone, M. T., and Creager, M. A. 1996. Impaired nitric oxide-mediated vasodilation in patients with non-insulin-dependent diabetes mellitus. *J. Am. Coll. Cardiol.* 27(3): 567–74.

Wilmink, H. W., Stroes, E. S., Erkelens, W. D., Gerritsen, W. B., Wever, R., Banga, J. D., and Rabelink, T. J. 2000. Influence of folic acid on postprandial endothelial dysfunction. *Arterioscler. Thromb. Vasc. Biol.* 20(1): 185–188.

Woo, C. W., Prathapasinghe, G. A., Siow, Y. L., and Karmin, O. 2006. Hyperhomocysteinemia induces liver injury in rat: Protective effect of folic acid supplementation. *Biochim. Biophys. Acta.* 1762(7): 656–665.

Woo, C. W., Siow, Y. L., and Karmin, O. 2008. Homocysteine induces monocyte chemoattractant protein-1 expression in hepatocytes mediated via activator protein-1 activation. *J. Biol. Chem.* 283(3): 1282–1292.

Woo, C. W., Siow, Y. L., Pierce, G. N., Choy, P. C., Minuk, G. Y., Mymin, D., and Karmin O. 2005. Hyperhomocysteinemia induces hepatic cholesterol biosynthesis and lipid accumulation via activation of transcription factors. *Am. J. Physiol. Endocrinol. Metab.*, 288(5): E1002–E1010.

Yang, Z.Z. and Zou, A. P. 2003. Homocysteine enhances TIMP-1 expression and cell proliferation associated with NADH oxidase in rat mesangial cells. *Kidney Int.* 63(3): 1012–1020.

Yi, F., Xia, M., Li, N., Zhang, C., Tang, L., and Li, P.L. 2009. Contribution of guanine nucleotide exchange factor Vav2 to hyperhomocysteinemic glomerulosclerosis in rats. *Hypertension* 53(1): 90–96.

Yi, F., Zhang, A. Y., Li, N., Muh, R. W., Fillet, M., Renert, A., and Li, P. L. 2006. Inhibition of ceramide-redox signaling pathway blocks glomerular injury in hyperhomocysteinemic rats. *Kidney Int.* 70(1): 88–96.

Zavadakova, P., Fowler, B., Zeman, J., Suormala, T., Pristoupilova, K., Kozich, V., and Zavadakova, P. 2002. CblE type of homocystinuria due to methionine synthase reductase deficiency: Clinical and molecular studies and prenatal diagnosis in two families. *J. Inherit. Metab. Dis.* 25(6): 461–76.

Zhang, R., Ma, J., Xia, M., Zhu, H., and Ling, W. 2004. Mild hyperhomocysteinemia induced by feeding rats diets rich in methionine or deficient in folate promotes early atherosclerotic inflammatory processes. *J. Nutr.* 134(4): 825–830.

6 Experimental and Clinical Evidence of Cardiovascular Benefits of Plant Sterols

Rgia A. Othman and Mohammed H. Moghadasian
University of Manitoba

CONTENTS

6.1 INTRODUCTION

Cardiovascular disease (CVD) is the leading cause of death in the Western societies. High total cholesterol (TC) and low-density lipoprotein cholesterol (LDL-C) levels are considered the major risk factors for coronary heart disease (CHD) (Steinberg and Gotto, 1999). Current evidence has determined a positive association between lifestyle and dietary factors as they correlate with blood lipid concentrations and CHD (Van Horn et al., 2008). It is well-documented that plasma TC levels are positively associated with ischemic heart disease (IHD) (Lewington et al., 2007), and a 1% decline in TC could be expected to reduce the risk of CHD by 2.7%. Similarly, a 10% decrease in LDL-C is associated with about 12% to 20% decline in the population incidence of IHD over 5 years (Katan et al., 2003). Hence, reducing blood cholesterol levels may be needed to lower risk of CVD. Therapeutic life-style changes, such as inclusion of dietary phytosterols, may reduce cardiovascular risk.

    Plant sterols (PS) have been shown in numerous studies to reduce the levels of TC, LDL-C, (Demonty et al., 2009), apolipoprotein B (apo-B) (Madsen et al., 2007), and non-high-density lipoproteins cholesterol (non-HDL-C) (Weidner et al., 2008), and C-reactive protein (CRP), interleukin-6 (IL-6), tumor necrosis factor-α (TNF-α), phospholipase A-1 (PLA-1), and fibrinogen (Bouic et al., 1999; Devaraj et al., 2006; Jones et al., 2007; Nashed et al., 2005). Hence, PS may reduce the risk of atherosclerosis (de Jong et al., 2003) and protect against CVD (Tapiero et al., 2003). The mechanisms involved in such effects remain unclear. However, PS may deter cholesterol absorption from the diet (Ohr, 2003) and, subsequently, lower plasma LDL-C (de Jong et al., 2003). The decline in TC and LDL-C could be an outcome of a decrease in cholesterol absorption and an alteration of enzymes involved in cholesterol metabolism and excretion (Kris-Etherton et al., 2002). Anti-inflammatory activity of PS may also be mediated through beneficial alterations in membrane composition, affecting membrane fluidity (Awad et al., 2004), sensitivity (Feigin et al., 1995), and signaling pathways. All of these can modulate the immune response by modifying eicosanoid, leukotrienes, and prostaglandin synthesis (Plat and Mensink, 2005). This chapter reviews the current knowledge of the cardiovascular benefits of PS as well as highlighting possible mechanisms, bringing into focus the lipid lowering, anti-inflammatory, and antiatherosclerotic activities.

6.2 DIETARY PHYTOSTEROLS

PS or phytosterols collectively indicate plant-derived sterols and stanols. PS are structurally related to cholesterol but the side chain contains a methyl (campesterol) or an ethyl (β-sitosterol and stigmasterol) group (Ostlund, 2002; Ohr, 2003) (Figure 6.1). β-sitosterol, campesterol, and stigmasterol are the principal molecular forms (Kochhar, 1983), while only sitosterol and campesterol are considered to be the most frequent PS in food constituting ~60% and 35%, respectively (Weingärtner et al., 2009). Saturated forms of PS are called stanols (sitostanol, campestanol, and stigmastanol) (Perisee, 2005). Humans cannot synthesize PS; thus, they always originate from the diet. While maximum amounts of PS can be sourced from plant oils, moderate and minimal levels can be found in nuts and seeds, and fruits and vegetables, respectively (Weihrauch and Gardner, 1978; Piironen et al., 2000). Tall oil, derived from the process of paper production from wood, is considered to be a high source of plant stanols than vegetable

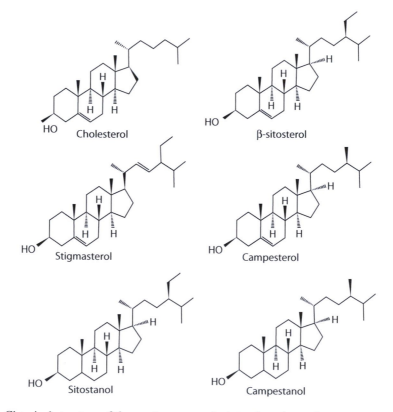

FIGURE 6.1 Chemical structure of the most common plant sterols and stanols.

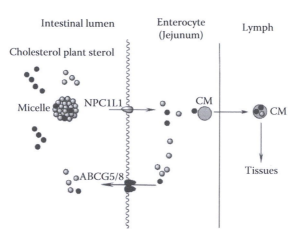

FIGURE 6.2 Cholesterol-lowering mechanism of phytosterols. Phytosterols binds to the mixed micelles, with a greater affinity than cholesterol, and are transported into the intestinal enterocyte through an NPC1L1-mediated pathway and efficiently pumped back out into the intestinal lumen by the ABCG5/8. Cholesterol is esterified and packaged into CM that are exported in the lymph. NPC1L1, Niemann-Pick C1 Like 1; ABCG5/8 = ATP-binding cassette transporter G5 and 8; CM, chylomicrons.

oils (Francisco and Resurreccion, 2008). With intestinal absorption rates ranging from 0.4% to 5% and 0.02% to 0.3%, respectively, plant sterols and stanols are considered to be poorly absorbed (Heinemann et al., 1993; Ostlund et al., 2002) compared to dietary cholesterol, which its absorption is estimated to range from 50% to 60% (Bosner et al., 1999). It is estimated that the dietary intake of PS generally do not exceed 200 mg/day in neither the American diet (Franz et al., 2003) nor in British diet (Morton et al., 1995) but to be upward of 373 mg/day in Japanese diet (Hirai et al., 1986), and 500 mg/day in vegetarian (Vuoristo and Miettinen, 1994; Franz et al., 2003) and Mediterranean diets (Rudkowska, 2008). PS in foods compete with cholesterol for uptake into mixed micelles, displacing cholesterol molecule from the micelles (Heinemann et al., 1991) and reducing intestinal cholesterol absorption (Richelle et al., 2004) (Figure 6.2). Low absorption rate of cholesterol may also be due to the active re-secretion of PS back into the intestinal lumen, which may be mediated by the ATP-binding cassette (ABC) half-transporters ABCG5 and ABCG8 (Berge et al., 2000). Increased PS absorption is extremely high in sitosterolemic patients, where the ABCG5 and/or ABCG8 are mutated (Oram and Vaughan, 2006).

After an extensive review of the scientific literature, a dose-response relationship was found with PS and a maximum effect of about 10% reduction in LDL-C levels at a dose of 2 g/day (Ostlund, 2002; Katan et al., 2003). This has been the impetus for the United States National Cholesterol Education Program (NCEP) (NCEP, 2001) to recommend the inclusion of PS (2 g/day) to the diet as a part of the therapeutic lifestyle changes to lower LDL-C in patients with elevated levels by about 10%. In similar, the FDA recommends a minimum of 800 mg/day of PS/stanols to assist reducing CHD risk through decreasing LDL-C (Retelny et al., 2008). Moreover, the FDA allowed a health claim stating that products containing phytosterols may reduce risk of CHD (Jenkins et al., 2005a; Retelny et al., 2008).

6.3 CHOLESTEROL-LOWERING EFFECTS

6.3.1 EXPERIMENTAL EVIDENCE

We previously showed that the addition of PS alone or with a combination with lipid-lowering agent to atherogenic diet reduced plasma cholesterol levels in apo-E-deficient mice (Moghadasian et al., 1997, 1999c, 2001; Lukic et al., 2003; Yeganeh et al., 2005; Nashed et al., 2005; Moghadasian, 2006a, 2006b). PS, in a dose-dependent manner, reduced serum lipids by 10% to 33% in various lipid fractions including very low-density lipoproteins (VLDL), intermediate density lipoproteins (IDL), LDL, hepatic cholesteryl esters (–62%), free cholesterol (–31%), and biliary cholesterol saturation index (–55%) in apo-E-deficient mice. However, they increased whole-body cholesterol synthesis as indicated by a 23% significant increase in serum lathosterol: cholesterol ratio with no significant changes in the LDL receptor, 3-hydroxy-3-methylglutaryl coenzyme A (HMG-CoA) synthase, cholesterol 7 α-hydroxylase (cyp7A1), and sterol 27-hydroxylase (Cyp27) at mRNA level in liver (Volger et al., 2001a). Feeding wild-type Kyoto (WKY) rats with diets containing PS (1%, w/w) for 4 weeks decreased plasma TC (21%) and hepatic cholesterol levels (34%) and increased the activity of the rate-limiting enzyme, HMG-CoA reductase, by 1.27-fold (Batta et al., 2005). Similarly, we have confirmed that long-term phytosterol treatment substantially upregulated the expression of HMG-CoA reductase, HMG-CoA synthase 1, and oxysterol 7β-hydroxylase (Cyp7B1) at the liver mRNA level in apoE-deficient mice (Xu et al., 2008). Dietary supplementation with stigmasterol (0.5%, w/w) for 6 weeks decreased plasma TC levels by 11% along with reductions in cholesterol and sitosterol absorption by 22% and 16% and by 23% and 30% in Wistar and WKY rats, respectively (Batta et al., 2006). These reductions were also associated with suppressions in the activity of HMG-CoA reductase by 44% and 77% and cyp7A1 by 71% and 39% in Wistar and WKY rats, respectively. The authors suggested that stigmasterol feeding may increase hepatocytes cholesterol levels, which could have suppressed HMG-CoA reductase and further cyp7A1.

Addition of stigmasterol decreased cholesterol synthesis, activated the liver X receptor (LXR) in a cell-based reporter assay, and suppressed SREBP-2 processing in cultured adrenal cells from ABCG5/8 knockout mice (Yang et al., 2004). Gavaging apo-E-deficient mice with plant sterol esters (PSE) of canola oil fatty acids once every 3 or 4 days (45 μL or 60 μL/day/mouse ~2.5 mg/day free PS) for 10 weeks reduced TG by 36% and TC by 21% relative to placebo (Fuhrman et al., 2007). The observed decline in TG levels could be related to the higher dosage of 1,3-diacylglycerol in PS of canola oil mixture. Nevertheless, the reduction in TG levels associated with PS treatment was also previously reported in mice (Lukic et al., 2003) and hamsters (Trautwein et al., 2002; Ebine et al., 2005). In agreement, feeding diet supplemented with PS mixture containing no sitostanol failed to reduce plasma TC levels in either hamsters (Ntanios and Jones, 1998) or rats (Ling and Jones, 1995). However, the decreases in plasma TC and LDL-C were attained when sitostanol was added to PS mixture (Ling and Jones, 1995). Ntanios et al. (1998) reported a similar observation in rabbits, suggesting that plant stanols might be more efficient in lowering cholesterol levels in rodents than PS. In apo-E-deficient mice, however, both nonhydrogenated phytosterols and saturated phytosterols had comparable cholesterol-lowering effects (Pritchard et al., 2003). Addition of either ferulate phytostanyl esters (FPE) or sitostanol to (0.1%, wt/wt) cholesterol diet significantly reduced plasma TC levels by 15% and 14%, respectively, in Golden hamsters after 6 weeks of treatment (Jain et al., 2008). These treatments did not alter the intestinal gene expression of sterol transporters including Niemann-Pick C1 like 1 (NPC1L1), ABCG5, or ABCG8 (Jain et al., 2008). This observation concurred with those in mice (Calpe-Berdie et al., 2005, 2006; Plosch et al., 2006).

Esterified phytostanols may exert more potent cholesterol-lowering effects than unesterified. In this regards, feeding disodium ascorbyl phytostanyl phosphate (DAPP) at either (0.7%, w/w) or (1.4%, w/w) induced 42% and 49% ($P < 0.05$) diminutions in plasma TG levels, respectively, in Golden Syrian hamsters fed (0.25%, w/w) cholesterol diet for 5 weeks compared to unesterified stanol (Ebine et al., 2006). Moreover, 1.4% DAPP significantly decreased body weights relative to noncholesterol and stanol diets. Since clinical evidence found a strong correlation between body fat mass and plasma TG (Pascot et al., 1999), it is plausible that reduced TG levels after DAPP treatment may be due to its lowering effect on body weight. Furthermore, relative liver weights were correlated with plasma TG, and reduced after DAPP treatment, suggesting less accumulation of TG in the liver and, subsequently, less secretion. Likewise, we previously showed that administration of DAPP by either food or drinking water contributed to 75% declines in TC levels relative to apo-E-deficient control mice (Lukic et al., 2003). Feeding Syrian golden hamsters an atherogenic diet containing 30% of energy as fat and cholesterol and supplemented with (0, 0.24%, 0.48%, 0.96%, 1.92%, and 2.84%, w/w) PSE for 12 weeks significantly reduced plasma TC and LDL-C levels compared to control (Ntanios et al., 2003). Consuming diet containing phytosterols sterified with fish oil fatty acids (25 g/kg diet) significantly reduced plasma TG, TC, and non-HDL-C levels compared to those fed no PS or fish oil (Ewart et al., 2002). Likewise, insulin resistant rats fed PS-fish oil esters (2.6 g/kg bw/day) showed significant decline in serum TG and TC compared to rats fed diet devoid of PS or fish oil (Russell et al., 2002). In contrast, PS esterified to fish oil (1.76% eicosapentaenoic acid (EPA) and docosahexaenoic acid (DHA) sterol esters, providing 1% PS) significantly reduced plasma TC levels by 20% and non-HDL-C by 29% in hamsters fed (0.25%, w/w) cholesterol diet for 5 weeks (Demonty et al., 2005).

Rasmussen et al. (2006) investigated the impact of the fatty acid moiety on cholesterol metabolism in male hamsters for 4 weeks, where the PSE esterified with fatty acids from soybean oil (SO), beef tallow (BT), or purified stearic acid (SA). The results revealed that hamsters fed BT and SA had significantly low cholesterol (LC) absorption and decreased levels of plasma non-HDL-C and liver esterified cholesterol (EC), and greater fecal sterol excretion compared to SO and control hamsters fed no PSE. Hayes et al. (2002) showed that nonesterified (free) phytosterols were as effective as esterified sterols and stanols in lowering plasma TC (58% vs. 54% and 52%) and hepatic TC (80% vs. 77% and 76%) and EC (91% vs. 88% and 88%), respectively, when compared to no PS-fed group. In parallel, fecal cholesterol excretion did not differ among these groups and was five times more than the control. Furthermore, while a 5:1 ratio of phytosterols: cholesterol decreased plasma TC by 27% and a 10:1 ratio reduced plasma TC by 17% in gerbils, both ratios similarly reduced hepatic TC by 57% and hepatic EC by 70%. A 5:1 low ratio was even more effective when consumed with each meal than receiving equal phytosterols in a 10:1 ratio every other day. Taken together, unesterified or esterified PS could have a comparable inhibitory influence on the cholesterol absorption as evidently supported by clinical and experimental data (Richelle et al., 2004; Meijer et al., 2003).

Hypocholesterolemic action of phytosterols/phytostanols is thought to occur, due to at least in part, a competition with dietary and biliary cholesterol for intestinal absorption in mixed micelles (Miettinen et al., 1990; von Bergmann et al., 2005). The precise mechanism of reduction in the rate of cholesterol absorption by PS remains to be clearly understood. However, it is thought that PSE may limit free cholesterol absorption rate by binding to cholesterol esterase, suppressing its activity (Trautwein et al., 2003) and preventing the esterification of free cholesterol into cholesterol esters (Child and Kuksis, 1986). If they remained intact in the intestine PSE could act as a lipophilic pool to attract both dietary and endogenous cholesterol to the lower part of the intestinal lumen where absorption is restricted (Trautwein et al., 2003). Increasing bile salt excretion has also been suggested (Gua et al., 1993). Because of their competition with cholesterol for solubilization in dietary mixed micelles, PS were shown to co-crystallize with cholesterol forming insoluble, complex crystal, which impedes the process of hydrolysis by lipases and cholesterol esterases (Trautwein et al., 2003). However, this mechanism needs further investigation since the formation of insoluble mixed crystals was not detected under *in vitro* lipolysis of model dietary emulsions (Mel'nikov et al., 2004).

Cholesterol-lowering effect of PS may be mediated through mechanisms other than suppressing cholesterol absorption. Indeed, PS may not be necessarily required to be in the intestinal lumen with cholesterol in order to exert their hypocholesterolemic effect since cholesterol-lowering effects of PS in chicks (Konlande and Fisher, 1969) and hamsters (Vanstone et al., 2001) were achieved with a subcutaneous (s.c.) injection. This may suggest other mechanism than blocking cholesterol absorption. PS seem to interrupt cholesterol homeostasis by affecting cholesterol efflux through ABC transporters. In this context, experimental evidence has shown that PS can be converted into a LXR agonist, which activates the expression of ABC proteins (Berger et al., 2004). In this regard, *in vitro* study with Caco-2 cells found that mixed micelles enriched with sitostanol were potent inducers of ABCA1 expression compared to free cholesterol study (Plat and Mensink, 2002). ABCA1 was found to pump free cholesterol out of the enterocytes back into the lumen (Repa et al., 2000). Furthermore, phytosterols may reduce cholesterol levels independently of the mRNA expression of ABCG5 and ABCG8 transporters (Calpe-Berdiel et al., 2006; Jia et al., 2007). Table 6.1 summarizes recent experimental studies that have been conducted regarding lipid-lowering effects of phytosterols.

TABLE 6.1

Recent Animal Studies of Lipid-Lowering Effects of Phytosterols Treatment

Reference	Model	Dose of Sterols/Stanols/Duration	Major Changes
Volger et al. (2001)	12-week-old female apoE *3-Leiden transgenic (n = 7)	Cholesterol containing diet (0.25%, w/w) plus 0.0%, 0.25%, 0.5%, 0.75%, or 1.0%, w/w) plant stanols (sitostanol 88%, campestanol 10%) (9 weeks)	↓ 10% to 33% (P < 0.05), mainly in VLDL-, IDL- and LDL-C; ↓ 62% in CE, ↓ 31% in free cholesterol and ↓ 38% in TG (hepatic contents) (all P < 0.05)
Hayes et al. (2002)	5- to 9-week-old male Mongolian gerbils (n = 5–8)	Cholesterol containing diet (0, 0.05, 0.1, 0.15, or 0.5%, g/100 g) plus 0.5 or 0.75% nonesterified (free), esterified sterols, esterified stanols (4–5 weeks)	↓ 58%, 54% and 52% in plasma TC; ↓ 80%, 77% and 76% in liver TC; ↓ 91%, 88% and 88% (all P < 0.05) in liver EC in free sterols, esterified sterols and esterified stanols, respectively versus no PS fed group
Batta et al. (2005)	7-week-old male WKY rats (n = 6)	Chow diet supplemented with (1%, w/w) PS with (4 weeks)	↓ 21% in TC; ↓ 34% hepatic cholesterol levels in WKY versus untreated rats (P < 0.05)
Demonty et al. (2005)	5- to 6-week-old male Golden Syrian hamsters weighing 80–100 g (n = 10)	Cholesterol containing diet (0.25%, w/w) plus EPA and DHA sterol esters (1.76%, providing 1% PS) (5 weeks)	↓ 20% in plasma TC levels (P = 0.001); ↓ 29% non-HDL-C (P < 0.0001) versus nonesterified PS
Batta et al. (2006)	6-week-old male Wistar or WKY rats (n = 6)	Chow diet enriched with (0.5%, w/w) stigmasterol (6 weeks)	↓ 11% in plasma TC (P < 0.05); ↓ 23 and 30% and ↓ 12 and 23% in cholesterol and sitosterol absorption (WKY and Wistar rats, respectively)
Ebine et al. (2006)	Male Golden Syrian hamsters weighing 90–110 g (n = 10)	Cholesterol containing diet (0.25, w/w) plus free phytostanols (1%, w/w), DAPP (0.7%, w/w) or DAPP (1.4%, w/w) (5 weeks)	↓ 45% in TG (DAPP 1.4%) (P < 0.05) versus cholesterol-control; ↓ 42% in TG (DAPP 0.7%) (P < 0.05) and ↓ 49% (P < 0.01) in TG in DAPP 1.4% versus stanol
Rasmussen et al. (2006)	Male F1B Syrian hamsters weighing 90–100 g (n = 8–9)	Diets containing 50 g/kg PSE esterified with fatty acids from SO, BT, or purified SA (4 weeks)	↓ 90% (SA) and 59% (BT) in cholesterol absorption; ↓ 99% (SA) and 96% (BT) in liver cholesterol; ↓73% (SA) and 64.4% (BT) in plasma non-HDL-C (all P < 0.05)
Fuhrman et al. (2007)	8-week-old apo E-deficient mice (n = 5)	PSE of canola oil fatty acids chow diet; 2.5 mg/day free PS mice were gavaged once in 3 or 4 days (45 μL/3 days/mouse or 60 μL/4 days/mouse) (10 weeks)	↓ in TC 21% (P < 0.0517); ↓ 36% in TG (P < 0.05)
Jain et al. (2008)	Male Golden Syrian hamsters weighing 80–110 g (n = 10–12)	Cholesterol containing diet (0.1%, w/w) plus sitostanol (0.5%, w/w) or FPE (0.73%, w/w) (4 weeks)	↓ 14% in TC (sitostanol) (P < 0.05); ↓ 15% in TC (FPE) (P < 0.02); ↓ in TG (sitostanol)(P = 0.041) and FPE (P = 0.049); ↓ 39% in HDL-C (sitostanol) (P = 0.001) and ↓ 22% (FPE) (P = 0.01)

6.3.2 CLINICAL EVIDENCE

The role of PS in the prevention of CVD, particularly LDL-C-lowering effects, has been the subject of numerous controlled clinical studies. Combining low-fat margarine and milk enriched with PS (2.3 g/day) with NCEP step 1 diet for 4 weeks contributed to significant decreases in TC (5.5%), LDL-C (7.7%), and apo-B (4.6%) levels (Madsen et al., 2007). The observed reduced LDL-C was previously reported after adding 2 g of plant stanol ester into the meat, pasta, low-fat yogurt drink (Salo and Wester, 2005), and low-fat hard cheese (Jauhiainen et al., 2006). Similarly, consuming chocolate snack bars containing 1.5 g PSE twice a day for 6 weeks contributed to 4.7%, 6%, and 7.4% significant reductions in the levels of TC, LDL-C, and TC:HDL-C ratio, respectively, in mild hypercholesterolemic subjects (Polagruto et al., 2006). Moreover, PS-group had significantly reduced lipid-adjusted serum β-carotene compared to control group (Polagruto et al., 2006). The decrease in the systemic antioxidant levels after PS intake may not affect LDL oxidation. In this regard, Hansel et al. (2007) reported reduced plasma oxidized LDL (oxLDL) and cholesterol levels without any significant changes to serum β-carotene levels after consuming low-fat yogurt containing (1.6 g/day) of PS for 6 weeks. Dietary PS may reduce LDL-C leading to a low number of circulatory LDL particles that are prone to oxidation. Consuming phytosterol-enriched drinkable yogurt (100 mL ~1.6 g/day) along with the main meal for 42 days reduced LDL-C levels by 10.6% (Plana et al., 2008). In contrast, incorporating phytosterols (1.8 g/day) into beverages containing either no fat or 1 g of fat failed to reduce TC and LDL-C levels (Jones et al., 2003). Similarly, consumption of phytosterol-supplemented nonfat and low-fat beverages for 3 weeks did not result in clinically meaningful modifications in the LDL particle size (Charest et al., 2005). Since C22-unsaturated sterols were found to potentially inhibit cholesterol synthesis by influencing $\Delta24$-reductase enzyme, an enzyme involves cholesterol biosynthesis (Fernandez et al., 2002), availability of PS in adequate amounts and sufficient dispersion in the fat phase of the digested food for best for solubilization in mixed micelles could be very crucial. Incorporating of PS (1 g/MJ) into portfolio diet, a diet high in PS, soy protein, viscous fiber, and almonds, reduced all the LDL fractions including small dense LDL as early as week 2 (Lamarche et al., 2004). Drinking milk tea supplemented with 2.3 or 1.5 g PS with the two fattiest meals of the day for 5 weeks reduced TC and LDL-C, however, to a lesser extent than was anticipated (Li et al., 2007). In disagreement, Weidner et al. (2008) showed significant diminutions in plasma levels of LDL-C (7%), TC (4%), and non-HDL-C (6%), compared to baseline levels, after 8 weeks of consuming 200 mL of soy drink enriched with 2.6 g PSE daily. Furthermore, linking the time of ingestion to a main meal is markedly more efficient than consumption not linked to meals (Poli et al., 2008). Doornbos et al., (2006) showed that single-dose yoghurt drink with PS (3 g/day) significantly attenuated LDL-C when was taken with a meal independent of its fat content.

A meta-analysis study conducted by AbuMweis et al. (2008) showed that the timing of administration of a single dose of PS might influence their cholesterol-lowering actions since consuming of single dose with main meal or lunch lowered LDL-C levels but not prior or with breakfast. Similarly, ingesting ground beef supplemented with 2.7 g of soybean phytosterols as a single dose for 1 month significantly attenuated the levels of TC (9.3%) and LDL-C (14.6%) in mildly hypercholesterolemic young men compared to those of baseline (Matvienko et al., 2002). Daily consumption of a relatively low-fat product enriched with 2 g of plant stanols esters significantly decreased TC by 3.8% and LDL-C by 4.9% (Seppo et al., 2007). The small decline in the LDL-C may be due to the low baseline LDL-C value as the magnitude appeared to be more pronounced when a single-shot yoghurt drink was consumed with lunch and the baseline LDL-C level was ≥3.4 mmol/L. The latter observation is supported by Mussner et al. (2002), AbuMweis et al. (2008), Naumann et al. (2008), and Demonty et al. (2009) but not by Noakes et al. (2005). Consuming plant stanol esters containing product at lunch time may inhibit the absorption of both dietary and biliary cholesterol (Miettinen et al., 1990; von Bergmann et al., 2005), and coincide with the diurnal rhythm of cholesterol and bile acid synthesis as cholesterol levels peaked at night and declined during day time, and bile acid synthesis showed the opposite (Galman et al., 2005). Ingesting 2.6 g of encapsulated phytosterol ester with a meal for 12 weeks resulted in a 5% decline in LDL-C, which was not as extensive as in food-based trials (Earnest et al., 2007). In contrast, a low dose of phytosterol ester 1.3 g/day lowered plasma LDL-C by 7% and 4% at both week 3 and week 4 in hypercholesterolemic subjects (Acuff et al., 2007).

Recent evidence suggests that decreases in plasma LDL-C increase with phytosterol doses, in the range from 0.7 to 2.0–2.5 g/day; however, high doses showed no additional benefits as to reducing plasma cholesterol (Poli et al., 2008). However, dose-dependent reduction in TC by phytosterols can be observed when dietary cholesterol intake increased (Volger et al., 2001a; Hayes et al., 2002). This may also explain, at least in part, variation in the range of LDL-C decline in the literatures. A meta-analysis by Demonty et al. (2009) showed that the higher baseline LDL-C values were related to greater LDL-C reductions whereas the effects of the dose–response curves established for PS versus stanols, fat-based versus nonfat-based food formats and dairy versus nondairy foods were not significantly different. However, solid foods compared to liquid foods tended to have a larger influence only at high doses of phytosterol (>2 g/day). Since the liquid portion of the meal undergoes fast gastric evacuating compared to solid portion (Maes et al., 1998), it is possible that delivering PS in solid portion of the meal could delay gastric emptying and prolong the time for micelle formation. Moreover, there was a tendency, but not statistically significant ($p = 0.054$), toward a greater influence of multiple daily intakes of phytosterols compared to single intakes. This observation conflicted with that of AbuMweis et al. (2008) and was not previously reported. However, since PS competes with cholesterol for micellar incorporation, it was suggested that a concurrent presence of phytosterols, cholesterol, and bile acids in repeated occasions during the day could lead to a larger efficacy than a single intake. However, this meta-analysis did not take into account the potential impact of the background diet on the cholesterol-lowering efficacy of phytosterols. Nevertheless, high intake of PS or stanols (2 g/day) reduced plasma TC and LDL-C levels by ~10–15% irrespective of baseline cholesterol levels or background diet (Ostlund, 2004; Perisee, 2005). Similarly, Kassis et al. (2008) revealed that the cholesterol content of the background diet did not influence the efficacy of PS in spite of independent impacts of PS and cholesterol intake on lipid levels.

PS may have an additive effect on reducing LDL-C levels when synergistically used with lipid-lowering agent. A 15.4% attenuation in LDL-C levels were noticed when PS (1.0 g/1000 kcal) were added into the portfolio diet in hyperlipidemic subjects (Jenkins et al., 2008). LDL-C was reduced by a 9.0%; however, after eliminating sterol-enriched margarine from the portfolio diet, a 6.3% of decline in LDL-C was ascribed to PS (Jenkins et al., 2008). Low magnitude of reduction in LDL-C in this study could be due to low saturated fat intakes (Mussner et al., 2002). In contrast, Cleghorn et al. (2003) provided 8.7% and 12.3% decreases in TC and LDL-C levels, respectively, after consuming low-fat diet containing 2 g/day of PS for 4 weeks. A 15% extra reduction in LDL-C levels were observed when plant stanols-enriched margarines were consumed (3 g/day) by hyperlipidemic patients treated with maximal doses of statins compared to 7.7% of control (only statins) (Castro Cabezas et al., 2006). Additional LDL-C reductions of 8.7% and 13.1% were observed in statins-treated patients who consumed margarine with added (2.5 g/day) PS or stanols for 85 weeks (de Jong et al., 2008a). Patch et al. (2006), de Jong et al. (2007), and Miettinen and Gylling (2009) concurred with the conclusion of this study but not Jakulj et al. (2005). In agreement, ingestion of bread (10 g/day) containing phytosterols dissolved in diacylglycerol at a concentration of (4%) for 6 months diminished serum TC and LDL-C, remnant-like lipoprotein particles-cholesterol and lipoprotein (a) levels, a putative risk factor for CHD among hyperlipidemic children where the drug therapy is restricted (Matsuyama et al., 2007). A similar finding was observed in adults with familial hypercholesterolemia (FH) (Moruisi et al., 2006). PS may work synergistically with exercise in treatment of dyslipidemia to favorably modulate lipid levels (Marinangeli et al., 2006).

Significant decreases in TC and LDL-C (13.3% and 12.5%) were observed after combining a phytosterol-enriched spread (2 g/day) with n-3 long-chain polyunsaturated fatty acids (LCPUFA) supplements (1.4 g/day) for 3 weeks (Micallef and Garg, 2008). Normén et al. (2004) and Demonty et al. (2006) agreed with this concept to treat lipid aberrations by such a combination. The efficacy of PS may vary dramatically among individuals due to a genetic component. In this regard, Sanchez-Muniz et al. (2009) showed that low-fat spreads containing PSE (1.1 g or 2.2 g/day) consumed with the NCEP-I diet for 5 weeks significantly decreased serum levels of TC, LDL-C, and Apo-B and TC: LDL-C and LDL-C: HDL-C ratios in only E2 and E3 subjects. Conversely, low-fat dairy products enriched with 2 g/day PS significantly attenuated TC and LDL-C when consumed for 6 weeks and neither influenced serum levels of 25(OH) vitamin D nor affected retinol by Apo-E phenotype (Korpela et al., 2006). In agreement, despite insignificant reductions in TC and LDL-C, daily ingestion of low-fat yoghurt enriched with PS (1–2 g/day) increased serum levels of campesterol and sitosterol (Niittynen et al., 2008) but remained within normal range and much lower than those seen in patients with sitosterolaemia (Kidambi and Patel, 2008).

Likewise, de Jong et al. (2008a) have also reported increased serum cholesterol-standardized campestanol levels after 45 weeks of plant stanols treatment. However, it should be mentioned that campesterol may preferentially be absorbed over sitosterol, since serum campesterol levels were higher than those of sitosterol in spite of low concentrations of campesterol in the diets (Plat et al., 2008). Serum phytosterol levels increased by more than 20% when heterozygous subjects consumed sterol-enriched margarine but decreased when stanol-enriched margarine was consumed (Kratz et al., 2007). A cohort study with 1242 subjects reported that plasma levels of PS were significantly elevated in patients without CHD (Fassbender et al., 2008). Furthermore, it should be pointed out that genetic variations including ATP-binding cassette half transporter G5/8 polymorphism could have an impact on the PS cholesterol-lowering response of subjects (Berge et al., 2000). Taken together, notable variations observed in the LDL-C responses to PS could be related to the diverse doses, the rate of esterification of sterols, the timing of administration and ingestion of PS with or without meal besides genotype variation of the subjects. Table 6.2 summarizes recent clinical studies that have been conducted regarding lipid-lowering effects of phytosterols.

6.4   ANTI-INFLAMMATORY EFFECTS

6.4.1   EXPERIMENTAL EVIDENCE

Inflammation plays a significant role in the etiology of atherosclerosis (Libby et al., 2002). We have documented the anti-inflammatory impacts of phytosterols in apo-E-deficient mice fed (2%, wt/wt) mixtures of phytosterols for 14 weeks (Nashed et al., 2005). These mice showed low proinflammatory cytokines, such as IL-6 and TNF-α production and elevated anti-inflammatory IL-10 levels following lipopolysaccharide (LPS)-stimulation as compared to the control group (Nashed et al., 2005). Phytosterols have shown to have an immunomodulatory effect by modifying cytokine profiles in favor of T-helper type1 (Th1-type) response and decreasing cytokines associated with the Th2-type cells (Bouic et al., 1996, 1999; Breytenbach et al., 2001). Feeding apo-E-deficient mice a (2%, w/w) phytosterol-supplemented diet increased IL-2 and interferon-γ (IFN-γ) secretion, and Th1 lymphocyte cytokines after stimulation with s.c. turpentine injection (Calpe-Berdiel et al., 2007). In contrast, spleen lymphocytes of turpentine-treated C57BL/6J mice fed with phytosterols had significant increases in IL-2 production, but not in IFN-γ, IL-4, or IL-10 production (Calpe-Berdiel et al., 2007). β-Sitosterol glycoside increased *in vitro* expression of Th1-type cytokines (IFN-γ and IL-2) in comparison to those of Th2-type cytokines (IL-4 and IL-10) (Lee et al., 2007), showing predominant induction of the Th1-type cytokine. These changes may explain the significant increases in mean survival times observed in mice challenged with an intravenous injection of live *Candida albicans* yeast cells and treated with intraperitoneal (i.p.) injection of β-sitosterol glycoside relative to untreated control. PS may interact with leukocyte function, inducing immunomodulatory activity by inhibition of classical and alternative complements pathways (Navarro et al., 2001).

β-Sitosterol glucoside significantly inhibited the ovalbumin-specific Ig-E in the bronchoalveolar lavage (BAL) fluid and blocked the survival rate of splenocytes incubated with 100 µg/mL

TABLE 6.2

Recent Clinical Studies of Lipid-Lowering Effects of Phytosterols Treatment

Reference	Study Design	Subjects	Dose of Phytosterols/Duration	Major Findings
Polagruto et al. (2006)	Randomized, double-blind, parallel arm	Hypercholesterolemic; (49 years, mean) ($n = 32$)	Cocoa flavanol-enriched snack bar containing 1.5 g phytosterol (6 weeks) ($2 \times$ /day)	$\downarrow$ 4.7% in TC ($P < 0.01$); $\downarrow$ 6% in LDL-C ($P < 0.01$);$\downarrow$ 7.4% in TC:HDL-C ratio ($P < 0.001$)
Castro et al. (2006)	Randomized single-blind	Patients on statins therapy at maximal doses (45.7 ± 11.7 years, mean) ($n = 20$)	3 g/day of plant stanols added to 30 to 35 g/day of margarine (6 weeks)	$\downarrow$ 15% in LDL-C versus $\downarrow$7.7% in statin without plant stanols
Hansel et al. (2007)	Randomized double-blind, parallel	Hypercholesterolemic ($n = 95$)	Low-fat fermented milk enriched with 0.8 g PSE/ portion($2 \times$ /day) (6 weeks)	$\downarrow$ 4.7% in TC; $\downarrow$7.8% in LDL-C ($P < 0.05$); $\downarrow$ in oxLDL versus control (−1.73 versus 1.40 U/L; $P < 0.03$)
Seppo et al. (2007)	Randomized, placebo, controlled, double-blind	Hypercholesterolemic ($n = 49.5 \pm 13.1$ years, mean) ($n = 102$)	2 g/day of stanols as stanol-ester-enriched low-fat milk product (5 weeks)	$\downarrow$ 3.8% in TC, $P < 0.001$;$\downarrow$ 4.9% in LDL-C, $p = 0.002$
Jenkins et al. (2008)	Intervention, single-phase	Hyperlipidemic (59.7 ± 1.5 years, mean) ($n = 42$)	PS-enriched margarine (1 g/1000 kcal) with portfolio diet (80 weeks); eliminating PS from the diet between weeks 52 and 62 weeks	$\downarrow$ 15.4% in LDL-C ($P < 0.001$) $\downarrow$ 9.0% in LDL-C ($P < 0.001$)
Weidner et al. (2008)	Randomized, placebo-controlled double-blind	Untreated moderate hypercholesterolemic (19–65 years) ($n = 25$)	200 mL of soy drink enriched with 2.6 g PSE (8 weeks)	$\downarrow$ 4% in TC; $\downarrow$ 7% in LDL-C; $\downarrow$ 6% in non-HDL-C ($P < 0.05$)
Kassis et al. (2008)	Semirandomized, double-blind, crossover	Hypercholesterolemic (45–85 years) ($n = 22$)	22 mg PS/kg of body weight (BW) with either LC- or high-cholesterol (HC) diets; four 28-day feeding phases each separated by a 4-week washout	$\downarrow$ 12.8% in TC; $\downarrow$ 11.9% in LDL-C(LC); $\downarrow$ 4.0% in TC; $\downarrow$ 2.5% in LDL-C(HC)

Micallef and Garg, (2008)	Randomized, double-blind, placebo-controlled	Hyperlipidemic (55.4 ± 1.0 years, mean) (n = 60)	25 g/day of a spread containing 2 g/day with 1.4 g/day (n–3) LCPUFA (3 weeks)	↓ 13.3% (P < 0.001) in TC; ↓ 12.5% (P < 0.002) in LDL-C; ↑ 8.6% (P < 0.04) in HDL-C
Niittynen et al. (2008)	Meta-analysis of two randomized double-blind crossover or parallel	Moderately hyperlipidem ic; study I: (41 years, mean) (n = 15); study II: (54 years, mean) (n = 27)	Study I: yoghurt containing 1 g PS 1 ×/day (4 weeks)-2-week run-in and 2-week wash-out periods; Study II: yoghurt containing 2 g PS 2 ×/day (8 weeks)	↓ 5.2% in TC P < 0.173; ↓ 5.8% in LDL-C (P < 0.261)
Plana et al., (2008)	Randomized, double-blind, placebo-controlled, parallel	Hypercholesterolemic (18–75 years) (n = 44)	100 mL phytosterol enriched (1.6 g 1 ×/day) drinkable yogurt along with the main meal for 42 days	↓ 10.6% in LDL-C; ↓ 14% in TG; ↑ in sterols:TC ratio
Sanchez-Muniz et al. (2009)	Randomized, double-blind, controlled	Hypercholesterolemic with varied apo-E genotype (21–75 years) (n = 120)	50% fat reduced spread as part of NCEP-I diet with PSE (1.1 g or 2.2 g/day)	↓ TC, LDL-C, apo-B TC:LDL-C and LDL: HDL-C ratios in only E2 and E3 subjects
Demonty et al. (2009)	Meta analysis, randomized controlled	Hypercholesterolemic (36–59 years) (n = 6–102)	2.15 g/day phytosterols provided in fat-based, nonfat-based, dairy, nondairy foods, solid, or liquid foods (≥3 weeks)	on average ↓ 0.34 mmol/L ~8.8% in LDL-C

ovalbumin. In parallel, PS suppressed synthesis of TNF-α, IL-6, IL-8, and the expression of cyclo-oxygenase-2 (COX-2) in human mast cells (Kim et al., 2007). Purified fungal and mushroom sterols showed inhibitory impact on LPS-induced TNF-α secretion, IL-1α/β expression, and DNA binding activity of nuclear factor-κB (NF-κB) in macrophage-like cells, and IFN-inducible genes in colorectal adenocarcinoma cells (Kobori et al., 2007). β-Sitosterol and campesterol treatments inhibited prostaglandin E2 release in macrophages by 68% and 55% and prostacyclin-I2 by 67% and 52%, respectively, relative to cholesterol-treated cells (Awad et al., 2004). Basal prostacyclin release was increased 43% by campesterol and 81% by β-sitosterol, whereas prostacyclin release increased 25% by campesterol and 54% by β-sitosterol (Awad et al., 2001). Long-term β-sitosterol treatment effectively inhibited cell growth, increased basal prostaglandin release, and induced apoptosis in human prostate cancer cells (Awad et al., 2005). Incorporation of these sterols into cell membrane may alter the enzyme activity involved prostaglandin synthesis pathways. Incubation of human lung cancer cells with PS inhibited NF-κB activation and downregulated the expression of inflammatory gene products including COX-2 and matrix metalloproteinase-9 (Shishodia and Aggarwal, 2004). These anti-inflammatory effects may be due to inhibition of NF-κB activation (Lv et al., 2008).

Administration of PS either i.p. (Park et al., 2001), orally (Al-Yousuf et al., 2002), or topically (Navarro et al., 2001) has shown anti-inflammatory effects as indicated by reducing pouch granuloma weight, edema thickness in the paws, and/or ear edema in mice, respectively. In contrast, β-sitosterol induced swelling in the carrageenan-induced paw edema when i.p. administered but its glucoside showed minimal anti-inflammatory effects (Villaseñor et al., 2002). β-Sitosterol and its glucoside at (100 mg/kg) reduced the number of squirms induced by acetic acid by 70% and 73.0% in Swiss Webster albino mice (Villaseñor et al., 2002). Incorporation of PS into cell membranes may modulate cellular membrane composition altering its fluidity (Awad et al., 2004) and sensitivity (Feigin et al., 1995) and influence signaling pathways involved apoptosis and immunological functions (Awad and Fink, 2000). In addition, PS could influence immune response by modulating eicosanoid, leukotrienes, and prostaglandin synthesis (Plat and Mensink, 2005). Table 6.3 summarizes recent experimental studies regarding anti-inflammatory effects of phytosterols.

6.4.2　Clinical Evidence

A daily consumption of camelina, rapeseed or sunflower oil spread containing 2 g plant stanols for 3 months reduced LDL-C by 9% but failed to improve carotid artery compliance (CAC) and brachial artery flow-mediated dilatation (FMD), markers of arterial health, compared to placebo in mild hypercholesterolemic subjects (Raitakari et al., 2008). However, plant stanols improved arterial elasticity and endothelial function in subjects with low baseline values for CAC and FMD, raising the possibility of enhancing vascular function in people with suboptimal values. A significant reduction in brachial artery diameter was observed in moderate hypercholesterolemic subjects who consumed PSE (2 g/day for 10 weeks) spread period compared to plant stanol ester period (Hallikainen et al., 2006). Although brachial artery diameter tended to be larger in patients with coronary artery disease (CAD) than in normal subjects (Holubkov et al., 2002), its clinical significance remains uncertain. Two grams of plant stanol esters from spread did not change brachial artery FMD in diabetic patients despite a 16.1% reduction in LDL-C (Hallikainen et al., 2008). de Jong et al. (2008b) showed that 16 weeks of PS or stanol (2.5 g/day) consumption did not affect soluble adhesion molecules, CRP and monocyte chemotactic protein-1 (MCP-1) levels regardless of a significant decline in LDL-C. It is possible that the effects of dietary phytosterols on endothelial dysfunction might not be cholesterol-dependent pathways, and the decrease in LDL-C levels may not be enough to modulate endothelial dysfunction or low-grade inflammatory markers.

In a head-to-head comparison with statin, considering PS (1.0 g/1000 kcal) as an integral part of the portfolio diet not only improved the atherogenic lipid profile but also decreased CRP levels by 28% (Jenkin et al., 2003) and by 23% (Jenkins et al., 2005b) in hyperlipidemic subjects. The reduction in CRP levels may be a result of cholesterol reduction; however, a significant correlation

TABLE 6.3
Recent Animal Studies of Anti-Inflammatory Effects of Phytosterols Treatment

Study	Model	Dose of Phytosterols/Duration	Major Findings
Park et al. (2001)	Male imprinting control region (ICR) mouse with induced chronic inflammation, weighing 27–35 g ($n = 5$)	200 mg/kg; i.p.; cactus extract containing β-sitosterol (5 days)	↓ 21.9% ($P < 0.05$) in adjuvant-induced pouch granuloma weight and ↓ 52.7% in its carmine content versus control (saline, 10 mL/kg/ i.p.)
Navarro et al. (2001)	Female Swiss mice with the carrageenan-induced paw edema ($n = 8$)	30 or 60 mg/kg (orally): 0.25, 0.5 and 1 mg/ear (topically) extract containing campesterol (7.6%), stigmasterol (28.4%), and β-sitosterol (61.1%) (4 h)	↓ 30.1 and 37.4% in hind paw swelling ↓ 41, 43, and 58.7% ($P < 0.01$) in inflammatory response; ↓ 52% in edema formation ($P < 0.01$) by β-sitosterol (0.5 mg/ear)
Villaseñor et al. (2002)	7–12 week-old Swiss Webster albino mice with induced paw edema weighing 20–25 g ($n = 5$)	100 mg/kg; i.p.; β-sitosterol and β-sitosterol-β-D-glucoside (3 h)	↑ swelling of the paw edema (β-sitosterol) and slightly ↓ edema (glucoside), (0.028 versus 0.20, change in volume); ↓ 70.0% and 73.0% in number of squirms;↑ 300% and 157% in pain tolerance
Al-Yousuf et al. (2002)	Male albino mice with induced paw edema weighing 25–30 g ($n = 10$)	5000, 1000, and 2000 mg/kg; or 250, 5000, 1000, and 2000 mg/kg of extract containing stigmasterol; oral rout (2–4 h)	↓ edema thickness in the paws ($P < 0.05$); ↓ formalin-induced pain
Nashed et al. (2005)	4 week-old apo-E-deficient mice ($n = 7$)	(2%, w/w) ~0.1 g/kg/day of soybean-derived phytosterol mixtures containing 58% β-sitosterol, 19% campesterol, 13% dihydrobrassicasterol and 10% stigmasterol (14 weeks)	↓ in plasma IL-6 and TNF-α ($P < 0.05$); ↔ in IL-12 p40;↑ 8–10 times in IL-10 levels versus control; ↑ 2–4 in Th2-associated IL-5 and IL-13 production; ↑ 6–8 times in OVA-specific IFN-γ responses versus control mice
Calpe-Berdiel et al. (2007)	8 week-old female apo-E-deficient and C57BL/6J mice ($n = 6–8$)	(2%, w/w) ~0.1 g/kg/day; mixture of 20% campesterol, 22% stigmasterol and 41% β-sitosterol (4 weeks)	↑ 1.9-fold in IL-2 and ↑ 3.3-fold in IFN-γ ($P < 0.05$); ↔ in IL-4 and IL-10 levels (apo-E-deficient mice); ↑ ~2-fold in IL-2 ($P < 0.05$); ↔ IFN-γ, IL-4 and IL-10; ↑ 2.9-fold and 2.1-fold in the Th1:Th2 ratio in apo-E-deficient and C57BL/6J mice
Lee et al. (2007)	6 week-old BALB/c female mice with candidiasis ($n = 5$)	200 µg/mL β-sitosterol glycoside; i.p.; (2 ×/day, 3 days)	↑ expression of IL-2 and IFN-γ levels versus IL-4 and IL-10 productions ($P < 0.01$); ↑ in mean survival times ($28.8 ± 10.7$ versus $12.8 ± 3.5$ in control, days) ($P < 0.01$)

between changes in both CRP and LDL-C was not found (Jenkin et al., 2003). Serum CRP levels were not changed in mild hypercholesterolemic subjects after consuming 2.3 g/day PS in low-fat margarine and low-fat milk for 4 weeks each (Madsen et al., 2007). Daily consumption of 1.6 g PS supplemented low-fat fermented milk for 6 weeks reduced CRP levels in hypercholesterolemic subjects but was not significantly different compared to the control fermented milk and baseline (Hansel et al., 2007). In contrast, PSE in capsule form (1.3 g/day) failed to alter CRP levels during a 4-week intervention period in hypercholesterolemic subjects (Acuff et al., 2007). Consumption of 1.7 g/day PS esterified to fish oil reduced plasminogen activator inhibitor-1 (PAI-1) levels by 49% relative to those esterified to sunflower oil, but not olive oil, after 28 days in mild hypercholesterolemic subjects (Jones et al., 2007). The observed effect on PAI-1 concentrations may be due to the presence of DAG in both fish- and olive oil-esterified PS. CRP levels tended to decrease upon increasing the PS dose from 1.6 g to 3.0 g/day for 3 weeks in free living mild hypercholesterolemic subjects (Clifton et al., 2008); however, the differences were not statistically significant compared to control. Drinking a low-calorie orange juice beverage enriched with PS (1 g/240 mL 2 × /day) for 8 weeks significantly reduced CRP concentrations (−12%) in 72 healthy subjects (Devaraj et al., 2006).

PS may have additional biological actions that include immunomodulatory properties. Bouic et al. (1996) revealed that T-cell proliferative responses increased both *in vivo* and *in vitro* by several hundred percent after the use of β-sitosterol and its glucoside. Bouic et al. (2001) showed that β-sitosterol and its glucoside mixture maintained a favorable Th1 response based on the analysis of the CD4 cell-type (Th1 vs. Th2-type) in HIV-infected patients with no antiretroviral drugs. Breytenbach et al. (2001) reported a beneficial Th1 response (IFN-γ) in HIV-infected patients who received a mixture of PS relative to HIV-infected patients on no therapy, who exhibited a predominant Th2 response (IL-4 secretion). Similarly, a double-blind placebo-controlled study showed that a PS-sterolin mixture was associated with less neutrophilia, lymphopenia, and leukocytosis compared to placebo group. PS-sterolin mixture capsules also decreased the plasma level of IL-6 in the runners (Bouic et al., 1999). Modulating cytokine profile of T cells toward Th1-type by phytosterol mixture contributed to less rhinonorea, less turbinate hypertrophy, less postnasal drip symptoms, and lower Ig-E levels in subjects with allergic conditions, in which immune abnormalities involved a Th2-predominant profile (excessive IL-4 secretion and hence Ig-E synthesis) (Bouic, 2002). These anti-inflammatory properties of phytosterol mixtures were also shown in patients with rheumatoid arthritis (Bouic, 2002). Table 6.4 summarizes recent experimental studies regarding anti-inflammatory effects of phytosterols.

6.5 ANTIATHEROSCLEROTIC EFFECTS

6.5.1 Experimental Evidence

Dietary supplementation with (0.8%, w/w) sitostanol substantially reduced lesion developments in ascending aorta and coronary arteries in atherogenic diet-fed rabbits (Ntanios et al., 1998). Phytosterols may decrease build up of fatty streaks by reducing circulating levels of atherogenic lipoproteins. In this context, comparable to the effects of the lipid-lowering drug atorvastatin, incubating HepG2 human liver cells and Caco2 human intestinal cells with 50 μmol/L of the stigmasterol, campesterol, and β-sitosterol for 24 h significantly reduced the secretion of apo-B100 by 30% and apo-B 48 by 15%, 16%, and 19%, respectively, compared to control (Ho and Pal, 2005). These reductions could be explained by limited lipid availability in the cell as indicated by the decline in the intracellular cholesteryl ester levels after phytosterol treatment. Maintaining a balance in proliferation and apoptosis of endothelial cells may play a significant role in the atherosclerosis prevention. In this regard, β-sitosterol showed a significantly stronger cytotoxic activity than cholesterol, apoptotic influence as indicated by inducing caspase-3 activity in the cells by 60%, and reduced cell viability with a concentration as low as 2 μM after 24 h incubation in the human abdominal aorta endothelial cells, HAAE-2 (Rubis et al., 2008). In addition, β-sitosterol and campesterol decreased growth of vascular

TABLE 6.4

Recent Clinical Studies of Anti-Inflammatory Effects of Phytosterols Treatment

Reference	Study Design	Subjects	Dose of Phytosterols/Duration	Major Findings
Jenkins et al. (2005 a,b)	Randomized crossover	Healthy hyperlipidemic (36–71 years) (n = 34)	1 g/day PS/1000 kcal diet as PS- enriched margarine (4 weeks)	↓ 23.8% in CRP ($P < 0.001$); ↓ 29.6% in LDL-C versus baseline
Jenkins et al. (2003)	Randomized controlled, parallel	Healthy hyperlipidemic (n = 46)	1 g/day PS/1000 kcal diet as PS- enriched margarine (4 weeks)	↓ 28.2% in CRP ($P < 0.02$); ↓ 28.6% in LDL-C ($P < 0.001$) versus baseline
Hallikainen et al. (2006)	Randomized double-blind cross-over	Moderate hypercholesterolemic (39.6 ± 2.4 years, mean) (n = 11)	Spread containing PSE and plant stanol ester (1.93–1.98 g/day) for 10 weeks each	↓ 9–12% in LDL-C versus control ($P < 0.05$); ↓ 2.2% in brachial artery diameter in PSE versus stanol ester ($p = 0.012$); ↔ CRP, IL-6, TNF-α, or FMD
Devaraj et al. (2006)	Randomized, double blind, placebo-controlled	Healthy subjects with LDL-C baseline levels 144 ± 30 to 145 ± 37 (mg/dL) (19–74 years) (n = 36)	Orange juice beverage containing 1 g PS /240 mL 2 ×/day (8 weeks)	↓ 12% ($P < 0.02$) in CRP levels; ↓ 5% in TC and 9.4% in LDL-C ($P < 0.05$) versus baseline and placebo; ↑ 6.6% in HDL-C ($P < 0.02$) versus baseline
Acuff et al. (2007)	Double-blind, placebo-controlled, nonrandomized	Hypercholesterolemic (25–72 years) (n = 16)	1 capsules 2 ×/day, ~1.3 g/day PSE (6 weeks)	↓ 4% in LDL-C; ↑ 9% in HDL-C ($P < 0.05$) at week 3 versus placebo; ↔ serum levels CRP
Jones et al. (2007)	Randomized cross-over	Mild overweight, hypercholesterolemic (n = 21)	1.7 g/day PS esterified to either fish oil, PS-FO, olive oil, PS-OO, sunflower oil PS-SO (28 days)	↓ 49% PAI-1 in PS-FO versus PS PS-SO ($P = 0.028$); ↓ TG in PS-FO versus PS-SO and PS-OO; ↔ TNF-α, IL-6, CRP
Madsen et al. (2007)	Double-blind, placebo-controlled cross-over	Mildly hypercholesterolemic (20–70 years) (n = 46)	2.3 g/day PS in low-fat margarine and milk, 69% β-sitosterol, 15% campesterol and 8% stigmasterol (8 weeks)	↓ 5.5% in TC and 7.7 in LDL-C; ↓ 4.6% in apo-B ($P < 0.05$); ↓ 3.4% in apo-B:apo-A I ratio; ↔ CRP levels
Hansel et al. (2007)	Randomized double-blind, randomized controlled	Moderate hypercholesterolemic (n = 95)	1.6 g/day PS in low-fat fermented milk, 75% β-sitosterol and 8.4% campesterol (6 weeks)	↓ 7.8% in LDL-C; ↓ in oxLDL (−1.73 vs. 1.40 U/L, $P < 0.05$) in control; ↔ in TG, HDL-C or CRP
Hallikainen et al. (2008)	Randomized, double blind, parallel	Type 1 diabetes (29–53 years) (n = 11)	2.0 g/day plant stanols (1.66 g sitostanol and 0.38 g campestanol) in spread (12 weeks)	↓ 10.8 in TC and ↓ 16.1% in LDL-C versus control ($P < 0.05$); ↔ in brachial artery diameter, FMD or endothelial function
de Jong et al. (2008b)	Randomized, double-blind, placebo-controlled	Patients on statin treatment (18–65 years) (n = 15)	2.5 g/day PS or plant stanol in margarine (16 weeks)	↓ LDL-C ($P = 0.026$); ↔ in MCP-1, CRP, soluble adhesion molecules
Clifton et al. (2008)	Randomized double-blind parallel	Mild hypercholesterolemic (20–69 years) (n = 40)	1.6 and 3.0 g/day PS as vegetable oil-based low-fat spread (3 weeks each dose)	↓ 10.4 and 14.7 in LDL versus control ($P < 0.05$); ↓ CRP ($P = 0.07$) versus control
Raitakari et al. (2008)	Randomized, double-blind, placebo-controlled	Mild hypercholesterolemic (20–50 years) (n = 68)	Camelina, rapeseed or sunflower oil spread with stanol (2 g/day) ester or sunflower oil spread (3 months)	↓ 9% in LDL-C versus control; ↔ CAC or FMD versus control; ↑ CAC from 1.23 to 1.59 and ↑ FMD from 6.9% to 8.6% in a subgroup analysis

smooth muscle cells (SMC) by 30% and 16%, respectively. This reduction could be attributable to inhibitory effects of PS on cholesterol metabolism, reducing cell membranes synthesis and cell proliferation (Awad et al., 2001). Decline in the number of endothelial cells after β-sitosterol treatment may also contribute to a lower blood coagulation, which in turn could have inhibited the proliferation of SMC (Awad et al., 2001). Antiatherogenic action of phytosterols may involve a reduction in the number of foam cells in the atherosclerotic plaque (de Jong et al., 2003). LDL oxidation stimulates macrophages to engulf oxLDL, which induce the secretion of proinflammatory cytokines and promote the recruitment of monocytes and accumulation of foam cells (Henriksen et al., 1981). Presence of β-sitosterol, however, enhanced the reversion of H_2O_2 production induced by oxLDL as well as arachidonic acid release and prostaglandin E2 synthesis in oxLDL-stimulated RAW 264.7 macrophages (Vivancos and Moreno, 2008). These effects of β-sitosterol might be attributed to the fact that β-sitosterol stimulates antioxidant enzymes such as Mn superoxide dismutase and glutathione peroxidase and consequently modulates the cellular redox state (Vivancos and Moreno, 2005).

Feeding female apoE*3-Leiden transgenic mice diets containing (1.0%, w/w) different derivatives of plant stanol esters for 38 weeks reduced atherosclerotic lesion area by 91% (vegetable oil), 97% (wood), and 78% (vegetable oil/wood) and the severity from regular intimal fatty streaks/mild plaques (type 2–3 lesions) in controls to individual intimal foam cells (<type 1 lesions) in the plant stanol esters groups (Volger et al., 2001b). Similarly, feeding LDL-r$^{+/-}$ mice with Western diets enriched with atorvastatin-attenuated serum TC by 22% and lesion area by 57%, whereas the addition of PS or stanols esters to statin for 35 weeks significantly lowered serum TC by 39% and 41% and atherosclerotic lesion size by 99% and 98%, respectively (Plat et al., 2006). Despite 4- to 11-fold increments in cholesterol standardized serum PS levels in the combination treatments, comparable antiatherogenic effect suggests that elevated serum levels of PS may not be atherogenic. This assumption was further confirmed by the second study, in which the mice LDLr$^{+/-}$ were fed a Western diet for 33 weeks, during which the lesions were formed. Adding PS or plant stanols to the diets for the next 12 weeks contributed to 66% and 64% significant declines in the lesion sizes compared to control but not atorvastatin groups ($P = 0.07$). While atorvastatin group had 60% type 1–2 and 40% type 3–5 lesions, both phytosterol groups showed mainly ~93% type 1–2, and 3–5 type lesions were hardly detected. Both studies even suggested that PS or stanols either alone or in combination with atorvastatin could reduce atherosclerotic lesions independent of serum PS levels. Concurrently, we showed that adding "tall oil"-derived phytosterol mixture (TODPM) at (2%, wt/wt) to (0.15%, w/w)-cholesterol supplemented diet for 18 weeks reduced the formation of atherosclerotic lesions in apo-E-deficient mice (Moghadasian et al., 1999a, 1999c). A strong positive correlation ($r = 0.69$, $P < 0.01$) was found between plasma TC levels and lesion area in the aortic sinuses (Moghadasian et al., 1999a). In contrast, after inducing atherosclerosis in apo-E-deficient mice by feeding them a Western-type diet (WTD) (9%, w/w) fat and (0.15%, w/w) cholesterol for 18 weeks, dietary enrichment with PS (2%, w/w) for the subsequent 25 weeks failed to hinder atherosclerotic lesions development. However, there was a tendency for the lesion size to increase in the PS group by 28% relative to a 40% increase in the control but was not statistically significant (Moghadasian et al., 1999b). This failure could not be interpreted by a lack of responsiveness for PS in this animal model in general. Indeed, using the same animal model, we compared the progression of atherosclerosis in groups treated with phytosterol, phytosterol and cyclosporine (CA), or CA to controls. Our results revealed that atherosclerotic lesion size and lesion: artery lumen ratios were significantly reduced in phytosterol by (64%, 63%) and (59%, 58%), phytosterol-CA combination by (47%, 46%) and (44%, 42%) relative to control and CA groups, respectively (Moghadasian 2006b). While probucol tended to decrease HDL-C by 64% and exacerbate development of atheroma by 163%, phytosterols treatment increased HDL-C by 66%, decreased atherosclerosis by 60% relative to control in apo-E-deficient mice fed atherogenic diet for 14 weeks (Moghadasian 2006a).

Addition of phytosterols to probucol reduced increase in TC levels by 59%. Such improvements in TC and HDL-C levels along with TC: HDL-C ratio by PS treatment may ameliorate proatherogenic impact of probucol. Furthermore, a strong positive correlation ($r = 0.607$) was found between atherosclerotic lesion size and TC: HDL-C ratio, suggesting that TC:HDL-C may be a reliable indicator for atherosclerosis risk. In another study with apo-E-deficient mice, we again revealed that phytosterol alone (Nashed et al., 2005) or in a synergy with niacin significantly diminished atherosclerotic lesion size and lesion: lumen ratio by 62% and 59.4% or by 50%, respectively, compared to control but not to fenofibrate (Yeganeh et al., 2005). Although supplementing diet with PSE, ezetimibe, lipid-lowering agent, or the combination significantly reduced atherosclerotic lesion formation compared to control animals, a significant trend toward more pronounced atherosclerotic lesion formation was observed in apo-E-deficient mice fed atherogenic diet supplemented with (2%, w/w) PSE compared to that supplemented with ezetimibe (Weingärtner et al., 2008). Furthermore, plasma PS were strongly correlated with increased atherosclerotic lesion formation ($r = 0.50$). However, additional effects of ezetimibe such as raising HDL-C, lowering TG, non-HDL-C, apo-B, and remnant-like particle cholesterol, reducing circulating PS, oxysterols, oxidative derivatives of cholesterol, and CRP levels (Bays et al., 2008), on atherogenesis can not be excluded. In contrast, in hypercholesterolemic female mice with >20-fold higher plasma levels of PS due to an inactivation of the two ABC half-transporters G5 and G8, no significant differences in aortic lesion were found after feeding with Western diets for 7 months (Wilund et al., 2004). In parallel, dietary PSE significantly reduced plasma TC and LDL-C, and attenuated foam cell area by 70% with a dietary dose as low as (0.24%, w/w) regardless of increase in plasma PS levels in hamsters fed an atherogenic diet for 12 weeks (Ntanios et al., 2003). The exact mechanism by which phytosterols induce antiatherogenic properties is yet to be elucidated; however, PS may demonstrate antiatherogenic property by lowering cholesterol absorption and decreasing hepatic lipase activity and plasma fibrinogen levels (Moghadasian et al., 1999a). PS may also reduce the accumulation of oxLDL in macrophages, and amount of serum peroxides (Summanen et al., 2003; Fuhrman et al., 2007), as well as preserve serum paraoxonase1 activity, an enzyme located on HDL and prevents LDL oxidation (Fuhrman et al., 2007). PS may also increase lecithin: cholesterol acyltransferase activity (Weisweiler et al., 1984) and hepatic bile salt secretion (Salen et al., 1970). Furthermore, it is also plausible that PS may not only inhibit intestinal absorption of cholesterol but also its oxidative derivatives, oxysterols, which come from thermal processed foods (Naruszewicz and Kozlowska-Wojciechowska, 2007). Incorporation of phytosterols into macrophages may protect against atherosclerosis by reducing prostaglandin release (Awad et al., 2004) and consequently atherosclerotic plaque formation, increasing prostacyclin production, and reducing vascular SMC proliferation (Awad et al., 2001). Table 6.5 summarizes recent experimental studies regarding antiatherosclerotic effects of phytosterols.

6.5.2 CLINICAL EVIDENCE

Phytosterol-enriched yogurt was associated with remarkable diminutions in CD36 and increases in LDL-receptor affinity expressions among polygenic hypercholesterolemic subjects, suggesting an important antiatherogenic effect (Ruiu et al., 2009). The activity of antithrombin-III, a potent inhibitor of coagulation, tended to increase in healthy subjects who consumed 4 g/day of wood-based stanol ester relative to control. Thus, phytosterols may attenuate atherogenesis through different mechanisms than cholesterol-lowering effects (Plat and Mensink, 2000). Consumption of PS-fortified margarine significantly prolonged the adhesion and aggregation time of blood platelets after collagen–epinephrine activation among 42 healthy male subjects, suggesting antiplatelet activity of PS in the prevention of CVD (Kozlowska-Wojciechowska et al., 2003). Short-term use of 2.0 g of plant stanols significantly reduced TC by 7.5% and LDL-C levels by 9.2%, but did not improve endothelial function as measured by FMD, the surrogate marker of atherosclerosis, in prepubertal children with FH (Jakulj et al., 2006). Since changes in LDL-C levels may determine the correlation between LDL-C levels and endothelial function (Tamai et al., 1997), a 9.2% decline in LDL in this study may not be large enough to improve endothelial function in those children. Similarly, the addition of plant stanol or PSE to spreads regardless of serum cholesterol reduction showed no additional improvement in vascular function (Gylling et al., 2009).

TABLE 6.5

Recent Animal Studies of Antiatherosclerotic Effects of Phytosterols Treatment

Reference	Model	Dose of Sterols/Stanols/ Duration	Major Changes
Moghadasian et al. (1999a)	5-week-old male apo-E-deficient mice (10)	Cholesterol-enriched diet (0.15%, wt/wt) plus TODPM (2%, wt/wt) (18 weeks)	↓ >50% in the average area of atheromata versus control (1.96 ± 0.8 vs. 4.08 ± 0.3 mm²; $P < 0.0001$)
Volger et al. (2001b)	12-week-old female apo-E*3-Leiden transgenic mice ($n = 10$)	Cholesterol-enriched diet (0.25%, w/w) plus (1.0%, w/w) plant stanol esters derived from either vegetable oil, wood or a mixture of both (38 weeks)	↓ 91% (vegetable oil), ↓ 97% (wood) and ↓ 78% (vegetable oil/wood) ($P < 0.0001$) in the atherosclerotic lesion area
Plat et al. (2006)	8-week-old female and male heterozygous LDLr +/− ($n = 6$–12)	Study I, Western diets enriched with atorvastatin (0.0025%, w/w) plus (1%, w/w) PS or stanols (35 weeks); Study II, Western diets (33 weeks and addition of atorvastatin (0.005%, w/w), (2%, w/w) PS or (2%, w/w) plant stanols for the subsequent 12 weeks	Study I: ↓ 99% (atorvastatin + PS); ↓ 98% (atorvastatin + stanol) in atheroma lesion size (all $P < 0.05$) versus controls Study II: ↓ 66% (PS); ↓ 64% (plant stanol) in atheroma lesion size versus control ($P < 0.03$)
Moghadasian et al. (2006a)	4-week-old male apo-E-deficient mice ($n = 8$)	Cholesterol-enriched diet (0.2%, w/w) plus (2%, w/w) soybean-derived phytosterol mixture with or without CA (0.02%, w/w) (14 weeks)	↓ (64, 63%) (phytosterol); ↓ (47, 46%) (phytosterol + CA) in atherosclerotic lesion size ratios; ↓ (59, 58%) (phytosterol); ↓ (44, 42%) (phytosterol + CA) in lesion:artery lumen ratios versus control and CA groups (all $P < 0.05$)
Moghadasian et al. (2006b)	4-week-old male apo-E-deficient mice ($n = 7$–8)	Cholesterol-enriched diet (0.2%, w/w) plus (2%, w/w) soybean-derived phytosterol mixture with or without (1%, w/w) probucol (14 weeks)	↓ 60% in atherosclerotic lesion area; ↑ 66% in HDL-C and ↓ 47% in TC:HDL ratio(phytosterol); ↓ 59% in TC (phytosterol + probucol) (all $P < 0.05$ vs. control)
Ntanios et al. (2003)	11-week-old male F1B hybrid Syrian golden hamsters weighing ~106 g ($n = 20$)	Basal diet containing (30%) of energy as fat enriched with (0.12%, w/w) cholesterol plus PSE (0, 0.24, 0.48, 0.96, 1.92 and 2.84%, w/w) (12 weeks)	~70, 90 and 100% in lipid-filled foam cell areas (0.24, 0.48 and 2.84% PSE); ↓19, 36, 51, 52 and 55% in TC(0.24, 0.48, 0.96, 1.92 and 2.84% PSE); ↓ 77, 50 and 47% in VLDL, LDL- & HDL-C (0.96% PSE) respectively (all $P < 0.001$ vs. control)
Yeganeh et al. (2005)	4-week-old male apo-E-deficient mice ($n = 7$–8)	Cholesterol-enriched diet (0.2%, w/w) plus (2%, w/w) soybean-derived phytosterol mixture with or without (0.1%, w/w) fenofibrate or (0.5%, w/w) niacin (14 weeks)	↓ 50% (phytosterol and phytosterol + niacin) in lesion size; ↓ 59 and 50% (phytosterol and phytosterol + niacin) in lesion:lumen ratio
Nashed et al. (2005)	4-week-old male apo-E-deficient mice	Cholesterol-enriched diet (0.2%, w/w) plus (2%, w/w) soybean-derived phytosterol mixture (14 weeks)	↓ 62% (phytosterol) in lesion size; ↓ 59.4% (phytosterol) in atherosclerotic lesion:lumen ratio versus control ($P < 0.05$)
Ntanios et al. (1998)	4–6-week-old male New Zealand White rabbits 80–100 g ($n = 6$)	Cholesterol-enriched diet (0.5%, w/w) plus PS mixtures (0.01, 0.2, or 0.8%, w/w) (2 months)	↓ 48.6% in TC; ↓ 63% in VLDL-C; ↓ plaque accretion in coronary arteries and ascending aorta in (0.8%, w/w) ($p < 0.005$ vs. control)
Weingärtner et al. (2008)	8–12-week-apo-E-deficient mice weighing 20–25 g ($n = 10$)	WTD containing either (2%, w/w) PSE (0.005%, w/w) ezetimibe or the combination (24 weeks)	↑ 20.4% in plaque sizes (WTD + PSE) versus 10.0% (WTD + ezetimibe); $p < 0.05$

There have been concerns with respect to the possible atherogenicity of PS in some people. These issues were brought up after reporting the formation of xanthomas and premature atherosclerosis in individuals with the autosomal-recessively inherited disease of sitosterolaemia who over absorb PS (Bhattacharyya and Connor, 1974). Increased serum stigmasterol and campesterol levels are thought to be associated with a family history of CAD in patients with hypercholesterolemia (Glueck et al., 1991), suggesting that slightly higher phytosterols were a heritable factor for increased CAD risk. However, like any observational study, no causal relationship can be proven. Similarly, in a nested case–control analysis, Assmann et al. (2006) found that elevated sitosterol concentrations or sitosterol: cholesterol ratios were associated with approximately 3-fold further raise in the CHD risk. Given that only univariate analysis was performed in this study, it is not clear if the positive correlation between plasma sitosterol levels and CHD risk would have still been significant if multivariate analyses had been used. Furthermore, phytosterols have been identified in atherosclerotic plaques biopsies (Miettinen et al., 2005) and stenotic aortic valves (Helske et al., 2008) obtained from patients with apparently normal PS absorption. These findings raised the possibility that phytosterols could be an independent risk marker for CHD. It should be mentioned that these observational studies are not comparable and the results are not conclusive (Patel and Thompson, 2006). Weingärtner et al. (2008) reported a 5-fold increment in sterol concentration in aortic valve tissue along with a rise in plasma PS in patients eating PSE-supplemented margarine (Weingärtner et al., 2008). However, no evidence of selective accumulation of phytosterols in diseased tissue has been found. Indeed, the distribution of PS across body tissues is virtually the same with that of cholesterol. Helske et al. (2008) found no significant differences in the valvular sterol contents between the stenotic and control valves. In parallel, no evidence supporting the association between plasma levels of sitosterol and campesterol and the family history of CHD was found after comparing plasma cholesterol, sitosterol, and campesterol levels in 2542 subjects who underwent coronary artery calcification scoring (Wilund et al., 2004). Windler et al. (2009) found no association between CHD and plasma phytosterol levels in women with incident symptomatic CHD, indicating that plasma PS levels in women with CHD were not higher than those of healthy women of the same age. Similarly, in a cohort of 1242 subjects older than 65 years, participating at the Longitudinal Aging Study Amsterdam (LASA), increased plasma levels of sitosterol were associated with a lowered risk for CHD, suggesting neutral or even protective effects on development of CHD (Fassbender et al., 2008). This was further supported by the observation that PS levels and their ratios to cholesterol were significantly increased in patients without CHD. Furthermore, neither stanols nor markers of cholesterol synthesis differed significantly in subjects with or without CHD (Fassbender et al., 2008). The relationship between plasma PS and the risk of CHD not only was examined in subjects with CHD but also in apparently healthy subjects. In this regard, Pinedo et al. (2007) have shown in a prospective study that the increased concentrations of PS, at least in the physiological range, did not appear to be adversely related to CAD in apparently healthy men and women. Silbernagel et al. (2009) measured plasma cholestanol, a metabolite of cholesterol, lathosterol, a cholesterol precursor, campesterol, and sitosterol levels in 2440 subjects who underwent angiography, and Friesinger scoring (FS) to assess the severity of CAD. The results revealed that while the campesterol: cholesterol ratio significantly associated with the FS ($P < 0.026$), sitosterol to cholesterol ratio showed no significant correlation with the FS in the whole group. The authors concluded that, in the absence of sitosterolemia, plasma PS seems less likely to have an atherogenic effect.

Weingärtner et al. (2009) suggested that increased plasma levels of PS could be an atherogenic risk factor. However, data from the available research showed no overall clear evidence suggesting involvement of PS in the development of atherosclerotic plaque (Chan et al. 2006). Indeed, epidemiological studies have revealed that a 4–5% reduction of LDL-C correlates with a 5–10% reduction in CHD risk in the first 5 years, and by 10% over a life time (Katan et al., 2003). Thus, atherogenic impact of PS seems unlikely, and LDL-C-lowering benefits of PS may far outweigh possible risks. However, more large epidemiological studies are needed to confirm their effect on the CHD risk. Table 6.6 summarizes recent clinical studies regarding antiatherosclerotic effect of phytosterols.

TABLE 6.6
Recent Clinical Studies of Antiatherosclerotic Effects of Phytosterols Treatment

Reference	Study Design	Subjects	Dose of Sterols/Stanols/ Duration	Major Findings
Jakulj et al. (2006)	Double-blind placebo-controlled crossover	Prepubertal children with FH (7–12 years) ($n = 20$)	500 mL of a low-fat yogurt enriched with 2.0 g/day of plant stanols (4 weeks)	↓ 7.5% in TC; ↓ 9.2% in LDL-C ($P < 0.001$); ↔ in FMD of the brachial artery versus placebo
Assmann et al. (2006)	Nested case-control analysis of the prospective cardiovascular münster	Patients with CHD in age, smoking status, and date of investigation-matched population based control (16–65 years) followed for 10 years ($n = 318$)	—	↑ in serum sitosterol levels or sitosterol:cholesterol ratio correlated with ~3-fold ↑ in the risk of CHD ($P < 0.030$)
Gylling et al. (2009)	Randomized, double-blind, parallel controlled	Mildly to moderately hypercholesterolaemic (25–70 years) ($n = 282$)	Plant stanol or PSE (2 g/day) containing spread (1-year)	↓ 4.2% (stanol ester) ($P < 0.01$) and ↓ 4.4 % (sterol ester) in TC ($P < 0.01$) group versus control;↔ in endothelial function
Helske et al. (2008)	Cross-sectional	Patients with clinically significant, symptomatic aortic valve stenosis (67 ± 10 years, mean) ($n = 82$)	—	Correlation of serum ratios of campesterol ($r = 0.88$; $P < 0.0001$ and sitosterol ($r = 0.84$; $P < 0.0001$):cholesterol with those of aortic valve campesterol and sitosterol
Windler et al. (2009)	Case-control study of CAD (CORA) study	Women with CHD in age-matched population-based controls (30–80 years) ($n = 200$)	—	No correlation between CHD and plasma phytosterol levels
Fassbender et al. (2008)	Cross-sectional	Subjects with CHD participating at the LASA (65–89 years) ($n = 1242$)	—	Correlation between ↑ in plasma sitosterol levels and ↓ in the risk for CHD (odd ratio 0.78, CI 0.62–0.98, $P < 0.05$)
Silbernagel et al. (2009)	Cohort study	Subjects with CAD participating in the Ludwigshafen Risk and Cardiovascular health aged study; mean age 58.1 ± 11.6 to 64.9 ± 9.3 years ($n = 2440$)	—	Correlation between high FS and ↑ in cholestanol and campesterol ($P < 0.006$ and $P < 0.026$):cholesterol ratios, but not with sitosterol; ↑ in campesterol, sitosterol and cholestanol:lathosterol ratios correlated with high FS ($P < 0.001$)
Ruiu et al. (2009)	Single-blind randomized crossover	Patients with polygenic Hypercholesterolemia (54.2 ± 7.3 years, mean) ($n = 15$)	Yogurt containing 1.6 g/day esterified phytosterols (equivalent to 1.0 g free phytosterol) (4 weeks)	↓ 4.3% in LDL-C ($P = 0.03$); ↑ ~10% in LDL-receptor affinity ($P = 0.01$); ↓ 18.2% in CD36 expression ($P = 0.01$)

TABLE 6.7
Food and Supplement Products in the Markets Fortified with Phytosterols

Product Brand Name	Matrix	Serving Size	Type and Dose of Phytosterols	Production Company
Benecol® Spreads[a] Benecol® Smart Chews[a]	Spreads chews	1 tbsp 1 chew	0.85 g of plant stanol esters, derived from tall oil, per serving 2 ×/day with meal	McNeil Nutritionals
Promise Take Control® spreads[a]	Spreads	1 tbsp	1 g of PS, derived from esterified SO, per serving 2 ×/day meal	Unilever
Promise activ® SuperShots[a]	Yogurts	3 oz bottle	2.0 g of PS/serving 2 ×/day with meal	Unilever
Nature valley healthy heart Granola bars[a]	Bars	1 bar	0.4 g of CoroWise™ PS 2 ×/day with meal	General Mills, Cargill
Lifetime low fat cheese[a]	Cheese	1 slice	0.65 g of CoroWise™ PS/serving 2 ×/day with meal	Lifeline Food Company, Cargill
[b]VitaTops™	Muffins	2 oz	0.4 g of CoroWise™ PS/serving 2 ×/day with meal	Cargill
[b]Centrum Cardio®	Multivitamins supplements	1 tablet	0.4 g of CoroWise™ phytosterols/serving 2 ×/day with meal	Cargill
Kroger active lifestyle milk[b]	Fat free milk	8 oz	0.4 g of CoroWise™ PS /serving 2 ×/day with meal	Kroger Company, Cargill
Giant Eagle® Fat free milk[b]	Fat free milk	8 oz	0.4 g of CoroWise™ PS/ serving 2 ×/day with meal	Cargill
Orowheat® Whole grain and oat[b]	Bread	1 slice	0.4 g of CoroWise™ PS/serving 2 ×/day with meal	Cargill
Active lifestyle bread from Kroger[b]	Bread	1 slice	0.4 g of CoroWise™ PS/serving 2 ×/day with meal	Cargill
Rice Dream® Heartwise[b]	Rice drink	8 oz	0.65 g of PSE/serving 2 ×/day with meal	Hain Celestial-Cargill
[b]Minute Maid® Premium Heart Wise™	Orange juice	8 oz	1 g of CoroWise™ PS/serving 2 ×/day with meal	Cargill, Coca-Cola Company
Cocoavia chocolate bars[c]	Chocolate bars	1 bar	1.1 to 1.5 g of PS/serving 2 ×/day with meal	Mars, Inc.
Yoplait healthy yogurt[d]	Yogurt	6 oz	0.4 g of CoroWise™ PS/serving 2 ×/day with meal	General Mills, Cargill
[e]Naturemade® Cholest-Off™	Dietary supplement	2 capsules	0.9 g of PS and stanols/serving 2 ×/day with meal	Forbes Medi-Tech, Pharmavite LLC

Source: http://findarticles.com/p/articles/mi_m0EIN/is_2003_March_4/ai_98320214 accessed February 26, 2009.

[a]   "More about Heart Health." October 03, 2007. http://www.highdesertslimdown.com/body?page = 4 accessed February 26, 2009.

[c]   "CocoaVia® Brand Heart Healthy Snacks." http://www.cocoavia.com/products/ accessed February 26, 2009.

[b]   "Foods Enriched with Plant Sterols." 2007. 2 December 2007. http://www.corowise.com/products.html accessed February 26, 2009.

[d]   "Health Publications, The culture wars: finding the best yogurts." Sept, 2005 http://findarticles.com/p/articles/mi_m0813/is_7_32/ai_n15342949 accessed February 26, 2009.

[e]   "Forbes Medi-Tech Announces Pharmavite Contract Extension." March 4, 2003.

6.6   PHYTOSTEROL-ENRICHED PRODUCTS ON MARKETS

The use of PS alone or in a combination with either low-saturated fat diet, drug therapy, or other functional food components has resulted in significant reductions in plasma TC and LDL-C levels. This encourages FDA and NCEP ATP III to recommend the use of phytosterol-enriched functional foods as part of an optimal dietetic prevention strategy in primary and secondary prevention of CVD. Phytosterol may have utmost potential impact to reduce the costs associated with the use of pharmacological approaches to cholesterol management. In fact, the use of fat spreads containing PS has been estimated to save $150 million annually in healthcare costs in the United Kingdom alone (Zawistowski and Kitts, 2004). FDA stated that the food must contain at least 0.65 g of PSE or at least 1.7 g of plant stanol esters/serving (2 × /day) with other foods to provide daily total intake of at least 1.3 g for PSE and 3.4 g for plant stanol esters as part of a diet low in saturated fat and cholesterol (FDA, 2000). On account of their solubility in oily food matrices, PS and stanols have been incorporated to margarines or dressings (Law, 2000). Food processing such as emulsification using lecithin improved texture, decreased calorie, and resulted in nonfat or low-fat food and beverages enriched with phytosterols, such as bread, breakfast cereal, snack bars, milk, and yoghurt (Ostlund, 2004; Clifton et al., 2004). Table 6.7 shows some commercially available food and supplement products fortified with phytosterols on the markets in many countries including the United States and Europe.

6.7   CONCLUSIONS

We have provided support, based on experimental and clinical studies that circulating cholesterol and proinflammatory cytokines levels can be reduced by ingestion of phytosterols, and thus may have a great potential in reducing cardiovascular risk. Further, clinical trials investigating the relationship between plasma PS levels and CHD (e.g., long-term trials or epidemiological studies) are certainly warranted.

ACKNOWLEDGMENT

Rgia A. Othman is grateful to the Libyan Scholarship Program and the Natural Sciences and Engineering Research Council of Canada (NSERC) for financial support.

REFERENCES

"FDA Authorizes New Coronary Heart Disease Health Claim for Plant Sterol and Plant Stanol Esters." FDA Talk Paper. September 5, 2000. Available at: http://www.cfsan.fda.gov/~lrd/tpsterol.html accessed February 26, 2009.

AbuMweis, S.S., Barake, R., Jones, P.J. 2008. Plant sterols/stanols as cholesterol lowering agents: A meta-analysis of randomized controlled trials. *Food Nutr Res.* **52**. Epub 2008 Aug 18.

Acuff, R.V., Cai, D.J., Dong, Z.P., Bell, D. 2007. The lipid lowering effect of plant sterol ester capsules in hypercholesterolemic subjects. *Lipids Health Dis.* **9**(6): 11.

Al-Yousuf, M.H., Ali, B.H., Bashir, A.K., Tanira, M.O., Blunden, G. 2002. Central nervous system activity of *Leucas inflata* Benth. in mice. *Phytomedicine* **9**: 3501–3507.

Assmann, G., Cullen, P., Erbey, J., Ramey, D.R., Kannenberg, F., Schulte, H. 2006. Plasma sitosterol elevations are associated with an increased incidence of coronary events in men: Results of a nested case–control analysis of the Prospective Cardiovascular Münster (PROCAM) study. *Nutr Metab Cardiovasc Dis.* **16**: 13–21.

Awad, A.B., Fink, C.S. 2000. Phytosterols as anticancer dietary components: Evidence and mechanism of action. *J Nutr.* **130**: 2127–2130.

Awad, A.B., Burr, A.T., Fink, C.S. 2005. Effect of resveratrol and β-sitosterol in combination on reactive oxygen species and prostaglandin release by PC-3 cells. *Prostaglandins Leukot Essent Fatty Acids.* **72**: 219–226.

Awad, A.B., Smith, A.J., Fink, C.S. 2001. Plant sterols regulate rat vascular smooth muscle cell growth and prostacyclin release in culture. *Prostaglandins Leukot Essent Fatty Acids.* **64**: 323–330.

Awad, A.B., Toczek, J., Fink, C.S. 2004. Phytosterols decrease prostaglandin release in cultured P388D(1)/MAB macrophages. *Prostaglandins Leukot Essent Fatty Acids.* **70**: 511–520.

Batta, A.K., Xu, G., Bollineni, J.S., Shefer, S., Salen, G. 2005. Effect of high plant sterol enriched diet and cholesterol absorption inhibitor, SCH 58235, on plant sterol absorption and plasma concentrations in hypercholesterolemic wild-type Kyoto rats. *Metabolism* **54**: 38–48.

Batta, A.K., Xu, G., Honda, A., Miyazaki, T., Salen, G. 2006. Stigmasterol reduces plasma cholesterol levels and inhibits hepatic synthesis and intestinal absorption in the rat. *Metabolism* **55**: 292–299.

Bays, H.E., Neff, D., Tomassini, J.E., Tershakovec, A.M. 2008. Ezetimibe: Cholesterol lowering and beyond. *Expert Rev Cardiovasc Ther.* **6**: 447–470.

Berge, K.E., Tian, H., Graf, G.A. et al. 2000. Accumulation of dietary cholesterol in sitosterolemia caused by mutations in adjacent ABC transporters. *Science* **290**: 1771–1775.

Berger, A., Jones, P.J., AbuMweis, S.S. 2004. Plant sterols: Factors affecting their efficacy and safety as functional food ingredients. *Lipids Health Dis.* **7**(3): 5.

Bhattacharyya, A.K., Connor, W.E. 1974. Beta-sitosterolemia and xanthomatosis. A newly described lipid storage disease in two sisters. *J Clin Invest.* **53**: 1033–1043.

Bosner, M.S., Lange, L.G., Stenson, W.F., Ostlund, R.E. Jr. 1999. Percent cholesterol absorption in normal women and men quantified with dual stable isotopic tracers and negative ion mass spectrometry. *J Lipid Res.* **40**: 302–308.

Bouic, P.J. 2002. Sterols and sterolins: New drugs for the immune system? *Drug Discov Today.* **15**(7): 775–778.

Bouic, P.J., Clark, A., Lamprecht, J. et al. 1999. The effects of β-sitosterol (BSS) and β sitosterol glucoside (BSSG) mixture on selected immune parameters of marathon runners: Inhibition of post marathon immune suppression and inflammation. *Int J Sports Med.* **20**: 258–262.

Bouic, P.J., Etsebeth, S., Liebenberg, R.W., Albrecht, C.F., Pegel, K., Van Jaarsveld, P.P. 1996. Beta-sitosterol and beta-sitosterol glucoside stimulate human peripheral blood lymphocyte proliferation: Implications for their use as an immunomodulatory vitamin combination. *Int J Immunopharmacol.* **18**: 693–700.

Bouic, P.J. Clark, A., Brittle, W. et al. 2001. Plant sterol/sterolin supplement use in a cohort of SA HIV infected patients: Effects on immunological and virological surrogate markers. *S Afr Med J.* **91**: 848–850.

Breytenbach, U., Clark, A., Lamprecht, J., Bouic, P. 2001. Flow cytometric analysis of the Th1-Th2 balance in healthy individuals and patients infected with the human immunodeficiency virus (HIV) receiving a plant sterol/sterolin mixture. *Cell Biol Int.* **25**: 43–49.

Calpe-Berdie, L., Escolà-Gil, J.C., Ribas, V., Navarro-Sastre, A., Garcés- Garcés, J., Blanco-Vaca, F. 2005. Changes in intestinal and liver global gene expression in response to a phytosterol-enriched diet. *Atherosclerosis.* **181**: 75–85.

Calpe-Berdiel, L., Escolà-Gil, J.C., Benítez, S. et al. 2007. Dietary phytosterols modulate T-helper immune response but do not induce apparent anti-inflammatory effects in a mouse model of acute, aseptic inflammation. *Life Sci.* **80**: 1951–1956.

Calpe-Berdiel, L., Escola-Gil, J.C., Blanco-Vaca, F. 2006. Phytosterol-mediated inhibition of intestinal cholesterol absorption is independent of ATP binding cassette transporter A1. *Br J Nutr.* **95**: 618–622.

Castro Cabezas, M., de Vries, J.H., Van Oostrom, A.J., Iestra, J., van Staveren, W.A. 2006. Effects of a stanol-enriched diet on plasma cholesterol and triglycerides in patients treated with statin. *J Am Diet Assoc.* **106**: 1564–1569.

Chan, Y.M., Varady, K.A., Lin, Y., Trautwein, E., Mensink, R.P., Plat, J., Jones, P.J. 2006. Plasma concentrations of plant sterols: Physiology and relationship with coronary heart disease. *Nutr Rev.* **64**: 385–402.

Charest, A., Vanstone, C., St-Onge, M.P., Parson, W., Jones, P.J., Lamarche, B. 2005. Phytosterols in nonfat and low-fat beverages have no impact on the LDL size phenotype. *Eur J Clin Nutr.* **59**: 801–804.

Child, P., Kuksis, A. 1986. Investigation of the role of micellar phospholipids in the preferential uptake of cholesterol over sitosterol by dispersed rat jejunal villus cells. *Biochem Cell Biol.* **64**: 847–853.

Cleghorn, C.L., Skeaff, C.M., Mann, J., Chisholm, A. 2003. Plant sterol—Enriched spread enhances the cholesterol-lowering potential of a fat-reduced diet. *Eur J Clin Nutr.* **57**: 170–176.

Clifton, P.M., Mano, M., Duchateau, G.S., van der knap, H.C., Trautwein, E. A. 2008. Dose–response effects of plant sterol sources in fat spreads on serum lipids and C reactive protein and on kinetic behavior of serum plant sterols. *Eur J Clin Nutr.* **62**: 968–977.

Clifton, P.M., Noakes, M., Sullivan, D. et al. 2004. Cholesterol-lowering effects of plant sterol esters differ in milk, yoghurt, bread and cereal. *Eur J Clin Nutr.* **58**: 503–509.

de Jong, A., Plat, J., Bast, A., Godschalk, R.W., Basu, S., Mensink, R.P. 2008b. Effects of plant sterol and stanol ester consumption on lipid metabolism, antioxidant status and markers of oxidative stress, endothelial function and low-grade inflammation in patients on current statin treatment. *Eur J Clin Nutr.* **62**: 263–273.

de Jong, A., Plat, J., Lütjohann, D., Mensink, R.P. 2008a. Effects of long-term plant sterol or stanol ester consumption on lipid and lipoprotein metabolism in subjects on statin treatment. *Br J Nutr.* **100**: 937–941.

de Jong, A., Plat, J., Mensink, R.P. 2003. Metabolic effects of plant sterols and stanols. *J Nutr Biochem.* **14**: 362–369.

de Jong, N., Zuur, A., Wolfs, M.C., Wendel-Vos, G.C., van Raaij, J.M., Schuit, A.J. 2007. Exposure and effectiveness of phytosterol/-stanol-enriched margarines. *Eur J Clin Nutr.* **61**: 1407–1415.

Demonty, I., Chan, Y.M., Pelled, D., Jones, P.J. 2006. Fish-oil esters of plant sterols improve the lipid profile of dyslipidemic subjects more than do fish-oil or sunflower oil esters of plant sterols. *Am J Clin Nutr.* **84**: 1534–1542.

Demonty, I., Ebine, N., Jia, X., Jones, P.J. 2005. Fish oil fatty acid esters of phytosterols alter plasma lipids but not red blood cell fragility in hamsters. *Lipids* **40**: 695–702.

Demonty, I., Ras, R.T., van der Knaap, H.C. et al. 2009. Continuous dose–response relationship of the LDL-cholesterol—lowering effect of phytosterol intake. *J Nutr.* **139**: 271–284.

Devaraj, S., Autret, B.C., Jialal, I. 2006. Reduced-calorie orange juice beverage with plant sterols lowers C-reactive protein concentrations and improves the lipid profile in human volunteers. *Am J Clin Nutr.* **84**: 756–7561.

Doornbos, A.M., Meynen, E.M., Duchateau, G.S., van der Knaap, H.C., Trautwein, E.A. 2006. Intake occasion affects the serum cholesterol lowering of a plant sterol enriched single-dose yoghurt drink in mildly hypercholesterolaemic subjects. *Eur J Clin Nutr.* **60**: 325–333.

Earnest, C.P., Mikus, C.R., Lemieux, I., Arsenault, B.J., Church, T.S. 2007. Examination of encapsulated phytosterol ester supplementation on lipid indices associated with cardiovascular disease. *Nutrition* **23**: 625–633.

Ebine, N., Demonty, I., Jia, X., Jones, P.J. 2006. Plant stanol ascorbate esters reduce body weight gain through decreased energy absorption in hamsters. *Int J Obes*(Lond). **30**: 751–757.

Ebine, N., Jia, X., Demonty, I., Wang, Y., Jones, P. J. 2005. Effects of a water-soluble phytostanol ester on plasma cholesterol levels and red blood cell fragility in hamsters. *Lipids* **40**: 175–180.

Ewart, H.S., Cole, L.K., Kralovec, J. et al. 2002. Fish oil containing phytosterol esters alters blood lipid profiles and left ventricle generation of thromboxane a(2) in adult guinea pigs. *J Nutr.* **132**: 1149–1152.

Expert Panel on Detection, Evaluation, and Treatment of High Blood Cholesterol in Adults. 2001. Executive Summary of the Third Report of the National Cholesterol Education Program (NCEP) Expert Panel on Detection, Evaluation, and Treatment of High Blood Cholesterol in Adults (Adult Treatment Panel III). *JAMA.* **285**: 2486–2497.

Fassbender, K., Lütjohann, D., Dik, M.G. et al. 2008. Moderately elevated plant sterol levels are associated with reduced cardiovascular risk—The LASA study. *Atherosclerosis.* **196**: 283–288.

Feigin, A.M., Teeter, J.H., Brand, J.G. 1995. The influence of sterols on the sensitivity of lipid bilayers to melittin. *Biochem Biophys Res Commun.* **211**: 312–317.

Fernandez, C., Suarez, Y., Ferruelo, A.J., Gomez-Coronado, D., Lasuncion, M.A. 2002. Inhibition of cholesterol biosynthesis by Delta22-unsaturated phytosterols via competitive inhibition of sterol Delta24-reductase in mammalian cells. *Biochem J.* **366**: 109–119.

Francisco, M.L., Resurreccion, A.V. 2008. Functional components in peanuts. *Crit Rev Food Sci Nutr.* **48**(8): 715–746.

Franz, M.J., Bantle, J.P., Beebe, C.A. et al. 2003. American Diabetes Association. Evidence-based nutrition principles and recommendations for the treatment and prevention of diabetes and related complications. *Diabetes Care.* **26**(suppl 1): S51–S61.

Fuhrman, B., Plat, D., Herzog, Y., Aviram, M. 2007. Consumption of a novel dietary formula of plant sterol esters of canola oil fatty acids, in a canola oil matrix containing 1,3-diacylglycerol, reduces oxidative stress in atherosclerotic apolipoprotein E-deficient mice. *J Agric Food Chem.* **55**: 2028–2033.

Galman, C., Angelin, B., Rudling, M. 2005. Bile acid synthesis in humans has a rapid diurnal variation that is asynchronous with cholesterol synthesis. *Gastroenterology.* **129**: 1445–1453.

Glueck, C.J., Speirs, J., Tracy, T., Streicher, P., Illig, E., Vandegrift, J. 1991. Relationships of serum plant sterols (phytosterols) and cholesterol in 595 hypercholesterolemic subjects, and familial aggregation of phytosterols, cholesterol, and premature coronary heart disease in hyperphytosterolemic probands and their first-degree relatives. *Metabolism.* **40**: 842–848.

Gua, J.K., Luke, A.H., Lee, W.P., Schoeller, D. 1993. Compound-specific carbon isotope ratio determination of enriched cholesterol. *Anal Chem.* **65**: 1954–1959.

Gylling, H., Hallikainen, M., Raitakari, O.T. et al. 2009. Long-term consumption of plant stanol and sterol esters, vascular function and genetic regulation. *Br J Nutr.* **101**: 1688–1695.

Hallikainen, M., Lyyra-Laitinen, T., Laitinen, T. et al. 2006. Endothelial function in hypercholesterolemic subjects: Effects of plant stanol and sterol esters. *Atherosclerosis.* **188**: 425–432.

Hallikainen, M., Lyyra-Laitinen, T., Laitinen, T., Moilanen, L., Miettinen, T.A., Gylling, H. 2008. Effects of plant stanol esters on serum cholesterol concentrations, relative markers of cholesterol metabolism and endothelial function in type 1 diabetes. *Atherosclerosis.* **199**: 432–439.

Hansel, B., Nicolle, C., Lalanne, F. et al. 2007. Effect of low-fat, fermented milk enriched with plant sterols on serum lipid profile and oxidative stress in moderate hypercholesterolemia. *Am J Clin Nutr.* **86**: 790–796.

Hayes, K.C., Pronczuk, A., Wijendran, V., Beer, M. 2002. Free phytosterols effectively reduce plasma and liver cholesterol in gerbils fed cholesterol. *J Nutr.* **132**: 1983–1988.

Heinemann, T., Axtmann, G., von Bergmann, K. 1993. Comparison of intestinal absorption of cholesterol with different plant sterols in man. *Eur J Clin Invest.* **23**: 827–831.

Heinemann, T., Kullak-Ublick, A., Pietruck, B., von Bergman, K. 1991. Mechanism of action of plant sterols on inhibition of cholesterol absorption. *Eur J Clin Pharmacol* **40**(suppl 1): 59S–63S.

Helske, S., Miettinen, T., Gylling, H. et al. 2008. Accumulation of cholesterol precursors and plant sterols in human stenotic aortic valves. *J Lipid Res.* **49**: 1511–1518.

Henriksen, T., Mahoney, E.M., Steinberg, D. 1981. Enhanced macrophage degradation of low density lipoprotein previously incubated with cultured endothelial cells: Recognition by receptors for acetylated low density lipoproteins. *Proc Natl Acad Sci USA.* **78**: 6499–6503.

Hirai, K., Shimazu, C., Takezoe, R. et al. 1986. Cholesterol, phytosterol and polyunsaturated fatty acid levels in 1982 and 1957 in Japanese diets. *J Nutr Sci Vitaminol.* **32**: 363–372.

Ho, S.S., Pal, S. 2005. Margarine phytosterols decrease the secretion of atherogenic lipoproteins from HepG2 liver and Caco2 intestinal cells. *Atherosclerosis.* **182**: 29–36.

Holubkov, R., Karas, R.H., Pepine, C.J. et al. 2002. Large brachial artery diameter is associated with angiographic coronary artery disease in women. *Am Heart J.* **143**: 802–807.

Jain, D., Ebine, N., Jia, X. et al. 2008. Corn fiber oil and sitostanol decrease cholesterol absorption independently of intestinal sterol transporters in hamsters. *J Nutr Biochem.* **19**: 229–236.

Jakulj, L., Trip, M.D., Sudhop, T., von Bergmann, K., Kastelein, J.J., Vissers, M.N. 2005. Inhibition of cholesterol absorption by the combination of dietary plant sterols and ezetimibe: Effects on plasma lipid levels. *J Lipid Res.* **46**: 2692–2698.

Jakulj, L., Vissers, M.N., Rodenburg, J., Wiegman, A., Trip, M.D., Kastelein, J.J. 2006. Plant stanols do not restore endothelial function in pre-pubertal children with familial hypercholesterolemia despite reduction of low-density lipoprotein cholesterol levels. *J Pediatr.* **148**: 495–500.

Jauhiainen, T., Salo, P., Niittynen, L., Poussa, T., Korpela, R. 2006. Effects of low-fat hard cheese enriched with plant stanol esters on serum lipids and apolipoprotein B in mildly hypercholesterolaemic subjects. *Eur J Clin Nutr* **60**: 1253–1257.

Jenkins, D.J., Kendall, C.W., Marchie, A. et al. 2003. Effects of a dietary portfolio of cholesterol-lowering foods vs. lovastatin on serum lipids and C-reactive protein. *JAMA.* **290**: 502–510.

Jenkins, D.J., Kendall, C.W., Marchie, A. et al. 2005a. Direct comparison of a dietary portfolio of cholesterol-lowering foods with a statin in hypercholesterolemic participants. *Am J Clin Nutr.* **81**: 380–387.

Jenkins, D.J., Kendall, C.W., Marchie, A. et al. 2005b. Direct comparison of dietary portfolio vs. statin on C-reactive protein. *Eur J Clin Nutr.* **59**: 851–860.

Jenkins, D.J., Kendall, C.W., Nguyen, T.H. et al. 2008. Effect of plant sterols in combination with other cholesterol-lowering foods. *Metabolism.* **5**: 130–139.

Jia, X., Ebine, N., Demonty, I. et al. 2007. Hypocholesterolaemic effects of plant sterol analogues are independent of ABCG5 and ABCG8 transporter expressions in hamsters. *Br J Nutr.* **98**: 550–555.

Jones, P.J., Demonty, I., Chan, Y.M., Herzog, Y., Pelled, D. 2007. Fish-oil esters of plant sterols differ from vegetable-oil sterol esters in triglycerides lowering, carotenoid bioavailability and impact on plasminogen activator inhibitor-1 (PAI-1) concentrations in hypercholesterolemic subjects. *Lipids Health Dis.* **6**: 28–32.

Jones, P.J., Vanstone, C.A., Raeini-Sarjaz, M., St-Onge, M.P. 2003. Phytosterols in low- and nonfat beverages as part of a controlled diet fail to lower plasma lipid levels. *J Lipid Res.* **44**: 1713–1719.

Kassis, A.N., Vanstone, C.A., AbuMweis, S.S., Jones, P.J. 2008. Efficacy of plant sterols is not influenced by dietary cholesterol intake in hypercholesterolemic individuals. *Metabolism* **57**: 339–346.

Katan, M.B., Grundy, S.M., Jones, P., Law, M., Miettinen, T., Paoletti, R. 2003. Efficacy and safety of plant stanols and sterols in the management of blood cholesterol levels. *Mayo Clin Proc.* **78**: 965–978.

Kidambi, S., Patel, S.B. 2008. Sitosterolaemia: Pathophysiology, clinical presentation and laboratory diagnosis. *J Clin Pathol.* **61**: 588–594.

Kim, S.J., Jeong, H.J., Yi, B.J. et al. 2007. Transgenic Panax ginseng inhibits the production of TNF-alpha, IL-6, and IL-8 as well as COX-2 expression in human mast cells. *Am J Chin Med.* **35**: 329–339.

Kobori, M., Yoshida, M., Ohnishi-Kameyama, M., Shinmoto, H. 2007. Ergosterol peroxide from an edible mushroom suppresses inflammatory responses in RAW 264.7 macrophages and growth of HT29 colon adenocarcinoma cells. *Br J Pharmacol.* **150**: 209–219.

Kochhar, S. 1983. Influence of processing on sterols of edible vegetable oils. *Prog Lipid Res.* **22**: 161–188.

Konlande, J.E., Fisher, H. 1969. Evidence for a nonabsorptive antihypercholesterolemic action of phytosterols in the chicken. *J Nutr.* **98**: 435–442.

Korpela, R., Tuomilehto, J., Högström, P. et al. 2006. Safety aspects and cholesterol lowering efficacy of low fat dairy products containing plant sterols. *Eur J Clin Nutr.* **60**: 633–642.

Kozlowska-Wojciechowska, M., Jastrzebska, M., Naruszewicz, M., Foltyńska, A. 2003. Impact of margarine enriched with plant sterols on blood lipids, platelet function, and fibrinogen level in young men. *Metabolism.* **52**: 1373–1378.

Kratz, M., Kannenberg, F., Gramenz, E. et al. 2007. Similar serum plant sterol responses of human subjects heterozygous for a mutation causing sitosterolemia and controls to diets enriched in plant sterols or stanols. *Eur J Clin Nutr.* **61**: 896–905.

Kris-Etherton, P.M., Hecker, K.D., Bonanome, A. et al. 2002. Bioactive compounds in foods: Their role in the prevention of cardiovascular disease and cancers. *Am J Med.* **113**: 71S–88S.

Lamarche, B., Desroches, S., Jenkins, D.J. et al. 2004. Combined effects of a dietary portfolio of plant sterols, vegetable protein, viscous fibre and almonds on LDL particle size. *Br J Nutr.* **92**: 657–663.

Law, M. 2000. Plant sterol and stanol margarines and health. *BMJ.* **320**: 861–864.

Lee, J.H., Lee, J.Y., Park, J.H. et al. 2007. Immunoregulatory activity by daucosterol, a beta-sitosterol glycoside, induces protective Th1 immune response against disseminated Candidiasis in mice. *Vaccine.* **25**: 3834–3840.

Lewington, S., Whitlock, G., Clarke, R. et al. 2007. Blood cholesterol and vascular mortality by age, sex, and blood pressure: A meta-analysis of individual data from 61 prospective studies with 55,000 vascular deaths. *Lancet.* **370**(9602): 1829–1839.

Li, N.Y., Li, K., Qi, Z. et al. 2007. Plant sterol-enriched milk tea decreases blood cholesterol concentrations in Chinese adults: A randomised controlled trial. *Br J Nutr.* **98**: 978–983.

Libby, P., Ridker, P.M., Maseri, A. 2002. Inflammation and atherosclerosis. *Circulation.* **105**: 1135–1143.

Ling, W.H., Jones, P.J.H. 1995. Enhanced efficacy of sitostanol-containing versus sitostanol-free phytosterol mixtures in altering lipoprotein cholesterol levels and synthesis in rats. *Atherosclerosis.* **118**: 319–331.

Lukic, T., Wasan, K.M., Zamfir, D., Moghadasian, M.H., Pritchard, P.H. 2003. Disodium ascorbyl phytostanyl phosphate reduces plasma cholesterol concentrations and atherosclerotic lesion formation in apolipoprotein E-deficient mice. *Metabolism.* **52**: 425–431.

Lv, N., Song, M.Y., Kim, E.K., Park, J.W., Kwon, K.B., Park, B.H. 2008. Guggulsterone, a plant sterol, inhibits NF-kappaB activation and protects pancreatic beta cells from cytokine toxicity. *Mol Cell Endocrinol.* **289**: 49–59.

Madsen, M.B., Jensen, A.M., Schmidt, E.B. 2007. The effect of a combination of plant sterol-enriched foods in mildly hypercholesterolemic subjects. *Clin Nutr.* **26**: 792–798.

Maes, B.D., Hiele, M.I., Guypens, B.J., Ghoos, Y.F., Rutgeerts, P.J. 1998. Gastric emptying of the liquid, solid and oil phase of a meal in normal volunteers and patients with Billroth II gastrojejunostomy. *Eur J Clin Invest.* **28**: 197–204.

Marinangeli, C.P., Varady, K.A., Jones, P.J. 2006. Plant sterols combined with exercise for the treatment of hypercholesterolemia: Overview of independent and synergistic mechanisms of action. *J Nutr Biochem.* **17**: 217–224.

Matsuyama, T., Shoji, K., Takase, H. et al. 2007. Effects of phytosterols in diacylglycerol as part of diet therapy on hyperlipidemia in children. *Asia Pac J Clin Nutr.* **16**: 40–48.

Matvienko, O.A., Lewis, D.S., Swanson, M., Arndt, B., Rainwater, D.L., Stewart, J., Alekel, D.L. 2002. A single daily dose of soybean phytosterols in ground beef decreases serum total cholesterol and LDL cholesterol in young, mildly hypercholesterolemic men. *Am J Clin Nutr.* **76**: 57–64.

Meijer, G.W., Bressers, M.A., de Groot, W.A., Rudrum, M. 2003. Effect of structure and form on the ability of plant sterols to inhibit cholesterol absorption in hamsters. *Lipids.* **38**: 713–721.

Mel'nikov, S.M., Seijen ten Hoorn, J.W., Bertrand, B. 2004. Can cholesterol absorption be reduced by phytosterols and phytostanols via a cocrystallization mechanism? *Chem Phys Lipids.* **127**: 15–33.

Micallef, M.A., Garg, M.L. 2008. The lipid-lowering effects of phytosterols and (n-3) polyunsaturated fatty acids are synergistic and complementary in hyperlipidemic men and women. *J Nutr.* **138**: 1086–1090.

Miettinen, T.A., Gylling, H. 2009. The effects of statins and sitosterols: Benefit or not? *Curr Atheroscler Rep.* **11**: 23–27.

Miettinen, T.A., Railo, M., Lepantalo, M., Gylling, H. 2005. Plant sterols in serum and in atherosclerotic plaques of patients undergoing carotid endarterectomy. *J Am Coll Cardiol.* **45**: 1794–1801.

Miettinen, T.A., Tilvis, R.S., Kesäniemi, Y.A. 1990. Serum plant sterols and cholesterol precursors reflect cholesterol absorption and synthesis in volunteers of a randomly selected male population. *Am J Epidemiol.* **131**: 20–31.

Moghadasian, M.H. 2006a. Dietary phytosterols reduce probucol-induced atherogenesis in apo E-KO mice. *Atherosclerosis.* **188**: 28–34.

Moghadasian, M.H. 2006b. Dietary phytosterols reduce cyclosporine-induced hypercholesterolemia in apolipoprotein E-knockout mice. *Transplantation.* **27**(81): 207–213.

Moghadasian, M.H., Godin, D.V., McManus, B.M., Frohlich, J.J. 1999b. Lack of regression of atherosclerotic lesions in phytosterol-treated apo E-deficient mice. *Life Sci.* **64**: 1029–1036.

Moghadasian, M.H., McManus, B.M., Godin, D.V., Rodrigues, B., Frohlich, J.J. 1999a. Proatherogenic and antiatherogenic effects of probucol and phytosterols in apolipoprotein E-deficient mice: Possible mechanisms of action. *Circulation.* **99**: 1733–1739.

Moghadasian, M.H., McManus, B.M., Pritchard, P.H., Frohlich, J.J. 1997. "Tall oil" derived phytosterols reduce atherosclerosis in ApoE-deficient mice. *Arterioscler Thromb Vasc Biol.* **17**: 119–126.

Moghadasian, M.H., Nguyen, L.B., Shefer, S., McManus, B.M., Frohlich, J.J. 1999c. Histologic, hematologic, and biochemical characteristics of apo E-deficient mice: Effects of dietary cholesterol and phytosterols. *Lab Invest.* **79**: 355–364.

Moghadasian, M.H., Nguyen, L.B., Shefer, S., Salen, G., Batta, A.K., Frohlich, J.J. 2001. Hepatic cholesterol and bile acid synthesis, low-density lipoprotein receptor function, and plasma and fecal sterol levels in mice: Effects of apolipoprotein E deficiency and probucol or phytosterol treatment. *Metabolism.* **50**: 708–714.

Morton, G.M., Lee, S.M., Buss, D.H. et al. 1995. Intakes and major dietary sources of cholesterol and phytosterols in the British diet. *J Human Nutr Diet.* **8**: 429–440.

Moruisi, K.G., Oosthuizen, W., Opperman, A.M. 2006. Phytosterols/stanols lower cholesterol concentrations in familial hypercholesterolemic subjects: A systematic review with meta-analysis. *J Am Coll Nutr.* **25**: 41–48.

Mussner, M.J., Parhofer, K.G., von Bergmann, K., Schwandt, P., Broedl. U., Otto. C. 2002. Effects of phytosterol ester–enriched margarine on plasma lipoproteins in mild to moderate hypercholesterolemia are related to basal cholesterol and fat intake. *Metabolism.* **51**: 189–194.

Naruszewicz, M., Kozlowska-Wojciechowska, M. 2007. Plant sterols beyond low-density lipoprotein-cholesterol. *Br J Nutr.* **98**: 454–455.

Nashed, B., Yeganeh, B., HayGlass, K.T., Moghadasian, M.H. 2005. Antiatherogenic effects of dietary plant sterols are associated with inhibition of proinflammatory cytokine production in apo E-KO mice. *J Nutr.* **135**: 2438–2444.

Naumann, E., Plat, J., Kester, A.D., Mensink, R.P. 2008. The baseline serum lipoprotein profile is related to plant stanol induced changes in serum lipoprotein cholesterol and triacylglycerol concentrations. *J Am Coll Nutr.* **27**: 117–126.

Navarro, A., De las Heras, B., Villar, A. 2001. Anti-inflammatory and immunomodulating properties of a sterol fraction from Sideritis foetens Clem. *Biol Pharm Bull.* **24**: 470–473.

Niittynen, L.H., Jauhiainen, T.A., Poussa, T.A., Korpela, R. 2008. Effects of yoghurt enriched with free plant sterols on the levels of serum lipids and plant sterols in moderately hypercholesterolaemic subjects on a high-fat diet. *Int J Food Sci Nutr.* **59**: 357–367.

Noakes, M., Clifton, P.M., Doornbos, A.M., Trautwein, E.A. 2005. Plant sterol ester enriched milk and yoghurt effectively reduce serum cholesterol in modestly hypercholesterolemic subjects. *Eur J Nutr.* **44**: 214–222.

Normén, L., Shaw, C.A., Fink, C.S., Awad, A.B. 2004. Combination of phytosterols and omega-3 fatty acids: A potential atrategy to promote cardiovascular health. *Curr Med Chem Cardiovasc Hematol Agents.* **2**: 1–12.

Ntanios, F.Y., Jones, P.J.H. 1998. Effects of variable dietary sitostanol concentrations on plasma lipid profile and phytosterol metabolism in hamsters. *Biochim Biophys Acta.* **1390**: 237–244.

Ntanios, F.Y., Jones, P.J., Frohlich, J.J. 1998. Dietary sitostanol reduces plaque formation but not lecithin cholesterol acyl transferase activity in rabbits. *Atherosclerosis.* **138**: 101–110.

Ntanios, F.Y., van de Kooij, A.J., de Deckere, E.A., Duchateau, G.S., Trautwein, E.A. 2003. Effects of various amounts of dietary plant sterol esters on plasma and hepatic sterol concentration and aortic foam cell formation of cholesterol-fed hamsters. *Atherosclerosis.* **169**: 41–50.

Ohr, L.M. 2003. Fats for healthy living. *Food Technol.* **57**: 91–96.

Oram, J.F., Vaughan, A.M. 2006. ATP-binding cassette cholesterol transporters and cardiovascular disease. *Circ Res.* **99**: 1031–1043.

Ostlund, R.E. Jr. 2002. Phytosterols in human nutrition. *Ann Rev Nutr.* **22**: 533–549.

Ostlund, R.E. Jr., McGill, J.B., Zeng, C.M. et al. 2002. Gastrointestinal absorption and plasma kinetics of soy Delta(5)-phytosterols and phytostanols in humans. *Am J Physiol Endocrinol Metab.* **282**: E911–E916.

Ostlund, R.E. Jr. 2004. Phytosterols and cholesterol metabolism. *Curr Opin Lipidol.* 15: 37–41.

Park, E.H., Kahng, J.H., Lee, S.H., Shin, K.H. 2001. An anti-inflammatory principle from cactus. *Fitoterapia.* **72**: 288–290.

Pascot, A., Lemieux, S., Lemieux, I. et al. 1999. Age-related increase in visceral adipose tissue and body fat and the metabolic risk profile of premenopausal women. *Diabetes Care.* **22**: 1471–1478.

Patch, C.S., Tapsell, L.C., Williams, P.G, Gordon, M. 2006. Plant sterols as dietary adjuvants in the reduction of cardiovascular risk: Theory and evidence. *Vasc Health Risk Manag.* **2**: 157–162.

Patel, M.D., Thompson, P.D. 2006. Phytosterols and vascular disease. *Atherosclerosis.* **186**: 12–19.

Perisee, D.M. 2005. Food fortification with plant sterol/stanol for hyperlipidemia: Management in free-living populations. *J Am Diet Assoc.* **105**: 52–53.

Piironen, V., Lindsay, D.G., Miettinen, T.A., Tovio, J., Lampi, A.M. 2000. Plant sterols: Biosynthesis, biological function and their importance to human nutrition. *J Sci Food Agric.* **80**: 939–966.

Pinedo, S., Vissers, M.N., von Bergmann, K. et al. 2007. Plasma levels of plant sterols and the risk of coronary artery disease: The prospective EPIC-Norfolk Population Study. *J Lipid Res.* **48**: 139–144.

Plana, N., Nicolle, C., Ferre, R. et al. 2008. Plant sterol-enriched fermented milk enhances the attainment of LDL cholesterol goal in hypercholesterolemic subjects. *Eur J Nutr.* **47**: 32–39.

Plat, J., Mensink, R.P. 2005. Food components and immune function. *Curr Opin Lipidol.* **16**: 31–37.

Plat, J., Mensink, R.P. 2000. Vegetable oil based versus wood based stanol ester mixtures: Effects on serum lipids and hemostatic factors in non-hypercholesterolemic subjects. *Atherosclerosis.* **148**: 101–112.

Plat, J. and Mensink, R.P. 2002. Increased intestinal ABCA1 expression contributes to the decrease in cholesterol absorption after plant stanol consumption. *FASEB J.* **16**: 1248–1253.

Plat, J., Beugels, I., Gijbels, M.J., de Winther, M.P., Mensink, R.P. 2006. Plant sterol or stanol esters retard lesion formation in LDL receptor-deficient mice independent of changes in serum plant sterols. *J Lipid Res.* **47**: 2762–2771.

Plat, J., de Jong, A., Volger, O.L., Princen, H.M., Mensink, R.P. 2008. Preferential campesterol incorporation into various tissues in apolipoprotein E*3-Leiden mice consuming plant sterols or stanols. *Metabolism.* **57**: 1241–1247.

Plosch, T., Kruit, J.K., Bloks, V.W. et al. 2006. Reduction of cholesterol absorption by dietary plant sterols and stanols in mice is independent of the ABCG5/8 transporter. *J Nutr.* **136**: 2135–2140.

Polagruto, J.A., Wang-Polagruto, J.F., Braun, M.M., Lee, L., Kwik-Uribe, C., Keen, C.L. 2006. Cocoa flavanol-enriched snack bars containing phytosterols effectively lower total and low-density lipoprotein cholesterol levels. *J Am Diet Assoc.* **106**: 1804–1813.

Poli, A., Marangoni, F., Paoletti, R. et al. 2008. Non-pharmacological control of plasma cholesterol levels. *Nutr Metab Cardiovasc Dis.* **18**: S1–S16.

Pritchard, P.H., Li, M., Zamfir, C., Lukic, T., Novak, E., Moghadasian, M.H. 2003. Comparison of cholesterol-lowering efficacy and anti-atherogenic properties of hydrogenated versus non-hydrogenated (Phytrol) tall oil-derived phytosterols in apo E-deficient mice. *Cardiovasc Drugs Ther.* **17**: 443–449.

Raitakari, O.T., Salo, P., Gylling, H., Miettinen, T.A. 2008. Plant stanol ester consumption and arterial elasticity and endothelial function. *Br J Nutr.* **18**: 1–6.

Rasmussen, H.E., Guderian, D.M. J.r., Wray, C.A., Dussault, P.H., Schlegel, V.L., Carr, T.P. 2006. Reduction in cholesterol absorption is enhanced by stearate-enriched plant sterol esters in hamsters. *J Nutr.* **136**: 2722–2727.

Repa, J.J., Turley, S.D., Lobaccaro, J.A. et al. 2000. Regulation of absorption and ABC1-mediated efflux of cholesterol by RXR heterodimers. *Science*. **289**: 1524–1529.

Retelny, V.S., Neuendorf, A., Roth, J.L. 2008. Nutrition protocols for the prevention of cardiovascular disease. *Nutr Clin Pract*. **23**: 468–476.

Richelle, M., Enslen, M., Hager, C., et al. 2004. Both free and esterified plant sterols reduce cholesterol absorption and the bioavailability of 1-carotene and a- tocopherol in normocholesterolemic humans. *Am J Clin Nutr*. **80**: 171–177.

Rubis, B., Paszel, A., Kaczmarek, M., Rudzinska, M., Jelen, H., Rybczynska, M. 2008. Beneficial or harmful influence of phytosterols on human cells? *Br J Nutr*. **100**: 1183–1191.

Rudkowska, I. 2008. Functional foods for cardiovascular disease in women. *Menopause Int*. **14**: 63–69.

Ruiu, G., Pinach, S., Veglia, F. et al. 2009. Phytosterol-enriched yogurt increases LDL affinity and reduces CD36 expression in polygenic hypercholesterolemia. *Lipids* **44**: 153–160.

Russell, J.C., Ewart, H.S., Kelly, S.E., Kralovec, J., Wright, J.L., Dolphin, P.J. 2002. Improvement of vascular dysfunction and blood lipids of insulin-resistant rats by a marine oil-based phytosterol compound. *Lipids*. **37**: 147–152.

Salen, G., Ahrens, E.H. J.r., Grundy, S.M. 1970. Metabolism of beta sitosterol in man. *Clin Invest*. **49**: 952–967.

Salo P., Wester, I. 2005. Low-fat formulations of plant stanols and sterols. *Am J Cardiol*. **96**: 51D–54D.

Sanchez-Muniz, F.J., Maki, K.C., Schaefer, E.J., Ordovas, J.M. 2009. Serum lipid and antioxidant responses in hypercholesterolemic men and women receiving plant sterol esters vary by apolipoprotein E genotype. *J Nutr*. **139**: 1–7.

Seppo, L., Jauhiainen, T., Nevala, R., Poussa, T., Korpela, R. 2007. Plant stanol esters in low-fat milk products lower serum total and LDL cholesterol. *Eur J Nutr*. **46**: 111–117.

Shishodia, S., Aggarwal, B.B. 2004. Guggulsterone inhibits NF-kappaB and IkappaBalpha kinase activation, suppresses expression of anti-apoptotic gene products, and enhances apoptosis. *J Biol Chem*. **279**: 47148–47158.

Silbernagel, G., Fauler, G., Renner, W. et al. 2009. The relationships of cholesterol metabolism and plasma plant sterols with the severity of coronary artery disease. *J Lipid Res*. **50**: 334–341.

Steinberg, D., Gotto, A.M. 1999. Preventing coronary artery disease by lowering cholesterol levels: Fifty years from bench to bedside. *JAMA*. **282**: 2043–2050.

Summanen, J., Yrjonen, T., Christiansen, L. et al. 2003. Effects of microcrystalline plant sterol suspension and a powdered plant sterol supplement on hypercholesterolemia in genetically obese Zucker rats. *J Pharm Pharmacol*. **55**: 1673–1679.

Tamai, O., Matsuoka, H., Itabe, H., Wada, Y., Kohno, K., Imaizumi, T. 1997. Single LDL apheresis improves endothelium-dependent vasodilatation in hypercholesterolemic humans. *Circulation*. **95**: 76–82.

Tapiero, H., Townsend, D.M., Tew, K.D. 2003. Phytosterols in the prevention of human pathologies. *Biomed Pharmacother*. **57**, 321–325.

Trautwein, E.A., Guus, S.M., Duchateau, J.E. et al. 2003. Proposed mechanisms of cholesterol-lowering action of plant sterols. *Eur J Lipid Sci Technol*. **105**: 171–185.

Trautwein, E.A., Schulz, C., Rieckhoff, D. et al. 2002. Effect of esterified 4 desmethylsterols and-stanols or 4,4′-dimethylsterols on cholesterol and bile acid metabolism in hamsters. *J Nutr*. **87**: 227–237.

Van Horn, L., McCoin, M., Kris-Etherton, P.M. et al. 2008. The evidence for dietary prevention and treatment of cardiovascular disease. *J Am Diet Assoc*. **108**: 287–331.

Vanstone, C.A., Raeini-Sarjaz, M., Jones, P.J. 2001. Injected phytosterols/stanols suppress plasma cholesterol levels in hamsters. *J Nutr Biochem*. **12**: 565–574.

Villaseñor, I.M., Angelada, J., Canlas, A.P., Echegoyen, D. 2002. Bioactivity studies on beta-sitosterol and its glucoside. *Phytother Res*. **16**: 417–421.

Vivancos, M., Moreno, J.J. 2005. β-Sitosterol modulates antioxidant enzyme response in RAW 264.7 macrophages. *Free Rad Biol Med*. **39**: 91–97.

Vivancos, M., Moreno, J.J. 2008. Effect of resveratrol, tyrosol and beta-sitosterol on\oxidised low-density lipoprotein-stimulated oxidative stress, arachidonic acid release and prostaglandin E2 synthesis by RAW 264.7 macrophages. *Br J Nutr*. **99**: 1199–1207.

Volger, O.L., Mensink, R.P., Plat, J., Hornstra, G., Havekes, L.M., Princen, H.M. 2001b. Dietary vegetable oil and wood derived plant stanol esters reduce atherosclerotic lesion size and severity in apoE*3-Leiden transgenic mice. *Atherosclerosis*. **157**: 375–381.

Volger, O.L., van der Boom, H., de Wit, E.C. et al. 2001a. Dietary plant stanol esters reduce VLDL cholesterol secretion and bile saturation in apolipoprotein E*3-Leiden transgenic mice. *Arterioscler Thromb Vasc Biol*. **21**: 1046–1052.

von Bergmann, K., Sudhop, T., Lutjohann, D. 2005.Cholesterol and plant sterol absorption: Recent insights. *Am J Cardiol.* **96**: 10D–14D.

Vuoristo, M., Miettinen, T.A. 1994. Absorption, metabolism, and serum concentrations of cholesterol in vegetarians: Effects of cholesterol feeding. *Am J Clin Nutr.* **59**: 1325–1331.

Weidner, C., Krempf, M., Bard, J.M., Cazaubiel, M., Bell, D. 2008. Cholesterol lowering effect of a soy drink enriched with plant sterols in a French population with moderate hypercholesterolemia. *Lipids Health Dis.* **7**: 35.

Weihrauch, J.L., Gardner, J.M. 1978. Sterol content of foods of plant origin. *J Am Diet Assoc.* **73**: 39–47.

Weingärtner, O., Lütjohann, D., Ji, S. et al. 2008.Vascular effects of diet supplementation with plant sterols. *J Am Coll Cardiol.* **51**(16): 1553–1561.

Weingärtner, O., Böhm, M., Laufs, U. 2009. Controversial role of plant sterol esters in the management of hypercholesterolaemia. *Eur Heart J.* **30**: 404–409.

Weisweiler, P., Heinemann, V., Schwandt, P. 1984. Serum lipoproteins and lecithin: Cholesterol acyltransferase (LCAT) activity in hypercholesterolemic subjects given beta-sitosterol. *Int Clin Pharmacol.* **22**: 204–206.

Wilund, K.R., Yu, L., Xu, F. et al. 2004. No association between plasma levels of plant sterols and atherosclerosis in mice and men. *Arterioscler Thromb Vasc Biol.* **24**: 2326–2332.

Windler, E., Zyriax, B.C., Kuipers, F., Linseisen, J., Boeing, H. 2009. Association of plasma phytosterol concentrations with incident coronary heart disease Data from the CORA study, a case-control study of coronary artery disease in women. *Atherosclerosis.* **203**: 284–290.

Xu, Z., Le, K., Moghadasian, M.H. 2008. Long-term phytosterol treatment alters gene expression in the liver of apo E-deficient mice. *J Nutr Biochem.* **19**: 545–554.

Yang, C., Yu, L., Li, W. et al. 2004. Disruption of cholesterol homeostasis by plant sterols. *J Clin Invest.* **114**: 813–822.

Yeganeh, B., Moshtaghi-Kashanian, G.R., Declercq, V., Moghadasian, M.H. 2005. Combination of dietary phytosterols plus niacin or fenofibrate: Effects on lipid profile and atherosclerosis in apoE-KO mice. *J Nutr Biochem.* **16**: 222–228.

Zawistowski, J., Kitts, D. 2004. Functional foods—A new step in the evolution of food development. *Clin Rounds.* **4**: 1–6.

7 Wine and Cardiovascular Benefits

Giuseppe Mazza
Mazza Innovation Ltd.

CONTENTS

7.1 INTRODUCTION

The word wine comes from the Latin "vinum," meaning vigor and strength. "Vita vinum est," life is wine, stated Gaius Petronious, a first-century Roman writer (~27–66 AD). Hippocrates (460–377 BC), known as the "Father of Medicine," recommends wine, mixed with water "in equal parts." Pasteur (1822–1895) called wine "the healthiest and most hygienic drink that man has produced." In 1979, St. Leger et al. drew attention to the protective effects of wine against ischemic heart disease (St. Leger et al., 1979).

In 1992, Renaud and de Lorgeril coined the expression "French Paradox," referring to the low mortality rate from ischemic heart disease and cardiovascular diseases (CVDs) displayed by French men despite a high level of risk factors, such as cholesterol, diabetes, hypertension, and a high intake of saturated fat (Renaud and de Lorgeril, 1992). More recent epidemiological studies have shown that moderate wine consumption, particularly of red wine, helps prevent CVDs and some cancers. CVDs are a group of disorders of the heart and blood vessels and include coronary heart disease (CHD) (heart attacks), cerebrovascular disease (stroke), elevated blood pressure (hypertension), peripheral arterial disease, rheumatic heart disease, congenital heart disease, and heart failure. The major causes of CVD are tobacco use, physical inactivity, and an unhealthy diet.

CHD is the leading cause of death in the developed world. Atherosclerosis, which damages the coronary arteries, is the primary disease mechanism of CHD. Wines, especially red wines, contain about 1800–4000 mg/L of polyphenolic compounds, most of which are potent antioxidants and are therefore thought to function as cardioprotectives and anticarcinogens. The association between wine phenolics and CHD has been ascribed in part to the presence of anthocyanins in red wine (Frankel et al., 1993; Kanner et al., 1994). In addition, several epidemiological studies have shown that CHD mortality can be reduced by moderate consumption of red wine (Rimon et al.,

1991; Klatsky, 1994). The primary mechanisms believed to be responsible for this reduced risk factor include reduced platelet coagulability (Elwood et al., 1991; Renaud et al., 1992), and higher circulatory high-density lipoprotein cholesterol (HDL-C) (Klatsky, 1994). Other mechanisms such as inhibition of lipoprotein oxidation, free-radical scavenging, and modulation of eicosanoid metabolism (Bors and Saran, 1987; Afanasev et al., 1989; Steinberg et al., 1989; Esterbauer et al., 1992; Mazza, 2007) are also thought to play a role in the reduction of atherosclerosis.

The focus of this chapter is to review the literature dealing with epidemiological and biological evidence, and mechanisms of action of red wine consumption on the risk of CVD.

7.2 PROTECTIVE COMPONENTS OF WINE

Regular, moderate consumption of red wine is linked to a reduced risk of CHD and to lower overall mortality. Wine consumers have approximately 5 years longer life expectancy compared with non-alcohol consumers (Streppel et al., 2009). The mechanisms for these reductions in CVD are not well established. However, wine's alcohol and polyphenol components are believed to be responsible for the reduced cardiovascular risk.

7.2.1 POLYPHENOLIC COMPOUNDS

Wine contains many phenolic compounds, most of which originate from the grapes. Red-wine polyphenols are a complex mixture of flavonoids (mainly anthocyanins and flavan-3-ols) and nonflavonoids (such as resveratrol and gallic acid). Flavan-3-ols are the most abundant, with oligomeric and polymeric procyanidins (condensed tannins) often representing 25–50% of the total phenolic constituents (Corder et al., 2006).

Anthocyanins and proacyanidins are among the most important compounds in determining the quality of red wine, because they greatly influence color, bitterness, astringency, and chemical stability toward oxidation (Dell'Agli et al., 2004). Anthocyanins are water-soluble plant pigments, localized in the skin of the berries of red grape cultivars. The term anthocyanins refers to the glycosides of anthocyanidins (aglycons). Anthocyanins may be acylated on the sugar moiety with aromatic and aliphatic acids. The 3-glucosides of cyanidin, peonidin, delphinidin, petunidin, and malvidin are the most abundant in *Vitis vinifera* and red wines (Figure 7.1) (Mazza and Miniati, 1993; Mazza, 1995; Dell'Agli et al., 2004).

The anthocyanins are basically responsible for all of the color differences between grapes and the resultant wines. The amount and composition of the anthocyanins present in red grapes varies greatly with the species, variety, maturity, seasonal conditions, production area, and fruit yield. Also, the conditions of fermentation and aging of wine such as temperature, duration, sulfur dioxide, and alcohol concentrations affect anthocyanin concentration in the wines (Gao et al., 1997). Furthermore, wine color (hue, brightness, and saturation) varies with the total concentration and composition of anthocyanin in the wine (Mazza et al., 1999).

Anthocyanins also contribute to the organoleptic and chemical qualities of wine because of their interaction with other phenolic compounds as well as with proteins and polysaccharides (Brouillard et al., 1989; Mazza and Brouillard, 1990; Davies and Mazza, 1993; Mazza, 1995).

In a study of 34,489 postmenopausal American women, the dietary intake of foods containing flavanones and anthocyanidins was associated with decreased cardiovascular and all-cause mortality. Consumption of red wine in that study was specifically associated with decreased risk of CHD (Mink et al., 2007).

A double-blind, randomized, placebo-controlled trial in which 120 dyslipidemic subjects (aged 40–65 years) were given 160 mg anthocyanins twice daily or a placebo for 12 weeks concluded that anthocyanin supplementation in humans improves low-density lipoprotein-cholesterol (LDL-C) and HDL-C concentrations and enhances cellular cholesterol efflux to serum (Qin et al., 2009). Anthocyanin consumption increased HDL-C (13.7% and 2.8%) and decreased LDL-C concentrations (13.6% and

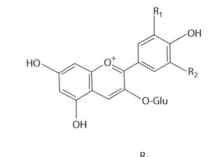

	R_1	R_2
Malvidin	OCH_3	OCH_3
Peonidin	OCH_3	H
Cyanidin	OH	H
Delphinidin	OH	OH
Petunidin	OH	OCH_3

FIGURE 7.1 Structure of the anthocyanins of red wines.

0.6%) significantly ($P < 0.001$) in the anthocyanin and placebo groups, respectively. Cellular choles-terol efflux to serum increased more in the anthocyanin group than in the placebo group, 20.0% and 0.2%, respectively ($P < 0.001$). Anthocyanin supplementation decreased the mass and activity of plasma cholesteryl ester transfer protein (CETP) by 7.4% and 6.3%, respectively, in the anthocyanin group and 23.5% and 1.1%, respectively, in the placebo group ($P < 0.001$). The change in HDL-C in the anthocyanin group, was negatively correlated ($r^2 = -0.330$) with the change in CETP activity; whereas the change in LDL-C was positively correlated ($r^2 = 0.354$) with the change in CETP mass.

Proacyanidins (or condensed tannins) are high-molecular weight polymers, made of flavan-3-ol units linked together by carbon–carbon bonds. Oxidative condensation occurs between carbon C4 of the heterocycle and C6 or C8 of the adjacent units. The flavan-3-ol unit may have a 3′, 4′ dihy-droxy substitution on the B ring (catechin and epicatechin) and 3′, 4′, 5′ trihydroxy substitution (gal-locatechin and epigallocatechin). Dimers, trimers (among which procyanidin C1 is the most abundant), tetramers, and oligomers up to eight units are present in grape (*V. vinifera* L.) seeds, stems, and skins. The procyanidin dimers B1–B4, characterized by the 4–8 linkage, are the most common in grapes. The corresponding 4–6-linked isomers B5–B8, may also occur (Figure 7.2). Until recently, complete characterization of procyanidins in grapes and wines has been impaired because of the difficulty in analyzing high-molecular weight compounds. However, newly devel-oped methods, based on high-performance liquid chromatography (HPLC) coupled with mass spec-trometry, allowed the characterization of complex mixture of grape seed extracts and in beverages (Vivas et al., 1996; Gabetta et al., 2000; Santos-Buelga and Scalbert, 2000; Dell'Agli et al., 2004).

Grape seeds are the main source of oligomeric procyanidins, but poor solubility, combined with oenological and viticultural factors, influence the amount of oligomeric procyanidins in wine. Corder et al. (2006) identified procyanidins as the principal vasoactive polyphenols in red wine and showed that they are present at higher concentrations in wines from areas of south western France and Sardinia, where traditional wine-making methods ensure that these compounds are efficiently extracted during vinification. These regions also happen to be associated with increased longevity in the population (Corder et al., 2006). Absorption of oligomeric procyanidins and their identifica-tion in plasma has been demonstrated *in vivo*, but little is known about their biological availability and metabolism.

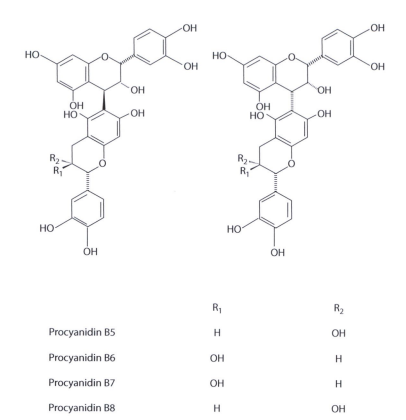

	R_1	R_2
Procyanidin B5	H	OH
Procyanidin B6	OH	H
Procyanidin B7	OH	H
Procyanidin B8	H	OH

FIGURE 7.2 Structure of procyanidins B5–B8.

The total amount of phenols found in a glass of red wine is around 200 mg compared to about 40 mg in a glass of white wine (Waterhouse, 2002). The protective effect of polyphenols is in part due to their ability to retard the development and progression of early atherosclerotic lesions to advanced atherosclerotic plaques. Antioxidant flavonoids found in red wine can reduce the oxidation of LDL-C, which is a key and early event of the atherogenic process (Frankel et al., 1993; Frei, 1995; Leifert and Abeywardena, 2008).

Flavonoids and other polyphenols have powerful antioxidant activities *in vitro*, able to scavenge a wide range of reactive species, including hydroxyl radicals, peroxyl radicals, hypochlorous acid, and superoxide radical (Fukomoto and Mazza, 2000). Flavonoids and other polyphenols can also inhibit biomolecular damage by peroxynitrite *in vitro* (Santos and Mira, 2004), although they are less effective in the presence of physiological levels of HCO_3^-/CO_2 (Ketsawatsakul et al., 2000). Many flavonoids chelate transition metal ions such as iron and copper, decreasing their ability to promote reactive species formation (Pannala et al., 1997). Other than antioxidant flavonoids and other phenolics have other potential actions, including modulation of the inflammatory cascade, improvement in vascular endothelial function (e.g., flow-mediated dilatation), and protection against atherothrombotic events including myocardial ischemia and inhibition of platelet aggregation (Wang and Mazza, 2002; Castilla et al., 2006).

Flavonoids may also interact with cellular drug transport systems, compete with glucose for transmembrane transport, interfere with cell cycle regulation, inhibit protein glycation, modulate paraoxonase, myeloperoxidase, and thyroid peroxidase activities, increase endothelial nitric oxide (NO) production and affect platelet function (Morris and Zhang, 2006; Singh and Agarwal, 2006). However, it is uncertain whether some of these effects occur *in vivo*, given the low concentration of bioavailable polyphenols (Halliwell, 2007; Mazza and Kay, 2008).

7.2.2 ALCOHOL

Excessive alcohol consumption is associated with cardiovascular disorders, including cardiomyopathy, hypertension, coronary artery disease, and stroke. However, more recent data suggest that moderate alcohol intake can actually provide a measure of cardioprotection, particularly against CHD and ischemia–reperfusion injury (Lucas et al., 2005).

Several epidemiological studies and small clinical trials have demonstrated that moderate consumption of alcohol raises HDL-C levels, and it is widely believed that HDL-C accounts for approximately 50% of the reduced risk of developing CHD (Gaziano et al., 1993; Hines and Rimm, 2001; Djousse et al., 2002).

HDL-C is a very important factor for maintaining appropriate concentrations of LDL-C in vascular and other cells throughout the body. Additionally, HDL-C reduces adhesion molecule expression, inhibits LDL-C oxidation, reduces thrombosis, and inhibits migration of inflammatory cells into the endothelial space (Lucas et al., 2005). Acting principally through apolipoprotein (apo)A1, HDL-C may also have a direct antioxidant effect. Moderate alcohol intake is associated with an increase in apoA1, the major HDL-C carrier protein. The synthesis and secretion of apoA1 by human liver and hepatoma cells in culture is stimulated by alcohol. *In vivo* studies also demonstrate increased transport rate of apoA1 and apoA2 in response to alcohol (Morgan et al., 2002). The dose effects of ethanol and potential mechanisms of action are shown in Figure 7.3. (Lucas et al., 2005).

Several studies have suggested that alcohol may affect blood clotting, either by causing the blood to clot less avidly through effects on coagulation factors and platelets or by enhancing the ability of the blood to break up clots when they form (Renaud and de Lorgeril, 1992). These studies are supported by epidemiological data suggesting that acute alcohol consumption causes short-term beneficial effect in protection against CHD in addition to long-term effects. Again, at least half of the

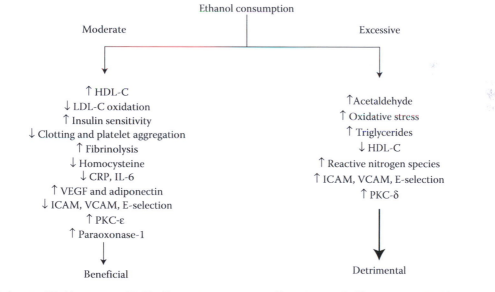

FIGURE 7.3 Dose effects of ethanol consumption and potential mechanisms of cardiovascular response. CRP, C-reactive protein; HDL-C, high-density lipoprotein cholesterol; ICAM, intercellular adhesion molecule; IL, interleukin; LDL-C, low-density lipoprotein cholesterol; PKC, protein kinase C; VCAM, vascular cell adhesion molecule; VEGF, vascular endothelial growth factor. (From Lucas, D. L. et al. 2005. *J. Am. Coll. Cardiol.* **45**(12): 1916–1924. With permission.)

inverse association between alcohol and CHD appears to be directly linked to alcohol through increased HDL-C levels (Pearson, 1996).

7.3 WINE CONSUMPTION AND CARDIOVASCULAR DISEASE

Many studies have demonstrated a U- or J-shaped relationship between alcohol intake and all-cause mortality. This association can be explained by a lower risk of CVD mortality in light-to-moderate drinkers (Pearson, 1996; Sesso and Gaziano, 1999; Sasaki, 2000; Corrao et al., 2004). The protective effect of light-to-moderate alcohol intake may be due to an increase in HDL-C and prevention of blood clotting and reduction in platelet aggregation (Rimm et al., 1999; Agarwal, 2002). Red wine consumption may have an additional health benefit because of its polyphenolic compounds (Burns et al., 2001; Wollin and Jones, 2001) that interfere with the initiation, progression, and rupture of the atherosclerotic plaques (Szmitko and Verma, 2005) and improve endothelial function (Leikert et al., 2002; Wallerath et al., 2003).

7.3.1 EPIDEMIOLOGICAL EVIDENCE

Studies of wine and its effects on health have a long history, ranging from anecdotal accounts in ancient times to more recent rigorous studies of populations with hundreds of thousands of participants (Rimm and Stampfer, 2002; de Gaetano et al., 2002; Britton et al., 2009; Streppel et al., 2009).

Most studies suggest that men and women who drink 1 to 2 drinks per day on average have lower total mortality rates, reflected in lower incidence of CHD (Di Castelnuovo et al., 2002), diabetes (Ajani et al., 2000), and ischemic stroke (Reynolds et al., 2003).

The benefit of moderate alcohol consumption on risk of coronary disease has been documented in about 100 studies (Rimm and Stampfer, 2002; Britton et al., 2009; Streppel et al., 2009). Evidence from a 2002 published meta-analysis of 13 studies (involving 209,418 subjects) on the relationship between wine consumption and risk of CVD has revealed an average significant reduction of 32% of overall vascular risk associated with moderate (1–2 drinks or 150–300 mL/day) versus no wine consumption (Di Castelnuovo et al., 2002).

There was strong evidence from 10 studies involving 176,042 persons to support a J-shaped relationship between different amounts of wine intake and vascular risk.

The best-fitting model includes a linear and a quadratic term and was used to construct an average dose–response curve. The complex relationship found was interpreted as a J-shaped curve because, after an initial progressive decrease in the vascular risk by increasing amounts of wine, the curve reaches a plateau at higher intake and tends to revert at the highest amounts explored. When only the seven prospective studies were considered, the fitting of the quadratic model considerably improved, and this was used to construct the average dose–response curve in Figure 7.4. A maximum reduction was predicted at 750 mL/day, but statistical significance was only reached up to the amount of 150 mL/day. In subgroup analysis, studies considering CHD or CVD or cardiovascular mortality as separate end points showed similar J-shaped curves that did not reach statistical significance. Interestingly, in studies with men only, the protection offered by wine was relatively small (13%) and not significant; in contrast in studies with both sexes the protection was 47%. Whether women are more susceptible to the benefit of wine or if they are more likely to drink lower amounts, thus captivating its maximal advantage, remains to be established (Di Castelnuovo et al., 2002).

Wine contains 8–15% ethanol by weight, and epidemiological evidence confirmed an association between moderate alcohol intake and a reduced risk of CHD in populations. A meta-analysis of 51 epidemiological studies (Corrao et al., 2000) concluded that the protective effects of alcohol were most pronounced at moderate doses. The risk of CHD decreased by 20% when 0–2 alcoholic drinks were consumed per day. One of the most important modifications with regular alcohol consumption is an increase in plasma levels of HDL (De Oliveira et al., 2000). A meta-analysis examining the effect of moderate alcohol intake on lipids (not differentiating between the type of alcoholic

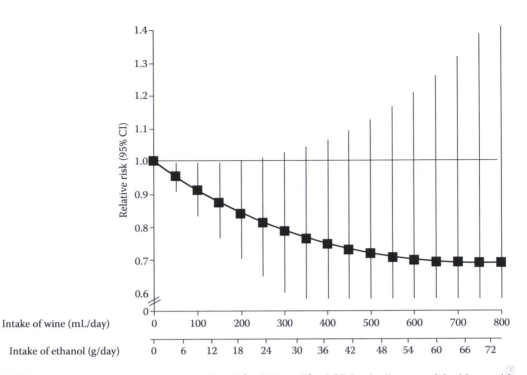

FIGURE 7.4 Best-fitting model for wine effect ($R^2 = 0.54$ vs. $R^2 = 0.27$ for the linear model with a positive linear term; $P = 0.34$), using dose-response curves in seven prospective studies. The best fitting model using data from the three case-control studies was a quadratic model that was not statistically significant with a positive linear term. Horizontal lines represent the 95% CI. (From Di Castelnuovo, A. et al. 2002. *Circulation* **105**(24): 2836-2844. With permission.)

beverage consumed) found that a 16.8% reduction in risk of CHD could be directly attributable to increased HDL concentration from the consumption of 30 g of alcohol (2.5 drinks) per day (Rimm et al., 1999). One to two drinks per day of any alcoholic beverage increases HDL by 12% on average (Linn et al., 1993).

A study of 1373 men by Streppel et al. (2009) concluded that long-term light alcohol intake lowered cardiovascular and all-cause mortality risk and increased life expectancy and light wine consumption was associated with 5 years longer life expectancy. More specifically, long-term light alcohol intake, that is <20 g/day, compared with no alcohol, was strongly and inversely associated with cerebrovascular (HR 0.43, 95% confidence interval (CI) 0.26–0.70), total cardiovascular (HR 0.70, 95% CI 0.55–0.89) and all-cause mortality. Independent of total alcohol intake, long-term wine consumption of, on average, less than half a glass per day was strongly and inversely associated with CHD (HR 0.61, 95% CI 0.41–0.89), total cardiovascular (HR 0.68, 95% CI 0.53–0.86) and all-cause mortality (HR 0.73, 95% CI 0.62–0.87) (Streppel et al., 2009).

A recent study by Latella et al. (2009) confirmed that the strongest effects of alcohol on cardiovascular risk factors were increases in HDL (both men and women) and blood pressure (men) and decreases in LDL (women). However, a primary gene for the metabolism of alcohol, alcohol dehydrogenase type 1C (ADH1C, also known as ADH3), had little effect on these associations. Variations in ADH1C modified the association between alcohol and measures of obesity in men consuming more than two typical drinks/day (especially those consuming more than four drinks/day), but not in women. The data presented show a significant interaction between the ADH1C genotype and alcohol consumption in relation to body mass index (BMI) and waist circumference in men, with substantial increase in both BMI and waist values for men homozygous for the gamma 2 allele who drank daily. No effects were seen for women, which may relate to their lower alcohol intake (about 1/4–1/2 of the amounts reported for men) or drinking pattern (not assessed). ADH1C variants did not interact with the effects of alcohol intake on HDL or blood pressure (Latella et al., 2009).

Similarly, a very recent meta-analysis by Costanzo et al. (2010), based on 16,351 subjects with CVD, showed that the relative risk (RR) of death for subjects who already had CVD was lower for all levels of drinking than it was for abstainers, although the reduction in risk was statistically significant only up to about two typical drinks/day. In comparison with nondrinkers, there was an approximately 20% lower risk of both cardiovascular mortality and total mortality for drinkers. Risk of death was reduced among those reporting as little as 5 g of alcohol per day (the equivalent of about 2½–3 typical drinks per week).

The overall association between alcohol consumption and cardiovascular mortality is shown in Figure 7.5. It clearly suggests that the lowest RR of cardiovascular death ("maximal protection") could be seen in subjects reporting as little as 5 g of alcohol per day, the equivalent of only about 2½–3 drinks/week. However, the RR of cardiovascular death remains lower than that of nondrinkers at all levels of alcohol intake; the 95% percentile estimate crosses that of nondrinkers.

Estimates of the association between alcohol and total mortality were very similar, with "maximal protection" 18–20% at between 5 and 10 g/day; the estimated RR remained lower than that of nondrinkers throughout the range of alcohol intake, with the upper 95% percentile reaching the risk of nondrinkers at about 24 g/day (Costanzo et al., 2010).

In a pooled analysis of eight prospective studies from North America and Europe including 192,067 women and 74,919 men free of CVDs, diabetes, and cancers at baseline, the average daily alcohol intake was assessed at baseline with a food frequency or diet history questionnaire. An inverse association between alcohol and risk of CHD was observed in all age groups; hazard ratios among moderately drinking men (5.0–29.9 g/day) 39–50, 50–59, and ≥60 years of age were 0.58 (95% CI, 0.36–0.93), 0.72 (95% CI, 0.60–0.86), and 0.85 (95% CI, 0.75–0.97) compared with abstainers. However, the analyses indicated a smaller incidence rate difference between abstainers and moderate consumers in younger adults (incidence rate difference, 45 per 100,000; 90% CI, 8–84) than in middle-aged (incidence rate difference, 64 per 100,000; 90% CI, 24–102) and older (incidence rate difference, 89 per 100,000; 90% CI, 44–140) adults. Similar results were observed

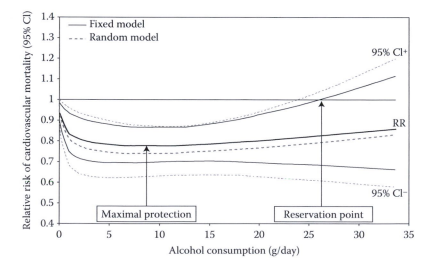

FIGURE 7.5 Pooled curves of RR of cardiovascular mortality and alcohol intake, extracted from seven independent relationships using fixed (solid lines) and random (dotted lines) models. RR, relative risk; 95% CI⁻, lower value of confidence interval; 95% CI⁺, upper value of confidence interval. (From Costanzo, S. et al. 2007. *J. Am. Coll. Cardiol.* **55**:1339–1347. With permission.)

in women. Thus, according to this study, alcohol is also associated with a decreased risk of CHD in younger adults; however, the absolute risk was small compared with middle-aged and older adults.

The importance of this study is in finding that moderate alcohol consumption is associated with lower risk of CHD regardless of age. Some may believe that this indicates that individuals should consider moderate drinking as a way of reducing their risk of heart disease at a younger age (e.g., before age 50). However, it must be kept in mind that the absolute risk of heart disease at this age is very low, so effects on other aspects of health (and social effects) must also be considered (Hvidtfeldt et al., 2010).

Recently several papers have dealt with the association between alcohol intake and blood pressure and between alcohol and the risk of CVD among hypertensives. Britton et al. (2009) presents an analysis of more than 5000 hypertensive subjects in the Physicians' Health Study with hypertension and alcohol intake assessed at baseline; potential changes in alcohol consumption during follow up were apparently not addressed. During 20 years of follow up, 623 cases of myocardial infarction (MI) occurred. The study confirms that alcohol intake is associated with lower risk of MI, as well as a lower risk of angina pectoris and total CHD, among subjects who are hypertensive. It is interesting that subjects consuming 1–4 drinks/day showed no effect, but decreases in risk were noted for 5–7 and 8 or more drinks/week, with the latter showing about 40% lower risk of CHD than was present for nondrinkers (Britton et al., 2009).

An interesting new association was reported by Wakabayashi (2009) regarding alcohol and blood pressure and serum lipids in healthy women. In his study among Japanese workers, an increase in blood pressure and risk of hypertension was observed only for leaner subjects, not among those in the highest tertile of body weight (Wakabayashi, 2009).

A meta-analysis by Taylor et al. (2009) reported slight differences in men and women in their blood pressure response to alcohol. In both genders, higher alcohol intake is associated with an increase in blood pressure (Taylor et al., 2009). In a new report by Rist et al. (2010) on alcohol and stroke from the Physicians' Health Study, there was no strong relationship between alcohol and stroke, or between alcohol and functional limitations from stroke. However, drinkers reporting 1 drink/week showed lower risk of stroke and of severe functional outcomes from stroke than subjects in the reference group reporting <1 drink/week. The authors noted that higher levels of alcohol consumption were not associated with a significant increased risk of transient ischemic attack or ischemic or hemorrhagic stroke. However, there were probably very few heavy drinkers in this cohort, so potential adverse health effects of heavy drinking could not be evaluated (Rist et al., 2010).

7.3.2 IN VITRO STUDIES

As delineated above, there is mounting evidence to indicate the potential cardioprotective effects of red wine, and this has been attributed to specific polyphenols and alcohol constituents. Numerous studies *in vitro* as well as in animals and humans demonstrate beneficial effects of wine polyphenols on traditional cardiovascular risk factors (Table 7.1).

In vitro studies with phenolics in red wine and normal human LDL showed that red wine inhibits the copper-catalyzed oxidation of LDL (Frankel et al., 1993). Two possible mechanisms for this action were advanced, that is, that phenolic compounds complex with Cu^{2+} to reduce it to Cu^+, which may in turn reduce hydroperoxides, and that during the LDL peroxidation, phenols in wine may act as self-regenerating reducing compounds. Therefore, these authors concluded that with regular ingestion of these antioxidant phenols via red wine consumption, a collective reduction in the oxidation of lipoproteins may occur and thus contribute to reduced atherosclerosis and mortality from CVD.

Grape flavonoids also protect and increase serum HDL paroxonase by reducing macrophage oxidative stress through inhibition of cellular oxygenases such as NADPH (nicotineamide adenine dinucleotide phosphate) oxidase, or myeloperoxidase (Fuhrman and Aviram, 2001).

TABLE 7.1

Effects of Red Wine/Grape Polyphenols on Traditional Cardiovascular Risk Factors

Risk Factor	Product	Study Outcome/Mechanisms
Hypertension	Red wine	Decreased systemic blood pressure in rats
	Flavanol-rich foods (wines), procyanidins	Inhibited angiotensin-converting enzyme activity
	Red wine-derived polyphenol extract	Reduced systemic blood pressure and improved aortic elasticity in stroke-prone spontaneously hypertensive rats
		Decreased blood pressure in NO-deficient hypertensive rats
		Prevented angiotensin II-induced hypertension in rats
	Grape juice	Reduced systolic blood pressure in hypertensive humans
	Grape seed-derived proanthrocyanidin extract	Decreased arterial pressure in estrogen-depleted female hypertensive rate
Diabetes	Grape seed-derived procyanidin extract	Antihyperglycemic effect in streptozotocin-induced diabetic rats
	Resveratrol	Enhanced insulin sensitivity in diabetic mice
Hypercholesterolemia	Polyphenol-enriched white wine, red wine	Lowered cholesterol concentrations and increased ratio of apoA1:apoB in hamsters[a]
	Grape juice-derived polyphenol extract	Increased both the activity and cell surface expression of the LDL receptor
	Dealcoholized red wine	Decreased expression and excretion of apoB in cultured human hepatic cells[a]
	Grape juice	Reduced LDL-C and apoB concentrations, decreased concentration of oxLDL, increased concentrations of HDL-C and apoA1 in healthy and hemodialysis-receiving humans[a]
Smoking	Dealcoholized red wine	Reduced lipid peroxidation in human male smokers
	Grape seed-derived polyphenol extract	Reduced susceptibility of LDL to oxidation in human male smokers

Source: Adapted from Dohadwala, M. M. and Vita, J. A. 2009. *J. Nutr.* **139**(9): 1788S–1793S.

[a] apo, apolipoprotein.

Rifici et al. (1999) compared the *in vitro* effects of red wine, white wine, and ethanol on cell-mediated oxidation of LDL and HDL by three frequently used assays. They reported that red wine (0.2 mg ethanol/mL) inhibited LDL oxidation as indicated by an 85.7% decrease in absorbance at 234 nm, a 96.5% decrease in thiobarbituric acid-reactive substances (TBARS) production and complete prevention of the decrease in trinitrobenzene sulfonic (TNBS) reactivity. White wine and ethanol did not have any significant effect at 0.2 mg/mL. White wine at 1 mg ethanol/mL inhibited TBARS production from LDL by 84%. Red wine (0.2 mg ethanol/mL) inhibited HDL oxidation as indicated by a 78.9% decrease in absorbance at 234 nm, an 81.7% decrease in TBARS production and by no change in TNBS acid reactivity. The authors concluded that red wine inhibits the cell-mediated oxidation of lipoproteins, white wine is not as effective as red wine and that the effect of the red wine is not due to its ethanol content.

Similarly, an *in vitro* study with J774.A1 macrophages and 2 and 4 μmol/L copper, in the absence and presence of polyphenols in ethanol at concentrations found in red wine revealed that red wine is more potent than white wine or pure ethanol in mediating lipoprotein oxidation.

A mixture of polyphenols in amounts found in red wine equivalent to 0.2 g/L ethanol and 0.05 g/L ethanol inhibited TBARS production from LDL by 91.7% and 45.9%, respectively, compared with ethanol controls ($P < 0.01$). HDL oxidation was inhibited 85% and 82.4% by the polyphenols at 0.2 and 0.05 g/L ethanol ($P < 0.01$). The effects of the polyphenol mixture on LDL oxidation were confirmed by measuring production of conjugated dienes and lipid peroxides, and TNBS acid reactivity. Catechin at the concentration found in red wine at an ethanol concentration equivalent to 0.2 g/L inhibited LDL oxidation by 83.2%, while epicatechin (0.56 µmol/L) and gallic acid (1.02 µmol/L) inhibited by 60.6% and 26.9%, respectively ($P < 0.05$). At 1 µmol/L, LDL oxidation was inhibited by epicatechin, catechin, and quercetin by 86.2%, 79.9%, and 69.4%, respectively ($P < 0.05$) (Rifici et al., 2002).

In cultured endothelial cells, wine, grape juice, grape seed extract, and specific polyphenols increase the activity of the endothelial isoform of NO synthase (NOS) and stimulate NO production (Leikert et al., 2002; Wallerath et al., 2002).

Platelets play a critical role in all phases of atherosclerosis, and flavonoids have been found to inhibit cyclooxygenase and reduce production of thromboxane A2. Red wine polyphenols (RWP) also decrease platelet production of hydrogen peroxide and inhibit activation of phospholipase C and protein kinase C (Pignatelli et al., 2000). Similarly, dilute grape juice inhibits platelet aggregation and this effect is associated with decreased production of superoxide anion and increased platelet NO production (Freedman et al., 2001).

Red wine and polyphenols also exhibit anti-inflammatory activity and inhibit activation of nuclear factor-κB and production of proinflammatory factors in endothelial cells and inflammatory cells (Blanco-Colio et al., 2000). Pretreatment of human aortic endothelial cells (HAEC) with (+)-catechin metabolites inhibited U937 cell adhesion to interleukin (IL)-1 β-stimulated cells, whereas pretreatment with intact (+)-catechin had no effect. Generation of reactive oxygen species (ROS) in hydrogen peroxide-stimulated HAEC was inhibited by (+)-catechin, its metabolites, and control plasma extract, whereas ROS generation in IL-1 β-stimulated HAEC was inhibited by (+)-catechin metabolites only. In contrast, quercetin inhibited U937 cell adhesion to IL-1 β-stimulated HAEC, whereas its metabolites were not effective. Thus, metabolic conversion of flavonoids such as (+)-catechin and quercetin modifies the flavonoids' biological activity. Metabolites of flavonoids, rather than their intact forms, may contribute to the reported effects of flavonoids on reducing the risk of CVD. Incubation of monocytes with catechin decreased their adhesion to endothelial cells (Koga and Meydani, 2001). Pretreatment of Jurkat T cells with the flavanols (−)-epicatechin, (+)-catechin, or B-type dimeric procyanidins oligomers also inhibit activation of nuclear factor-κB in T lymphocyte cell lines (Mackenzie et al., 2004). NO released from endothelial cells via the endothelial NOS (eNOS) is a pivotal vasoprotective molecule (Li and Förstermann, 2000). In addition to its vasodilating feature, endothelial NO has antiatherosclerotic properties, such as inhibition of platelet aggregation, leukocyte adhesion, smooth muscle cell proliferation, and expression of genes involved in atherogenesis (Li and Förstermann, 2000). Thus, eNOS is a significant target in cardiovascular pharmacology. The eNOS enzyme is regulated posttranslationally but can also be influenced on the transcriptional level (Förstermann et al., 1998). Red wine contains unique polyphenolic constituents that may augment eNOS expression and thus endothelial NO output. Increased active eNOS levels may antagonize the development of endothelial dysfunction and subsequent atherosclerosis (Leikert et al., 2002). Also, resveratrol, at concentrations as low as 1 mmol/L and 100 nmol/L, significantly inhibited intracellular adhesion molecule 1 (ICAM-1) and vascular cell adhesion molecule 1 (VCAM-1) expression by stimulated endothelial cells expression by tumor necrosis factor α-stimulated human umbilical vein endothelial cells and lipopolysaccharide-stimulated human saphenous vein endothelial cells, respectively. Thus, resveratrol has been shown to have anti-inflammatory effects, including inhibition of adhesion molecule expression (Ferrero et al., 1998).

A 2011 study, published in the *Journal of Biological Chemistry*, reported that resveratrol stimulates the expression and protein clustering (multimerization) of adiponectin in specialized animal fat cells through the activation of a protein known as disulfide bond-A oxidoreductase-like protein

(DsbA-L). The researchers also reported that the stimulatory effect of resveratrol was not affected by knocking out Sirt1, thus confirming a novel, Sirt1 independent mechanism for the actions of resveratrol; but was reduced by the suppression of DsbA-L expression (Wang et al., 2011).

7.3.3 Animal Studies

Studies with dogs, monkeys, rabbits, and hamsters have shown that red wine may inhibit the initiation of atherosclerosis by one or more of the following mechanisms: platelet activation, oxidative modification of LDL, endothelial dysfunction, and inflammation (Folts, 2002). Demrow and Folts (1995) used a coronary artery platelet aggregation model that mimics acute coronary syndromes to demonstrate platelet inhibition following oral administration of red wine to dogs. Similar effects observed in monkeys (Osman et al., 1998) have been shown to depend on NO production (Wollny et al., 1992).

The effect of consuming red wine, or its major polyphenol constituents catechin or quercetin, on the development of atherosclerotic lesions was studied in atherosclerotic apo E-deficient (E°) mice. Forty E° mice at the age of 4 weeks were divided into four groups, 10 mice in each group, and were supplemented for up to 6 weeks in their drinking water with placebo (1.1% alcohol); catechin or quercetin (50 µg/day per mouse), or red wine (0.5 mL/day per mouse). Consumption of catechin, quercetin, or red wine had no effect on plasma LDL-C or HDL-C levels. The atherosclerotic lesion area was smaller in the treated mice by 39%, 46%, and 48%, respectively, in comparison with E° mice that were treated with placebo. In accordance with these findings, cellular uptake of LDL derived after catechin, quercetin, or red wine consumption was found to be reduced by 31%, 40%, and 52%, respectively. These results were associated with reduced susceptibility to oxidation of LDL isolated after red wine or quercetin and, to a lesser extent after catechin consumption, compared with LDL isolated from the placebo group. Similar results were obtained when LDL was preincubated *in vitro* with red wine or with the polyphenols prior to its oxidation. These results demonstrated that the susceptibility of LDL to aggregation is reduced in comparison with placebo-treated mice, by 63%, 48%, or 50% by catechin, quercetin, and red wine consumption, respectively, and this effect could be also shown *in vitro*. The inhibition of LDL oxidation by polyphenols could be related, at least in part, to a direct effect of the polyphenols on the LDL, since both quercetin and catechin bind to the LDL particle via the formation of an ether bond. Thus, dietary consumption by E° mice of red wine or its polyphenolic flavonoids quercetin and, to a lesser extent, catechin leads to attenuation in the development of the atherosclerotic lesion, and this effect is associated with reduced susceptibility to LDL oxidation and aggregation (Hayek et al., 1997).

The effects of a white wine enriched with polyphenols from Chardonnay grapes and sparkling red wine (SRW) from Pinot Noir and Chardonnay grapes on early atherosclerosis in weanling male Syrian golden hamsters were studied by Auger et al. (2005). Hamsters were fed a semipurified atherogenic diet for 12 weeks in which the cholesterol content had been set at 0.5% and which was supplemented with 15% lard at the expense of starch and sucrose; no selenium, vitamin C, and vitamin E were added to this diet. The animals of each group were additionally force-fed daily either tap water (control), 12% ethanol (group ETH), or phenolics-enriched white wine (group PEWW) or SRW (mimicking a moderate consumption of approximately two red wine glasses per meal for a 70 kg human). Plasma cholesterol concentrations were lower in groups that consumed white wine enriched with polyphenols and SRW accompanied by an increase in the ratio apoA1/apoB. Liver-specific activities of superoxide dismutase (SOD) and catalase increased significantly by (38% and 16%, respectively) and by (48% and 15%, respectively). White wine enriched with polyphenols and ETH significantly increased plasma antioxidant capacity and vitamin A concentrations. Aortic fatty streak area (AFSA) was significantly strongly reduced in the groups receiving white wine enriched with polyphenols (85%) and SRW (89%) in comparison with the control. AFSA was reduced by ethanol to a lesser extent (58%). These data suggest that tannins from the phenolics-enriched white wine induce a protective effect against early atherosclerosis comparable to that produced by SRW containing tannins and anthocyanins and dissociated from the antioxidant action of these compounds (Auger et al., 2005).

A study by Pal et al. (2003) on the effect of red wine polyphenolics on hepatic lipoprotein metabolism revealed that the polyphenolics decreased the intracellular levels of cholesterol, which may trigger a feedback mechanism involving the upregulation of LDL receptor and 3-hydroxy-3-methylglutaryl coenzyme A reductase expression. Limited cholesterol availability also appears to increase the degradation of apoB100 in cells, resulting in an attenuation of apoB100 secretion from cells. These results provide an explanation of the attenuation of circulating very low density lipoprotein (VLDL) and LDL levels in animal supplemented with red wine polyphenolics.

Diebolt et al. (2001) determined the effects of short-term oral administration of red wine polyphenolic compounds on hemodynamic parameters and on vascular reactivity in rats. Endothelial function and vascular smooth muscle contractility were studied in association with the induction of gene expression in the vascular wall. Rats were treated daily for 7 days by intragastric administration of either 5% glucose or red wine polyphenolic compounds (20 mg/kg). Administration of these compounds produced a progressive decrease in systolic blood pressure, which became significantly different on day 4. Aortas from rats treated with red wine polyphenolic compounds displayed increased endothelium-dependent relaxation to acetylcholine which was related to an increase in endothelial NO activity and involved a mechanism sensitive to superoxide anion scavengers. However, no increase in whole-body oxidative stress has been observed in rats treated with red wine polyphenolic compounds, as shown by plasma glutathione assay. Also, in the aorta, red wine polyphenolic compounds increased the expression of cyclooxygenase-2 and increased the release of endothelial thromboxane A_2, which compensated for the extraendothelial NO-induced hyporeactivity in response to norepinephrine, resulting from enhanced inducible NOS expression. This study provides evidence that short-term oral administration of red wine polyphenolic compounds produces a decrease in blood pressure in normotensive rats. This hemodynamic effect was associated with an enhanced endothelium-dependent relaxation and an induction of gene expression (of inducible NOS and cyclooxygenase-2) within the arterial wall, which together maintain unchanged agonist-induced contractility. These effects of red wine polyphenolic compounds may be a potential mechanism for preventing CVDs.

The effects of the red wine polyphenolic compounds (Provinol) on hypertension, left ventricular hypertrophy, myocardial fibrosis, and vascular remodeling were investigated after chronic inhibition of NOS by administration of NG-nitro-L-arginine methyl ester (L-NAME) to rats. Rats were divided into four groups: a control group, a group treated for 4 weeks with L-NAME (40 mg/kg/day), and two groups treated with L-NAME followed by 3 weeks of either spontaneous recovery or recovery with Provinol treatment (40 mg/kg/day). Provinol produced a greater decrease in blood pressure than that in the spontaneous recovery group. It significantly depressed myocardial fibrosis and accelerated the decrease in contraction of the aorta and aortic cross-sectional area, and increased the endothelium-dependent relaxation. These effects of Provinol were associated with a greater increase of NOS activity in the left ventricle and the aorta. This study provides evidence that Provinol accelerates the regression of blood pressure and improves structural and functional cardiovascular changes produced by chronic inhibition of NO synthesis (Bernatova et al., 2002).

Recently, Chalopin et al. (2010) used mice bred to be without estrogen receptors to demonstrated that estrogen receptor α plays an essential role in the beneficial effects of certain wine polyphenols on endothelial function. Endothelial function determines the ability of blood vessels to relax, and is a key factor in the development of atherosclerosis and vascular disease. This study demonstrates that estrogen receptor α plays an important, perhaps the most important, role in the metabolic pathway by which these polyphenols help reduce the risk of vascular disease. Mice bred to be without these estrogen receptors could not utilize polyphenols to increase NO production that leads to vaso relaxation. Also, when this estrogen receptor was blocked in normal mice, there was no improvement in vascular function from these polyphenols. These findings provide important new mechanisms by which wine and other sources of polyphenols may prevent CVD (Chalopin et al., 2010).

RWP and a grape skin extract also reduced blood pressure in several models of experimental hypertension, which has been related to a combination of vasodilator and antioxidant actions (Soares de Moura et al., 2002; Pechanova et al., 2004; Sarr et al., 2006; Jimenez et al., 2007).

Recently Lopez-Sepulveda et al. (2008) investigated the possible *in vivo* protective effects of RWP on blood pressure and endothelial function in female spontaneously hypertensive rats and demonstrated that RWP treatment reduces elevated blood pressure, endothelial dysfunction, and vascular oxidative stress in this model of genetic hypertension. These effects seem to be independent of ovarian function and were related to the increased NO bioactivity, resulting from reduced NADPH oxidase-mediated O_2^- production.

Further evidence that polyphenol content in wine accounts for cardiovascular benefits may be derived from studies comparing different types of wine. The highest concentrations of grape polyphenols are found in the skin, stems, and seeds. The longer contact with these components during the production of red wine increases polyphenolic content up to 10-fold compared with white wine (Sparwel et al., 2009). Investigators suggest that this difference in phytochemical content explains the reported additional health benefit of red wine over white wine or grape juice (Opie and Lecour, 2007). In support of this possibility, numerous human studies suggest that red wine has greater antioxidant effects and more favorable effects on lipid metabolism than white wine (van Velden et al., 2002). However, it must be acknowledged that several observational studies from North American cohorts did not reveal differential effects of red and white wines (Klatsky et al., 2003; Stampfer et al., 2005).

7.3.4 CLINICAL EVIDENCE

Moderate red wine consumption is inversely associated with CVD risk, and red wine contains flavonoids with antioxidant and antiplatelet properties believed to be protective against cardiovascular events. Acute cardiac events are also associated with decreased platelet-derived NO release. Both alcohol and polyphenolic antioxidant components contribute to the cardioprotective effects of wine compared to other alcoholic beverages.

Although many epidemiological and *in vitro* studies associate wine intake with reduced risk of CVD, the number of the reliable controlled clinical trials that have studied and confirmed these findings is limited. Reasons for the limited number of clinical trials are that studying the metabolic fate of wine and other beverages with complex phytochemical ingredients is challenging, because the exact composition and active molecules are not known, and because the absorption and metabolism of these phytochemicals in humans may be highly variable (Mazza et al., 2002; Mazza and Kay, 2008).

Nigdikar et al. (1998) compared red wine (375 mL/day), white wine (375 mL/day), RWP (1 g/day, equivalent to 375 mL red wine/day) in capsules, RWP (1 g/day) dissolved in white wine, and a control alcoholic drink (40 g ethanol/day) on LDL oxidation in 6–9 healthy men for 2 weeks. Analyses of the results (Table 7.2) showed no significant difference among any of the groups treated with the various RWP forms. There was, however, a significant difference observed between the groups treated with white wine and the control drink versus those treated with the various RWP forms. These results led the authors to conclude that red wine consumption increases polyphenols in plasma and LDL; in addition to enhancing the antioxidant activity that was shown by decreased plasma total peroxides, increased lag time and decreased lipid peroxides in the copper-catalyzed peroxidation of LDL-conjugated dienes. It can therefore be extrapolated that decreasing LDL oxidation through the consumption of red wine may prevent the development of CVD.

Stein et al. (1999) demonstrated a reduction in the susceptibility of LDL to copper-mediated oxidation following consumption of purple grape juice for 2 weeks in patients with coronary artery disease. A further study (Abu-Amsha Caccetta et al., 2000) examined 12 healthy male nonsmokers who consumed red wine, phenol-stripped red wine, dealcoholized red wine, or water, each at a separate visit, in random order and 1 week apart. Beverages were consumed over 30 min and blood was

TABLE 7.2

Comparison of Red and White Wines, Red Wine Polyphenols, and an Alcoholic Drink on Plasma and LDL-Associated Antioxidant Effects

Supplement	Plasma Polyphenols	Plasma Lipid Peroxides	LDL Polyphenols	LDL Peroxidation Lag Time	LDL Conjugated-Diene Formation	LDL Lipid Peroxides	LDL Peroxidation Lag Time
Red wine	↑ 38%	↓ 32%	↑ 26%	↑ 31%	↓ 15%	↓ 22%	↑ 31%
White wine	No change	↓ 23%	Not reported	Not reported	↓ 14%	Not reported	Not reported
White wine plus polyphenol powder	↑ 27%	↓ 29%	↑ 62%	↑ 21%	↓ 11%	↓ 23%	↑ 21%
Polyphenol powder capsules	↑ 28%	↓ 28%	↑ 29%	↑ 27%	↓ 12%	↓ 25%	↑ 27%
Alcoholic drink	No oxidative or antioxidative effects were observed after the control drink						

Source: Data adapted from Nigdikar, S. V. et al., 1998. *Am. J. Clin. Nutr.* **68**: 258–265; From Wollin, S. D. and Jones, P. J. H. 2001. *J. Nutr.* **131**(5): 1401–1404. With permission.

sampled just before beverage consumption and 1, 2, and 4 h after consumption. Copper-induced serum and LDL oxidizability *ex vivo*, together with serum uric acid, and plasma caffeic, protocatechuic, and 4-*O*-methylgallic acids were measured. The results showed that consumption of red wine or dealcoholized red wine significantly increased plasma phenolic acid concentrations. Red wine (whether dealcoholized, phenol stripped, or as is) also caused a significant elevation in serum uric acid. Despite these changes, there was no effect on *ex vivo* lipoprotein oxidation over a 4 h time period. The results are not in agreement with other research findings in which the consumption of red wine decreased LDL oxidation in humans (Frankel et al., 1993; and Nigdikar et al., 1998).

Red wine consumption in healthy subjects also reduced urinary levels of prostaglandin F2-a, a marker of systemic lipid peroxidation (Pignatelli et al., 2006). A similar effect on urinary isoprostane concentrations were observed in pre and postmenopausal women following treatment with lyophilized grape powder (LGP) for 4 weeks (Zern et al., 2005). At the present time, no study, to our knowledge, has shown a relation between polyphenol consumption and reduced atherosclerosis in humans (Dohadwala and Vita, 2009).

Human studies have also demonstrated antiplatelet effects of grape-derived beverages. Freedman et al. (2001) showed that grape juice consumption for 14 days decreased platelet aggregation and superoxide production and increased NO production in healthy volunteers. In that study, grape juice also inhibited protein kinase C and spared cellular antioxidants.

Another human study demonstrated a decrease in platelet aggregation, increase in platelet-derived NO release, and a decrease in superoxide formation, both *in vitro* and after oral supplementation with purple grape juice, confirming the absorption and bioavailability of the bioactives from purple grape juice (Freedman et al., 2001).

In a study involving only 10 subjects, the effects of drinking purple grape juice, grapefruit juice, or orange juice for 1 week were examined (Keevil et al., 2000). Platelet aggregation responses to collagen were significantly reduced in the grape juice group only and appear to reflect the total phenolic contents of the test components. For instance, the total phenolics (gallic acid equivalents) were 2.26, 0.75, and 0.86 g/L for purple grape juice, orange juice, and grapefruit juice, respectively. In addition, purple grape juice contained flavonols, anthocyanidins, and proanthocyanidins (PAs), but there was no detectable levels of these components in the orange or grapefruit juices (Leifert and Abeywardena, 2008).

In humans, treatment with LGP for 4 weeks was associated with a reduction in tissue necrosis factor-α, but not C-reactive protein (CRP) or IL-6 (Zern et al., 2005). Wine and gin consumption for 4 weeks also reduced systemic markers of inflammation in healthy men and the effect was more marked following wine consumption (Estruch et al., 2004). Thus, anti-inflammatory effects might be a contributing mechanism for the benefits of grape polyphenols against CVD (Dohadwala and Vita, 2009).

Tsang et al. (2005) investigated the effects of moderate red wine consumption on the antioxidant status and indices of lipid peroxidation and oxidative stress associated with CHD. They performed a randomized, controlled study with 20 free-living healthy volunteers in which subjects in the red wine group consumed 375 mL red wine (young vatted Cabernet Sauvignon, 12% alcohol) daily for 2 weeks, and measured the total concentration of phenolics and analyzed the individual phenolics in the wine and plasma by HPLC with tandem mass spectrometry. The antioxidant capacity of plasma was measured with electron spin resonance spectroscopy while homocysteine and fasting plasma lipids were also determined. The production of conjugated dienes and TBARS were measured in Cu-oxidized LDL. Plasma total phenolic concentrations increased significantly after 2 weeks of daily red wine consumption ($P < 0.001$) and trace levels of metabolites, mainly glucuronides and methyl glucuronides of (+)-catechin and (−)-epicatechin, were detected in the plasma of the red wine group. These flavan-3-ol metabolites were not detected in plasma from the control group. The maximum concentrations of conjugated dienes and TBARS in Cu-oxidized LDL were reduced ($P < 0.05$) and HDL-C concentrations increased ($P < 0.05$) following red wine consumption. These findings provide some evidence for potential protective effects of moderate consumption of red wine in healthy volunteers.

A comparison of the *in vivo* effect of red versus white wine consumption, by six female and seven male volunteers, who consumed red and then white wine for 28 days respectively, revealed that diet and red wine had a synergistic effect in decreasing platelet aggregation; and red wine had a significant effect on the fibrinolytic factors than white wine (Mansvelt et al., 2002).

A randomized, cross-over, single-blind trial by Estruch et al. (2004) evaluated the effects of wine and gin on inflammatory biomarkers of atherosclerosis. Forty healthy men (mean age, 37.6 years) consumed 30 g ethanol per day as either wine or gin for 28 days. Before and after each intervention, they measured the expression of lymphocyte function-associated antigen 1 (LFA-1), Mac-1, very late activation antigen 4 (VLA-4), and monocyte chemoattractant protein (MCP-1) in monocytes, as well as the soluble VCAM-1, ICAM-1, IL-1α, hs-CRP (high-sensitivity C-reactive protein) and fibrinogen. The results showed that after either gin or wine consumption, plasma fibrinogen decreased by 5% and 9%, respectively, and cytokine IL-1α by 23% and 21%. The expression of LFA-1 (−27%), Mac-1 (−27%), VLA-4 (−32%), and MCP-1 (−46%) decreased significantly after wine, but not after gin. Wine reduced the serum concentrations of hs-CRP (−21%), VCAM-1 (−17%) and ICAM-1 (−9%). Thus, both wine and gin showed anti-inflammatory effects by reducing plasma fibrinogen and IL-1α levels. However, wine had the additional effect of decreasing hs-CRP, as well as monocyte and endothelial adhesion molecules (Estruch et al., 2004).

In 24 pre and 20 postmenopausal women, treatment with LGP for 4 weeks was associated with a reduction in tissue necrosis factor-α, but not CRP or IL-6. The subjects were randomly assigned to consume 36 g of a LGP or a placebo for 4 weeks. The LGP consisted of 92% carbohydrate and was rich in flavans, anthocyanins, quercetin, myricetin, kaempferol, and resveratrol. After a 3-week washout period, subjects were assigned to the alternate treatment for an additional 4 weeks. The placebo consisted of an equal ratio of fructose and dextrose and was similar in appearance and energy content (554 kJ) to LGP. Plasma triglyceride concentrations were reduced by 15% and 6% in pre and postmenopausal women, respectively ($P < 0.01$) after LGP supplementation. In addition, plasma LDL-C and apos B and E were lower due to LGP treatment ($P < 0.05$). Further, cholesterol ester transfer protein activity decreased by ~15% with intake of LGP ($P < 0.05$). In contrast to these beneficial effects on plasma lipids, LDL oxidation was not modified by LGP treatment. However, whole-body oxidative stress as measured by urinary F_2-isoprostanes was significantly reduced after LGP supplementation. LGP also decreased the levels of plasma tumor necrosis factor-α, which plays a major role in the inflammation process. Through alterations in lipoprotein metabolism, oxidative stress, and inflammatory markers, LGP intake beneficially affected key risk factors for CHD in both pre and postmenopausal women (Zern et al., 2005).

Other studies have shown that red wine prevents nuclear factor-κB activation in peripheral blood mononuclear cells of healthy volunteers during postprandial lipemia. These data are significant because the monocytes/macrophages and the nuclear transcription factor κB are implicated in the pathogenesis of atherosclerotic lesions (Blanco-Colio et al., 2000).

A recent European randomized cross-over trial of high-PA in red dealcoholized wine (DAW) (500 mL/die, PA dose = 7 mg/kg b.w.) versus low-PA rose DAW (500 mL/die, PA dose = 0.45 mg/kg) was conducted in 21 postmenopausal women in Florence, Italy (Giovannelli et al., 2011). Oxidative DNA damage by the comet assay and gene expression by microarray were measured in peripheral blood lymphocytes, collected during the study period. Blood samples were also collected for the evaluation of hematological, hemostatic, hemorheological, and inflammatory parameters.

The results of this study provide evidence that consumption of substantial amounts of DAW for 1 month does not exert a protective activity toward oxidative DNA damage, or modifies significantly the gene-expression profile of peripheral lymphocytes, whereas it shows blood-thinning effect, expressed as a significant decrease in blood viscosity. However, this effect does not correlate with the dosage of polyphenols of the DAW (Giovannelli et al., 2011). Thus, more intervention studies are needed to provide further evidence for the health-protective effects of wine PAs.

The effects of a moderate intake of an alcoholic beverage with high polyphenol (red wine) and without polyphenol content (gin) on plasma antioxidant vitamins, lipid profile, and oxidability of LDL was compared by Estruch et al. (2009). In this study, 40 healthy men (mean age, 38 years) were included in a randomized cross-over trial. After a 15-day washout period, subjects received 30 g/ethanol/day as either wine or gin for 28 days. Diet and exercise were monitored. Before and after each intervention, serum vitamins, malondialdehyde (MDA), SOD and glutathione peroxidase activities, lipid profile, oxidized LDL, and LDL resistance to ex $vivo$ oxidative stress were measured. Compared to gin intervention, wine intake reduced plasma SOD activity [-8.1 U/g of hemoglobin (U/g Hb) (95% CI, -138 to -25; $P = 0.009$)] and MDA levels [-11.9 nmol/L (CI, -21.4 to -2.5; $P = 0.020$)]. Lag-phase time of LDL oxidation analysis also increased 11.0 min (CI, 1.2–20.8; $P = 0.032$) after wine, compared to gin, whereas no differences were observed between the two interventions in oxidation rate of LDL particles. Peroxide concentration in LDL particles also decreased after wine [-0.18 nmol/mL (CI, -0.3 to -0.08; $P = 0.020$)], as did plasma oxidized LDL concentrations [-11.0 U/L (CI, -17.3 to -6.1; $P = 0.009$)]. Thus, according to this study, red wine intake compared to gin has greater antioxidant effects, probably due to its high polyphenolic content (Estruch et al., 2009).

Red wine has more potent antiplatelet effects than white wine (Gresele et al., 2008). In that study, 20 healthy volunteers were examined before and after 15 days of controlled white or red wine intake (300 mL/day). Plasma resveratrol and the release of NO by stimulated platelets increased significantly after wine intake. Resveratrol, at the concentrations detected in plasma after wine intake, was incubated in $vitro$ with washed platelets and several variables related to NO production and to signal transduction were measured. Resveratrol in $vitro$ significantly enhanced the production of NO by stimulated platelets, the activity of platelet NOS, phosphorylation of protein kinase B, an activator of the eNOS, and phosphorylation of vasodilator-activated protein, an expression of the biologic activity of NO in platelets. Simultaneously, they observed decreased phosphorylation of P38 mitogen-activated protein kinase (p38MAPK), a proinflammatory pathway in human platelets, a reduction of the activity of NADPH oxidase, a major source of ROS and of the generation of O_2^-

radicals, as detected by cytochrome C reduction. The conclusion is that resveratrol, at concentrations attainable after moderate wine intake, activates platelet eNOS and in this way blunts the pro-inflammatory pathway linked to p38MAPK, thus inhibiting ROS production and ultimately platelet function. According to the authors, this activity may contribute to the beneficial effects of moderate wine intake on ischemic CVD (Gresele et al., 2008).

Human studies support a benefit of wine on endothelial function. Flesch et al. (1998) investigated whether the vasodilatory activity involves the endothelium and is specific for certain wines. The effects of different red and white wines and phenolic ingredients on vascular tension and cyclic guanosine monophosphate (cGMP) content were studied in human coronary arteries and rat aortic rings *in vitro*. Only French and Italian red wines aged in wooden barrels (1:1000, vol/vol), quercetin (1–100 μM), and tannic acid (1–100 μg/mL) decreased tension of precontracted vascular rings and increased vascular cGMP content (both $P < 0.001$). The effects were abolished after endothelial denudation and reversible by NOS inhibition. Red wines not produced en barrique, white wines, and ethanol did not affect vascular tension or cGMP content. Thus, endothelium-dependent vasodilatory effects may be specific for red wines aged in wooden barrels, and thus high in phenolic substances.

In a study by Serafini et al. (1998), 10 healthy subjects (six women and four men) consumed 113 mL of tap water (control) or alcohol-free red and white wine at 1 week intervals. Both alcohol-free wines possessed an *in vitro* dose-dependent peroxyl-radical activity, but red wine, with a poly-phenol concentration of 363 ± 48.0 mg/L quercetin equivalent (QE), was 20 times more active (40.0 ± 0.1 mmol/L) than white wine (1.9 ± 0.1 mmol/L), which had a polyphenol concentration of 31 ± 1 mg QE/L. The ingestion of alcohol-free red wine significantly increased plasma total radical-trapping antioxidant parameter values and polyphenol concentrations 50 min after ingestion. Alcohol-free white wine and water had no effects on either of the plasma values. The parallel and prompt increase of antioxidant status and of circulating levels of polyphenols in fasting subjects after ingestion of a moderate amount of alcohol-free red wine suggests that polyphenols are absorbed in the upper gastrointestinal tract and might be directly involved in the *in vivo* antioxidant defenses.

A study with 12 healthy subjects, less than 40 years of age without known cardiovascular risk factors showed that consumption of 250 mL of red wine with alcohol dilated the brachial artery and increased blood flow (Agewall et al., 2000). These changes were not observed following the dealcoholized red wine and were thus attributable to ethanol. These hemodynamic changes may have concealed an effect on flow-mediated brachial artery dilatation which did not increase after drinking red wine with alcohol. Flow-mediated dilatation of the brachial artery increased significantly after dealcoholized red wine and this finding may support the hypothesis that antioxidant qualities of red wine, rather than ethanol in itself, may protect against CVD (Agewall et al., 2000).

Interestingly, red wine consumption also prevents the acute impairment of endothelial function that occurs following cigarette smoking (Papamichael et al., 2004) or consumption of a high-fat meal (Cuevas et al., 2000).

Recently, van Dorsten et al. (2010) studied the metabolic impact of polyphenol-rich red wine and grape juice consumption in 58 men and women, and showed that 4-week consumption of polyphenol-rich wine and grape supplements results in the elevated excretion of a wide range of phenolic acids, which is in line with extensive gut microbial metabolism of grape/wine polyphenols. The metabolomics approach was able to detect marginally different impacts on urine metabolic profiles, following consumption of red wine and red grape juice extracts or only a red grape juice dry extract, although they only had a slightly different polyphenol composition. Thus, a change in phytochemical composition of the diet can induce shifts in local and/or systemic profiles of phenolic metabolites with potential significance to human health. Metabolomics can play an important role in nutritional intervention studies to help unravel the complex interactions between food bioactives and human metabolism and health (van Dorsten et al., 2010).

Longer term exposure to red wine extracts or resveratrol stimulates an increase in enzyme expression and activity (Leikert et al., 2002). The effects of resveratrol on endothelial function

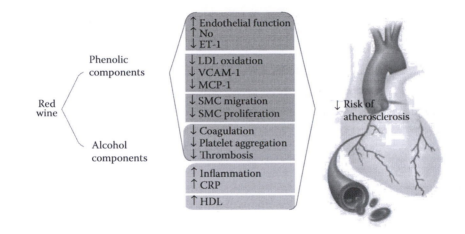

FIGURE 7.6 Both the alcohol and phenolic components found in red wine are believed to decrease the risk of atherosclerotic disease via several different mechanisms. CRP, C-reactive protein; ET-1, endothelin-1; HDL, high-density lipoprotein; LDL, low-density lipoprotein; MCP-1, monocyte chemoattractant protein-1; NO, nitric oxide; SMC, smooth muscle cell; VCAM-1, vascular adhesion molecule-1. (From Szmitko, P. E. and Verma, S. 2005. *Am. J. Physiol. Heart Circ. Physiol.* **288**(5): H2023–H2030. With permission.)

may be mediated through an effect on Sirtuin-1 protein, which regulates the gene expression related to cell survival and stress response (Baur and Sinclair, 2006). Furthermore, activation of Sirtuin-1 decreases the activity of p53, a regulator of apoptosis and cell cycle, and activates AMP-dependent protein kinase, a regulator of cellular energy status (Dohadwala and Vita, 2009; Suchankova et al., 2009).

From the above it is apparent that *in vitro* and *in vivo* experimental research support the biological plausibility of red wine, both the alcohol and phenolic components found in red wine are believed to decrease the risk of atherosclerotic disease via several different mechanisms. Red wine may promote the maintenance of a healthy endothelium and inhibit atherosclerotic plaque formation, progression and rupture (Szmitko and Verma, 2005).

In vivo, platelet aggregation was inhibited after healthy human volunteers consumed purple grape juice, suggesting grape derived flavonoids and not just ethanol, may contribute to the apparent antithrombotic effect of red wine (Freedman et al., 2001) (Figure 7.6).

7.4   CONCLUDING REMARKS

There is increasing evidence that regular and moderate consumption of red wine is linked to a reduced risk of CVD and overall mortality, and this is due to both the alcohol and phenolic components found in red wine. This is supported by data from epidemiological studies and *in vitro*, *ex vivo*, and *in vivo* animal studies and, albeit limited, human trials. The beneficial effects of wine polyphenols and alcohol appear to be mediated via an overabundance of biochemical pathways and signaling mechanisms acting either independently or synergistically. The pleiotropic (many effects) nature of the reported benefits of wine polyphenols tends to suggest the modulation of multiple mechanisms and may explain their physiological efficacy.

Red wine, which has a higher content of phenolics appears to be superior to white wine and other alcoholic beverages protecting against CHD and stroke. *In vivo* and *in vitro* studies indicate that the polyphenolic compounds in red wine, in addition to ethanol, may play an active role in limiting the initiation and progression of atherosclerosis by a number of mechanisms, including inhibition of LDL oxidation and other favorable effects on cellular redox state, improvement of endothelial function, lowering blood pressure, inhibition of platelet aggregation, reduction of inflammation, and activation of novel proteins that prevent cellular senescence, for example, Sirtuin 1. Studies in humans also support these beneficial effects. However, in this era of evidence-based medicine clinical evidence is insufficient to firmly conclude that the consumption of wine prevents CVD. Although biologically plausible and epidemiologically convincing, the cardiovascular protection afforded by red wine will remain unknown until randomized, clinical trials are performed.

REFERENCES

Abu-Amsha Caccetta, R., Croft, K. D., Beilin, L. J., and Puddey, I. B. 2000. Ingestion of red wine significantly increases plasma phenolic acid concentrations but does not acutely affect *ex vivo* lipoprotein oxidizability. *Am. J. Clin. Nutr.* **71**: 67–74.

Afanasev, I. B., Dorozhko, A. I., Brodskii, A. V., Kostyuk, V. A., and Potapovitch, A. I. 1989. Chelating and free radical scavenging mechanisms of inhibitory actions of rutin and quercetin in lipid peroxidation. *Biochem. Pharmacol.* **38**(11): 1763–1769.

Agarwal, D. P. 2002. Cardioprotective effects of light–moderate consumption of alcohol: A review of putative mechanisms. *Alcohol Alcohol.* **37**(5): 409–415.

Agewall, S., Wright, S., Doughty, R. N., Whalley, G. A., Duxbury, M., and Sharpe, N. 2000. Does a glass of red wine improve endothelial function? *Eur. Heart J.* **21**(1): 74–78.

Ajani, U. A., Hennekens, C. H., Spelsberg, A., and Manson, J. E. 2000. Alcohol consumption and risk of type 2 diabetes mellitus among US male physicians. *Arch. Intern. Med.* **160**(7): 1025–1030.

Auger, C., Rouanet, J. M., Vanderlinde, R., Bornet, A., Decorde, K., Lequeux, N., Cristol, J. P., and Teissedre, P. L. 2005. Polyphenols-enriched Chardonnay white wine and sparkling Pinot Noir red wine identically prevent early atherosclerosis in hamsters. *J. Agric. Food Chem.* **53**(25): 9823–9829.

Baur, J. A. and Sinclair, D. A. 2006. Therapeutic potential of resveratrol: The *in vivo* evidence. *Nat. Rev. Drug Discov.* **5**(6): 493–506.

Bernatova, I., Pechanova, O., Babal, P., Kysela, S., Stvrtina, S., and Andriantsitohaina, R. 2002. Wine polyphenols improve cardiovascular remodeling and vascular function in NO-deficient hypertension. *Am. J. Physiol. Heart Circ. Physiol.* **282**(3): H942–H948.

Blanco-Colio, L. M., Valderrama, M., Alvarez-Sala, L. A., Bustos, C., Ortego, M., Hernandez-Presa, M. A., Cancelas, P., Gomez-Gerique, J., Millan, J., and Egido, J. 2000. Red wine intake prevents nuclear factor-kappaB activation in peripheral blood mononuclear cells of healthy volunteers during postprandial lipemia. *Circulation* **102**(9): 1020–1026.

Bors, W. and Saran, M. 1987. Radical scavenging by flavonoid antioxidants. *Free Radical Res. Commun.* **2**(4–6): 289–294.

Britton, K. A., Gaziano, J. M., Sesso, H. D., and Djoussé, L. 2009. Relation of alcohol consumption and coronary heart disease in hypertensive male physicians (from the Physicians' Health Study). *Am. J. Cardiol.* **104**(7): 932–935.

Brouillard, R., Mazza, G., Saad, Z., Albrecht-Gary, A. M., and Cheminat, A. 1989. The copigmentation reaction of anthocyanins: A microprobe for the structural study of aqueous solutions. *J. Am. Chem. Soc.* **111**(7): 2604–2607.

Burns, J., Crozier, A., and Lean, M. E. 2001. Alcohol consumption and mortality: Is wine different from other alcoholic beverages? *Nutr. Metab. Cardiovasc. Dis.* **11**(4): 249–258.

Castilla, P., Echarri, R., Davalos, A., Cerrato, F., Ortega, H., Teruel, J. L., Lucas, M. F., Gomez-Coronado, D., Ortuno, J., and La suncion, M. A. 2006. Concentrated red grape juice exerts antioxidant, hypolipidemic, and antiinflammatory effects in both hemodialysis patients and healthy subjects. *Am. J. Clin. Nutr.* **84**(1): 252–262.

Chalopin, M., Tesse, A., Martınez, M. C., Rognan, D., Arnal, J. F., and Andriantsitohaina, R. 2010. Estrogen receptor alpha as a key target of red wine polyphenols action on the endothelium. *PLoS ONE* **5**(1): e8554. doi:7.1371/journal.pone.0008554.

Corder, R., Mullen, W., Khan, N. Q., Marks, S. C., Wood, E. G., Carrier, M. J., and Crozier, A. 2006. Oenology: Red wine procyanidins and vascular health. *Nature* **444**: 566. doi:7.1038/44456a.

Corrao, G., Rubbiati, L., Bagnardi, V., Zambon, A., and Poikolainen, K. 2000. Alcohol and coronary heart disease: A meta-analysis. *Addiction* **95**(10): 1505–1523.

Corrao, G., Bagnardi, V., Zambon, A., and La Vecchia, C. 2004. A meta-analysis of alcohol consumption and the risk of 15 diseases. *Prev. Med.* **38**(5): 613–619.

Costanzo, S., Di Castelnuovo, A., Donati, M. B., Iacoviello, L., and de Gaetano, G. 2010. Alcohol consumption and mortality in patients with cardiovascular disease. A meta-analysis. *J. Am. Coll. Cardiol.* **55**: 1339–1347.

Cuevas, A. M., Guasch, V., Castillo, O., Irribarra, V., Mizon, C., San Martin, A., Strobel, P., Perez, D., Germain, A. M., and Leighton, F. 2000. A high-fat diet induces and red wine counteracts endothelial dysfunction in human volunteers. *Lipids* **35**(2): 143–148.

Davies, A. J. and Mazza, G. 1993. Copigmentation of simple and acylated anthocyanins with colorless phenolic compounds. *J. Agric. Food Chem.* **41**(5): 716–720.

de Gaetano, G., Di Castelnuovo, A., Rotondo, S., Iacoviello, L., and Donati, M.B. 2002. A meta-analysis of studies on wine and beer and cardiovascular disease. *Pathophysiol. Haemost. Thromb.* **2002**(32): 353–355.

Dell'Agli, M., Busciala, A., and Bosisio, E. 2004. Vascular effects of wine Polyphenols. *Cardiovasc. Res.* **63**(4): 593–602.

Demrow, H. S. and Folts, J.D. 1995. Administration of wine and grape juice inhibits *in vivo* platelet activity and thrombosis in stenosed canine coronary arteries. *Circulation* **91**(4): 1182–1188.

De Oliveira, E., Silva, E. R., Foster, D., McGee Harper, M., Seidman, C. E., Smith, J. D., Breslow, J. L., and Brinton, E. A. 2000. Alcohol consumption raises HDL cholesterol levels by increasing the transport rate of apolipoproteins A-I and A-II. *Circulation* **102**(19): 2347–2352.

Di Castelnuovo, A., Rotondo, S., Iacoviello, L., Donati, M.B., and de Gaetano, G. 2002. Meta-analysis of wine and beer consumption in relation to vascular risk. *Circulation* **105**(24): 2836–2844.

Diebolt, M., Bucher, B., and Andriantsitohaina, R. 2001. Wine polyphenols decrease blood pressure, improve NO vasodilatation and induce gene expression. *Hypertension* **38**(2): 159–165.

Djousse, L., Ellison, R. C., Beiser, A., Scaramuccii, A., and D'Agostino, R. B. 2002. Alcohol consumption and risk of ischemic stroke: The Framingham Study. *Stroke* **33**(4): 907–912.

Dohadwala, M. M. and Vita, J. A. 2009. Grapes and cardiovascular disease. *J. Nutr.* **139**(9): 1788S–1793S.

Elwood, P. C., Renaud, S., Sharp, D. S., Beswick, A. D., O'Brien, J. R., and Yarnell, J. W. G. 1991. Ischemic heart disease and platelet aggregation. *Circulation* **83**(1): 38–44.

Esterbauer, H., Gebicki, J., Puhl, H., and Jurgens, G. 1992. The role of lipid peroxidation and antioxidants in oxidative modification of LDL. *Free Radic. Biol. Med.* **13**(4): 341–390.

Estruch, R., Sacanella, E., Badia, E., Antunez, E., Nicolas, J. M., Fernandez-Sola, J., Rotilio, D., de Gaetano, G., Rubin, E., and Urbano-Marquez, A. 2004. Different effects of red wine and gin consumption on inflammatory biomarkers of atherosclerosis: A prospective randomized crossover trial. Effects of wine on inflammatory markers. *Atherosclerosis* **175**(1): 117–123.

Estruch, R., Sacanella, E., Mota, F., Chiva-Blanch, G., Antunez, E., Casals, E., Deulofeu, R. et al., 2009. Moderate consumption of red wine, but not gin, decreases erythrocyte superoxide dismutase activity: A randomised cross-over trial. *Nutr. Metab. Cardiovasc. Dis.* **21**(1): 46–53.

Ferrero, M. E., Bertelli, A. E., Fulgenzi, A., Pellegatta, F., Corsi, M. M., Bonfrate, M., Ferrara, F., De Caterina, R., Giovannini, L., and Bertelli, A. 1998. Activity *in vitro* of resveratrol on granulocyte and monocyte adhesion to endothelium. *Am. J. Clin. Nutr.* **68**(6): 1208–1214.

Flesch, M., Schwarz, A., and Bohm, M. 1998. Effects of red and white wine on endothelium-dependent vasorelaxation of rat aorta and human coronary arteries. *Am. J. Physiol.* **275**(4): H1183–H1190.

Folts, J. D. 2002. Potential health benefits from the flavonoids in grape products on vascular disease. *Adv. Exp. Med. Biol.* **505**: 95–111.

Förstermann, U., Boissel, J.P., and Kleinert, H. 1998. Expressional control of the constitutive isoforms of nitric oxide synthase (NOS I and NOS III). *FASEB J.* **12**(10): 773–790.

Frankel, E. N., Kanner, J., German, J. B., Parks, E., and Kinsella, J. E. 1993. Inhibition of oxidation of human low-density lipoprotein by phenolic substances in red wine. *Lancet* **341**(8843): 454–457.

Freedman, J.E., Parker, C., Liqing, L., Perlman, J. A., Frei, B., Ivanov, V., Deak, L. R., Iafrati, M. D., and Folts, J. D. 2001. Select flavonoids and whole juice from purple grapes inhibit platelet function and enhance nitric oxide release. *Circulation* **103**(23): 2792–2798.

Frei, B. 1995. Cardiovascular disease and nutrient antioxidants: Role of low density lipoprotein oxidation. *Crit. Rev. Food Sci. Nutr.* **35**(1–2): 83–98.

Fuhrman, B. and Aviram, M. 2001. Flavonoids protect LDL from oxidation and attenuate atherosclerosis. *Curr. Opin. Lipidol.* **12**(1): 41–48.

Fukomoto, L. and Mazza, G. 2000. Assessing antioxidant and prooxidant activity of phenolic compounds. *J. Agric. Food Chem.* **48**(8): 3597–3604.

Gabetta, B., Fuzzati, N., Griffini, A., Lolla, E., Pace, R., Ruffilli, T., and Peterlongo, F. 2000. Characterization of proanthocyanidins from grape seeds. *Fitoterapia* **71**(2): 162–175.

Gao, L., Girard, B., Mazza G., and Reynolds, A. G. 1997. Changes in anthocyanins and color characteristics of Pinot noir wines during different vinification processes. *J. Agric. Food Chem.* **45**(6): 2003–2008.

Gaziano, J. M., Buring, J. E., Breslow, J. L.,Goldhaber, S. Z., Rosner, B., VanDenburgh, M., Willett, W., and Hennekens, C. H. 1993. Moderate alcohol intake, increased levels of HDL and its subfractions, and decreased risk of myocardial infarction. *N. Engl. J. Med.* **329**(25): 1829–1834.

Giovannelli, L., Pitozzi, V., Luceri, C., Giannini, L., Toti, S., Salvini, S. Sera, et al., 2011. Effects of de-alcoholised wines with different polyphenol content on DNA oxidative damage, gene expression of peripheral lymphocytes, and haemorheology: An intervention study in post-menopausal women. *Eur. J. Nutr.* **50**(1): 19–29.

Gresele, P., Pignatelli, P., Guglielmini, G., Carnevale, R., Mezzasoma, A. M., Ghiselli, A., Momi, S., and Violi, F. 2008. Resveratrol, at concentrations attainable with moderate wine consumption, stimulates human platelet nitric oxide production. *J. Nutr.* **138**(9): 1602–1608.

Halliwell, B. 2007. Dietary polyphenols: Good, bad, or indifferent for your health? *Cardiovasc. Res.* **73**(2): 341–347.

Hayek, T., Fuhrman, B., Rosenblat, M., Vaya, J., Belinky, P., Coleman, R., Elis, A., and Aviram, M. 1997. Reduced progression of atherosclerosis in apolipoprotein E-deficient mice following consumption of red wine, or its polyphenols quercetin or catechin, is associated with reduced susceptibility of LDL to oxidation and aggregation. *Arterioscler. Thromb. Vasc. Biol.* **17**(11): 2744–2752.

Hines, L. M. and Rimm, E. B. 2001. Moderate alcohol consumption and coronary heart disease: A review. *Postgrad. Med. J.* **77**(914): 747–752.

Hvidtfeldt, U. A., Tolstrup, J. S., Jakobsen, M. U., Heitmann, B. L., Gronbaek, M., O'Reilly, E., Balter, K. et al., 2010. Alcohol intake and risk of coronary heart disease in younger, middle-aged, and older adults. *Circulation* **121**(14): 1589–1597.

Jimenez, R., Lopez-Sepulveda, R., Kadmiri, M., Romero, M., Vera, R,. Sanchez, M., Vargas, F. et al., 2007. Polyphenols restore endothelial function in DOCA-salt hypertension: Role of endothelin-1 and NADPH oxidase. *Free Radic. Biol. Med.* **43**(3): 462–473.

Kanner, J., Frankel, E., Granit, R., German, B., and Kinsella, J. E. 1994. Natural antioxidants in grapes and wines. *J. Agric. Food Chem.* **42**(1): 64–69.

Keevil, J. G., Osman, H. E., Reed, J. D., and Folts, J. D. 2000. Grape juice, but not orange juice or grapefruit juice, inhibits human platelet aggregation. *J. Nutr.* **130**(1): 53–56.

Ketsawatsakul, U., Whiteman, M., and Halliwell, B. 2000. A reevaluation of the peroxynitrite scavenging activity of some dietary phenolics. *Biochem. Biophys. Res. Commun.* **279**(2): 692–699.

Klatsky, A. L. 1994. Epidemiology of coronary heart disease-influence of alcohol. *Alcohol. Clin. Exp. Res.* **18**(1): 88–96.

Klatsky, A. L., Friedman, G. D., Armstrong, M. A., and Kipp, H. 2003. Wine, liquor, beer, and mortality. *Am. J. Epidemiol.* **158**(6): 585–595.

Koga, T. and Meydani, M. 2001. Effect of plasma metabolites of (+)-catechin and quercetin on monocyte adhesion to human aortic endothelial cells. *Am. J. Clin. Nutr.* **73**(5): 941–948.

Latella, M. C., Di Castelnuovo, A., de Lorgeril, M., Arnoute, J., Cappuccio, F. P., Krogh, V., Siani, A. et al., 2009. On behalf of the European Collaborative Group of the IMMIDIET Project. Genetic variation of alcohol dehydrogenase type 1C (ADH1C), alcohol consumption, and metabolic cardiovascular risk factors: Results from the IMMIDIET study. *Atherosclerosis* **207**(1): 284–290.

Leifert, W. R. and M, Y. Abeywardena. 2008. Cardioprotective actions of grape polyphenols. *Nutr. Res.* **28**(11): 729–737.

Leikert, J. F., Rathel, T. R., Wohlfart, P., Cheynier, V., Vollmar, A. M., and Dirsch, V. M. 2002. Red wine polyphenols enhance endothelial nitric oxide synthase expression and subsequent nitric oxide release from endothelial cells. *Circulation* **106**(13): 1614–1617.

Li, H. and Förstermann, U. 2000. Nitric oxide in the pathogenesis of vascular disease. *J. Pathol.* **190**(3): 244–254.

Linn, S., Carroll, M., Johnson, C., Fulwood, R., Kalsbeek, W., and Briefel, R. 1993. High-density lipoprotein cholesterol and alcohol consumption in US white and black adults: Data from NHANESII. *Am. J. Public Health* **83**(6): 811–816.

Lopez-Sepulveda, R., Jimenez, R., Romero, M., Zarzuelo, M. J., Sanchez, M., Gomez-Guzman, M., Vargas, F. et al., 2008. Wine polyphenols improve endothelial function in large vessels of female spontaneously hypertensive rats. *Hypertension* **51**(4): 1088–1095.

Lucas, D. L., Brown, R. A., Wassef, M., and Giles, T. D. 2005. Alcohol and the cardiovascular system: Research challenges and opportunities. *J. Am. Coll. Cardiol.* **45**(12): 1916–1924.

Mackenzie, G. G., Carrasquedo, F., Delfino, J. M., Keen, C. L., Fraga, C. G., and Oteiza, P. I. 2004. Epicatechin, catechin, and dimeric procyanidins inhibit PMA-induced NF-kappaB activation at multiple steps in Jurkat T cells. *FASEB J.* **18**(1): 167–169.

Mansvelt, E. P., van Velden, D. P., Fourie, E., Rossouw, M., van Rensburg, S. J., and Smuts, C. M. 2002. The *in vivo* antithrombotic effect of wine consumption on human blood platelets and hemostatic factors. *Ann. N. Y. Acad. Sci.* **957**: 329–332.

Mazza, G. 1995. Anthocyanins in grapes and grape products. *Crit. Rev. Food Sci. Nutr.* **35**(4): 341–371.

Mazza, G. 2007. Anthocyanins and heart health. *Ann. Ist Super. Sanita* **43**(4): 369–374.

Mazza, G. and Kay, C.D. 2008. Bioactivity, absorption, and metabolism of anthocyanins. In *Recent Advances in Polyphenols Research*, Daayf, F. and Lattanzio, V. (eds), Vol. I, Chapter 10, Oxford, UK: Blackwell Publishing, pp. 228–262.

Mazza, G. and Brouillard, R. 1990. The mechanism of co-pigmentation of anthocyanins in aqueous solutions. *Phytochem.* **29**(4): 1097–1102.

Mazza, G. and Miniati, E. 1993. *Anthocyanins in Fruits, Vegetables and Grains*. Boca Raton, FL: CRC Press Inc. 362 pp. ISBN 0-8493-0172-6.

Mazza, G., Fukumoto, L., Delaquis, P., Girard, B., and Ewert, B. 1999. Anthocyanins, phenolics, and color of Cabernet Franc, Merlot and Pinot Noir wines from British Columbia. *J. Agric. Food Chem.* **47**(10): 4009–4017.

Mazza, G., Kay, C. D., Cottrell, T., and Holub, B. J. 2002. Absorption of glycosylated and acetylated anthocyanins from blueberries and serum antioxidant status in humans. *J. Agric. Food Chem.* **50**(26): 7731–7737.

Mink, P. J., Scrafford, C. G., Barraj, L. M., Harnack, L., Hong, C. P., Nettleton, J. A., and Jacobs, D. R. Jr. 2007. Flavonoid intake and cardiovascular disease mortality: A prospective study in postmenopausal women. *Am. J. Clin. Nutr.* **85**(3): 895–909.

Morgan, K., French, A. W., and Morgan, T. R. 2002. Production of a cytochrome P450 2E1 transgenic mouse and initial evaluation of alcoholic liver damage. *Hepatology* **36**(1): 122–134.

Morris, M. E. and Zhang, S. 2006. Flavonoid-drug interactions: Effects of flavonoids on ABC transporters. *Life Sci.* **78**(18): 2116–2130.

Nigdikar, S. V., Williams, N. R., Griffin, B. A., and Howard, A. N. 1998. Consumption of red wine polyphenols reduces the susceptibility of low-density lipoproteins to oxidation *in vivo*. *Am. J. Clin. Nutr.* **68**: 258–265.

Opie, L. H. and Lecour, S. 2007. The red wine hypothesis: From concepts to protective signaling molecules. *Eur. Heart J.* **28**(14): 1683–1693.

Osman, H. E., Maalej, N., Shanmuganayagam, D., and Folts, J. D. 1998. Grape juice but not orange or grapefruit juice inhibits platelet activity in dogs and monkeys. *J. Nutr.* **128**(12): 2307–2312.

Pal, S., Ho, N., Santos, C., Dubois, P., Mamo, J., Croft, K., and Allister, E. 2003. Red wine polyphenolics increase LDL receptor expression and activity and suppress the secretion of ApoB 100 from human Hep G2 cells. *J. Nutr.* **133**(3): 700–706.

Pannala, A. S., Rice-Evans, C. A., Halliwell, B., and Singh, S. 1997. Inhibition of peroxynitrite-mediated tyrosine nitration by catechin polyphenols. *Biochem. Biophys. Res. Commun.* **232**(1): 164–168.

Papamichael, C., Karatzis, E., Karatzi, K., Aznaouridis, K., Papaioannou, T., Protogerou, A., Stamatelopoulos, K., Zampelas, A., Lekakis, J., and Mavrikakis, M. 2004. Red wine's antioxidants counteract acute endothelial dysfunction caused by cigarette smoking in healthy nonsmokers. *Am. Heart J.* **147**(2): E5.

Pearson, T.A. 1996. Alcohol and heart disease. *Circulation* **94**(11): 3023–3025.

Pechanova, O., Bernatova, I., Babal, P., Martinez, M. C., Kysela, S., Stvrtina, S., and Andriantsitohaina, R. 2004. Red wine polyphenols prevent cardiovascular alterations in L-NAME-induced hypertension. *J. Hypertens.* **22**(8): 1551–1559.

Pignatelli, P., Pulcinelli, F. M., Celestini, A., Lenti, L., Ghiselli, A., Gazzaniga, P. P., and Violi, F. 2000. The flavonoids quercetin and catechin synergistically inhibit platelet function by antagonizing the intracellular production of hydrogen peroxide. *Am. J. Clin. Nutr.* **72**(5): 1150–1155.

Pignatelli, P., Ghiselli, A., Buchetti, B., Carnevale, R., Natella, F., Germano, G., Fimognari, F., Di Santo, S., Lenti, L., and Violi, F. 2006. Polyphenols synergistically inhibit oxidative stress in subjects given red and white wine. *Atherosclerosis* **188**(1): 77–83.

Qin, Y., Xia, M., Ma, J., Hao, Y., Liu, J., Mou, H., Cao, L., and Ling, W. 2009. Anthocyanin supplementation improves serum LDL- and HDL-cholesterol concentrations associated with the inhibition of cholesteryl ester transfer protein in dyslipidemic subjects. *Am. J. Clin. Nutr.* **90**(3): 485–492.

Renaud, S. and de Lorgeril, M. 1992. Wine, alcohol, platelets, and the French paradox for coronary heart disease. *Lancet* **339**(8808): 1523–1526.

Renaud, S. C., Beswick, A. D., Fehily, A. M., Sharp, D. S., and Elwood, P.C. 1992. Alcohol and platelet aggregation: The Caerphilly prospective heart disease study. *Am. J. Clinical Nutr.* **55**: 1012–1017.

Reynolds, K., Lewis, L. B., Nolen, J. D. L., Kinney, G. L., Sathya, B., and He, J. 2003. Alcohol consumption and risk of stroke: A meta-analysis. *JAMA* **289**(5): 579–588.

Rifici, V. A., Stephan, E. M., Schneider, S. H., and Khachadurian, A. K. 1999. Red wine inhibits the cell-mediated oxidation of LDL and HDL. *J. Am. Coll. Nutr.* **18**: 137–143.

Rifici, V. A., Schneider, S. H., and Khachadurian, A. K. 2002. Lipoprotein oxidation mediated by J774 murine macrophages is inhibited by individual red wine polyphenols but not by ethanol. *J. Nutr.* **132**(9): 2532–2537.

Rimm, E. B., Williams, P., Fosher, K., Criqui, M., and Stampfer, M. J. 1999. Moderate alcohol intake and lower risk of coronary heart disease: Meta-analysis of effects on lipids and haemostatic factors. *BMJ* **319**(7224): 1523–1528.

Rimm, E. B. and Stampfer, M. J. 2002. Wine, beer, and spirits: Are they really horses of a different color? *Circulation* **105**(24): 2806–2807.

Rimon, E. B., Giovanucci, E. L., and Willett, W. C. 1991. Prospective study of alcohol consumption and risk of coronary disease in men. *Lancet* **338**(8765): 464–468.

Rist, P. A., Berger, K., Buring, J. E., Kase, C. S., Gaziano, J. M., and Kurth, T. 2010. Alcohol consumption and functional outcome after stroke in men. *Stroke* **41**(1): 141–146.

Santos-Buelga, C. and Scalbert, A. 2000. Proanthocyanidins and tannin-like compounds—Nature, occurrence, dietary intake and effects on nutrition and health. *J. Sci. Food Agric.* **80**(7): 1094–1117.

Santos, M. R. and Mira, L. 2004. Protection by flavonoids against the peroxynitrite-mediated oxidation of dihydrorhodamine. *Free Radic. Res.* **38**(9): 1011–1018.

Sarr, M., Chataigneau, M., Martins, S., Schott, C., El Bedoui, J., Oak, M. H., Muller, B., Chataigneau, T., and Schini-Kerth, V. B. 2006. Red wine Polyphenols prevent angiotensin II-induced hypertension and endothelial dysfunction in rats: Role of NADPH oxidase. *Cardiovasc. Res.* **71**(4): 794–802.

Sasaki, S. 2000. Alcohol and its relation to all-cause and cardiovascular mortality. *Acta. Cardiol.* **55**(3): 151–156.

Serafini, M., Maiani, G., and Ferro-Luzzi, A. 1998. Alcohol-free red wine enhances plasma antioxidant capacity in humans. *J. Nutr.* **128**(6): 1003–1007.

Sesso, H. D. and Gaziano, J. M. 1999. Alcohol intake and cardiovascular morbidity and mortality. *Curr. Opin. Nephrol. Hypertens.* **8**(3): 353–357.

Singh, R. P. and Agarwal, R. 2006. Natural flavonoids targeting deregulated; cycle progression in cancer cells. *Curr. Drug Targets* **7**(3): 345–354.

Soares de Moura, R., Costa Viana, F. S., Souza, M. A. V., Kovary, K., Guedes, D. C., Oliviera, E. P., Rubenich, L. M. et al., 2002. Antihypertensive, vasodilator and antioxidant effects of vinifera grape-skin extract. *J. Pharm. Pharmacol.* **54**(11): 1515–1520.

Sparwel, J., Vantler, M., Caglayan, E., Kappert, K., Fries, J. W., Dietrich, H., Bohm, M., Erdmann, E., and Rosenkranz, S. 2009. Differential effects of red and white wines on inhibition of the platelet-derived growth factor receptor: Impact of the mash fermentation. *Cardiovasc. Res.* **81**(4): 758–770.

Stampfer, M. J., Kang, J. H., Chen, J., Cherry, R., and Grodstein, F. 2005. Effects of moderate alcohol consumption on cognitive function in women. *N. Engl. J. Med.* **352**(3): 245–253.

Stein, J. H., Keevil, J. G., Wiebe, D. A., Aeschlimann, S., and Folts, J. D. 1999. Purple grape juice improves endothelial function and reduces the susceptibility of LDL cholesterol to oxidation in patients with coronary artery disease. *Circulation* **100**(10): 1050–1055.

Steinberg, D., Parsatharathy, S., Carew, T. E., Khoo, J. C., and Witztum, J. L. 1989. Beyond cholesterol. Modifications of low-density lipoprotein that increase its atherogenicity. *N. Engl. J. Med.* **320**(14): 915–924.

St Leger, A.S., Cochrane, A. L., and Moore, F. 1979. Factors associated with cardiac mortality in developed countries with particular reference to the consumption of wine. *Lancet* **1**(8124): 1017–1020.

Streppel, M. T., Ocke, M. C., Boshuizen, H. C., Kok, F. J., and Kromhout, D. 2009. Long-term wine consumption is related to cardiovascular mortality and life expectancy independently of moderate alcohol intake: The Zutphen Study. *J. Epidemiol. Community Health* **63**(7): 534–540.

Suchankova, G., Nelson, L. E., Gerhart-Hines, Z., Kelly, M., Gauthier, M. S., Saha, A. K., Ido, Y., Puigserver, P., and Ruderman, N. B. 2009. Concurrent regulation of AMP-activated protein kinase and SIRT1 in mammalian cells. *Biochem. Biophys. Res. Commun.* **378**(4): 836–841.

Szmitko, P. E. and Verma, S. 2005. Anti atherogenic potential of red wine: Clinician update. *Am. J. Physiol. Heart Circ. Physiol.* **288**(5): H2023–H2030.

Taylor, B., Irving, H. M., Baliunas, D., Roerecke, M., Patra, J., Mohapatra, S., and Rehm, J. 2009. Alcohol and hypertension: Gender differences in dose–response relationships determined through systematic review and meta-analysis. *Addiction* **104**(12): 1981–1990.

Tsang, C., Higgins, S., Duthie, G. G., Duthie, S. J., Howie, M., Mullen, W., Lean, M. E. J., and Crozier, A. 2005. The influence of moderate red wine consumption on antioxidant status and indices of oxidative stress associated with CHD in healthy volunteers. *Br. J. Nutr.* **93**(2): 233–240.

van Dorsten, F. A., Grun, C. H., van Velzen, E. J. J., Jacobs, D. M., Draijer, R., and van Duynhoven, J. P. M. 2010. The metabolic fate of red wine and grape juice polyphenols in humans assessed by metabolomics. *Mol. Nutr. Food Res.* **54**(7): 897–908.

van Velden, D. P., Mansvelt, E. P., and Troup, G. J. 2002. Red wines good, white wines bad? *Redox Rep.* **7**(5): 315–316.

Vivas, N., Bourgeois, G., Vitry, C., Glories, Y., and de Freitas, V. 1996. Determination of the composition of commercial tannin extracts by liquid secondary ion mass spectrometry (LSIMS). *J. Sci. Food Agric.* **72**(3): 309–317.

Wakabayashi, I. 2009. Influence of body weight on the relationships of alcohol drinking with blood pressure and serum lipids in women. *Prev. Med.* **49**(5): 374–379.

Wallerath, T., Deckert, G., Ternes, T., Anderson, H., Li, H., Witte, K., and Forstermann, U. 2002. Resveratrol, a polyphenolic phytoalexin present in red wine, enhances expression and activity of endothelial nitric oxide synthase. *Circulation* **106**(13): 1652–1658.

Wallerath, T., Poleo, D., Li, H., and Forstermann, U. 2003. Red wine increases the expression of human endothelial nitric oxide synthase: A mechanism that may contribute to its beneficial cardiovascular effects. *J. Am. Coll. Cardiol.* **41**(3): 471–478.

Wang, J. and Mazza, G. 2002. Inhibitory effects of anthocyanins and other phenolic compounds on nitric oxide production in LPS/IFN-γ-activated RAW 264.7 macrophages. *J. Agric. Food Chem.* **50**(4): 850–857.

Wang, A., Liu, M., Liu, X., Dong, L. Q., Glickman, R. D., Slaga, T. J., Zhou, Z., and Liu, F. 2011. Up-regulation of adiponectin by resveratrol: The essential roles of the Akt/Fox01 and AMP-activated protein kinase signaling pathways and DsbA-L. *J. Biol. Chem.* **286**(1): 60–66.

Waterhouse, A. L. 2002. Wine phenolics. *Ann. N. Y. Acad. Sci.* **957**: 21–36.

Wollin, S. D and Jones, P. J. H. 2001. Alcohol, red wine and cardiovascular disease. *J. Nutr.* **131**(5): 1401–1404.

Wollny, T., Aiello, L., Di Tommaso, D., Bellavia, V., Rotilio, D., Donati, M. B., de Gaetano, G., and Iacoviello, L. 1992. Modulation of haemostatic function and prevention of experimental thrombosis by red wine in rats: A role for increased nitric oxide production. *Br. J. Pharmacol.* **127**(3): 747–755.

Zern, T. L., Wood, R. J., Greene, C., West, K. L., Liu, Y., Aggarwal, D., Shachter, N. S., and Fernandez, M. L. 2005. Grape polyphenols exert a cardioprotective effect in pre and postmenopausal women by lowering plasma lipids and reducing oxidative stress. *J. Nutr.* **135**(8): 1911–1917.

8 Role of Garlic Products in Reducing Cardiovascular Risks

Atif B. Awad and Peter G. Bradford
State University of New York

CONTENTS

8.1 INTRODUCTION

Cardiovascular disease is responsible for increased number of deaths in Western societies more than any other cause. Despite long-term decreasing trends, the latest data from the Center for Disease Control and Prevention estimated that more than 806,000 Americans died of major cardiovascular diseases in 2007 (Xu et al., 2010). One of the major pathologies underlying cardiovascular disease is atherosclerosis or hardening of large blood vessels. The progression of atherosclerosis particularly in coronary artery disease involves damage to the endothelium, deposition and oxidation of low-density lipoprotein (LDL) cholesterol, formation of detectable fibrous plaque, and ultimately to microthrombotic lesions and infarct (Hansson, 2005). Numerous conventional risk factors for heart disease have been identified through extensive epidemiological analysis and include smoking, hypertension, diabetes, and hyperlipidemia (Khot et al., 2003). However, several positive protective factors have also been identified such as elevated high-density lipoprotein (HDL) cholesterol and reduction in lifestyle stress, but also dietary considerations such as consumption of fruits and vegetables and of other foods containing natural antioxidants and cardioprotective compounds

(Kromhout et al., 2002). Among these foods with positive cardioprotective activity is garlic and the evidence supporting this contention is summarized in this chapter.

8.2 PREPARATIONS AND BIOACTIVE COMPONENTS

Garlic (*Allium sativum*) has a rich history in medicinal and dietary therapeutics. Garlic was referenced in the Egyptian *Codex Ebers*, perhaps the oldest preserved medical document and dated to over 35 centuries ago, as a strength-giving supplement and a remedy for numerous ailments including heart disorders (Rivlin, 2001). Its therapeutic use is additionally documented in biblical references, in archives from ancient India, China, and Japan, and in handwritten and early typeset books dating to the European medical renaissance. Today, garlic is used as a flavoring agent, a functional food, and as a component of complementary medicine. The major producers of garlic are China, India, Korea, and the United States. China accounts for about 77% of worldwide production, whereas 1–2% of the world's garlic is harvested in the United States (Boriss, 2006). Most of the garlic raised in the United States is grown in California. The per capita consumption of garlic in the United States is estimated to be 2.6 pounds (farm weight) (Boriss, 2006).

Garlic consumption is associated with a reduction in risk factors of cardiovascular disease. Such risk factors include elevated reactive oxygen species (ROS), hypertension, increased platelet reactivity, and accelerated blood coagulation. The health benefits of garlic are supported and substantiated by intense investigative research as reflected in the nearly 3200 Medline citations since 1950. Despite its long history, the active components in garlic and their mechanisms of action are still being characterized. Various modes of garlic preparation differentially affect the formation and longevity of several of the important sulfur-based compounds which are believed to be among the bioactive components (Table 8.1).

Commercial garlic preparations include whole garlic cloves, crushed raw garlic, garlic oil macerates, garlic essential oils or steam-distilled garlic oil, aged garlic extracts (AGEs), as well as dried garlic formulations including marketed products such as Garlicin, Kwai, Pure-Gar, and Kyolic-100. These preparations differ in the type and amounts of the various organosulfur and nonsulfur compounds, but are often standardized according to allicin content, sulfur content, or γ-glutamylcysteine content. More detailed summaries of the chemical compounds present in various garlic preparations can be found in recent reviews (Amagase et al., 2001; Amagase, 2006; Butt et al., 2009).

Crushed raw garlic is in essence an aqueous extract of garlic in which allicin (diallyl thiosulfinate) is one of the principal sulfur compounds (Banerjee and Maulik, 2002). Upon crushing or macerating, activated endogenous alliinase enzyme converts precursor alliin to allicin. However, pharmacokinetic analyses suggest that little allicin can be found in serum following ingestion of crushed raw garlic. Rather, because of its extreme instability, allicin decomposes readily to other organo- and nonorganosulfur volatiles including diallyldisulfide (DADS), diallylsulfide (DAS), diallyltrisulfide (DAT), (E,Z)-ajoenes, allylmercaptan, and sulfur dioxide. Likewise, little allicin is found in any processed garlic preparations. Aqueous and alcoholic garlic extracts do contain S-allyl-L-cysteine (SAC) which is derived enzymatically from γ-glutamyl-S-allyl-cysteines. Garlic powder is derived from dehydrated garlic cloves and thus its composition is similar to that of fresh crushed raw garlic. Ajoenes are stable organic disulfides formed when garlic cloves are crushed or chopped and are chemically derived from the condensation of two allicin molecules. Ajoenes are found in garlic extracts, chopped garlic, and garlic oil.

AGE is prepared naturally by storing sliced raw garlic in 15–20% ethanol for up to 20 months (Banerjee and Maulik, 2002). This process renders the garlic less pungent and, chemically, promotes the decomposition of volatile substances and the enrichment of a number of water-soluble organosulfur compounds believed to promote unique health benefits. Organosulfur compounds include γ-glutamylcysteine, SAC, S-allylmercaptocysteine, and S-methylcysteine. Other preparations of garlic include garlic oil and oil-macerated garlic extract. Garlic oil is prepared by steam distillation of crushed garlic and by capturing the resultant released oil. This oil is enriched in organosulfur components including DAS, DAT, and other allyl di- and tri-sulfides (El-Sabban,

TABLE 8.1

Garlic Preparations and Principal Bioactive Constituents

Garlic Preparations	Active Compounds	Structures
Crushed raw garlic, garlic powder	Alliin (SAC sulfoxide)	
	Allicin (diallylthiosulfinate)	
	Diallyl sulfide (DAS)	
	Diallyl disulfide (DADS)	
	Diallyl trisulfide (DAT)	
	E-, Z-ajoenes	
	γ-Glutamyl-S-allyl-cysteines	
	S-Allyl-L-cysteine (SAC)	
	S-allyl mercaptocysteine	
	S-methyl cysteine	
Aged garlic extract	γ-Glutamylcysteine	
	S-allyl cysteine (SAC)	
	S-allyl mercaptocysteine	
	S-methylcysteine	
Garlic oil	Diallyl sulfide (DAS)	
	Diallyl disulfide (DADS)	
	Diallyl trisulfide (DAT)	

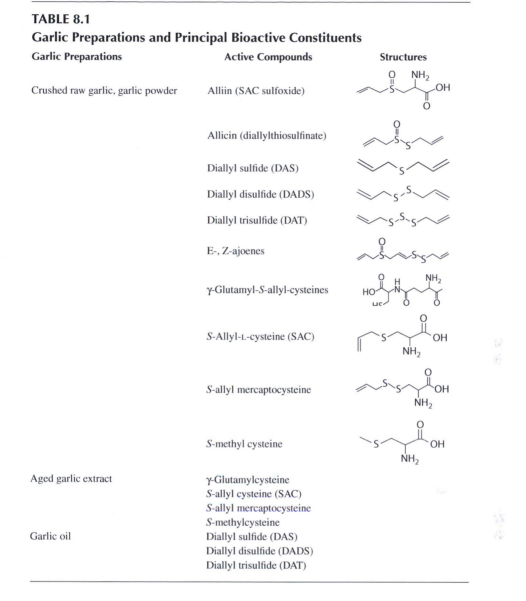

2009). Analyses of typical commercial garlic oil products show enrichments in DADS (26%), DATS (19%), allyl methyl trisulfide (15%), and allyl methyl disulfide (13%) (Lawson, 1998). Oil-macerated garlic extract, which is distributed commercially in gel capsules, is prepared by maceration or finely chopping of garlic, soaking the resultant in oil, and then straining out solids leaving just the garlic extract. This extract is depleted of DADS and DAT but is enriched in ajoenes and dithiins.

8.3 GARLIC ABSORPTION AND METABOLISM

8.3.1 SHORT AND LONG HALF-LIFE COMPONENTS

The most important compounds reported in intact garlic are the primary sulfur compounds including the nonvolatile γ-glutamyl-alkyl cysteines, which comprise >80% of the sulfur content, and the alkyl-cysteine sulfoxides, of which alliin is the principal component (WHO, 1999). Once garlic is cut, crushed, or chewed, dozens of organosulfur compounds are generated and each of these has varying stability and capacities to be absorbed. Alliin is rapidly converted into the thiosulfinate compound allicin by the activated vacuolar enzyme alliinase. Allicin, in turn, is unstable and spontaneously converted to additional thiosulfinate compounds including ajoenes and polysulfides, specifically allylsulfides. The latter compounds are more stable and include DAS, DADS, and DAT. Both allicin and ajoene are converted to allyl mercaptan in the blood (WHO, 1999). Similarly, γ-glutamyl-allyl-cysteine is rapidly hydrolyzed, being converted to the stable compound SAC. The results from controlled studies with human indicate that the bioavailability of SAC is high, estimated to be 60–70%. Plasma concentrations of SAC after oral administration of 0.67–0.82 mg garlic preparation to healthy volunteers peaked at 1 h, exhibiting a plasma $t\frac{1}{2}$ of 10 h and a clearance time of more than 30 h (Kodera et al., 2002a). SAC is stable in plasma as recovery of SAC from plasma in these same controlled studies was almost 100% after 3 h; and recovery of SAC from the red blood cell fraction was up to 87% (Kodera et al., 2002b).

8.3.2 EFFECTS ON DRUG METABOLISM

Garlic preparations exhibit a number of drug interactions. Patients on warfarin should be informed that garlic supplements may increase bleeding times. The allyl sulfides from garlic, particularly DADS and DAT, affect hepatic phase II drug detoxification enzymes. In experimental rodent systems, i.p. administration of DADS and DAT increased the activities of glutathione-S-transferase, quinine reductase, and glutathione peroxidase; however, the same treatment significantly reduced hepatic injury when the rats were given oral carbon tetrachloride, presumably due to increased metabolism of this chlorinated hydrocarbon (Fukao et al., 2004). In human volunteers, daily administration of allicin capsules for 14 d affected subsequent metabolism of drugs, including, as shown in one specific study, the proton pump inhibitor drug omeprazole; however, this was observed only in those individuals with a particular CYP2C19 genotype (Yang et al., 2009). Oral allicin administration reduced the CYP2C19 dependent-metabolism of omeprazole in individuals homozygous for the *1 or *3 genotype but not those homozygous for the *2 genotype. No effect was observed on CYP3A4 activity. In rodent studies, DADS and DAS significantly decreased hepatic CYPE1 protein levels, an enzyme induced by ethanol and by exposure to cleaning agents and recently shown to be important in the progression of colorectal cancer (Davenport and Wargovich, 2005).

8.3.3 HYDROGEN SULFIDE: AN IMPORTANT METABOLITE

Two interesting and recent experimental observations are that garlic-derived polysulfides can be converted by red blood cells and other components of the vascular system into hydrogen sulfide gas (H_2S) and that H_2S promotes vascular smooth muscle relaxation and potential cardioprotection (Benavides et al., 2007; Lefer, 2007; Calvert et al., 2010). The enzyme cystathione γ-lyase (CSE), found in vascular components such as endothelium-free aorta and pulmonary artery converts cystine to pyruvate, ammonia, and thiocysteine (Pryor et al., 2006; Elsey et al., 2010). Thiocysteine reacts with other thiols such as glutathione and also sulfur compounds including components of garlic to promote H_2S production. In controlled investigational studies, the aortic relaxant effects of garlic-derived polysulfides are synchronous with H_2S production and the potencies of DADS and DAT to elicit aortic relaxation correlates with their abilities to promote H_2S production (Benavides et al., 2007). The production of H_2S from organic polysulfides such as DADS and DAT requires glucose and involves reaction with other biological thiols (Benavides et al., 2007). In the rat, bolus injections of H_2S promoted a transient decreases in blood pressure through a mechanism inhibited by the K_{ATP} channel blocker glibenclamide and mimicked by ATP and pinacidil, the K_{ATP} channel opener (Zhao et al., 2001). The mechanism of how H_2S promotes vasorelaxtion or the attenuation of hypertension is distinct from the vasorelaxant effects of nitric oxide and has been proposed to involve, in part, vascular smooth muscle hyperpolarization via activation of K_{ATP} channels and perhaps mechanisms involving the S-sulfhydration of a subset of proteins (Mustafa et al., 2009). In an *in vivo* murine model of myocardial ischemia reperfusion, delivery of H_2S at the time of cardiac reperfusion limited infarct size and preserved left ventricular function (Elrod et al., 2007). Interestingly, H_2S was shown to reduce oxygen demand in awake, spontaneously breathing mice and rats (however, not piglets and perhaps limiting extension to large animals) by promoting a metabolic status characterized as "suspended animation-like" (Baumgart et al., 2009; Sivarajah et al., 2009; Derwall et al., 2010). Thus, one of the important cardiovascular-protecting metabolites of garlic is H_2S.

8.4 EFFECT ON CARDIOVASCULAR ACTIVITIES

8.4.1 PLASMA CHOLESTEROL AND LIPOPROTEINS

Review of the published studies of the effects of garlic on plasma cholesterol indicates that in many early studies a hypocholesterolemic effect was observed (Stevinson et al., 2000; Rahman and Lowe, 2006; Gorinstein et al., 2007). The majority of studies published prior to 2007 attest to this hypocholesterolemic effect of garlic. However, later studies failed to confirm these earlier observations. In earlier animal studies, the form of garlic affected the outcome. For example, using garlic preparations boiled for more than 20 min eliminated any hypocholesterolemic potency (Gorinstein et al., 2006a,b). Similarly, steam-distilled garlic oil preparation was ineffective in lowering plasma cholesterol. However, in one placebo-controlled, double-blinded study with 42 men, analysis of the effects of time-released garlic allicor tablets showed significant benefits on plasma lipoproteins. After the daily consumption of 600 mg allicor by mild hypercholesterolemic patients for 8–12 weeks, the total cholesterol decreased by 7–8% and LDL cholesterol was reduced to 12–14% versus control (Sobenin et al., 2008). The basal cholesterol levels in the experimental subjects appeared to affect the outcomes, as no significant effects were observed in normocholesterolemic individuals. On the other hand, a larger study involving nearly 200 participants failed to show an effect of garlic on LDL-cholesterol or other plasma lipid concentrations (Gardner et al., 2007). In the latter study, garlic was given to moderate hypercholesterolemic adults in raw, powdered, or aged extract forms in approximate doses corresponding to 4 g clove per day, yet no statistically or clinically significant effects on plasma lipid concentrations were observed at any monthly interval up to the 6-month study limit. Moreover, results from a meta-analysis which included 13 separate trials and involved over a thousand subjects indicated that there was no significant effect of garlic on plasma cholesterol (Khoo and Aziz, 2009). Thus, it appears that there is variability in published outcomes and this lack of consistency does not appear to stem from variations in basal plasma cholesterol level of participating subjects, the duration of the studies, or the form and dose of garlic. Despite this, most studies appear to show less of a lipid-lowering effect of garlic than once believed.

8.4.2 ANTIOXIDANT ACTIVITY

ROS play major roles in many diseases, including cardiovascular diseases (Petersen et al., 2005). In myocardial ischemia and following heart failure, intracellular ROS rise rapidly in cardiac myoctyes and endothelial cells and apoptosis ensues. Antioxidants can down regulate ROS generation and protect against coronary dysfunction. Early studies show that garlic possesses such antioxidant activities (Borek and Jaskolski, 2000). Using isolated human LDL and challenge with a range of different oxidants, it was observed that a 10% aqueous preparation of AGE completely inhibited the oxidative modification of LDL, impaired superoxide production and reduced lipid peroxide formation (Dillon et al., 2003). *Ex vivo* LDL oxidation, as assessed by the Cu^{2+}-dependent appearance of thiobarbituric acid reactive substances, was inhibited in a concentration-dependent way by AGE (Lau, 2001). More recently, Vazquez-Prieto et al. (2010) demonstrated that aqueous garlic extract administration to rats supplemented with 10% fructose in water to induce metabolic syndrome resulted in reductions of oxidative stress and vascular remodeling as assayed by the plasma biomarkers. As another assessment of the antioxidative potential of garlic, the antioxidant capacity of individual serum was determined before and after administration of standardized commercial garlic tablets to 17 healthy volunteers (Koseoglu et al., 2010). Total antioxidant capacity of serum was increased significantly by approximately 10% after 30 d garlic treatment. Garlic was also observed to preserve intracellular glutathione level which serves as a defense against free radicals, particularly in endothelial cells (Ide and Lau, 2001). Furthermore, garlic may inhibit the uptake of LDL by macrophages, an important step in atherosclerosis development (Gonen et al., 2005). In a murine model of cardiac hypertrophy, oral gavage with the garlic sulfur compound allicin not only improved cardiac performance but also inhibited the development of cardiac hypertrophy (Liu et al., 2010). In the same study, isolated myocytes were treated with or without 10 µM allicin, before incubation with angiotensin II to induce hypertrophy and to increase intracellular ROS. Allicin significantly reduced ROS production as well as ROS-dependent ERK1/2, JNK1/2, AKT, NF-κB and Smad signaling (Liu et al., 2010). In summary, garlic and its constituents have prominent antioxidative properties and clear potential in combating cardiovascular diseases.

8.4.3 ANTI-INFLAMMATORY ACTION

Inflammation is central to both the initiation and progression of atherothrombotic events and atherosclerosis. Garlic and its numerous active ingredients have been observed to affect these events and to affect the inflammatory process in particular. Aqueous extracts of garlic were observed to inhibit inflammatory cytokine-induced expression of leukocyte adhesion molecules on endothelial cells *in vitro* (Rassoul et al., 2006). Incubation of cultured primary human coronary artery endothelial cells with aqueous garlic extracts (0.25–4 mg/mL) for 24 h significantly decreased the IL-1α-driven expression of intercellular adhesion molecule-1 and vascular cell adhesion molecule (VCAM-1) by the endothelial cells. The presence of the garlic extract also significantly inhibited the adhesion of monocytic U937 cells to the IL-1α-treated endothelial cells. In a separate investigation, the effectiveness of thiacremonone, a novel cyclic sulfur compound isolated from garlic, as an anti-inflammatory agent was demonstrated using two separate animal models of inflammation and edema, as well as by the observation that thiacremonone inhibited NF-κB activation and DNA binding (Ban et al., 2009). The garlic sulfur compound DAS was observed to decrease cyclooxygenase-2 expression in models of joint inflammation (Lee et al., 2009). Numerous additional biochemical markers of inflammation in several separate cellular and animal systems have been observed to be inhibited by garlic and its extracts (Lang et al., 2004; Makris et al., 2005; Chiang et al., 2006; Keophiphath et al., 2009; Sohn et al., 2009). Overall, beneficial effects of dietary garlic as an anti-inflammatory mediator are broadly observed by experiments.

8.4.4 EFFECTS ON BLOOD CLOTTING

Effects of garlic on blood clotting and platelet function are established. Platelets play an important role in the development of atheroma and in the progression of atherosclerosis. Platelets aggregate at the site of atheroma to form a thrombus and may ultimately block the vessel and prevent blood flow (Gawaz and Favaloro, 2010). It is thus of significance that *in vitro* and *in situ* studies have demonstrated that garlic has antithrombotic, fibrinolytic, as well as antiplatelet activities (El-Sabban, 2009). Dietary supplementation with AGE for 13 weeks to human volunteers slowed ADP-induced aggregation of the platelet-rich plasma derived from drawn blood (Rahman and Billington, 2000). Addition of an ethanolic extract of garlic powder inhibited ADP-driven human platelet aggregation, suggesting a direct effect on the ADP-dependent pathway (Hiyasat et al., 2009). Analysis of garlic oil constituents identified methyl allyl trisulfide as the most active principal in inhibiting platelet aggregation both *in vitro* and *in vivo* (Ariga and Seki, 2006). Administration of methyl allyl trisulfide to rats in amounts achieving 1 µM concentrations in the blood markedly inhibited laser-induced thrombosis formation in aortic vessels. Methyl allyl trisulfide directly inhibited platelet cyclooxygenase; however, at slightly higher concentrations, this sulfide also inhibited prostacyclin production by aortic endothelial cells (Ariga and Seki, 2006). Overall, several biochemical mechanisms have been shown to be involved in the inhibition of platelet aggregation by garlic, including inhibition of cyclooxygenase; impairment of intraplatelet calcium mobilization; increases in cAMP, nitric oxide, and antioxidants; and inhibitory effects on the gpIIb/IIIa fibrinogen receptor (Rahman, 2007).

8.4.5 EFFECTS ON BLOOD PRESSURE

As high blood pressure is considered a risk factor for cardiovascular disease, several studies were conducted to examine any potential antihypertensive effect of garlic and its products. Reinhart et al. (2008) conducted a meta-analysis of qualified clinical studies available through 2008. Data from 10 clinical trials that met criteria and used subjects with elevated systolic pressures indicated that garlic has significant antihypertensive action. Similarly, results were reported of a meta-analysis which included 11 qualified studies published in Medline and Embase databases between 1955 and 2007 (Ried et al., 2008). The conclusion of this meta-analysis was that garlic preparations are superior to placebo in reducing blood pressure in individuals with hypertension. More recently, results of a randomized controlled study were published and suggested that AGE lowers blood pressure in patients with treated but uncontrolled hypertension (Karin et al., 2010). On the other hand, a comparable meta-analysis which included fewer studies but studies which met more rigid criteria concluded that an antihypertensive effect of garlic on blood pressure cannot be certain (Simons et al., 2009).

Experiments with animals demonstrated that garlic or its bioactive compounds used in combination with antihypertensive medications such as ACE inhibitors can synergistically lower blood pressure (Asdaq and Inamdar, 2010). Several mechanisms have been offered, including direct inhibition of ACE, inhibition of thromboxane and prostaglandin synthesis, enhancement of nitric oxide production, and suppression of peroxynitrite levels (Ku et al., 2002; Al-Qattan et al., 2003; Sharifi et al., 2003; Medina-Campos et al., 2007; Chen et al., 2009).

8.4.6 IMPROVEMENT OF ENDOTHELIAL FUNCTION

Endothelial dysfunction is considered the first step in the pathogenesis of developing atherosclerosis (Hansson, 2005). Damage to the endothelium can be initiated by hypertension, smoking, and hyperlipidemia, and the response to this injury and progression of damage involves platelet and macrophage adherence and generation of ROS, inflammatory cytokines, and oxidized lipoproteins. In a randomized crossover study of men with coronary artery disease, Williams et al. (2005) found that AGE improved endothelial dysfunction. At the end of the 4-week crossover periods, brachial artery flow-mediated endothelium-dependent dilation was significantly greater in the AGE treatment group compared to placebo. They attributed this beneficial outcome to the antioxidant properties of garlic. However, markers of oxidative stress, systemic inflammation and endothelial VCAM-1 were unchanged. Although, this study was short term, impaired endothelium function in men with coronary artery disease was improved by consumption of the garlic extract. In a separate placebo-controlled, double-blind, randomized trial involving 58 asymptomatic patients, the daily consumption for 1 year of commercially available AGE (250 mg) along with vitamins B6, B12, and L-arginine resulted in significant improvements in several cardiovascular outcomes versus placebo (Budoff et al., 2009). These outcomes included coronary artery calcium scanning, oxidative markers (oxidized apolipoprotein B-100 particles), vascular reactivity, and overall reduced progression of subclinical atherosclerosis (Budoff et al., 2009). Furthermore, in an *in vitro* study using human endothelial cell cultures, Lei et al. (2010) observed that a 16 h-treatment with either of the garlic components DADS and DAT protected endothelial nitric oxide synthase (eNOS) activity in the cells against oxidized LDL insult. No production was effectively restored by treatment with DADS or DAT. The authors suggest that the protection was due to the action of these sulfide compounds on PI 3-kinase-protein kinase B signaling with resultant inhibition of eNOS degradation.

8.4.7 Cardiac Arrhythmia

Garlic was tested for its ability to promote antiarrhythmic effects and to improve defibrillation status in a porcine model. Ventricular fibrillation thresholds and the upper limits of vulnerability, a measure of acute defibrillation threshold, were determined in pigs before and after intravenous administration of solutions containing garlic (20–40 mg/kg, 1.35% allicin). The defibrillation threshold was unchanged in the 20 mg/kg group but was significantly lower than control in the 40 mg/kg group. Although these are very limited data, an electrophysiological effect of garlic on the heart like that observed by Sungnoon et al. (2008a,b) may be beneficial in promoting terminations of spontaneous ventricular fibrillations and in the prevention of sudden cardiac death.

8.5 EFFECTS ON RELATED CARDIOVASCULAR DISEASES

8.5.1 Gallstones

Gallstones that arise from cholesterol supersaturation of the bile are by far the most common type. Garlic has been used in experimental animal systems to treat gallstones (Vidyashankar et al., 2010). Cholesterol gallstones were induced in mice by feeding a lithogenic diet containing 0.25% of bile salts and 0.5% cholesterol for 10 weeks. Animals were then fed basal diets containing 0.6% garlic powder for further 10 weeks. Dietary garlic resulted in up to 53% regression in gallstone formation compared to only a 10% drop in control animals and this regression was associated with lowered cholesterol saturation index in the bile and decreased serum and liver cholesterol levels. The study indicated that dietary garlic effectively accelerated the regression of preformed cholesterol gallstones by promoting cholesterol desaturation in bile (Vidyashankar et al., 2010).

8.5.2 Obesity

Obesity is a risk factor for cardiovascular disease. According to the WHO there are more than 1 billion overweight adults worldwide with at least 300 million of them clinically obese. A study by Keophiphath et al. (2009) demonstrated the effectiveness of garlic 1,2-vinyldithiin in inhibiting the differentiation of human preadipocytes in culture. Similarly, treatment of preadipocytes and mature 3T3-L1 adipocytes with 100–200 µM ajoene inhibited adipogenesis and induced apoptosis, suggesting antiobesity effects (Ambati et al., 2009). However, in an independent study in which the same murine 3T3-L1 adipocytes were treated with 50–100 µM of the garlic sulfur compound DADS, terminal differentiation into fully mature adipocytes and accumulation of cellular triglycerides were accelerated and this occurred in as short an exposure as 48 h (Lee et al., 2007). Differences among these studies could be due to species and/or the garlic compounds used.

8.5.3 Diabetes

WHO estimates that more than 220 million people worldwide have diabetes and that this number is likely to more than double by 2030 without intervention. Animal research suggests that diets enriched in garlic or garlic products are effective in reducing diabetic markers such as serum glucose and triglyceride levels (Liu et al., 2005; Eidi et al., 2006). Among many mechanisms suggested for this effect of garlic, two experimental observations of interest are that garlic and its products stimulate residual insulin secretion from the pancreatic β-cells and that garlic improves insulin sensitivity in insulin target tissues (Augusti and Sheela, 1996; Liu et al., 2005; Kim et al., 2010). In addition, studies *in vitro* showed that AGE and *S*-allyl-cysteine inhibited glucose-derived glycation of serum albumin, perhaps indicating that dietary garlic might delay or prevent complications of diabetes such as advanced glycation end products which cause many of the debilitating complications of diabetes (Ahmad et al., 2007).

8.6 CONCLUSION

Despite the fact that recent investigative studies support less of a lipid-lowering effect of garlic as once thought, controlled clinical and experimental studies show that garlic and its biocomponents are effective in promoting healthy cardiovascular function. Active biocomponents of garlic include allyl-polysulfides and numerous other sulfur-containing metabolites. There are strong research data showing that these garlic metabolites possess vascular antioxidant activity, suppress inflammation, slow platelet activation, and overall promote aortic relaxation, protect arteries from plaque formation, and improve endothelial function. In addition, preliminary studies suggest that garlic may also provide benefits in terminating spontaneous ventricular fibrillations and in promoting improvement in the cardiovascular-related maladies of gallstone disease, obesity, and diabetes.

REFERENCES

Ahmad, M.S., Pischetsrieder, M., and Ahmed, N. 2007. Aged garlic extract and S-allyl cysteine prevent formation of advanced glycation end products. *Eur. J. Pharmacol.* **561**(1–3): 32–38.

Al-Qattan, K.K., Khan, L., Alnaqeeb, M.A., and Ali, M. 2003. Mechanism of garlic (*Allium sativum*) induced reduction of hypertension in 2K-1C rats: A possible mediation of Na/H exchanger isoform-1. *Prostaglandins Leukot Essent Fatty Acids.* **69**(4): 217–222.

Amagase, H. 2006. Clarifying the real bioactive constituents of garlic. *J. Nutr.* **136**(3 Suppl.): 716S–725S.

Amagase, H., Petesch, B.L., Matsuura, H., Kasuga, S., and Itakura, Y. 2001. Intake of garlic and its bioactive components. *J. Nutr.* **131**(3s): 955S–962S.

Ambati, S., Yang, J.-Y., Rayalam, S., Park, H.J., Della-Fera, M.A., and Baile, C.A. 2009. Ajoene exerts potent effects in 3T3-L1 cells. *Phytother. Res.* **23**(4): 513–518.

Ariga, T. and Seki, T, 2006. Antithrombotic and anticancer effects of garlic-derived sulfur compounds: A review. *Biofactors.* **26**(2): 93–103.

Asdaq, S.M. and Inamdar, M.N. 2010. Potential of garlic and its active constituent, S-allyl cysteine, as antihypertensive and cardioprotective in presence of captopril. *Phytomedicine.* **17**(13): 1016–1026.

Augusti, K.T. and Sheela, C.G. 1996. Antiperoxide effect of S-allyl cysteine sulfoxide, an insulin secretagogue, in diabetic rats. *Experientia.* **52**(2): 115–120.

Ban, J.O., Oh, J.H., Tim, T.M., Kim, D.J., Jeong, J.-S., Ban, S.B., and Hong, J.T. 2009. Anti-inflammatory and arthritic effects of thiacremonone, a novel sulfur compound isolated from garlic via inhibition of NF-κB. *Arthritis Res. Ther.* **11**(5): R145.

Banerjee, S.K. and Maulik, S.K. 2002. Effect of garlic on cardiovascular disorders: A review. *Nutr. J.* **1**: 4.

Baumgart, K., Georgieff, M., Radermacher, P., and Calzia, E. 2009. Cardioprotection by hydrogen sulfide: Suspended animation, inflammation, and apoptosis. *Shock.* **31**(2): 218–219.

Benavides, G.A., Squadrito, G.L., Mills, R.W., Patel, H.D., Scott Isbell, T., Patel, R.P., Darley-Usmar, V.M., Doeller, E., and Kraus, D.W. 2007. Hydrogen sulfide mediates the vasoactivity of garlic. *Proc. Natl. Acad. Sci. USA.* **104**(46): 17977–17982.

Borek, D. and Jaskolski, M. 2000. Crystallization and preliminary crystallographic studies of a new L-asparaginase encoded by the *Escherichia coli* genome. *Acta. Crystallogr. D Biol. Crystallogr.* **56**(Pt 11): 1505–1507.

Boriss, H. 2006. *Commodity Profile: Garlic*, A.M.R. Center, Editor. http://aic.ucdavis.edu/profiles/Garlic-2006B.pdf.

Budoff, M.J., Ahmadi, M., Gul, K.M., Liu, S.T., Flores, F.R., Tiano, J., Takasu, J., Miller, E., and Tsimikas, S. 2009. Aged garlic extract supplemented with B-vitamins, folic acid and l-arginine retards the progression of subclinical atherosclerosis: A randomized clinical trial. *Prev. Med.* **49**(2–3): 107–117.

Butt, M.S., Sultan, M.T., and Iqbal, J. 2009. Garlic: Nature's protection against physiological threats. *Crit. Rev. Food Sci. Nutr.* **49**(6): 538–551.

Calvert, J.W., Coetzee, W.A., and Lefer, D.J. 2010. Novel insights into hydrogen sulfide-mediated cytoprotection. *Antioxid. Redox Signal.* **12**(10): 1203–1217.

Chen, Z.Y., Peng, C., Jiao, R., Wong, Y.M., Yang, N., and Huang, Y. 2009. Anti-hypertensive nutraceuticals and functional foods. *J. Agric. Food Chem.* **57**(11): 4485–4499.

Chiang, Y.H., Jen, L.N., Su, H.Y., Lii, C.K., and Liu, C.T. 2006. Effects of garlic oil and two of its major organosulfur compounds, diallyl disulfide and diallyl trisulfide, on intestinal damage in rats injected with endotoxin. *Toxicol. Appl. Pharmacol.* **213**(1): 46–54.

Davenport, D.M. and Wargovich, M.J. 2005. Modulation of cytochrome P450 enzymes by organosulfur compounds from garlic. *Food Chem. Toxicol*, **43**(12): 1753–1762.

Derwall, M., Westerkamp, M., Lower, C., Deike-Glindemann, J., Schnorrenberger, N.K., Coburn, M., Nolte, K.W. et al., 2010. Hydrogen sulfide does not increase resuscitability in a porcine model of prolonged cardiac arrest. *Shock*. **34**(2): 190–195.

Dillon, S.A., Burmi, R.S., Lowe, G.M., Billington, D., and Rahman, K. 2003. Antioxidant properties of aged garlic extract: An *in vitro* study incorporating human low density lipoprotein. *Life Sci*. **72**(14): 1583–1594.

Eidi, A., Eidi, M., and Esmaeli, E. 2006. Antidiabetic effect of garlic (*Allium sativum* L.) in normal and strep-tozotocin-induced diabetic rats. *Phytomedicine*. **13**(9–10): 624–629.

El-Sabban, F.M. 2009. Current stand on supplementation with antioxidant vitamins in cardiovascular disease. *Saudi Med J*. **30**(7): 969–970.

Elrod, J.W., Calvert, J.W., Morrison, J., Doeller, J.E., Kraus, D.W., Tao, L., Jiao, X. et al., 2007. Hydrogen sulfide attenuates myocardial ischemia-reperfusion injury by preservation of mitochondrial function. *Proc. Natl. Acad. Sci. USA*. **104**(39): 15560–15565.

Elsey, D.J., Fowkes, R.C., and Baxter, G.F. 2010. Regulation of cardiovascular cell function by hydrogen sul-fide (H(2)S). *Cell Biochem. Funct*. **28**(2): 95–106.

Fukao, T., Hosono, T., Misawa, S., Seki, T., and Ariga, T. 2004. The effects of allyl sulfides on the induction of phase II detoxification enzymes and liver injury by carbon tetrachloride. *Food Chem. Toxicol*. **42**(5): 743–749.

Gardner, C.D., Lawson, L.D., Block, E., Chetterjee, L.M., Kiazand, R., Balise, R.R., and Kraemer, H.C. 2007. Effect of raw garlic vs commercial garlic supplements on plasma lipid concentrations in adults with moderate hypercholesterolemia: A randomized clinical trial. *Arch. Intern. Med*. **167**(4): 346–353.

Gawaz, M. and Favaloro, E.J. 2010. Platelets, inflammation and cardiovascular diseases. New concepts and therapeutic implications. *Semin. Thromb. Hemost*. **36**(2): 129–130.

Gonen, A., Shaish, A., and Harats, D. 2005. The antiatherogenic effect of allicin: Possible mode of action. *Pathobiol*. **72**(6): 325–334.

Gorinstein, S., Leontowicz, H., Leontowicz, M., Drzewiecki, J., Najman, K., Katrich, L., Barasch, D., Yamamoto, K., and Trakhtenberg, S. 2006a. Raw and boiled garlic enhances plasma antioxidant activity and improves plasma lipid metabolism in cholesterol-fed rats. *Life Sci*. **78**(6): 655–663.

Gorinstein, S., Leontowicz, M., Leontowicz, H., Jastrzebski, Z., Drzewiecki, J., Namieskin, J., Zachwieja, Z. et al., 2006b. Dose-dependent influence of commercial garlic (*Allium sativum*) on rats fed cholesterol-containing diet. *J. Agric. Food Chem*. **54**(11): 4022–4027.

Gorinstein, S., Jastrzebski, Z., Namieskin, J., Leontowicz, H., Leontowicz, M., and Trakhtenberg, S. 2007. The atherosclerotic heart disease and protecting properties of garlic: Contemporary data. *Mol. Nutr. Food Res*. **51**(11): 1365–1381.

Hansson, G.K. 2005. Inflammation, atherosclerosis, and coronary artery disease. *N. Engl. .J. Med*. **352**(16): 1685–1695.

Hiyasat, B., Sabha, D., Grotzinger, K., Kempfert, J., Rauwald, J.W., Mohr, F.W., and Dhein, S. 2009. Antiplatelet activity of *Allium ursinum* and *Allium sativum*. *Pharmacology*. **83**(4): 197–204.

Ide, N. and Lau, B.H.S, 2001. Garlic compounds minimize intracellular oxidative stress and inhibit nuclear factor-{{kappa}}B activation. *J. Nutr*. **131**(3): 1020S–1026S.

Karin, R., Oliver, R.F., and Nigel, P.S. 2010. Aged garlic extract lowers blood pressure in patients with treated but uncontrolled hypertension: A randomised controlled trial. *Maturitas*. **67**(2): 144–150.

Keophiphath, M., Priem, F., Jacquemond-Collet, I., Clement, K., and Lacasa, D. 2009. 1,2-vinyldithiin from garlic inhibits differentiation and Inflammation of human preadipocystes. *J. Nutr*. **139**(11): 2055–2060.

Khoo, Y.S. and Aziz, Z. 2009. Garlic supplementation and serum cholesterol: A meta-analysis. *J. Clin. Pharm. Ther*. **34**(2): 133–145.

Khot, U.N., Khot, M.B., Bajzer, C.T., Sapp, S.K., Ohman, E.M., Brener, S.J., Ellis, S.G., Lincoff, A.M., and Topol, E.J. 2003. Prevalence of conventional risk factors in patients with coronary heart disease. *JAMA*. **290**(7): 898–904.

Kim, J., Kim, J., Kang, M., Han, J., and Kang, Y. 2010. Aged black garlic improves insulin sensitivity in fruc-tose fed rats. *FASEB J*. **24**(1 Meeting Abstracts): 722.4.

Kodera, Y., Suzuki, A., Imada, O., Kasuga, S., Sumioka, I., Kanezawa, A., Taru, N. et al., 2002a. Physical, chemical and biological properties of *S*-allyl-cysteine, an amino acid derived from garlic. *J. Agric. Food Chem*. **50**(3): 622–632.

Kodera, Y., Ishikawa, M., Yoshida, J., Kashimoto, N., Uda, N., Sumioka, I., Ide, N., and Ono, K. 2002b. Pharmacokinetic study of allixin, a phytoalexin produced by garlic. *Chem. Pharm. Bull* (Tokyo). **50**(3): 354–363.

Koseoglu, M., Isleten, F., Atay, A., and Kaplan, Y.C. 2010. Effects of acute and subacute garlic supplement administration on serum total antioxidant capacity and lipid parameters in healthy volunteers. *Phytother. Res.* **24**(3): 374–378.

Kromhout, D., Menotti, A., Kesteloot, H., and Sans, S. 2002. Prevention of coronary heart disease by diet and lifestyle: Evidence from prospective cross-cultural, cohort, an intervention studies. *Circulation.* **105**(7): 893–898.

Ku, D.D., Abdel-Razek, T.T., Dai, J., Kim-Park, S., Fallon, M.B., and Abrams, G.A. 2002. Garlic and its active metabolite allicin produce endothelium- and nitric oxide-dependent relaxation in rat pulmonary arteries. *Clin. Exp. Pharmacol. Physiol.* **29**(1–2): 84–91.

Lang, A., Lahav, M., Sakhnini, E., Barshack, I., Fidder, H.H., Avidan, B., Bardan, E., Hershkoviz, R., Bar-Meir, S., and Chowers, Y. 2004. Allicin inhibits spontaneous and TNF-alpha induced secretion of proinflamma- tory cytokines and chemokines from intestinal epithelial cells. *Clin. Nutr.* **23**(5): 1199–1208.

Lau, B.H. 2001. Suppression of LDL oxidation by garlic. *J. Nutr.* 131(3s): 985S-Please provide the complete page range in Lau, 2001.

Lawson, L.D. 1998. Garlic: A review of its medicinal effects and indicated active Compounds. In *Phytomedicines of Europe. Chemistry and Biological Activity.* Series 691 (L.D. Lawson and R. Baur, eds), American Chemical Society, Washington, DC, pp. 176–209.

Lee, H.S., Lee, C.H., Tsai, H.C., and Salter, D.M. 2009. Inhibition of cyclooxygenase 2 expression by diallyl sulfide on joint inflammation induced by urate crystal and IL-1beta. *Osteoarthritis Cartillage.* **17**(1): 91–99.

Lee, J.H., Kim, K.A., Kwon, K.B., Kim, E.K., Lee, Y.R., Song, M.Y., Koo, J.H., Ka, S.O., Park, J.W., and Park, B.H. 2007. Dially disulfide accelerates adipogenesis in 3T3-L1 cells. *Int. J. Mol. Med.* **20**(1): 59–64.

Lefer, D.J. 2007. A new gaseous signaling molecule emerges: Cardioprotective role of hydrogen sulfide. *Proc. Natl. Acad. Sci. (USA).* **104**(46): 17907–17908.

Lei, Y.P., Liu, C.T., Sheen, L.Y., Chen, H.W., and Lii, C.K. 2010, Diallyl disulfide and diallyl trisulfide protect endothelial nitric oxide synthase against damage by oxidized low-density lipoprotein. *Mol. Nutr. Food Res.* **54**(Suppl. 1): 542–552.

Liu, C., Cao, F., Tang, Q.Z., Yan, L., Dong, Y.G., Zhu, L.H., Wang, L., Bian, Z.Y., and Li, H. 2010. Allicin protects against cardiac hypertrophy and fibrosis via attenuating reactive oxygen species-dependent sig- nalling pathways. *J. Nutr. Biochem.* **21**(12): 1238–1250.

Liu, C.T., Hse, H., Lii, C.K., Chen, P.S., and Sheen, L.Y. 2005. Effects of garlic oil and diallyl trisulfide on glycemic control in diabetic rats. *Eur. J. Pharmacol.* **516**(2): 165–173.

Makris, A., Thornton, C.E., Xu, B., and Hennessy, A. 2005. Garlic increases IL-10 and inhibits TNFalpha and IL-6 production in endotoxin-stimulated human placental explants. *Placenta.* **26**(10): 828–834.

Mustafa, A.K., Gadalla, M.M., Sen, N., Kim, S., Mu, W., Gazi, S.K., Barrow, R.K., Yang, G., Wang, R., and Solomon, H.M. 2009. H_2S signals through protein S-sulfhydration. *Sci. Signal.* **2**(96): ra72.

Medina-Campos, O.N., Barrera, D., Segoviano-Murillo, S., Rocha, D., Maldonado, P.D., Mendoza-Patino, N., and Pedraza-Chaverri, J. 2007. S-allylcysteine scavenges singlet oxygen and hypochlorous acid and pro- tects LLC-PK(1) cells of potassium dichromate-induced toxicity. *Food Chem. Toxicol.* **45**(10): 2030–2039.

Petersen, O.H., Spat, A., and Vekhasty, A. 2005. Introduction: Reactive oxygen. *Philos. Trans. Royal Soc. B: Biol. Sci.* **360**(1464): 2197–2199.

Pryor, W.A., Houk, K.N., Foote, C.S., Ignarro, L.J., Squadrito, G.L., and Davies, K.J. 2006. Free radical biol- ogy and medicine: It's gas, man! *Am. J. Physiol. Regul. Integr. Comp. Physiol.* 291(3): R491–R511.

Rahman, K., and Billington, D. 2000. Dietary supplementation with aged garlic extract inhibits ADP-induced platelet aggregation in humans. *J. Nutr.* **130**(11): 2662–2665.

Rahman, K., and Lowe, G.M. 2006. Garlic and cardiovascular disease: A critical *J, Nutr.* **136**(3 Suppl.): 736S–740S.

Rahman, K 2007. Effects of garlic on platelet biochemistry and physiology. *Mol. Nutr. Food Res.* **51**(11): 1335–1344.

Rassoul, F., Salvetter, J., Reissig, D., Schneider, W., Theiry, J., and Richter, V. 2006. The influence of garlic (*Allium sativum*) extract on interleukin 1alpha-induced expression of endothelial intercellular adhesion molecule-1 and vascular cell adhesion molecule 1. *Phytomedicine.* **13**(4): 230–235.

Ried, K., Frank, O.R., Stocks, N.P., Fakler, P., and Sullivan, T. 2008. Effect of garlic on blood pressure: A sys- tematic review and meta-analysis. *BMC Cardiovascular Disorders.* **8**: 13.

Reinhart, K.M., Coleman, C.L., Teevan, C., Vachhani, P., and White, C.M. 2008. Effects of garlic on blood pressure in patients with and without systolic hypertension: A meta-analysis. *Ann. Pharmacother.* **42**(12): 1766–1771.

Rivlin, R.S. 2001.Historical perspectives on the use of garlic. *J. Nutr.* **131**(3s): 9515–9245.

Sharifi, A.M., Darabi, R., and Akbarloo, N. 2003. Investigation of antihypertensive Rat. *J. Ethnopharmacol.* **86**(2–3): 219–224.

Simons, S., Wollersheim, H., and Thien, T. 2009. Asystematic review on the influence of trial quality on the effect of garlic on blood pressure. *Neth. J. Med.* **67**(6): 212–219.

Sivarajah, A., Collino, M., Yasin, M., Benetti, E., Gallicchio, M., Mazzon, E., Cuzzocrea, S., Fantozzi, R., and Thiemermann, C. 2009. Anti-apoptotic and anti-inflammatory effects of hydrogen sulfide is a rat model of a regional myocardial 1/R. *Shock.* **31**(3): 267–274.

Sobenin, I.A., Andrianova, I.V., Demidova, O.N., Gorchakova, T., and Orekhov, A.N. 2008. Lipid lowering effects of a time-released garlic powder Tablets in double-blinded placebo-controlled randomized study. *J. Atheroscler. Thromb.* **15**(6): 334–338.

Sohn, D.W., Han, C.H., Jung, Y.S., Kim, S.I., Kim, S.W., and Cho, Y.-H. 2009. Anti-inflammatory and antimicrobial effects of garlic and synergistic effect between garlic and ciprofoxa in a chronic bacterial prostatitis rat model. *Int. J. Antimicrob. Agents.* **34**(3): 215–219.

Stevinson, C., Pittler, M.H., and Ernst, E. 2000. Garlic for treating hypercholesterolemia. A meta-analysis of randomized clinical trials. *Annals of Internal Medicine* **133**(6): 420–429.

Sungnoon, R., Kanlop, N., Chattipakorn, S.C., Tawan, R., and Chattipakorn, N. 2008a. Effects of garlic on the induction of ventricular fibrillation. *Nutrition* **24**(7–8): 711–716.

Sungnoon, R., Shinlapawittayatorn, K., Chattipakorn, S.C., and Chattipakorn, N. 2008b. Effects of garlic on defibrillation efficacy. *Int. J. Cardiol.* **126**(1): 143–144.

Vazquez-Prieto, M.A., Gonzalez, R.E., Renna, N.F., Galmarini, C.N., and Miatello, R.M. 2010. Aqueous garlic extracts prevent oxidative stress and vascular remodeling of an experimental model of metabolic syndrome. *J. Agric. Food Chem.* **58**(11): 6630–6635.

Vidyashankar, S., Sambaiah, S.K., and Srinivasan, K. 2010. Regression of preestablished cholesterol gall stones by dietary garlic and onion in experimental mice. *Metabolism.* **59**(10): 1402–1412.

WHO. *Monograph on Selected Medicinal Plants.* 1999. http://apps.who.int/medicinedocs/pdf/s2200e/s2200e.pdf to the citation.

Williams, M.J., Sutherland, W.H., McCormick, M.P., Yeoman, D.J., and de Jong, S.A. 2005. Aged garlic extract improves endothelial function in men with coronary artery disease. *Phytother. Res.* **19**(4): 314–319.

Xu, J., Kochanek, K.D., Murphy, S.L., and Tejada-Vera, B. 2010. Final Data for 2007. *National Vital Statistics Report.* **58**: 1–135.

Yang, L.J., Fan. L., Liu, Z.Q., Mao, Y.M., Guo, D., Liu, L.H., Tan, Z.R. et al., 2009. Effects of allicin on CYP2C19 and CYP3A4 activity in healthy volunteers with different CYP3C19 genotypes. *Eur. J. Clin. Pharmacol.* **65**(6): 601–608.

Zhao, W., Zhang, J., Lu, Y., and Wang, R. 2001. The vasorelaxant effect of H(2)S as a novel endogenous gaseous K(ATP) channel opener. *EMBO J.* **20**(21): 6008–6016.

9 Impact of Egg Consumption in Development or Prevention of Heart Disease

Donald J. McNamara
Eggs for Health Consulting

CONTENTS

9.1 INTRODUCTION

For over 40 years there has been continuous debate regarding the relationship between dietary cholesterol intake and its impact on blood cholesterol levels and coronary heart disease (CHD) risk. The 1968 American Heart Association recommendation that dietary cholesterol be limited to not more than 300 mg/day, and that egg intake be limited to not more than 3 egg yolks/week, initiated a scientific debate that continues to this day. When this recommendation was originally proposed there was a limited understanding of endogenous cholesterol metabolism and its regulation, and of the impact of dietary factors on blood cholesterol levels and CHD risk. From a purely logical perspective it does seem reasonable to assume that dietary cholesterol would affect blood cholesterol levels and there was epidemiological evidence suggesting a relationship between blood cholesterol levels and CHD risk. Forty years later it is clear that, while this assumed relationship may have been logical in 1968, it has not withstood the test of time.

9.2   BASIS OF THE DIETARY CHOLESTEROL: HEART DISEASE HYPOTHESIS

In 1918 Russian scientists fed rabbits milk, meat, and eggs and observed that the animals developed atherosclerotic lesions (Anitschkow and Chalatow, 1913). The fact that rabbits do not normally consume milk, meat, and eggs was not a consideration in the study design nor in its interpretation. Other animal studies have utilized massive doses of dietary cholesterol to induce hypercholesterolemia and atherosclerosis in various animal species with varying degrees of success; however, for omnivores and carnivores, intake of cholesterol within physiological ranges has little effect on plasma cholesterol levels or plaque development (McNamara, 1990). This is due to effective feedback regulatory mechanisms by which endogenous cholesterol synthesis is suppressed and fecal bile acid excretion increased to compensate for the increase in absorbed dietary cholesterol (Dietschy, 1984). Only when these compensatory mechanisms are overwhelmed by feeding pharmacological levels of cholesterol do most nonherbivore animal species develop hypercholesterolemia and atherosclerotic plaques.

A major contributor to the *dietary cholesterol–plasma cholesterol–heart disease risk* hypothesis was the observation from epidemiological studies of a simple correlation between dietary cholesterol and CHD incidence across and within populations. These same studies also reported significant correlations between calories from saturated fat and CHD incidence. What these early studies failed to account for was the highly significant colinearity between cholesterol and saturated fatty acids found in most animal products (Hegsted and Ausman, 1988). Once this colinearity confounder was accounted for using multiple regression analysis, dietary cholesterol was no longer found to be correlated with CHD risk (McNamara, 2000a). This has been found in numerous epidemiological surveys and readily explains the fallacy of relying on simple correlations between dietary cholesterol and heart disease incidence reported in the early stages of nutritional epidemiology in determining dietary limitations (Kromhout et al., 1995).

Early clinical cholesterol feeding studies often relied on administering excessive amounts of dietary cholesterol in order to obtain measurable changes in plasma total cholesterol levels (McNamara, 1990). Often the test doses exceeded the body's production of cholesterol thus overwhelming any feedback regulatory mechanisms that might exist resulting in an expanded blood cholesterol pool. Studies over the last three decades have used more physiological ranges of cholesterol intakes and documented relatively modest changes in plasma cholesterol levels. It was also assumed in these early studies that any change in plasma total cholesterol content was a surrogate marker for changes in CHD risk since epidemiological studies indicated a direct relationship between plasma total cholesterol levels and CHD incidence. Analyses of the effects of dietary cholesterol on the plasma concentrations and properties of specific lipoprotein subfractions have shown that dietary cholesterol affects both the atherogenic low-density lipoprotein (LDL) levels as well as the antiatherogenic high-density lipoprotein (HDL) cholesterol concentrations with little if any change in an important determinant of CHD risk, the LDL:HDL cholesterol ratio (Herron and Fernandez, 2004; Fernandez and Webb, 2008).

In order to understand the basis of the conflict it is essential to understand the complexities of cholesterol metabolism (McNamara, 1987). On a cholesterol-free diet, endogenous cholesterol

TABLE 9.1

Cholesterol Metabolism in a 70 kg Adult with Three Different Cholesterol Intakes

	Sterols (mg/day)		
Dietary cholesterol	0	300	1500
Biliary cholesterol	1400	1400	1400
Total GI cholesterol	**1400**	**1700**	**2900**
Absorbed cholesterol (60%)	840	1020	1740
Fecal cholesterol	560	680	1160
Fecal bile acids (bile acid synthesis)	350	350	350
Total fecal steroids	**910**	**1030**	**1510**
Endogenous synthesis	910	750	500
Total input	**910**	**930**	**2010**
Δ Plasma cholesterol (mg/dL)		+3	+15

Source: Adapted from McNamara, D. J. et al. 1987. *J. Clin. Invest.* **79**: 1729–1739.

synthesis averages 11–13 mg/kg/day. For a hypothetical 70 kg subject, endogenous cholesterol synthesis would be around 940 mg/day. Each day this subject would secrete ~1400 mg of cholesterol into the gastrointestinal (GI) tract as biliary cholesterol which mixes with exogenous dietary cholesterol. On average, humans absorb 60% of the cholesterol in the GI tract, although individual variations range from 20% to 80% absorption (McNamara et al., 1987). Another 350 mg/day of cholesterol is converted into bile acids to compensate for daily fecal loss. As shown in Table 9.1, an increase in dietary cholesterol of 300 mg/day actually results in a very small change in overall endogenous cholesterol metabolism due to the relatively small contribution of dietary cholesterol to the total daily mass dynamics of cholesterol, and the fact that most individuals have effective feedback control mechanisms which are able to compensate for an increase in dietary cholesterol by a reduction in endogenous synthesis (McNamara, 2000a). This ability to balance the two input sources results in little change in plasma cholesterol levels when physiological levels of cholesterol are fed. On the contrary, when the dietary cholesterol challenge overwhelms the metabolic controls, there is a significant increase in plasma cholesterol levels when a challenge dose of cholesterol equal to 1500 mg/day is used (Table 9.1).

9.3 THE DIETARY CHOLESTEROL–HEART DISEASE RISK RELATIONSHIP: EPIDEMIOLOGICAL EVIDENCE

A number of reviews on the epidemiological evidence for the dietary cholesterol–CHD relationship have been published over the last decade (McNamara and Howell, 1992; McNamara, 2000a; Kritchevsky and Kritchevsky, 2000; Kritchevsky, 2004; Lee and Griffin, 2006; Gray and Griffin, 2009) and all have reached a similar conclusion: dietary cholesterol intake is not a significant independent risk factor for either elevated plasma cholesterol levels or CHD incidence.

Ravnskov (1995) published a review of 13 case–control studies carried out between 1968 and 1985 which measured dietary cholesterol intakes and CHD incidence. The mean cholesterol intake in CHD patients was 223 ± 11 mg/1000 kcal versus controls with an average intake of 216 ± 11 mg/1000 kcal. The mean difference between CHD cases and controls of 6.4 mg/1000 kcal is equivalent to 16 mg/day for someone on a 2500 kcal diet. Based on these data, Ravnskov (1995) concluded that there was no evidence for an independent effect of dietary cholesterol on CHD relative risk.

The epidemiological results from cross-cultural and within population survey studies have failed to document a significant relationship between cholesterol intakes and CHD incidence when using multivariant analyses. The results of an analysis of the Twenty Countries database by Hegsted and Ausman (1988) and the Seven Countries Study by Kromhout et al. (1995) reported that dietary cholesterol was not a contributing factor to CHD incidence. Numerous other epidemiological studies have reached the same conclusion (McNamara, 2000a).

The following studies have all reported a nonsignificant relationship between dietary cholesterol and CHD risk.

- Twenty Countries Study (Hegsted and Ausman, 1988)
- Seven Countries Study (Kromhout et al., 1995)
- Thirteen different case–control studies (reviewed in reference (Ravnskov, 1995)
- Lipid Research Clinics Prevalence Follow-Up Study (Esrey et al., 1996)
- Health Professionals Follow-Up Study (Ascherio et al., 1996)
- Nurses' Health Study (Hu et al., 1997)
- ATBC Cancer Prevention Study (Pietinen et al., 1997)
- Framingham Heart Study (Millen et al., 1996)

9.4 EGGS AND HEART DISEASE RISK

Of all the animal products routinely consumed, eggs present a unique mixture of high cholesterol (215 mg/large egg) and low saturated fat (1.5 g). Compared to broiled ground beef with 5.2 g saturated fat and 70 mg cholesterol or a cup of whole milk with 4.6 g saturated fat and 24 mg cholesterol, eggs have a unique cholesterol–saturated fat relative content for an animal product. Thus, the egg was a specific target for dietary cholesterol restrictions as compared to other animal products in the original dietary recommendations, and continues so today in some countries even though epidemiological studies of the association between egg intake and CHD risk have consistently shown a nonsignificant relationship.

One of the earliest studies of the relationship between egg consumption and plasma cholesterol levels and CHD incidence was carried out using data from the Framingham Heart Study and indicated that there was no significant relationship (Dawber et al., 1982). Since then numerous epidemiological studies have failed to document an effect of egg intake on CHD risk.

- Framingham Heart Study (Dawber et al., 1982)
- Health Professional Follow-Up Study (Hu et al., 1999)
- Nurses' Health Study (Hu et al., 1999)
- NHANES (Qureshi et al., 2007)
- Hiroshima/Nagasaki Life Span Study (Sauvaget et al., 2003, 2004)
- Japan Public Health Center Prospective Study (Nakamura et al., 2006)
- Other smaller epidemiological trials (reviewed in McNamara, 2000a and Kritchevsky, 2004)

There is a complete lack of evidence for a relationship between dietary cholesterol, whether from eggs alone or total intake from all animal products, and CHD risk from epidemiological studies. Once the colinearity between dietary saturated fat and dietary cholesterol is accounted for, dietary cholesterol is no longer significantly related to risk (Hegsted and Ausman, 1988; Kromhout et al., 1995; McNamara, 2000a). An interesting example of this is the finding reported by Hu et al. (1999) that egg consumption in males in the Health Professionals Follow-Up Study was found to be unrelated to heart disease risk only after correction for bacon intake. While clearly a case of guilt by association, this is not evidence of eggs as an independent risk factor.

9.5   THE DIETARY CHOLESTEROL–HEART DISEASE RISK RELATIONSHIP: CLINICAL EVIDENCE

Earlier clinical studies of the impact of cholesterol feeding on plasma cholesterol levels did indicate that high intakes of cholesterol (1500 mg/day in some studies, six eggs per day in others) did in fact increase plasma total cholesterol levels. And at that time, changes in plasma total cholesterol levels served as a surrogate marker for changes in CHD risk. What is clear today is that these pharmacological cholesterol feeding studies increased plasma total cholesterol levels simply because they overwhelmed the endogenous feedback mechanisms since more cholesterol was absorbed than the body produced. Cholesterol feeding studies within more physiological ranges (adding 200–600 mg/day) indicate modest changes in plasma total cholesterol levels (McNamara, 1990; Clarke et al., 1997; Howell et al., 1997; Weggemans et al., 2001). Data from two reported meta-analyses of the effects of dietary cholesterol on plasma cholesterol levels by Clarke et al. (1997) and Howell et al. (1997) reported plasma cholesterol changes of 2.5 mg/dL and 2.2 mg/dL per 100 mg/day dietary cholesterol, respectively. The analyses indicate that when there is a measurable change, the increase occurs in both the atherogenic LDL cholesterol and the antiatherogenic HDL cholesterol levels (Clarke et al., 1997; McNamara, 2000b). While it has been argued that the small changes in the LDL:HDL ratio observed represent an increase in CHD risk, this very much depends on the baseline lipoprotein cholesterol levels (McNamara, 2002). As shown in Table 9.2, addition of an egg a day to the diet of individuals with low LDL levels, and low CHD risk, does increase the LDL:HDL ratio slightly, whereas in someone with high LDL levels, the increase is virtually undetectable (Greene et al., 2005). In either case there is little or no change in the CHD risk profile.

Other studies have shown that any dietary cholesterol mediated increases in LDL cholesterol levels are due to increases in LDL particle size, not the particle number (Ballesteros et al., 2004; Herron et al., 2004; Greene et al., 2006; Mutungi et al., 2010). Given that egg intake does not change either the LDL:HDL ratio or the number of LDL particles, the evidence indicates that dietary cholesterol does not change cardiovascular disease risk. Furthermore, studies indicate that dietary cholesterol intake does not alter markers of inflammation (Ratliff et al., 2008), another indicator of CHD risk.

There have been numerous reports of the heterogeneity of the plasma cholesterol responses to a dietary cholesterol challenge (Beynen et al., 1987; McNamara et al., 1987; McNamara, 1990). One of the major causes for this variability is responses as illustrated in Table 9.3, showing what impacts differences in body weight and differences in fractional cholesterol absorption can have on the total cholesterol input. Since endogenous cholesterol synthesis is a function of body weight, the dietary

TABLE 9.2
Theoretical Changes in Plasma Lipoprotein Cholesterol Levels and LDL:HDL Ratio with Addition of an Egg a Day to the Diet

	Cholesterol (mg/dL)		LDL:HDL Ratio	
	LDL	HDL	LDL:HDL	% Change
Baseline (low risk)	130	50	2.60	+1.2%
+1 egg/day	134	51	2.63	
Baseline (mid risk)	150	50	3.00	+0.7%
+1 egg/day	154	51	3.02	
Baseline (high risk)	170	50	3.40	+0.3%
+1 egg/day	174	51	3.41	

Source: Adapted from McNamara, D. J. 2000b. *J. Am. Coll. Nutr.* **19**: 540S–548S.

TABLE 9.3

Dietary Cholesterol, Body Weight, and Endogenous Cholesterol Metabolism

Cholesterol Metabolism (mg/day)	50 kg Female		75 kg Male		100 kg Male	
Dietary intake	250	750	250	750	250	750
Endogenous synthesis	600	600	900	900	1200	1200
Percent absorption	65%	65%	50%	50%	35%	35%
Absorbed	162	487	125	375	87	262
% Endogenous	27	81	14	42	7	22
Total input	762	1087	1025	1275	1287	1462
Total input (mg/kg/day)	15	22	14	18	13	15

cholesterol challenge needs to be adjusted for differences in body weights between study subjects. It is evident that adding 500 mg of cholesterol per day to the diet will have very different effects on plasma cholesterol levels for a 50 kg female as compared to a 100 kg male given that their endogenous cholesterol synthesis rates differ twofold. While this variable is easy to adjust for (i.e., Δ mg/dL per Δ 100 mg/70 kg/day), very few studies have actually normalized the data. A more complicated issue is the fact that few studies have measured fractional cholesterol absorption rates (McNamara et al., 1987) which can vary threefold (25–75%). As shown in Table 9.3, differences in body weights and differences in fractional absorption of intestinal cholesterol can result in very significant differences in total cholesterol input resulting in highly variable plasma cholesterol changes even though the same dietary cholesterol challenge is tested.

When body-weight-adjusted dose responses are calculated, the data indicate that the plasma cholesterol response to a dietary cholesterol challenge can be divided into two distinct groups—hyporesponders who exhibit little, if any, change in plasma cholesterol levels, and hyperresponders who exhibit a small, but measurable, change in their plasma cholesterol levels when cholesterol is increased in the diet (McNamara et al., 1987; Herron et al., 2004). Most analyses suggest that the distribution of these two groups in the population is 15–20% hyperresponders and 80–85% hyporesponders. No detailed studies have been carried out to determine whether hyper- and hyporesponders differ in terms of fractional cholesterol absorption although there is evidence that ATP-binding cassette G5 (ABCG5) polymorphisms does play a role in the response to dietary cholesterol (Herron et al., 2006). The existence of hyperresponders in the population has been used as a rationale for dietary cholesterol restrictions; however, data indicate that even this group has little, if any, change in CHD risk associated with dietary cholesterol.

The available data indicate that the dose-adjusted plasma cholesterol response to a 100 mg/day dietary cholesterol challenge in hyperresponders is 3.9 ± 0.6 mg/dL ($n = 10$, 95% CI 2.5–5.3), compared to a response of 1.4 ± 0.2 mg/dL ($n = 13$, 95% CI 1.0–1.9) in hyporesponders ($p = 0.0002$) (McNamara, 2000b). The difference in the plasma cholesterol response between hypo- and hyperresponders to dietary cholesterol is almost threefold. As might be expected, the plasma lipoprotein responses to dietary cholesterol in hyporesponders and hyperresponders differ primarily in the LDL cholesterol response, with the LDL response being 0.76 ± 0.25 ($n = 5$) versus 2.84 ± 0.66 ($n = 5$) mg/dL per 100 mg/day in hyporesponders versus hyperresponders ($p = 0.0185$). The plasma HDL cholesterol changes with a 100 mg/day change in dietary cholesterol were 0.50 ± 0.14 ($n = 5$) and 0.69 ± 0.16 ($n = 5$) in hyporesponders and hyperresponders, respectively ($p = 0.05$). All responses are variable with the degree of unsaturation of dietary fat with the highest responses associated with a high saturated fat intake (Clarke et al., 1997; McNamara, 2000b; Weggemans et al., 2001).

What the majority of published studies indicate is that egg intake does not increase the atherogenic profile of the plasma lipoproteins based on the observation that there is little, if any, measurable change in the LDL:HDL cholesterol ratio (McNamara, 2000a; Weggemans et al., 2001; Knopp et al., 2003; Ballesteros et al., 2004; Greene et al., 2005; Fernandez, 2006) nor is there an increase in atherogenic small, dense LDL particles (Herron and Fernandez, 2004; Greene et al., 2006; Fernandez, 2006). The evidence indicates that dietary cholesterol increases the size, not the number, of LDL particles, and the larger LDL particles are less atherogenic than the small, dense particles. Thus, while the clinical evidence that dietary cholesterol does result in a small increase in plasma total cholesterol, the increase is in both the LDL and HDL cholesterol fractions and in LDL size, not number. Hence, the earlier interpretation that changes in plasma total cholesterol levels were an appropriate surrogate marker for changes in cardiovascular disease risk must be reconsidered in view of the more current interpretations of changes in risk associated with changes in the LDL:HDL ratio and in LDL size.

9.6 A FAILED HYPOTHESIS

There are usually three lines of scientific evidence used to relate a nutrient, or a specific food item, to disease risk: animal feeding studies, epidemiological survey data, and clinical trials. The case against dietary cholesterol, as well as eggs, as a contributor to CHD risk is not substantiated by any of these lines of evidence.

Animal studies testing the effect of physiological intakes of cholesterol on plasma lipoprotein cholesterol levels and atherogenesis in omnivores are species dependent and highly variable depending on the overall composition of the diet (animal versus vegetable protein, type and amount of dietary fat, type and amount of dietary fiber, etc.). It is virtually impossible to argue for or against a dietary cholesterol–heart disease risk relationship based on results from animal model studies.

Epidemiological surveys originally suggested a positive relationship between dietary cholesterol and CHD risk with simple regression analyses; yet this association vanishes once the colinearity between dietary cholesterol and saturated fat intake is accounted for. Numerous studies have documented a null relationship between CHD incidence and egg intake, a high cholesterol food which has modest saturated fat content. To date there are at least a dozen large major and a number of minor surveys indicating no relationship between egg intake and heart disease risk.

In debates on the dietary cholesterol–heart disease relationship it is always emphasized that in well-controlled clinical studies there is, on average, a small, but measurable, increase in plasma total and LDL cholesterol levels and that some individuals are "hyperresponders" to dietary cholesterol. Further to above mentioned information, a couple of points are significant in considering the relevance of these arguments. First, there is little, if any, measurable change in the LDL:HDL ratio (McNamara, 2000b, 2002); second, there is no change in the number of LDL particles, and finally, there is no evidence that the atherogenicity of the LDL particle is altered.

The rationale conclusion from these various lines of investigation is that dietary cholesterol, whether from eggs or other animal products, is not a contributor to CHD risk in the population.

9.7 CONTRIBUTION OF EGGS TO HEALTH PROMOTION AND DISEASE PREVENTION

While there is little, if any, evidence that egg consumption increases CHD risk, there is accumulating evidence that nutrients and components in the egg do contribute to health promotion as well as facilitating disease prevention. Studies published over the past 20 years have shown that egg intake has a number of positive effects on a wide range of health issues ranging from fetal brain development to eye health to minimizing sarcopenia in the elderly. The data indicate that the range of health benefits, in terms of health promotion and disease prevention, are quite significant.

9.8 PROTEIN AND HEALTH

Eggs provide an affordable source of high-quality animal protein in the diet. In fact, eggs are the standard by which other dietary proteins are evaluated (Layman and Rodriguez, 2009). As an affordable source of high-quality protein, egg intake is associated with the many benefits of high-quality protein in the diet.

9.8.1 SARCOPENIA

The degenerative loss of skeletal muscle mass and strength associated with aging is a significant health issue for elderly subjects. In the beginning of the fourth decade of life, adults lose 3–5% of muscle mass per decade, a rate of decline that increases to 1–2% per year after 50 years of age. Loss of skeletal muscle is associated with declining health and can be a contributor to disability and disease progression. The estimated direct health care cost attributable to sarcopenia in the United States in 2000 was $18.5 billion (Janssen et al., 2004). In a recent analysis of the relationship between protein intake and lean mass loss with aging, Houston et al. (2008) reported that, over a three-year period, participants in the Health, Aging, and Body Composition study with the highest quintile of protein intake lost 40% less lean mass than did those in the lowest quintile of protein intake. The authors found significant associations between animal protein intake and changes in lean mass, but no such association with vegetable protein intake.

It has been known for many years that intake of high-quality animal protein facilitates optimal protein synthesis even in elderly individuals (Campbell et al., 1999; Pannemans et al., 1998). To maintain or build muscle mass in elderly subjects it has been shown that the use of a protein/calorie supplement was associated with greater gains in strength and muscle mass when combined with a strength training program compared with strength training alone (Evans, 2004).

9.8.2 WEIGHT CONTROL

Studies have shown that eggs, primarily egg yolk (Villaume et al., 1986; Pelletier et al., 1996), have a significant effect on satiety and can facilitate weight loss on a hypocaloric diet (Vander Wal et al., 2005, 2008). In a series of studies comparing two breakfasts, investigators found that, compared to an isocaloric, equal weight bagel-based breakfast, an egg-breakfast induced greater satiety and significantly reduced food intake both at lunch on the day of the test as well as over the subsequent day. In a subsequent study these same investigators reported that for individuals on a hypocaloric diet, consumption of the egg breakfast 5 days a week for 8 weeks resulted in a twofold greater weight loss as compared to those consuming the bagel breakfast 5 days a week over the same time period (Vander Wal et al., 2008). In the groups on a eucaloric intake there was no difference in body weight changes between the egg and bagel breakfasts. The investigators concluded that "The egg breakfast enhances weight loss, when combined with an energy-deficit diet, but does not induce weight loss in a free-living condition. The inclusion of eggs in a weight management program may offer a nutritious supplement to enhance weight loss" (Vander Wal et al. 2008). Interestingly, it also appears that the timing of protein intake affects satiety during energy restriction as shown by the studies of Leidy et al. (2009), indicating that both the initial and the sustained feelings of fullness following protein consumption is greatest when the protein is consumed at breakfast. These studies suggest that eggs can play a significant role in weight loss and weight control programs based on unique satiety effects associated with egg yolk consumption (Villaume et al., 1986; Pelletier et al., 1996).

9.9 CHOLINE AND HEALTH

In 1998, the Institute of Medicine of the National Academy of Sciences established choline as an essential nutrient setting Adequate Intake (AI) levels for all age groups and for pregnant and lactating women. The recommended AI for choline has been set at 425 mg/day for women, 450 mg/day for pregnant women, 550 mg/day for lactating women, and 550 mg/day for men (Food and Nutrition Board, Institute of Medicine, 1998).

Choline serves various functions in the body including the structure of cell membranes, protecting the liver from accumulating fat, as a precursor for the neurotransmitter acetylcholine, and functions in methyl transfer. Because of rapid development in fetuses and infants, they have a higher need for choline during early development and human breast milk has high levels of choline, hence the higher AI values for pregnant and lactating women.

There is a significant variation in the dietary requirement for choline that can be explained by common genetic polymorphisms (daCosta et al., 2006). Understanding dietary choline requirements and their modulation by genetic polymorphism has public health significance, especially with regard to its role in brain development (Zeisel, 2006). Current recommended intakes do not take into consideration these genetic variations as a modulator of dietary requirement.

9.9.1 Choline and Fetal Brain Development

Studies indicate that choline plays important roles in fetal and neonatal brain development. Researchers found that fetal rats whose mothers did not get enough choline in their diets had less brain development and poorer memories after birth than those whose mothers who ate adequate amounts of the nutrient. Investigators have also found that choline intake is associated with a reduced risk of neural tube defects (NTDs) and that the risk for having an infant with an NTD was 2.4 times greater in women who had the lowest blood levels of choline, compared to women who had average choline levels.

Research has shown that pregnancy and lactation result in especially high demand for choline, and that providing choline to the developing fetus and nursing infant is critical for optimal development which is why the recommended AI levels are increased to 450 mg/day for pregnant women and 550 mg/day for lactating women. Large amounts of choline are delivered to the fetus across the placenta and the choline concentration in amniotic fluid is 10-fold greater than maternal blood (Zeisel and Niculescu, 2006). Plasma choline concentrations are six- to sevenfold higher in the fetus and newborn than levels found in adults (Ozarda et al., 2002). The high transport of choline from the mother to fetus depletes maternal plasma choline in humans despite enhanced capacity to synthesize choline during pregnancy (Zeisel, 2006). Similarly, since human milk is rich in choline, lactation further exacerbates maternal demand, resulting in extended depletion of tissue stores (Steegers-Theunissen et al., 1994). This increased choline demand during pregnancy and lactation is the basis for the recommended increased dietary intake.

During later periods of pregnancy the memory center of the brain (the hippocampus) is developing and choline supplementation or depletion in rodents causes lifelong changes in brain structure and function (Zeisel, 2006). Adult rodents typically experience a decline in memory as they age; yet offspring exposed to extra choline *in utero* do not show this change with age (Meck and Williams, 2003).

The evidence suggests that choline supplementation during development results in improved performance of offspring in cognitive or behavioral tests, and in changes in a variety of neurological functional indicators: (1) enhanced performance, particularly of more difficult tasks; (2) increases (choline supplementation) or decreases (choline deficiency) are observed in electrophysiological responsiveness and size of neurons in offspring; and (3) supplementation results in some protection against adverse effects of several neurotoxic agents (including alcohol) in offspring (McCann et al., 2006; Mellott et al., 2007).

Recent studies indicate that during development, choline controls the epigenetic switches that support brain development in the fetus. In one set of studies, mice were fed a diet that contained choline while another group was given no choline, and brain tissue was sampled during the period of time when a fetus develops its hippocampus, the part of the brain responsible for memory. The insolated cells from the developing fetuses' brains were grown in cell cultures and the investigators determined that the expression of genes for two proteins that regulate neuronal cell creation and maturation were more prevalent in mice that received choline (Mehedint et al., 2010).

9.9.2 Choline and NTD Risk

Choline is not only involved in development of memory centers during fetal and early postnatal development; recent studies have shown that, like folate, choline intake is associated with reduced risk of NTDs. Shaw et al. (2004) found that women in the lowest quartile for dietary choline intake had four times the risk of giving birth to a child with an NTD, compared with women in the highest quartile of intake. Decreased risks of NTD-affected pregnancies were found for higher periconceptional intakes of choline for all NTDs as well as for spina bifida and anencephaly separately. Shaw et al. (2009) subsequently reported that reduced NTD risk was associated with higher levels of plasma choline. Specifically, they observed an odds ratio of 2.4 (95% CI = 1.3–4.7) associated with the lowest decile and an odds ratio of 0.14 (0.02–1.0) associated with the highest decile of plasma choline, both relative to the 25th and 74th percentiles of the control distribution.

9.9.3 Choline and Alzheimer's Disease

Choline intake is not only associated with fetal and early postnatal brain development but has also been shown to interact with other nutrients to impact traits associated with Alzheimer's disease. A study was conducted in 225 Alzheimer's patients who were given either a control beverage or a nutrient combination containing uridine, choline, and the omega-3 fatty acid docosahexaenoic acid (DHA). These compounds were selected because they are all precursors to molecules that make up brain cell membranes which form the brain connections, called synapses, and one of the features of a brain with Alzheimer's disease is the loss of synapses. The patients who had been given the nutrient combination showed a statistically significant improvement compared with controls: 40% of the treated patients improved on verbal memory compared with 24% in the control group. Among the treated patients, those who had the mildest stage of Alzheimer's showed the most improvement (Scheltens et al., 2010a,b).

9.9.4 Choline and Inflammation

Low-grade inflammation is generally recognized as a key component in the pathogenesis of atherosclerosis, and inflammatory biomarkers such as C-reactive protein (CRP), interleukin-6 (IL-6), homocysteine (tHcy), and tumor necrosis factor-α (TNF-α) have been associated with risk of cardiovascular events. Upon development of quantitative values for the choline content of foods, epidemiological studies have been carried out relating choline intake and inflammation showing an inverse relationship between dietary choline and plasma levels of inflammatory markers.

Findings from the ATTICA study indicated that subjects whose diets were rich in choline and betaine had the lowest levels of several inflammatory markers, including CRP, tHyc, IL-6, and TNF-α (Detopoulou et al. 2008). These findings were significant even after adjusting for various sociodemographic, lifestyle, and clinical characteristics of the participants. In a similar manner, Cho et al. (2006) found that among 1960 participants in the Framingham Offspring Study that the combined dietary intakes of choline and betaine were associated with lower plasma tHcy concentrations. Another study reported that in a Norwegian adult and elderly population not taking vitamin supplements, plasma tHcy concentrations were lowered with a diet rich in complex carbohydrates, proteins, and B-vitamins. The authors noted that such a diet includes vegetables, fruits, whole-grain bread and cereals, as well as fish, nonprocessed meat, chicken, and eggs (Konstantinova et al., 2007).

In clinical studies, Olthof et al. (2005) demonstrated that a high daily dose of choline (2.6 g choline/day), supplemented as phosphatidylcholine, lowered fasting as well as postmethionine-loading plasma total tHcy concentrations in healthy men with mildly elevated plasma tHcy concentrations. Other studies have reported similar findings (see Verhoef and de Groot, 2005 for review). Ratliff et al. (2008) reported that daily intake of three eggs while following a carbohydrate-restricted diet resulted in a significant decrease in CRP and a more pronounced increase in adiponectin, thus, improving the inflammatory profile. The effect of egg intake on inflammatory markers could be due to the choline content of eggs as well as the highly bioavailable zanthophylls which have also been shown to have anti-inflammatory effects (Dwyer et al., 2001).

9.9.5 Choline and Breast Cancer Risk

A number of recent studies have suggested a relationship between egg intake and reduced breast cancer risk as well as a negative relationship between dietary choline and breast cancer incidence and mortality. In support of these relationships are findings from animal model studies of a significant effect of dietary choline early in the development on later susceptibility to breast cancer carcinogens.

Frazier et al. (2003) reported findings from the Nurses' Health Study, indicating that women who had, during adolescence, a higher consumption of eggs had a lower risk of breast cancer. In this study population, the median serving of eggs was 0.43 egg/day and the relative risk for breast cancer was 0.82 (95% CI 0.67–0.99) for women consuming 1 egg/day. Two years later, Shannon et al. (2005) reported data from a case-control study of breast cancer incidence of women in Shanghai China showing that egg consumption was significantly inversely associated with risk of breast cancer (odds ratio for ≥6.0 eggs/week versus ≤2.0 eggs/week was 0.56; 95% CI 0.35–0.91).

Utilizing a population-based study of 1508 cases and 1556 controls, Xu et al. (2008) investigated the association of dietary intake of choline and two related micronutrients, methionine and betaine, and risk of breast cancer. The highest quintile of choline consumption was associated with a lower risk of breast cancer (odds ratio 0.76; 95% CI 0.58–1.00) compared with the lowest quintile. In another study, it was reported that there was an indication that a higher intake of free choline was associated with reduced risk of breast cancer (P(trend) = 0.04). Higher intakes of betaine, phosphocholine, and free choline were associated with reduced all-cause as well as breast cancer-specific mortality in a dose-dependent fashion (Xu et al., 2009).

Animal model studies provide a possible mechanism for these observations. In one study, pregnant rats were fed either a control, a choline-supplemented, or a choline-deficient diet (8, 36, and 0 mmol/kg of choline, respectively) during gestational days 11–17. On postnatal day 65, the female offspring received the breast cancer carcinogen 7,12-dimethylbenz[α]anthracene. The tumor growth rate was inversely related to choline content in the prenatal diet. This was accompanied by distinct expression patterns of genes in tumors derived from the three dietary groups. Tumors from the prenatally choline-supplemented rats overexpressed genes that confer favorable prognosis in human cancers and underexpressed those associated with aggressive disease. DNA methylation within the tumor suppressor gene, stratifin was proportional to the prenatal choline supply and correlated inversely with the expression of its mRNA and protein in tumors, suggesting that an epigenetic mechanism may underlie the altered molecular phenotype and tumor growth (Kovacheva et al., 2009).

9.9.6 Inadequate Choline Intake

A recent analysis of data from NHANES 2003–2004 revealed that for older children, men, women, and pregnant women, mean choline intakes are far below the AI. Ten percent or fewer had usual choline intakes at or above the AI (Jensen et al., 2007). Additional analysis of NHANES 2003–2004 data found that choline intake decreases with age and that adults aged 71 and older consumed an average of about 264 mg/day, about one-half of the AI for choline (Keast, 2007).

Eggs are one of the few concentrated food sources of choline. Though eggs are a more concentrated source of choline, in the Nurses' Health Study and Nurses' Health Study 2, milk provided the largest percentage of dietary choline, because it was consumed more frequently. However, NHANES 2003–2004 data showed that eggs contributed a relatively higher share of total choline intake for those whose intake was at or above the AI, compared to others (Jensen et al., 2007). Eggs also provide more choline per kilocalorie compared to most other foods, including milk. To get the same amount of choline found in a single egg (125 mg/72 calories), one would need to consume 3¼ cups of nonfat milk (270 calories) or 3½ ounces of wheat germ (366 calories). One egg provides ~125 mg of choline, all of which is found in the egg yolk.

9.10 XANTHOPHYLLS AND HEALTH

The xanthophyll carotenoids lutein and its stereoisomer zeaxanthin have a critical function in the maintenance of visual function. These polar compounds are the predominant carotenoids in the macula of the eye and the high concentrations of these carotenoids result in the yellowish color of the macula lutea ("yellow spot"). Similar to the macula, the predominant carotenoids found in the lens are lutein and zeaxanthin. The xanthophylls act as antioxidants to protect tissues against damage induced by reactive oxygen species. Xanthophyll intakes have been associated with a reduced risk of age-related macular degeneration (AMD) and cataracts (Moeller et al., 2000) as well as reduced risk for breast cancer and carotid artery atherosclerosis (McNamara 2005). Major sources of lutein are green leafy vegetables and corn is the primary source of zeaxanthin. These xanthophylls are also found in egg yolks.

AMD is the leading cause of irreversible vision loss in the elderly in the Western world. It is estimated that 1.6% of the population in the 50–65-year-old age group is affected, rising to 30% in the over-75-year-old age group. AMD risk has been shown in numerous studies to be related to dietary intakes and to serum xanthophyll levels as well as low macular pigment optical density (MPOD). While eggs do not normally contain a high lutein and zeaxanthin content, these xanthophylls have high bioavailability (Chung et al., 2004) and eggs are a significant contributor of xanthophylls in the diet (Granado et al., 2003). Studies have shown that addition of eggs to the diet increases plasma lutein levels (Handelman et al., 1999; Goodrow et al., 2006) and xanthophyll deposition in the macula as determined from measurement of MPOD (Wenzel et al., 2006; Vishwanathan et al., 2009). Lutein intake is also associated with reduced risk of cataracts and data from the Beaver Dam Eye Study indicated that cataract risk was 60% lower in the highest egg consumers as compared to the lowest egg consumers (Lyle et al., 1999).

Lutein has also been associated with reduced risk of carotid artery intimal medial thickening. Dwyer et al. (2001) reported the results of a multifaceted study of the relationship between lutein and atherogenesis, and concluded that the epidemiological, *in vitro*, and mouse model findings provided strong support for the hypothesis that increased dietary intake of lutein is protective against the development of early atherosclerosis. Monitoring 480 men and women between 40 and 60 years old participating in the Los Angeles Atherosclerosis Study with no history of heart disease or stroke by using ultrasound technology, measurements were made of the thickness of the walls of the carotid (neck) arteries once at the beginning of the study and again 18 months later and results correlated to levels of lutein in participants' blood over the same time span. Participants whose blood carried the highest levels of lutein averaged only a 0.004 mm increase in the artery thickness over 18 months, whereas those with the lowest levels of lutein increased an average of 0.021 mm. Interestingly, Sauvaget et al. (2003) reported that egg intake was negatively associated with stroke mortality; those that ate eggs daily had a 30% lower relative risk for stroke mortality than those who never ate eggs.

Egg lutein content can be increased by addition of marigold extract to the diet and there are lutein-enriched eggs available in various markets in the United States and internationally.

9.11 THE "FUNCTIONAL" EGG

One of the unique properties of the egg is that the nutrient composition of the egg can be naturally enhanced by varying the composition of the feed given to the birds. Omega-3-enriched eggs (both alpha-linolenic acid (ALA) and DHA enriched) are currently available in most markets. In addition, eggs enriched with vitamin E, lutein, selenium, and vitamin D are commercially available in many parts of the world. The potential for nutrient-enriched eggs is seen in one French brand which has increased the content of eight different nutrients. It is reported that 100 g of Benefic® eggs contain six times more of omega-3 fatty acid ALA (15% of the French recommended daily allowance (RDA)), three times more DHA (100% of RDA), three times more vitamin D (30% of RDA), four times more folic acid (70% of RDA), six times more vitamin E (66% of RDA), six times more lutein and zeaxanthin (70% of international recommendation), 2.5 times more iodine (100% RDA), and four times more selenium (45% RDA) (Bourre and Galae, 2006).

9.12 INTERNATIONAL PERSPECTIVES

Since 1977 the United States has included dietary cholesterol limits as part of its Dietary Guidelines for Americans. On the contrary, many countries have reviewed the evidence regarding dietary cholesterol and heart disease risk and have reached completely different conclusions. In fact, most countries do not have a dietary cholesterol recommendation as part of their dietary guidance.

9.12.1 CANADA

Health Canada does not have a dietary cholesterol recommendation for healthy individuals. In Canada, eggs carry the Heart Check of the Heart and Stroke Foundation of Canada. As noted on the Foundation's web site: *Research from the 1970s reported that high-cholesterol foods, especially eggs, raise blood cholesterol levels. These early studies included foods that were rich in both cholesterol and saturated fat (such as butter), so scientists incorrectly believed that cholesterol was the main culprit. When researchers recently re-evaluated the data, they learned that diets high in saturated or trans fat—not dietary cholesterol—are mostly responsible for increases in blood cholesterol levels.* (http://www.heartandstroke.com/site/apps/nlnet/content2.aspx?c=ikIQLcMWJtE&b= 4869055&ct=7511425)

9.12.2 AUSTRALIA AND NEW ZEALAND

The Heart Foundation of Australia has given eggs the Tick "because they are a nutritious food" and states that "You can enjoy up to six eggs each week as part of a healthy balanced diet. We recommend that one serve of eggs (two eggs per serve) be included in two to three meals each week." In addition, similar to the Heart and Stroke Foundation of Canada, they state that "The dietary cholesterol in eggs has only a small insignificant effect on blood cholesterol, especially when compared with the much greater effects of saturated and trans fats on blood cholesterol." (http://www.heartfoundation.org.au/Healthy_Living/Eating_and_Drinking/Fats_and_Cholesterol/About_eggs/Pages/default.aspx). The National Heart Foundation of New Zealand has also done away with its recommendation to restrict eggs in the diet.

9.12.3 GREAT BRITAIN

In 2009, following publication of a review of the egg–heart disease relationship by Gray and Griffin, the British Heart Foundation responded to the report by dispensing with its recommendation of limiting eggs to three or four a week, and the Food Standards Agency advised that most people do not need to restrict their egg intake if they eat a balanced diet.

9.12.4 IRELAND

"Nutrition guidelines recommend that a healthy individual can have up to seven eggs a week and those on a cholesterol lowering diet can have four to six eggs a week." (http://www.bordbia.ie/aboutfood/eggs/Pages/default.aspx) A review commissioned by Bord Bría (Irish Food Board) titled "An Overview of the Nutritional Role of Eggs in the Diet" concluded that eggs provide many essential nutrients in the diet.

9.13 PRIMUM NON-NOCERE

Given the current state of knowledge, perhaps, it is time to ask whether the recommended dietary cholesterol and egg restrictions have in fact done harm to the health of the public. Too often a food is viewed only from the perspective of a single component in that food, such as eggs as a source of cholesterol, without appropriate consideration of the other nutrients that it contains. For example, eggs are an excellent source of dietary choline (120 mg per large egg); yet due to egg restrictions, it is almost impossible for an individual to attain the recommended AI for choline, given its limited content in other food sources. Has harm been done to the elderly who need a source of high-quality protein in the diet which is affordable, convenient, nutrient dense, and easy to chew and digest in order to minimize the risk of excessive sarcopenia?

9.14 THE COST OF EGG RESTRICTIONS

A recent analysis of the economic impact of egg restrictions on health care costs concluded that public health campaigns promoting limiting egg consumption as a means to reduce CHD risk are not cost-effective from a societal perspective when other benefits are considered (Schmier et al., 2009). As shown in Table 9.4, the potential yearly reductions in health care costs from adding one egg a day to the diet would be quite significant, estimates at over $3 billion. It should be noted that these estimated cost reductions do not include reductions in breast cancer morbidity and mortality which has been shown to be reduced by both egg and choline intake. In addition, the impact of xanthophyll-enriched eggs on AMD and cataracts incidence cannot be estimated at this time. The cost of adding an egg a day to the US diet would be ~$750 million annually.

9.15 SUMMARY

There is more to an egg than its cholesterol content; yet for many consumers and health professionals that is the first thing they think about. After years of being ostracized as a contributor to CHD incidence, the egg has slowly begun its rehabilitation with the establishment of a large body of

---

TABLE 9.4
Estimate of Health Care Cost Benefits from Adding an Egg a Day to the Diet

Condition[a]	Cost Benefit	Minimum–Maximum	Comments
AMD	−$958 M	−$7.95 M to −$2.99B	Medical and nonmedical (caregiving, assistive devices) costs
Cataract	−$2.21B	−$151 M to −$5.28B	Medical costs only, includes two common complications
Sarcopenia	−$129 M	−$60.4 M to −$227 M	Medical costs only
NTD	−$4.68 M	−$2.63 M to −$7.31 M	Hospital charges

Source: Data from Schmier, J. K., Baraj, L. M., and Tran, N. L. 2009. *Cost Eff. Resource Alloc.* 7: 7.

[a] AMD: age-related macular degeneration; NTD: neural tube defects.

research documenting its various contributions to disease prevention and health promotion. It is ironic to consider the findings that eggs actually seem to contribute to CHD prevention: choline lowers inflammatory markers which are associated with CHD risk; increased plasma lutein is associated with slower progression of carotid artery intimal medial thickening; and the satiety effect of eggs contributes to weight control and obesity is a contributor to the metabolic syndrome and diabetes which are associated with increased CHD risk. In addition, egg restrictions have inadvertently led to inadequate choline intake in the population as a whole and more importantly in pregnant and lactating women where choline plays such an important role in reducing NTD risk and in fetal and postnatal brain development. The number of elderly who fear eating eggs as a source of high-quality protein because of dietary cholesterol concerns no doubt also plays a role in sarcopenia and associated infirmities. Clearly there is more to an egg than just its cholesterol content (Ruxton et al., 2010).

REFERENCES

Anitschkow, N. and Chalatow, S. 1913. Ueber Experimentelle Cholesterinsteatose und ihre Bedeutung fur die Entstehung einiger pathologischer Prozesse. *Zentralbl Allg Pathol Anat.* **24**: 1–9.

Ascherio, A., Rimm, E. B., Giovannucci, E. L., Spiegelman, D. Stampfer M., and Willett, W.C. 1996. Dietary fat and risk of coronary heart disease in men: Cohort follow up study in the United States. *BMJ.* **313**: 84–90.

Ballesteros, M. N., Cabrera, R. M., Saucedo, M. D., and Fernandez, M. L. 2004. Dietary cholesterol does not increase biomarkers for chronic disease in a pediatric population from northern Mexico. *Am. J. Clin. Nutr.* **80**: 855–861.

Beynen, A. C., Katan, M. B., and Van Zutphen, L. F. 1987. Hypo- and hyperresponders: Individual differences in the response of serum cholesterol concentration to changes in diet. *Adv. Lipid Res.* **22**: 115–171.

Bourre, J. M. and Galea, F. 2006. An important source of omega-3 fatty acids, vitamins D and E, carotenoids, iodine and selenium: A new natural multi-enriched egg. *J. Nutr. Health Aging.* **10**: 371–376.

Campbell, W. W., Barton, Jr., M. L., Cyr-Campbell, D., Davey, S. L., Beard, J. L., Parise, G., and Evans, W. J. 1999. Effects of an omnivorous diet compared with a lactoovovegetarian diet on resistance-training-induced changes in body composition and skeletal muscle in older men. *Am. J. Clin. Nutr.* **70**: 1032–1039.

Cho, E. S. H., Zeisel, S. H., Jacques, P., Selhub, J., Dougherty, L., Colditz, G. A., and Willett, W. C. 2006. Dietary choline and betaine assessed by food-frequency questionnaire in relation to plasma total homocysteine concentration in the Framingham Offspring Study. *Am. J. Clin. Nutr.* **83**: 905–911.

Chung, H. Y., Rasmussen, H. M., and Johnson, E. J. 2004. Lutein bioavailability is higher from lutein-enriched eggs than from supplements and spinach in men. *J. Nut.* **134**: 1887–1893.

Clarke, R., Frost, C., Collins, R., Appleby, P., and Peto, R. 1997. Dietary lipids and blood cholesterol: Quantitative meta-analysis of metabolic ward studies. *BMJ.* **314**: 112–117.

Da Costa, K. A., Kozyreva, O. G., Song, J., Galanko, J. A., Fischer, L.M., and Zeisel, S.H. 2006. Common genetic polymorphisms affect the human requirement for the nutrient choline. *FASEB J.* **20**: 1336–1344.

Dawber, T. R., Nickerson, R. J., Brand, F. N., and Pool, J. 1982. Eggs, serum cholesterol, and coronary heart disease. *Am. J. Clin. Nut.* **36**: 617–625.

Detopoulou, P., Panagiotakos, D. B., Antonopoulou, S., Pitsavos, C., and Stefanadis, C. 2008. Dietary choline and betaine intakes in relation to concentrations of inflammatory markers in healthy adults: ATTICA study. *Am. J. Clin. Nutr.* **87**: 424–430.

Dietschy, J. M. 1984. Regulation of cholesterol metabolism in man and in other species. *Klin. Wochenschr.* **62**: 338–345.

Dwyer, J. H., Navab, M., Dwyer, K. M., Hassan, K., Sun, P., Shircore, A., Hama-Levy, S. et al. 2001. Oxygenated carotenoid lutein and progression of early atherosclerosis: The Los Angeles atherosclerosis study. *Circulation.* **103**: 2922–2927.

Esrey, K. L., Joseph, L., and Grover, S. A. 1996. Relationship between dietary intake and coronary heart disease mortality: Lipid research clinics prevalence follow-up study. *J. Clin. Epidemiol.* **49**: 211–216.

Evans, W. J. 2004. Protein nutrition, exercise and aging. *J. Am. Coll. Nutr.* **23**: 601S–609S.

Fernandez, M. L. 2006. Dietary cholesterol provided by eggs and plasma lipoproteins in healthy populations. *Curr. Opin .Clin. Nutr. Metab .Care.* **9**: 8–12.

Fernandez, M. L. and Webb, D. 2008. The LDL to HDL cholesterol ratio as a valuable tool to evaluate coronary heart disease risk. *J. Am. Coll. Nutr.* **27**: 1–5.

Food and Nutrition Board, Institute of Medicine, 1998. *Dietary Reference Intakes: Thiamin, Riboflavin, Niacin, Vitamin B-6, Vitamin B012, Pantothenic Acid, Biotin, and Choline. National Academy of Sciences*, Washington, DC, pp. 390–422.

Frazier, A. L., Ryan, C. T., Rockett, H., Willett, W. C., and Colditz, G. A. 2003. Adolescent diet and risk of breast cancer. *Breast Cancer Res.* **5**: R59–R64.

Goodrow, E. F., Wilson, T. A., Houde, S. C., Vishwanathan, R., Scollin, P. A., Handelman, G., and Nicolosi, J. 2006. Consumption of one egg per day increases serum lutein and zeaxanthin concentrations in older adults without altering serum lipid and lipoprotein cholesterol concentrations. *J. Nutr.* **136**: 2519–2524.

Greene, C. M., Zern, T. L., Wood, R. J., Shrestha, S., Aggarwal, D., Sharman, M. J., Volek, J. S., and Fernandez, M. L. 2005. Maintenance of the LDL cholesterol:HDL cholesterol ratio in an elderly population given a dietary cholesterol challenge. *J .Nutr.* **13**: 2793–2798.

Greene, C. M., Waters, D., Clark, R. M., Contois, J. H., and Fernandez, M. L. 2006. Plasma LDL and HDL characteristics and carotenoid content are positively influenced by egg consumption in an elderly population. *Nutr. Metab (Lond).* **3**: 6.

Granado, F., Olmedilla, B., and Blanco, I. 2003. Nutritional and clinical relevance of lutein in human health. *Br. J. Nutr.* **90**: 487–502.

Gray, J. and Griffin, B. 2009. Eggs and dietary cholesterol—Dispelling the myth. *Br. Nutr. Found. Nutr. Bull.* **34**: 66–70.

Handelman, G. J., Nightingale, Z. D., Lichtenstein, A. H., Schaefer, E. J., and Blumberg, J. B. 1999. Lutein and zeaxanthin concentrations in plasma after dietary supplementation with egg yolk. *Am. J. Clin. Nutr.* **70**: 247–251.

Hegsted, D. M. and Ausman, L. M. 1988. Diet, alcohol and coronary heart disease in men. *J. Nutr.* **118**: 1184–1189.

Herron, K. L. and Fernandez, M. L. 2004. Are the current dietary guidelines regarding egg consumption appropriate? *J. Nutr.* **134**: 187–190.

Herron, K. L., Lofgren, I. E., Sharman, M., Volek, J. S., and Fernandez, M. L. 2004. High intake of cholesterol results in less atherogenic low-density lipoprotein particles in men and women independent of response classification. *Metabolism.* **53**: 823–830.

Herron, K. L., McGrane, M. M.,Waters, D., Lofgren, I. E., Clark, R. M., Ordovas, J., and Fernandez, M. L. 2006. The ABCG5 polymorphism contributes to individual responses to dietary cholesterol and carotenoids in eggs. *J. Nutr.* **136**: 1161–1165.

Houston, D. K., Nicklas, B. J., Ding, J., Harris, T. B., Tylavsky, F. A., Newman, A. B., Lee, J. S., Sahyoun, N. R., Visser, M., and Kritchevsky, S.B. for the Health ABC Study. 2008. Dietary protein intake is associated with lean mass change in older, community-dwelling adults: The Health, Aging, and Body Composition (Health ABC) Study. *Am. J. Clin. Nutr.* **87**: 150–155.

Howell, W. H., McNamara, D. J., Tosca, M. A., Smith, B. T., and Gaines, J. A. 1997. Plasma lipid and lipoprotein responses to dietary fat and cholesterol: A meta-analysis. *Am. J. Clin. Nut.* **65**: 1747–1764.

Hu, F. B., Stampfer, M. J., Manson, J. E., Colditz, G. A., Rosner, B., Speizer, F. E., Hennekens, C. H., and Willett, W. C.1999. Egg consumption and risk of cardiovascular disease in women. *Circulation.* **99**: 1121.

Hu, F. B., Stampfer, M. J., Manson, J. E., Rimm, E., Colditz, G. A., Rosner, B. A., Hennekens, C. H., and Willett, W. C. 1997. Dietary fat intake and the risk of coronary heart disease in women. *N. Engl. J. Med.* **337**: 1491–1499.

Janssen, I., Shepard, D. S., Katzmarzyk, P. T., and Roubenoff, R. J. 2004. The healthcare costs of sarcopenia in the United States. *Am. Geriatr. Soc.* **52**: 80–85.

Jensen, H., Batres-Marques, Carriquiry, A., and Schalinske, K. 2007. Choline in the diets of the U.S. Population: NHANES, 2003–2004. *National Nutrient Data Bank Conference*.

Keast, D. 2007. Food sources of choline in the diets of US older adults: NHANES, 2999–2004. *National Nutrient Data Bank Conference*.

Knopp, R. H., Retzlaff, B., Fish, B., Walden, C., Wallick, S., Anderson, M., Aikaw, K., and Kahn, S. E. 2003. Effects of insulin resistance and obesity on lipoproteins and sensitivity to egg feeding. *Arterioscler. Thromb. Vasc. Biol.* **23**: 1437–1443.

Konstantinova, S. V., Vollset, S. E., Berstad, P., Ueland, P. M., Drevon, C. A., Refsum, H., and Tell, G. S. 2007. Dietary predictors of plasma total homocysteine in the Hordaland Homocysteine Study. *Br. J. Nutr.* **98**: 201–210.

Kovacheva, V. P., Davison, J. M., Mellott, T. J., Rogers, A. E., Yang, S., O'Brien, M. J., and Blusztajn, J. K. 2009. Raising gestational choline intake alters gene expression in DMBA-evoked mammary tumors and prolongs survival. *FASEB J.* **23**: 1054–1063.

Kritchevsky, S. B. 2004. A review of scientific research and recommendations regarding eggs. *J. Am. Coll. Nutr.* **23**(6): 596S–600S.

Kritchevsky, S. B. and Kritchevsky, D. 2000. Egg consumption and coronary heart disease: An epidemiologic overview. *J. Am. Coll. Nutr.* **19**: 549S–555S.

Kromhout, D., Menotti, A., Bloemberg, B., Aravanis, C., Blackburn, H., Buzina, R., Dontas, A. S. et al. 1995. Dietary saturated and trans fatty acids and cholesterol and 25-year mortality from coronary heart disease: The Seven Countries Study. *Prev. Med.* 24: 308–315.

Layman, D. K. and Rodriquez, N. R. 2009. Egg protein as a source of power, strength, and energy. *Nutr. Today.* **44**: 43–48.

Lee, A. and Griffin, B. 2006. Dietary cholesterol, eggs and coronary heart disease risk in perspective. *Br. Nutr. Found. Nutr. Bull.* **31**: 21–27.

Leidy, H. J., Bossingham, M. J., Mattes, R. D., and Campbell, W. W. 2009. Increased dietary protein consumed at breakfast leads to an initial and sustained feeling of fullness during energy restriction compared to other meal times. *Br. J. Nutr.* **101**: 798–803.

Lyle, B. J., Mares-Perlman, J. A., Klein, B. E., Klein, R., and Greger, J. L. 1999. Antioxidant intake and risk of incident age-related nuclear cataracts in the Beaver Dam Eye Study. *Am. J. Epidemiol.* **149**: 801–809.

McCann, J. C., Hudes, M., and Ames, B. N. 2006. An overview of evidence for a causal relationship between dietary availability of choline during development and cognitive function in offspring. *Neurosci. Biobehav. Rev.* **30**: 696–712.

McNamara, D. J. 1987. Effects of a fat modified diet on cholesterol and lipoprotein metabolism in man. *Ann. Rev. Nutr.* **7**: 273–290.

McNamara, D. J. 1990. Relationship between blood and dietary cholesterol. In *Meat and Health. Advances in Meat Research.* A. M. Pearson and T. R. Dutson, eds. Elsevier, New York. Vol. 6, pp. 63–87.

McNamara, D. J. 2000a. Dietary cholesterol and atherosclerosis. *Biochim. Biophys. Acta.* **1529**: 310–320.

McNamara, D. J. 2000b. The impact of egg limitations on coronary heart disease risk: Do the numbers add up? *J. Am. Coll. Nutr.* **19**: 540S–548S.

McNamara, D. J. 2002. Eggs and heart disease risk: Perpetuating the misperception. *Am. J. Clin. Nutr.* **75**: 333–335.

McNamara, D. J. 2005. Egg xanthophylls and health implications. In *Egg Nutrition for Health*, J. S. Sim and H. H Sunwoo, eds. University of Alberta Canada, pp. 95–110.

McNamara, D. J. and Howell, W. H. 1992. Epidemiological data linking diet to hyperlipidemia and arteriosclerosis. *Semin. Liver Dis.* **12**: 347–355.

McNamara, D. J., Kolb, R., Parker, T. S., Batwin, H., Samuel, P., Brown, C. D., and Ahrens, Jr., E. H. 1987. Heterogeneity of cholesterol homeostasis in man. Response to changes in dietary fat quality and cholesterol quantity. *J. Clin. Invest.* **79**: 1729–1739.

Meck, W. H. and Williams, C. L. 2003. Metabolic imprinting of choline by its availability during gestation: Implications for memory and attentional processing across the lifespan. *Neurosci. Biobehav. Rev.* **27**: 385–399.

Mehedint, M. G., Niculescu, M. D., Craciunescu, C. N., and Zeisel, S. H. 2010. Choline deficiency alters global histone methylation and epigenetic marking at the Re1 site of the calbindin 1 gene. *FASEB J.* **24**: 184–195.

Mellott, T. J., Follettie, M. T., Diesl, V., Hill, A. A., Lopez-Coviella, I., and Blusztajn, J. K. 2007. Prenatal choline availability modulates hippocampal and cerebral cortical gene expression. *FASEB J.* **21**: 1311–1333.

Millen, B. E., Franz, M. M., Quatromoni, P. A., Gagnon, D. R., Sonnenberg, L. M., Ordovas, J. M., Wilson, P. W. F., Schaefer, E. J., and Cupples, L. A. 1996. Diet and plasma lipids in women .1. Macronutrients and plasma total and low-density lipoprotein cholesterol in women: The Framingham nutrition studies. *J. Clin. Epidemiol.* **49**: 657–663.

Moeller, S. M., Jacques, P. F., and Blumberg, J. B. 2000. The potential role of dietary xanthophylls in cataract and age-related macular degeneration. *J. Am. Coll. Nutr.* **19**: 522S–527S.

Mutungi, G., Waters, D., Ratliff, J., Puglisi, M., Clark, R. M., Volek, J. S., and Fernandez, M. L. 2010. Eggs distinctly modulate plasma carotenoid and lipoprotein subclasses in adult men following a carbohydrate-restricted diet. *J. Nutr. Biochem.* **21**: 261–267.

Nakamura, Y., Iso, H., Kita, Y., Ueshima, H., Okada, K., Konishi, M., Inoue, M., and Tsugane, S. 2006. Egg consumption, serum total cholesterol concentrations and coronary heart disease incidence: Japan Public Health Center-based prospective study. *Br. J. Nutr.* **96**: 921–928.

Olthof, M. R., Brink, E. J., Katan, M. B., and Verhoef, P. 2005. Choline supplemented as phosphatidylcholine decreases fasting and postmethionine-loading plasma homocysteine concentrations in healthy men. *Am. J. Clin. Nutr.* **82**: 111–117.

Ozarda Ilcol, Y., Uncu, G., and Ulus, I. H. 2002. Free and phospholipid-bound choline concentrations in serum during pregnancy, after delivery and in newborns. *Arch. Physiol. Biochem.* **110**: 393–399.

Pannemans, D. L., Wagenmakers, A. J., Westerterp, K. R., Schaafsma, G., and Halliday, D. 1998. Effect of protein source and quantity on protein metabolism in elderly women. *Am. J. Clin. Nutr.* **68**: 1228–1235.

Pelletier, X., Thouvenot, P., Belbraouet, S., Chayvialle, J. A., Hanesse, B., Mayeux, D., and Debry, G. 1996. Effect of egg consumption in healthy volunteers: Influence of yolk, white or whole-egg on gastric empty-ing and on glycemic and hormonal responses. *Ann. Nutr. Metab.* **40**: 109–115.

Pietinen, P., Ascherio, A., Korhonen, P., Hartman, A. M., Willett, W. C., Albanes, D., and Virtamo, J. 1997. Intake of fatty acids and risk of coronary heart disease in a cohort of Finnish men—The alpha-tocopherol, beta-carotene cancer prevention study. *Am. J. Epidemiol.* **145**: 876–887.

Qureshi, A. I., Suri, F. K., Ahmed, S., Nasar, A., Divani, A. A., and Kirmani, J. F. 2007. Regular egg consump-tion does not increase the risk of stroke and cardiovascular diseases. *Med. Sci. Monit.* **13**: CR1–CR8.

Ratliff, J. C., Mutungi, G., Puglisi, M. J., Volek, J. S., and Fernandez, M. L. 2008. Eggs modulate the inflam-matory response to carbohydrate restricted diets in overweight men. *Nutr. Metab. (Lond).* **5:** 6–14.

Ravnskov, U. 1995. Quotation bias in reviews of the diet-heart idea. *J. Clin. Epidemiol.* **48**: 713–719.

Ruxton, C. H. S., Derbyshire. E., and Gibson, S. 2010. The nutritional properties and health benefits of eggs. *Nutr. Food Sci.* **40**: 263–279.

Sauvaget, C., Nagano, J., Allen, N., Grant, E. J., and Beral, V. 2003. Intake of animal products and stroke mor-tality in the Hiroshima/Nagasaki Life Span Study. *Int. J. Epidemiol.* **32**: 536–543.

Sauvaget, C., Nagano, J., Hayashi, M., and Yamada, M. 2004. Animal protein, animal fat, and cholesterol intakes and risk of cerebral infarction mortality in the adult health study. *Stroke.* **35**: 1531–1537.

Scheltens, P., Kamphuis, P. J., Verhey, F. R., Olde Rikkert, M. G., Wurtman, R. J., Wilkinson, D., Twisk, J. W., and Kurz, A. 2010a. Efficacy of a medical food in mild Alzheimer's disease: A randomized, controlled trial. *Alzheimers Dement.* **6**: 1–10 e1.

Scheltens, P., Kamphuis, P. J., Verhey, F. R., Olde Rikkert, M. G., Wurtman, R. J., Wilkinson, D., Twisk, J. W., and Kurz, A. 2010b. Efficacy of a medical food in mild Alzheimer's disease: A randomized, controlled trial. *Cost Eff. Resour. Alloc.* **7**: 7.

Schmier, J. K., Baraj, L. M., and Tran, N. L. 2009. Single food focus dietary guidance: Lessons learned from economic analysis of egg consumption. *Cost Eff. Resour. Alloc.* 7: 7.

Shannon, J., Ray, R., Wu, C., Nelson, Z., Gao, D. L., Li, W., Hu, W. et al. 2005. Food and botanical groupings and risk of breast cancer: A case–control study in Shanghai, China. *Cancer Epidemiol. Biomark. Prev.* **14**: 81–90.

Shaw, G. M., Carmichael, S. L., Yang, W., Selvin, S., and Schaffer, D. M. 2004. Periconceptional dietary intake of choline and betaine and neural tube defects in offspring. *Am. J. Epidemiol.* **160**: 102–109.

Shaw, G. M., Finnell, R. H., Blom, H. J., Carmichael, S. L.,Vollset, S. E., Yang, W., and Ueland, P. M. 2009. Choline and risk of neural tube defects in a folate-fortified population. *Epidemiol.* **20**: 714–719.

Steegers-Theunissen, R. P., Boers, G. H., Trijbels, F. J., Finkelstein, J. D., Blom, H. J., Thomas, C. M., Borm, G. F., Wouters, M. G., and Eskes, T. K. 1994. Maternal hyperhomocysteinemia: A risk factor for neural-tube defects? *Metabolism.* **43**: 1475–1480.

Vander Wal, J. S., Gupta, A., Khosla, P., and Dhurandhar, N. V. 2008. Egg breakfast enhances weight loss. *Int. J. Obes. (Lond).* **32**: 1545–1551.

Vander Wal, J. S., Marth, J. M., Khosla, P., Jen, K. L., and Dhurandhar, N. V. 2005. Short-term effect of eggs on satiety in overweight and obese subjects. *J. Am. Coll. Nutr.* **24**: 510–515.

Verhoef, P. and de Groot, L. C. 2005. Dietary determinants of plasma homocysteine concentrations. *Semin. Vasc. Med.* **5**: 110–123.

Villaume, C., Beck, B., Rohr, R., Pointel, J. P., and Debry, G. 1986. Effect of exchange of ham for boiled egg on plasma glucose and insulin responses to breakfast in normal subjects. *Diabetes Care.* **9**: 46–49.

Vishwanathan, R., Goodrow-Kotyla, E. F., Wooten, B. R.,Wilson, T. A., and Nicolosi, R. J,. 2009. Consumption of 2 and 4 egg yolks/d for 5 wk increases macular pigment concentrations in older adults with low macu-lar pigment taking cholesterol-lowering statins. *Am. J. Clin. Nutr.* **90**: 1272–1279.

Weggemans, R. M., Zock, P. L., and Katan, M. B. 2001. Dietary cholesterol from eggs increases the ratio of total cholesterol to high-density lipoprotein cholesterol in humans: A meta-analysis. *Am. J. Clin. Nutr.* **73**: 885–891.

Wenzel, A. J., Gerweck, C., Barbato, D., Nicolosi, R. J., Handelman, G. J., and Curran-Celentano, J. 2006. A 12-wk egg intervention increases serum zeaxanthin and macular pigment optical density in women. *J. Nutr.* **136**: 2568–2573.

Xu, X., Gammon, M. D., Zeisel, S. H., Bradshaw, P. T., Wetmur, J. G., Teitelbaum, S. L., Neugut, A. I., Santella, R. M., and Chen, J. 2009. High intakes of choline and betaine reduce breast cancer mortality in a population-based study. *FASEB J.* **23**: 4022–4028.

Xu, X., Gammon, M. D., Zeisel, S. H., Lee, Y. L., Wetmur, J. G., Teitelbaum, S. L., Bradshaw, P. T., Neugut, A. I., Santella, R. M., and Chen, J. 2008. Choline metabolism and risk of breast cancer in a population-based study. *FASEB J.* **22**: 2045–2052.

Zeisel, S. H. 2006. Choline: Critical role during fetal development and dietary requirements in adults. *Ann. Rev. Nutr.* **26**: 229–250.

Zeisel, S. H. and Niculescu, M. D. 2006. Perinatal choline influences brain structure and function. *Nutr. Rev.* **64**: 197–203.

10 Fibers and Prevention of Cardiovascular Disease

Amy Noto, Peter Zahradka, Tabitha Marshall,
and Carla Taylor
University of Manitoba

CONTENTS

10.1   INTRODUCTION

Cardiovascular disease (CVD) is the major cause of death, accounting for more than one-third of all deaths in the United States and Canada (AHA 2009, HSFC 2005). CVD encompasses a wide range of conditions that affect either the functioning of the heart or blood flow to critical organs of the body, and includes those that originate due to genetic abnormalities and infectious diseases. The more prevalent diseases such as coronary heart disease (CHD), cerebrovascular disease, hypertension, and peripheral arterial disease that occur due to environment (i.e., diet, lifestyle, tobacco use) are typically recognized as CVD (AHA 2009). This chapter will illustrate the role of fiber intake in the prevention of CVD according to the epidemiological, clinical, and experimental data, and provide evidence that the increased incidence of CVD is in part due to the fact that most people do not meet the adequate intake (AI) for total fiber intake.

It is estimated that 90% of the population displays at least one risk factor for CVD (HSFC 2005). Risk factors that may be modified by fiber intake include obesity, abnormal glucose and insulin metabolism, inflammation, hypertension, dyslipidemia, dyslipoproteinemia, and thrombosis. Several possible mechanisms related to these risk factors that may contribute to the protective effects of dietary fiber for CVD are discussed. Additionally, the emerging role of nutrigenomic and nutrigenetic approaches to examine the role of fiber in modulating processes that affect cardiovascular function is considered.

National diet recommendations including Canada's Food Guide (Health Canada 2007a) and MyPyramid (USDA 2009a), as well as other dietary patterns such as Portfolio, Mediterranean, Dietary Approaches to Stop Hypertension (DASH) and related Optimal Macronutrient Intake Trial to Prevent Heart Disease (OmniHeart) that emphasize whole grains, fruits, vegetables, nuts, and legumes may help individuals meet the Dietary Reference Intake (DRI) for dietary fiber. Additionally, several functional/novel fibers are under investigation for their health benefits and they may help people meet fiber requirements.

10.2   DEFINITIONS OF FIBER

10.2.1   DIETARY FIBER

Dietary fiber is defined by the American Association of Cereal Chemists (AACC) as "the edible parts of plants or analogous carbohydrates that are resistant to digestion and absorption in the human small intestine with complete or partial fermentation in the large intestine. Dietary fiber includes polysaccharides, oligosaccharides, lignin, and associated plant substances. Dietary fibers promote beneficial physiological effects including laxation, and/or blood cholesterol attenuation, and/or blood glucose attenuation" (AACC 2001).

In the most recent DRI documents, the definition of fiber is simply, "nondigestible carbohydrates and lignin that are intrinsic and intact in plants" (IOM 2001, p. 339).

10.2.2   FUNCTIONAL/NOVEL FIBER

Functional (the United States) or novel (Canada) fibers are isolated, purified, synthetic fibers that provide physiological benefits (IOM 2001). Health Canada (1985) defines novel fiber or a novel fiber source as a "food that has been manufactured to be a source of dietary fiber and has not been used for human consumption to any significant extent; or has been chemically or physically processed so as to modify the properties of the fiber; or has been highly concentrated from its plant source." Examples of functional/novel fibers include isolated sources of the fiber types (discussed in Section 10.3) such as psyllium, β-glucan, inulin, and fructooligosaccharides (FOSs). The American Association of Cereal Chemists International opposes the use of the term functional fiber on food labels as defined by the Institute of Medicine (IOM) since "current analytical methods cannot discriminate between dietary fiber that is naturally present in a food and isolated fiber that is added to a food. The IOM definition may also confuse consumers who perceive functional fiber to be healthier than dietary fiber due to confusion with the term functional foods" (AACC 2008).

10.2.3 Codex Allimentarius Definition

There is not a single, agreed-upon definition of fiber worldwide; however, the proposed Codex Allimentarius definition of dietary fiber, put forth by the Codex Committee on Nutrition and Foods for Special Dietary Uses, includes both food and isolated sources. This definition reads: "Dietary fiber means carbohydrate polymers* with ten or more monomeric units,† which are not hydrolyzed by the endogenous enzymes in the small intestine of humans and belong to the following categories: (i) Edible carbohydrate polymers naturally occurring in the food as consumed; (ii) Carbohydrate polymers which have been obtained from food raw material by physical, enzymatic or chemical means and which have been shown to have a physiological effect of benefit to health as demonstrated by generally accepted scientific evidence to competent authorities; (iii) Synthetic carbohydrate polymers which have been shown to have a physiological effect of benefit to health as demonstrated by generally accepted scientific evidence to competent authorities. These substances are included in the definition of fiber insofar as they are actually associated with the poly- or oligosaccharidic fraction of fiber. However, when extracted or even re-introduced into a food containing non-digestible polysaccharides, they cannot be defined as dietary fiber. When combined with polysaccharides, these associated substances may provide additional beneficial effects (pending adoption of Section on Methods of Analysis and Sampling)." (ALINORM 09/32/26 2009).

10.3 FIBER TYPES

Carbohydrates and noncarbohydrates that may be defined as fiber include (AACC 2001, Buttriss and Stokes 2008, Nugent 2005):

1. *Celluloses* are linear, closely packed, insoluble glucose polymers that are part of plant cell walls. They make up about one-quarter to one-third of the fiber in grains, fruit, vegetables, and nuts.
2. *β-Glucans* are glucose polymers that have a branched structure, which differentiates them from celluloses, and makes them soluble and highly viscous. They are the major component of oat and barley cell walls and found in small amounts in wheat.
3. *Hemicelluloses* are polysaccharides made up of sugars other than glucose, associated with cellulose in plant cell walls and may be insoluble or soluble. They make up about one-third or more of the fiber in cereal grains, vegetables, fruits, legumes, and nuts.
4. *Pectins* are polysaccharides made up of galacturonic acid and variety of sugars. They are soluble in hot water and form gels when cooled. They are found in high amounts in the cell walls and intracellular tissue of fruits and some vegetables (e.g., sugar beet, potatoes), and to a lesser extent in other vegetables, legumes, and nuts.
5. *Oligosaccharides* are made up of 3–10 sugar units and occur naturally in vegetables, cereals, and nuts. FOSs and inulins (3–60 fructose units) are used as functional, prebiotic fibers and are found in onions, chicory, and Jerusalem artichokes.

---

* When derived from a plant origin, dietary fiber may include fractions of lignin and/or other compounds when associated with polysaccharides in the plant cell walls and if these compounds are quantified by the [Association of Analytical Communities (AOAC)] gravimetric analytical method for dietary fiber analysis: Fractions of lignin and the other compounds (proteic fractions, phenolic compounds, waxes, saponins, phytates, cutin, phytosterols, etc.) intimately "associated" with plant polysaccharides are often extracted with the polysaccharides in the AOAC 991.43 method.

† Decision on whether to include carbohydrates from 3 to 9 monomeric units should be left to national authorities.

6. *Gums* are hydrocolloids derived from plant exudates (arabic, tragacanth), seeds (guar, locust bean), and seaweed (agar, carageenan, alginates). Gums are used as gelling, thickening, stabilizing, and emulsifying agents.

7. *Mucilages* are found in the cell walls of some seeds such as psyllium. They are used similarly to gums and in the case of psyllium, as a functional fiber.

8. *Resistant starches* (*RS*) and starch degradation products are not absorbed in the small intestine and can be fermented in the large intestine. There are four types of RS. RS1 are found in whole or partly milled grains, seeds, legumes, and pasta. RS2 are found in raw potatoes, unripe bananas, and some legumes. High-amylase starches produced by the food industry are also considered RS2. RS3 are found in cooked and cooled potatoes, bread, cornflakes, and food products with prolonged and/or repeated moist heat treatment. RS4 are found in some fiber-rich drinks and foods that have modified starch as an ingredient. Processing, storage, and mastication can lead to the production or degradation of RS in various foods, and so they can be difficult to quantify.

9. *Lignans* are noncarbohydrates that are chemically bound to hemicelluloses in plant cell walls and can be found in, for example, celery and the outer layer of cereal grains.

10. *Other* noncarbohydrates that may or may not classify as fiber, depending on the definition used, include fatty acid derivatives such as *waxes*, *cutin*, *saponins*, and *suberin*; animal "fibers" such as *chitan* and *chitosan*; as well as *phytate* and *tannins* associated with cereal fibers.

10.4 FIBER CLASSIFICATIONS

Traditionally, fiber has been classified based on water solubility, being either insoluble (e.g., cellulose, most hemicellulose, lignin) or soluble (e.g., pectins, gums, mucilages). More recently, fibers have also been classified based on their viscosity and ability to be fermented. Most food sources of fiber contain a mix of fiber types but some are higher in either soluble/viscous or insoluble/nonviscous fibers. Many cereal grains, such as wheat, rye, and rice contain mostly insoluble, low viscosity, and low fermentable fibers and are beneficial for laxation. Foods that contain half or more of their fiber content as soluble, viscous, and highly fermentable fibers include oats, legumes, fruits, and vegetables, and they may be more beneficial in reducing CVD risk (Marlett et al. 2002, Suter 2005). The effect of molecular weight is less established in determining the functionality of fiber. For example, low- and high-molecular-weight barley β-glucan reduced blood cholesterol to similar extents in two human trials, although only the high-molecular-weight barley β-glucan reduced circulating triglycerides (TG) at a 5 g/day dose (Pins et al. 2002, Queenan et al. 2007).

10.5 SOURCES OF DIETARY FIBER

Dietary fiber is found in fruits, vegetables, and grains, in amounts of 1–3% of fresh weight, while nuts, legumes, and high-fiber grains typically contain more (IOM 2001). Sources and quantities of dietary fiber are shown in Table 10.1. In the diet of American male health professionals, vegetables, cereals, wheat products, and fruits contributed the greatest proportion of dietary fiber (Rimm et al. 1996). In that study, intake from vegetables and breakfast cereals accounted for about one-third each, while wheat products and fruits accounted for about one-quarter and one-seventh, respectively, of total dietary fiber intake. Oats and cruciferous foods were classified separately and contributed to a lesser extent to dietary fiber intake, providing 2–5% of dietary fiber intake.

10.6 FACTORS AFFECTING DIETARY FIBER CONTENT

Fiber content of foods may vary by crop and processing, and functionality may vary by solubility and viscosity. Ames and Rhymer (2008), using the example of barley as a fiber source, discuss that

TABLE 10.1
Sources of Dietary Fibers

10.1–14.0 g Fiber/Serving

Legumes (175 mL serving)
Kidney beans, light red; pinto beans, boiled; baked beans, cooked
Cereals and grains (30 g serving)
All-Bran Buds® cereal, All-Bran Original® cereal, 100% Bran® cereal
Flaxseed, whole, ground

6.1–10.0 g Fiber/Serving

Legumes (175 mL serving)
Great Northern beans; navy beans; kidney beans, dark red; soybeans, dry; Lima beans, boiled
Vegetables (125 mL serving)
Yellow beans; french beans, boiled

2.0–6.0 g Fiber/Serving

Legumes (175 mL serving)
Chickpeas (garbonzo beans), boiled
Peas, green, frozen, boiled
Vegetables (125 mL serving)
Sweet or white potato, baked without peeling the skin
Brussels sprouts; snow peas, boiled, drained
Yams, boiled or baked
Carrots; okra (gumbo), boiled
Cereals and grains (30 g serving)
Bran flakes cereal; Shredded Wheat® cereal; Grape-nuts® cereal; puffed wheat cereal
Bulgur, cooked
Corn, sweet, frozen or fresh, boiled
Oatmeal, cooked
Barley, pearled, cooked
Fruits (1 medium or 125 mL serving)
Pear, raspberries, gooseberries, orange, kiwifruit, apple, strawberries, blueberries, raw, with skin
Nuts and Seeds (60 mL serving)
Sesame seeds, whole; almonds, dried
Breads, Pastas, and Rice (1 slice or 125 mL serving):
Whole-wheat bread or pita
Whole-wheat pasta, cooked
Pumpernickel bread
Rice, brown, medium grain, cooked
Rye bread

Source: Adapted from United States Department of Agriculture (USDA). 2009b. Agricultural Research Service, *Nutrient Data Laboratory. USDA National Nutrient Database for Standard Reference, Release 21. Content of Selected Foods per Common Fiber, Total Dietary g, Measure, Sorted by Nutrient Content.* Available at http://www.nal.usda.gove/fnic/foodcomp/Data/SR21/nutrlist/sr21w291.pdf: Health Canada 2007b, *Canadian Nutrient File.* Available at http://webprod.hc-sc.gc.ca.proxy2.lib.umanitoba.ca/cnf-fce/index-eng.jsp.

the soluble fiber content of a crop or food type can vary by 3–23%. They also point out that processing of grains via milling, extraction, and temperature treatment can alter the structure and viscosity of fiber, which may in turn influence physiological response.

There may be some discrepancies in the fiber content of foods reported in food composition tables because of the lack of a global definition of fiber, as well as differing methods for determining the fiber content of foods (IOM 2001). The various enzymatic–gravimetric and enzymatic–chemical methods are described in detail in the IOM report, Dietary Reference Intakes: Proposed Definition of Dietary Fiber (IOM 2001). AOAC 985.29, developed by Prosky et al. (1985) is an enzymatic–gravimetric method of determining total fiber content that is used by many governments for nutrition labeling purposes. Other AOAC methods include 991.42 for insoluble dietary fiber; 991.43 for total, soluble, and insoluble dietary fiber; 993.19 for soluble dietary fiber; as well as several methods specific to food types (AOAC 2009). There are concerns however with the use of multiple methods and whether these methods are appropriate based on the evolving definitions of fiber (Betteridge 2009). For example, the AOAC 985.29 method used for food labeling measures nonstarch polysaccharides and lignin, only some RS, inulin, chitin, and other noncarbohydrates, but does not measure oligosaccharides, polydextrose, or resistant maltodextrose (IOM 2001). Therefore, the total fiber content may be underrepresented by this method according to the latest definitions. McCleary (2007) has developed a method which measures total dietary fiber, including RS, nondigestible oligosaccharides and available carbohydrates that is in the final stages of colab testing with AOAC (Betteridge 2009). Clearly, globally agreed-upon definitions and methods for fiber determination are required.

10.7 DIETARY REFERENCE INTAKES

The DRI for total fiber (dietary plus novel/functional fiber) is based on an AI of 14 g/1000 kcal/day for people aged 1 to >70 years. Important to the current discussion, the AIs are based primarily on the level observed to protect against CVD. Based on this, 19–50-year-old adults have an AI of 38 g/day for men and 25 g/day for women (IOM 2006). In reality, the actual dietary fiber intake for men and women in this age range is ~19 and 15 g/day, respectively, or on average about half of the AI (CDC 2009, Statistics Canada 2007). For men and women over 50, the AI recommendation is for 30 and 21 g/day, respectively (IOM 2006), while the actual intake is ~18 and 15 g/day, respectively, or about two-thirds of the AI (CDC 2009, Statistics Canada 2007). It should be noted that dietary sources of fiber are also sources of vitamins, minerals, and phytochemicals that contribute health benefits. When examining the food sources of dietary fiber (Table 10.1), it is clear that choosing legumes, high-fiber cereals, whole grains, nuts, vegetables and fruits as part of the diet, for example, by following MyPyramid/Canada's Food Guide recommendations and/or high-fiber dietary patterns (discussed in Section 10.12), will aid individuals in meeting the AI for total fiber.

10.8 FOOD LABELING

A "high-fiber" product in the United States must contain 5 g of fiber or more, per serving (USFDA 2009a). In Canada, a product that is a "source of fiber" must contain at least 2 g of fiber while high fiber and very high-fiber sources contain at least 4 and 6 g of fiber per serving, respectively (Health Canada 2009).

10.9 BENEFITS OF FIBER FOR CARDIOVASCULAR DISEASE

10.9.1 EPIDEMIOLOGICAL DATA

The benefit of dietary fiber for CVD prevention has been shown in several cohort studies. Data from the National Health and Nutrition Examination Survey (NHANES) follow-up study showed that participants in the highest quartile of dietary fiber intake (20.7 g/day) had an adjusted relative risk of 0.88 and 0.89 for CHD and CVD events, respectively, compared with the lowest quartile of dietary fiber intake (5.9 g/day), over an average follow-up of 19 years (Bazzano et al. 2003). In the elderly, the relative risk reduction for CVD events was 0.79 with high cereal fiber intake versus low cereal fiber intake (>6.3 vs. <1.7 g/day), based on an 11 year follow-up (Mozaffarian et al. 2003). For women specifically, Wolk et al. (1999) documented a 0.53 relative risk reduction for CVD with high fiber versus low fiber intake (22.9 vs. 11.5 g/day), after an average follow-up of 10 years. Similar comparisons in men showed relative risk for myocardial infarction and CHD death was 0.59 and 0.69, respectively, after a 6 year follow up when comparing high total dietary fiber intake versus low total dietary fiber intake (34.8 vs. 16.1 g/day) (Pietinen et al. 1996, Rimm et al. 1996). Streppel et al. (2008) have demonstrated that every additional 10 g of dietary fiber intake per day reduced CHD mortality by 17% in men.

Whole grain intake as a source of dietary fiber, but also containing other protective constituents, is inversely related to carotid artery atherosclerosis (Mellen et al. 2007), CHD in women (Liu et al. 1999) and CVD risk factors including body mass index (BMI), waist-to-hip ratio, total cholesterol (TC), low-density lipoprotein cholesterol (LDL-C) and fasting insulin (McKeown et al. 2002). Lairon et al. (2005) specifically looked at fiber sources and their effect on individual CVD risk factors and reported that fibers from cereals, vegetables, and fruits were associated with reduced blood pressure; fibers from cereals, dried fruits, and nuts/seeds were associated with lower BMI; fibers from cereals and vegetables were associated with lower homocysteine concentrations (see Chapter 5 for further discussion on homocysteine); fibers from fruits and dried fruits or nuts/seeds were associated with a lower waist-to-hip ratio, and the latter was also associated with lower fasting apoB and glucose.

There are limitations, however, to epidemiological data as it is dependent on diet self-reporting, usually through food frequency questionnaires, and their analysis, which relies primarily on fiber values in nutrient databases. Additionally, the inability to delineate which fiber type is present in the diet using this approach limits the ability to identify specific fiber types with benefits for CVD. Regardless, the epidemiological studies show risk reduction in the order of 11–41% when comparing relatively high fiber intakes (20.7–34.1 g/day) to low fiber intakes (5.9–16.1 g/day). The benefits of dietary fibers are therefore known and their effects on CVD risk reduction are being delineated by examining individual risk factors.

10.9.2 EXPERIMENTAL AND CLINICAL DATA

The following sections examine the experimental and clinical studies which have investigated the effects of dietary fiber on specific risk factors for CVD.

10.9.2.1 Obesity

Central obesity is a major risk factor for CVD. For example, waist-to-hip ratio and waist circumference predict death from CVD, while intraabdominal adipose loss appears to reduce CVD risk (Dhaliwal and Welborn 2009, Katsoulis et al. 2009). Thus, dietary strategies such as a high-fiber diet that may aid in weight management are relevant. Viscous fiber in particular may promote satiety by delaying gastric emptying which is theorized to attenuate energy intake and reduce the risk of obesity (Spiller 1994, Slavin 2008).

Observational data have shown an inverse relationship between dietary fiber or whole grain intake and body weight, fat mass, or waist circumference in adults and children (Appleby et al. 1998, Nelson and Tucker 1996, Liu et al. 2003, Koh-Banerjee et al. 2004, Ventura et al. 2008). The benefits of fiber for obesity appear to be in a preventative capacity according to these data and the World Health Organization (WHO/FAO 2003).

Many clinical trials have failed to show a direct effect of fiber intake on reducing body weight in adults, including those using oats or β-glucan, psyllium, pectin, guar gum, inulin, and plantago ovate husk (Table 10.2: Anderson et al. 1990, Wolever et al. 1994, Blake et al. 1997, Brighenti et al. 1999, Saltzman et al. 2001, Jenkins et al. 2002, Keogh et al. 2003, Schwab et al. 2006, Forcheron and Beylot 2007, Queenan et al. 2007, Sola et al. 2007). However, Reyna-Villasmil et al. (2007) demonstrated that dyslipidemic men following the American Heart Association Step II diet plus 6 g β-glucan/day for 8 weeks, lost more weight than those without the fiber supplementation (5.8 kg as opposed to 3.8 kg weight loss).

TABLE 10.2

Summary of Clinical Randomized Controlled Trials with No Effect on Body Weight

Dose/Day and Duration	Control	Subjects	Body Weight	Reference
Oats, Barley, or β-Glucan				
25 g Oat bran × 2 weeks	Cornflakes	$n = 12$ Mildly dyslipidemic adults	NS	Anderson et al. (1990)
8.1–11.9 g β-Glucan × 4 weeks	Glucose	$n = 18$ Mildly dyslipidemic men	NS	Keogh et al. (2003)
6 g β-Glucan × 6 weeks	Dextrose	$n = 90$ Dyslipidemic adults	NS	Queenan et al. (2007)
45 g Oats × 4 weeks (2 weeks energy restriction prior and during)	No oats	$n = 43$ Healthy adults	NS	Saltzman et al. (2001)
Psyllium				
8 g Soluble fiber from psyllium or β-glucan × 4 weeks	No psyillium or β-glucan	$n = 68$ Dyslipidemic adults	NS	Jenkins et al. (2002)
54 g Psyllium × 2 weeks	Wheat bran	$N = 18$ Moderately dyslipidemic adults	NS	Wolever et al. (1994)
Pectin				
4 dL Sugar beet pectin providing 16 g fiber/day × 12 weeks	Polydextrose	$n = 66$ Adults with impaired glucose tolerance	NS	Schwab et al. (2006)
Guar Gum				
≤16 g Guar gum × 3 weeks	Wheat bread	$n = 12$ Moderately dyslipidemic men	NS	Blake et al. (1997)
Inulin				
9 g Inulin × 4 weeks	Rice cereal	$n = 12$ Normolipidemic men	NS	Brighenti et al. (1999)
10 g Inulin × 6 months	Unspecified placebo	$n = 17$ Healthy adults	NS	Forcheron and Beylot (2007)
Other				
10.5 g Plantago ovata husk × 8 weeks	Plantago ovata seed	$n = 28$ Men with ischemic heart disease	NS	Sola et al. (2007)

Note: NS = not statistically different from control intervention.

In summary, high-fiber diets appear beneficial for obesity prevention, while more data are required to say that they also aid in clinically meaningful weight loss.

10.9.2.2   Postprandial Glucose and Insulin Metabolism

Hyperglycemia, hyperinsulinemia, and insulin resistance (IR) are also major risk factors for CVD that are often associated with obesity (Jiamsripong et al. 2008). IR is defined as the diminished ability of cells to respond to the action of insulin in transporting glucose into tissues and is measured by various calculations based on circulating glucose and insulin levels. Postprandial measurements of glucose and insulin are useful because they are indications of how effectively insulin is providing glucose to tissues. Postprandial glucose is typically measured at 2 h post-ingestion or as part of an oral glucose tolerance test, as this is the time period when blood glucose levels usually begin to normalize. However, if there is a degree of IR, glucose may stay elevated postprandially. Postprandial hyperglycemia is associated with increased risk of CVD in people with diabetes or impaired glucose tolerance, while treatment of hyperglycemia decreases the risk of CVD (Hanefeld et al. 1996a,b, Chiasson et al. 2003, Hanefeld and Schaper 2004, Esposito et al. 2004a, Zeymer et al. 2004 Cavalot et al. 2006). Thus, fiber-containing foods that are able to attenuate postprandial glucose and insulin are useful for metabolic control.

Clinical trials have shown little effect of fibers such as oat bran, β-glucan, and flaxseed on *fasting* glucose or insulin in nondiabetic adults (Table 10.3: Queenan et al. 2007, Saltzman et al. 2001, Kestin et al. 1990, Lovegrove et al. 2000, Dodin et al. 2008, Behall et al. 2004b). An exception to this was a significant attenuation of fasting insulin levels at 4 weeks in dyslipidemic adults supplemented with 10 g inulin/day for 8 weeks (Jackson et al. 1999). As well, Bloedon et al. (2008) showed that 40 g flaxseed/day for 10 weeks improved IR in adults as assessed by homeostasis model assessment (HOMA), which is based on fasting measures of glucose and insulin. In adults with well-controlled type 2 diabetes, flaxseed incorporated into the diet did not alter glycemia or fasting insulin levels (Taylor et al. 2010).

There has been more evidence for positive effects of fiber on postprandial metabolism. In nondiabetic relatives of people with type 2 diabetes, intake of dietary fiber, assessed by 3-day food records, was inversely associated with IR, based on oral glucose tolerance testing, HOMA, and incremental 30-min insulin/glucose (Ylonen et al. 2003). In overweight or obese, normoglycemic women, 31.2 g cereal fiber/day for 3 days improved whole-body insulin sensitivity, assessed by steady-state analysis, that is, calculating whole-body glucose disposal ($M = $ mg/min/kg), as well as M/serum insulin (Weickert et al. 2006). Dubois et al. (1995) demonstrated that 40 g oat bran/day for 2 weeks attenuated the postmeal insulin rise by 40% in dyslipidemic men. Biorklund et al. (2005) showed that

TABLE 10.3

Summary of Clinical Randomized Controlled Trials with No Effect on Fasting Glucose or Insulin

Dose/Day and Duration	Control	Subjects	Glucose or Insulin	Reference
		Oats, Barley or β-Glucan		
3 or 6 g β-Glucan × 5 weeks + STEP 1 diet 17 weeks	0 g β-Glucan	$n = 25$ Mildly dyslipidemic adults	NS fasting glucose, OGTT	Behall et al. (2004b)
~10 g oat bran × 4 weeks	Wheat or rice bran	$n = 24$ Mildly dyslipidemic men	NS fasting insulin, glucose or AUC	Kestin et al. (1990)
20 g Oat bran concentrate (~3 g β-glucan) × 8 weeks	Wheat bran	$n = 62$ Healthy adults	NS fasting glucose or insulin	Lovegrove et al. (2000)
6 g β-Glucan × 6 weeks	Dextrose	$n = 90$ Dyslipidemic adults	NS fasting glucose	Queenan et al. (2007)
45 g Oats × 4 weeks (2 weeks energy restriction prior and during)	None	$n = 43$ Healthy adults	NS fasting glucose, insulin or HOMA	Saltzman et al. (2001)
		Flaxseed		
40 g Milled flaxseed × 12 months	Wheat germ	$n = 179$ Postmenopausal women	NS fasting glucose, insulin	Dodin et al. (2008)

Note: AUC = area under the curve; HOMA = homeostasis model assessment; NS = not statistically different from control intervention; OGTT = oral glucose tolerance test; STEP 1 diet = 55% carbohydrate, 30% fat (<10% saturated fat, <300 mg cholesterol), 15% protein as previously endorsed by the American Heart Association.

5 g oat β-glucan/day for 5 weeks significantly lowered 30-min postmeal glucose and insulin in dys-lipidemic adults. Panahi et al. (2007) demonstrated that enzymatically processed, but not aqueously processed, β-glucan from oats lowered the area under the curve (AUC) for glucose in healthy adults. RS also appear to have a positive effect on postprandial glucose and, to a greater degree, insulin response, although the results are mixed (Nugent 2005). One study, however, showed a negative effect of 16 g of fiber from beet pectin or polydextrose taken for 12 weeks on hemoglobin A1c, a measure that is proportional to the average blood sugar over the previous 1–3 months, in adults with impaired fasting glucose (Schwab et al. 2006). However, the actual changes were small in this study (mean increases ~0.1–0.2%), and there were no acute affects on fasting glucose, insulin, or postpran-dial glucose (Schwab et al. 2006). Meta-analysis has shown that overall, diets high in dietary fiber have a favorable effect on glycemic control, including hemoglobin A1c (Anderson et al. 2004).

Therefore, the majority of the evidence shows that total fiber, and fiber from cereals, oats, or isolated β-glucan can improve postprandial glucose and insulin metabolism.

10.9.2.3 Adipokines and Inflammatory Markers

Chronic, low-grade inflammation is one proposed mechanism for the link between obesity, insulin/glucose dysregulation, and CVD. Adipose tissue has a recognized role in endocrine function and proteins such as adiponectin that are secreted from adipose tissue may play an important anti-inflammatory role (Sun et al. 2009). Adiponectin is often reduced in those with the metabolic syndrome and diabetes (Kadowaki et al. 2006), while higher circulating adiponectin levels are associated with lower cardiovascular risk (Han et al. 2007). Some of the emerging functions of adiponectin include reducing circulating free fatty acids and improving vascular endothelial function (Combs et al. 2001, Mantzoros et al. 2005, Giannessi et al. 2007).

Additionally, obesity is characterized by large adipocytes and infiltration by macrophages, both of which are capable of releasing inflammatory cytokines such as the interleukins and tumor necro-sis factor-α (DeClercq et al. 2008). Several circulating acute-phase proteins, such as C-reactive protein (CRP) have also been associated with the inflammation associated with obesity (Jiamsripong et al. 2008). Therefore, prevention of obesity or weight reduction, as discussed in the previous sec-tion, may modify inflammation.

Limited data show that dietary fiber may favorably modify both adiponectin and the interleukins. Cross-sectional analyses by Qi et al. (2005, 2006) showed that men and women with diabetes in the Nurses' Health Study and Health Professionals Follow Up Study who consumed the highest amount of cereal fiber (10.0 g cereal fiber/day and 30.9 g total fiber/day) had greater circulating adiponectin levels, even after adjustment for BMI. In clinical trials, serum concentrations of interleukin-6 were lower and adiponectin were higher at breakfast following an evening meal with barley-kernel bread containing 10.7 g fiber compared with white wheat flour bread containing 2.6 g fiber (Nilsson et al. 2008). In people with type 2 diabetes, a high-fiber meal containing 16.8 g whole-wheat flour versus a low-fiber, low-carbohydrate meal lowered serum interleukin-8 but did not affect adiponectin com-pared to high-fat and low-fiber meals (Esposito et al. 2003). Therefore, fiber may favorably reduce inflammation, possibly by increasing anti-inflammatory proteins (e.g., adiponectin) and lowering proinflammatory mediators (e.g., interleukins).

Other markers of inflammation have also been favorably modified by fiber intake. Following a high-fiber (>40 g/day from mixed sources), low fat diet, for 3 weeks, plasma lipid hydroperoxides were reduced and the anti-inflammatory properties of HDL were improved in overweight or obese adults (Roberts et al. 2006). Interestingly, the high-fiber DASH diet, which included either dietary or supplemental fiber sources, reduced circulating CRP in lean subjects, but not overweight subjects (King et al. 2007). In a longitudinal analysis, Ma et al. (2006) showed that healthy adults with the highest quartile of total fiber intake (32 g/day) were at less risk for elevated CRP levels and there was an inverse relationship between total dietary fiber and circulating CRP concentrations. Milled flaxseed (40 g/day) had no effect on circulating CRP, interleukin-6, oxidized LDL or urinary isoprostanes in healthy menopausal women, postmenopausal women, or men (Bloedon et al. 2008, Dodin et al. 2008).

Overall, there exist interesting data to suggest that cereal fiber or high total fiber intake may favorably affect adiponectin, interleukins, and CRP, and this requires further investigation. Adiponectin may also provide benefits via mechanisms that are independent of inflammation (discussed in Section 10.10).

10.9.2.4   Hypertension

Hypertension, especially elevated systolic blood pressure, is a major risk factor for CVD events (Kannel 2009, Pencina et al. 2009). There have been mixed results for the effect of fiber on hypertension. Systolic blood pressure was improved by approximately 5% in overweight adults consuming dietary oats (45 g/day) with 3.3–4.2 MJ energy restriction, compared to energy restriction alone for 8 weeks (Saltzman et al. 2001). Hypertensive adults with a BMI of >31.5 who consumed oat products containing 7.7 g β-glucan/day and increased their total fiber intake by 12 ± 1.6 g/day had lower systolic (−5.6 mmHg) and diastolic (−2.1 mmHg) blood pressure compared to low-fiber controls after 12 weeks (Maki et al. 2007). Supplementation with 10.5 g psyllium fiber/day, for 6 months, led to reductions in both systolic and diastolic blood pressure of 5.6 and 2.2 mmHg, respectively, in hypertensive overweight subjects (Cicero et al. 2007). Guar gum (7.5–21 g/day with meals) reduced systolic and diastolic blood pressure by 6 and 3 mmHg, respectively, in healthy men and diastolic blood pressure by 4 mmHg in people with type 2 diabetes (Landin et al. 1992, Uusitupa et al. 1984). However, in other studies of various durations, dietary oats, β-glucan, psyllium, or pectin have shown no beneficial effect on blood pressure (Table 10.4) (Kestin et al. 1990, Wolever et al. 1994, Jenkins et al. 2002, Keogh et al. 2003, Schwab et al. 2006, Cicero et al. 2007).

The potential of fiber to reduce systolic blood pressure, even modestly, is an important aspect of CVD prevention. However, the effects of fibers on blood pressure appear inconclusive at this time

TABLE 10.4

Summary of Clinical Randomized Controlled Trials with No Effect on Blood Pressure

Dose/Day and Duration	Control	Subjects	Blood Pressure	Reference
Oats, Barley, or β-Glucan				
8.1–11.9 g β-Glucan × 4 weeks	Glucose	$n = 18$ Mildly dyslipidemic men	NS	Keogh et al. (2003)
~10 g Oat bran × 4 weeks	Wheat or rice bran	$n = 24$ Mildly dyslipidemic men	NS	Kestin et al. (1990)
Psyllium				
8 g Soluble fiber from psyllium or β-glucan × 4 weeks	No psyllium or β-glucan	$n = 68$ Dyslipidemic adults	NS	Jenkins et al. (2002)
54 g Psyllium × 2 weeks	Wheat bran	$n = 18$ Moderately dyslipidemic adults	NS	Wolever et al. (1994)
Pectin				
4 dL Sugar beet pectin providing 16 g fiber × 12 weeks	Polydextrose	$n = 66$ Adults with impaired glucose tolerance	NS	Schwab et al. (2006)

Note: NS = not statistically different from control intervention.

and are likely intertwined with multiple other CVD risk factors even though the positive effects of oats, pysllium, and guar gum discussed above were independent of weight loss.

10.9.2.5 Lipidemia

The bulk of clinical research on fiber and CVD has been largely focused on lipidemia. The Framingham Heart and Framingham Offspring Studies have provided important data on CVD risk factors as well as algorithms for predicting up to 30-year CHD risk, and blood cholesterol concentrations are an important part of those equations. According to the most recent Framingham data, TC and high-density lipoprotein cholesterol (HDL-C) have hazard ratios of 1.33 and 0.78, respectively (Pencina et al. 2009). Target LDL levels are based on risk, with the highest risk patients striving for an LDL-C of <2.0 mmol/L, or a 50% reduction from baseline (NCEP Adult Treatment Panel III 2002, Genest et al. 2009). However, as discussed in Section 10.13.2, it should also be noted that CVD occurs in individuals with blood cholesterol in the recommended range. Early experimental work showed a marked reduction in serum TC of rats fed with oats (de Groot et al. 1963), and subsequently several trials in people have shown that various fibers can favorably modify serum TC and LDL-C status which is paramount to reducing CVD risk.

Several studies have demonstrated that oat intakes of 25–110 g/day reduce serum TC and LDL-C concentrations. In dyslipidemic men, oat bran or oatmeal at fairly high intakes (70–110 g/day) for 10–21 days reduced serum TC and LDL-C by 9–18% and 9–24%, respectively, with no effect on HDL-C or TG (Kirby et al. 1981, Anderson et al. 1990, Davidson et al. 1991, Gerhardt and Gallo 1998, Davidson and Maki 1999). In mildly dyslipidemic adults, with most trials being in men, similar levels of oat bran intakes for 28–56 days showed more modest reductions of 4.9–6.0% and 3.0–8.5%, respectively, in serum TC and LDL-C, while again there was no effect on serum TG or HDL-C in most studies (Anderson et al. 1990, 1991, Kestin et al. 1990, Van Horn et al. 1991). Congruently, meta-analyses have shown that oats, providing 3 g soluble fiber/day, reduce TC by 0.13 mmol/L (Ripsin et al. 1992). When oat consumption (45 g/day) was coupled with weight loss by energy restriction, healthy adults were able to lower serum TC and LDL-C by 18–19% (Saltzman et al. 2001). Two studies did not find any effect of oat bran in adults with dyslipidemia after 14–28 days (Leadbetter et al. 1991, Dubois et al. 1995). In nondyslipidemic adults, 87 g oat bran/day for 6 weeks had no effect on plasma cholesterol compared to a low-fiber wheat product (Swain et al. 1990).

The effective hypolipidemic compounds in oats and barley may be the β-glucans. Dyslipidemic men or healthy adults who consumed products containing 3.8–6.0 g β-glucan/day (oat milk, orange juice, fruit drink) or concentrated β-glucan from oats or barley experienced reductions in plasma TC and LDL of 5–8%, but there was usually no effect on HDL-C or TG (McIntosh et al. 1991, Nicolosi et al. 1999, Onning et al. 1999, Kerckhoffs et al. 2003, Biorklund et al. 2005, Karmally et al. 2005, Naumann et al. 2006, Keenan et al. 2007, Queenan et al. 2007). Two trials with barley products containing up to 8 g β-glucan/day have shown more dramatic reductions of 12–15% and 14–24% in TC and LDL-C, respectively, after 5 weeks in men and women with normal cholesterol or mild hypercholesterolemia (Newman et al. 1991, Behall et al. 2004a,b). Also in dyslipidemic men, 5 g β-glucan/day of oat muesli for 3 weeks lowered plasma LDL-C by 5%, and when consumed with plant stanols, plasma LDL-C was lowered by 10% (Theuwissen and Mensink 2007). When an American Heart Association Step II diet was paired with 6 g β-glucan/day in bread for 8 weeks, mildly to moderately dyslipidemic men were able to lower their circulating TC (16% vs. 13%) and LDL-C (27% vs. 17%) and raise HDL-C (28% vs 2%) to a greater degree than with the Step II diet alone (Reyna-Villasmil et al. 2007). Ames and Rhymer (2008) have studied the physiological effects of barley β-glucan, some of which have been mentioned here, and they concluded that barley β-glucan is effective, and can reduce TC and LDL-C by 5–24%. Again, a few studies found no effect of concentrated sources of β-glucan (oat bran concentrate, cookies, and bread baked with β-glucan) on circulating lipids in healthy adults or mildly lipidemic adults (Lovegrove et al. 2000, Keogh et al. 2003, Kerckhoffs et al. 2003). It is logical that when lipidemia is within normal ranges, there is limited effect of fiber, although the studies by Newman et al. (1991) and Li et al. (2003) using barley β-glucan dispute this notion, showing its effects on normolipidemia. There are several other factors that may explain discrepancies in the data including amount of fiber consumed, source of fiber, effects of processing, molecular weight and viscosity of fiber, as well as the study duration.

In dyslipidemic adults, 20–40 g milled flaxseed/day reduced plasma TC and LDL in the short term (3 and 5 weeks) but not with slightly greater duration (10 weeks) compared to wheat bran (Bloedon et al. 2008, Jenkins et al. 1999). Similar levels of daily milled flaxseed had no effect on lipidemia in postmenopausal women after 12 months compared to wheat germ (Dodin et al. 2008).

Meta-analysis has shown that on average, 10.1 g/day psyllium with a low fat diet may reduce TC by 4% and LDL-C by 7% (Anderson et al. 2000). Trials with 1.8–6.7 g/day psyllium incorporated into various test foods have reduced TC and LDL by 8–21% in dyslipidemic adults compared to a wheat bran control (Wolever et al. 1994, Jenkins et al. 2002). In these two trials, the study by Jenkins et al. (2002) also found a beneficial effect of psyllium on plasma TG (reduced by 5%), while the study by Wolever et al. (1994) found a small negative effect on plasma HDL-C (reduced by 7%).

Pectin from sugar beets reduced LDL-C by 8% after 12 weeks compared to polydextrose in adults with impaired glucose tolerance (Schwab et al. 2006). Similarly, a grape product (7.5 g/day) fed for 16 weeks lowered total LDL-C by 9% in adults (Jimenez et al. 2008). Again, neither product showed an effect on HDL-C or TG. According to meta-analysis, oats, psyllium, and pectin are all effective in reducing TC and LDL-C by 0.045 and 0.057 mmol/L/g of soluble fiber, respectively (Brown et al. 1999).

Guar (glactomannan) gum (15–30 g/day) effectively lowered TC and LDL-C in the range of 10–14% and 10–18%, respectively, in dyslipidemic adults compared to those fed placebos in studies lasting 3, 6, or 12 weeks and up to 24 months (Niemi et al. 1988, Turner et al. 1990, Salenius et al. 1995, Blake et al. 1997). Once again, no effect on HDL-C or TG was observed.

Supplementation with inulin (18 g/day for 6 weeks) lowered TC and LDL-C by 7% and 12%, respectively, in healthy adults and, in agreement with other dietary and functional fiber data, did not improve HDL-C or TG (Davidson and Maki 1999). However, inulin supplementation (9–14 g/day for 4–14 weeks) to healthy or moderately dyslipidemic adults had no effect on blood cholesterol, although three trials reported a TG-lowering effect compared to placebo (Pedersen et al. 1997, Brighenti et al. 1999, Jackson et al. 1999, Letexier et al. 2003, Forcheron and Beylot 2007).

RS do not appear to affect lipidemia in humans as they do in animal models (reviewed in Nugent 2005).

In summary, dietary fibers including oats and milled flaxseed, as well as functional fibers such as concentrated β-glucan, psyllium, pectin, guar gum, and inulin, reduce plasma total and LDL-C in the range of ~5–15%, with greater efficiency seen in combination with lower fat diets or energy restriction, and for those individuals with a greater degree of dyslipidemia. The majority of clinical trials do not demonstrate a beneficial effect of fiber on circulating HDL-C or TG, although inulin may lower blood TG.

10.9.2.6 Lipoproteinemia

Apolipoprotein Bs (apoB; subtypes apoB48 and apoB100) are structural components of the athero-genic lipoproteins LDL, intermediate-density lipoprotein (IDL) and very low-density lipoprotein (VLDL) (Grundy 2002). Apolipoprotein As (apoA; subtypes apoA-I, apoA-II, apoA-IV, and apoA-V) are similarly associated with HDL. Thus a reduction in apoB, or a reduction in the ratio of apoB:apoA, is favorable for reducing CVD risk.

A handful of studies have demonstrated trends or significant reductions in apoB without affect-ing apoAI when dyslipidemic adults consumed 25–84 g oats/day or 3 g β-glucan/day for 2–6 weeks (Anderson et al. 1990, Kestin et al. 1990, Gerhardt and Gallo 1998, Karmally et al. 2005). Milled flaxseed reduced both circulating apoB and apoA-I in dyslipidemic subjects compared to wheat bran or wheat germ in both short-term and long-term trials of 3 weeks to 12 months (Jenkins et al. 1999, Dodin et al. 2008). Lupton et al. (1994) showed that barley flour and oil both reduced apoA, but only the oil decreased apoB100. Meta-analysis has shown that the ratio of apoB:apoA was reduced by 6% with 10 g of psyllium supplementation/day (Anderson et al. 2000). Guar gum supplementation reduced apoB by 22% after 6 weeks in a small trial of hyperlipidemic patients (Turner et al. 1990) but had no effect on apoB, apoA-I, or lipoprotein (a) in another larger trial lasting 12 weeks (Salenius et al. 1995).

In summary, fiber sources such as oats, psyllium, and guar gum may lower apoB or apoB:apoA. The data are limited but would be expected given the LDL-lowering effects seen with many different fibers, as discussed above.

10.9.2.7 Atherosclerosis and Thrombosis

All the risk factors discussed above are believed to impact the progression of atherosclerosis which is narrowing of blood vessels due to the buildup of fatty materials on the vessel walls. Wu et al. (2003) studied men and women aged between 40 and 60 years and found a significant inverse association between intima-media thickness (IMT) of the common carotid arteries and viscous fiber as well as pectin intake. The authors postulated that this may have been mediated by a favorable impact of fiber on plasma lipids which they also reported, since oxidized LDL is a primary factor in the atherosclerotic process. In Spanish adults with the average age of 67 years, the mean common carotid IMT was also inversely associated with energy-adjusted fiber intake (Buil-Cosiales et al. 2009). Similarly, in postmenopausal women with carotid artery disease, Erkkila et al. (2005) found that those who consumed more than 3 g fiber/1000 kcal or >6 servings of whole grains/week had less carotid artery atherosclerosis as assessed by a decline in mean minimum coronary artery diameter.

With regard to thrombosis, or the formation of a blood clot inside a blood vessel, multiple regression analysis revealed that higher fiber intake (29.2 ± 5.4 g/day in the highest quintile versus 9.7 ± 3.7 g/day in the lowest quintile) was inversely associated with plasminogen activator inhibitor type 1 (PAI-1) in the Heart, Lung, and Blood Institute Family Heart Study (Djousse et al. 1998). Generally speaking, PAI-1 inhibits blood clotting and is inversely associated with ischemic heart disease (Hamsten et al. 1987, Meade et al. 1993). Fiber intakes did not, however, have an association with fibrinogen, a blood clotting factor, in the same report or in adults who consumed diets containing 19 g of cereal fiber or 40 g of milled flaxseed per day (Dodin et al. 2008, Fehily et al. 1986).

The evidence for the effect of fiber on atherosclerosis and thrombosis is limited, but given the enormity and particular relevance of these two parameters in CVD, these data showing a possible favorable effect are quite important.

10.10 MECHANISMS OF ACTION

Individual fiber types may have specific effects but overall there is good evidence to suggest that various fiber sources can attenuate circulating LDL-C, apoB, and postprandial circulating glucose and insulin concentrations. There is also evidence for a beneficial effect of fibers on the prevention or treatment of obesity, hypertension, inflammation, atherosclerosis, and thrombosis, as described in the previous sections. The presence of metabolic syndrome substantially raises CVD risk and is defined generally as central obesity, IR, dyslipidemia, hypertension, and inflammation (Alberti et al. 2006). People with metabolic syndrome and diabetes often display dyslipidemia in the form of elevated circulating LDL-C and TG and low HDL-C, along with markers of inflammation and obesity. Possible interrelated mechanisms of action of fiber consumption on these risk factors are summarized in Figure 10.1 and explained next.

Possible positive effects of fiber on obesity (discussed in Section 10.9.2.1) and postprandial metabolism (discussed in Section 10.9.2.2) may be due to the fact that (1) fiber-containing foods are often less-energy-dense than foods that do not contain fiber and (2) fiber modifies transit time in the gastrointestinal tract, thus increasing satiety by delaying gastric emptying and slowing absorption (Howarth et al. 2001). These two points are related to the glycemic index (GI), which is a measure of the effect of carbohydrate-containing foods on blood glucose levels (Jenkins et al. 1981). In

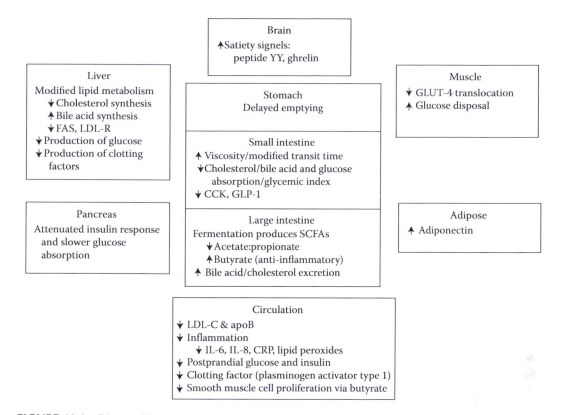

FIGURE 10.1 Dietary fiber reduces CVD risk factors: Possible mechanisms. Fiber ingestion slows gastric emptying and creates greater viscosity in small intestine, reducing cholesterol/bile acid absorption in the small intestine and increasing cholesterol/bile excretion from the large intestine, as well as slower glucose absorption in the small intestine, and attenuating the postprandial rise in blood glucose and the pancreatic insulin response. Fiber fermentation in the large intestine favorably modifies the ratio of short-chain fatty acids (SCFAs) produced and those entering circulation favorably modify hepatic cholesterol, bile acid, fatty acid (e.g., via fatty acid synthase (FAS)), and glucose metabolism, as well as the production of clotting factors. Cholecystokinin (CCK), glucagon-like peptide-1 (GLP-1), peptide YY, and ghrelin are reduced in circulation implying increased satiety. Favorable effects on circulation may include reduced LDL-cholesterol (LDL-C), apolipoprotein B (apoB), inflammatory markers (interleukins-6 and 8 (IL-6, IL-8), C-reactive protein (CRP), lipid peroxides), clotting factors (plasminogen activator inhibitor type 1 (PAI-1)), and smooth muscle cell proliferation. Possible effects on peripheral metabolism include reduced glucose transporter-4 translocation in muscle and improved adiponectin function from adipose (see references in Section 10.10).

general, epidemiological studies support the conclusion that a higher intake of dietary fiber, especially cereal fiber, is associated with a lower risk of diabetes (Salmeron et al. 1997, Meyer et al. 2000, Stevens et al. 2002), but few studies have examined the role of GI or specific fiber compositions over the long term. A study by Schulze et al (2004) was one of the first to report that a higher dietary GI, of all carbohydrate foods consumed, was significantly associated with increased risk of diabetes based on participants in The Nurses' Health Study II. They also reported that cereal fiber intake was associated with decreased risk of diabetes and that carbohydrate quality, not quantity, was an important factor. Low-GI diets have also been linked to a lower risk of CVD and improvement in CVD risk factors (Brand-Miller et al. 2007, Philippou et al. 2008).

Looking at the effects of fiber on digestion more specifically, certain fibers may improve postprandial satiety, circulating glucose and insulin via cholecystokinin (CCK), glucagon-like peptide-1 (GLP-1), peptide YY, ghrelin, propionate, and glucose transporter-4 (GLUT-4) regulation (Anderson and Bridges 1984, Holt et al. 1992, Massimino et al. 1998, Bourdon et al. 1999, Song et al. 2000,

Pereira and Ludwig 2001, Cani et al. 2004). CCK is secreted from the small intestine and functions to regulate gastric emptying and stimulate the exocrine pancreas which provides digestive enzymes and bicarbonate (Liddle 1997). Holt et al. (1992) and Bourdon et al. (1999) have demonstrated sustained CCK in the circulation following fiber-rich meals, compared to energy-matched, low-fiber meals. Ingestion of inulin has been associated with increased plasma GLP-1, peptide YY, and ghrelin concentrations, all functioning to regulate appetite (Massimino et al. 1998, Cani et al. 2004). In the large intestine, production of propionate (a short-chain fatty acid (SCFA) discussed below) may inhibit excess hepatic glucose production, a characteristic of IR and diabetes mellitus, as shown in rat hepatocytes *in vitro* (Anderson and Bridges 1984). Additionally, as shown in rats, viscous fiber may increase translocation of GLUT-4 receptors to the muscle cell membrane resulting in greater rates of glucose disposal (Song et al. 2000).

Inflammation is now a central theory of the metabolic syndrome (DeClercq et al. 2008), and so the fact that fiber has been shown to reduce proinflammatory markers such as CRP and interleukin-6 and -8 (discussed in Section 10.9.2.3) may also explain reduced CVD risk. Colonic fermentation of fiber to produce butyrate, another SCFA, may play an anti-inflammatory role, as it reduces inflammation in macrophages, monocytes, and endothelial cells (Saemann et al. 2002, Zapolska-Downar et al. 2004). A possible association between adiponectin and cereal fibers, as discussed above (Qi et al. 2005, 2006), although observational at this time, may also partially explain anti-inflammatory effects. Although adiponectin has a major endocrine role as an anti-inflammatory adipokine (Scherer et al. 1995), hypoadiponectinemia is also associated with atherosclerosis and endothelial dysfunction (Kadowaki and Yamauchi 2005), possibly in part because adiponectin is a mediator of nitric oxide production, adhesion molecules, and scavenger receptor gene expression (Zhu et al. 2008). Adiponectin inversely correlates with hypertension and can be increased by certain antihypertensive medications (Chang et al. 2009). Adiponectin may thus operate through multiple mechanisms to protect the vasculature and represent a plausible target for dietary fibers.

Fiber may have possible antithrombotic effects (discussed in Section 10.9.2.7) by reducing PAI-1 (Djousse et al. 1998). Galisteo et al. (2008) speculate that the SCFAs produced in the colon may directly inhibit the hepatic synthesis of coagulation factors. Additionally, they point out that PAI-1 and insulin sensitivity have a positive association, and so, if fiber does in fact improve adiponectin and insulin sensitivity, this may be an underlying mechanism for the antithrombotic effects.

Any positive effects of fiber on fat mass, glycemia/insulinemia, and inflammation (discussed in Sections 10.9.2.1 through 10.9.2.3, respectively) may also mediate benefits on blood pressure (discussed in Section 10.9.2.4), and blood pressure reduction has been observed in the absence of weight loss or improvements in insulin sensitivity (Saltzman et al. 2001). Other possible mechanisms with regard to hypertension are speculative at this time; however, it would be interesting to explore how the renin–angiotensin system is affected by fiber intake. Shin et al. (2005) have described angiotensin converting enzyme inhibition *in vitro* by an oat β-glucan derivative.

The mechanisms for LDL-C lowering (discussed in Section 10.9.2.5) by dietary fiber appear to involve increased excretion, decreased absorption or reabsorption, and/or altered metabolism of bile acids and cholesterol. Viscous fibers may inhibit bulk diffusion of cholesterol by increasing the resistance of the unstirred water layer lining on enterocytes (Salas-Salvado et al. 2006). For example, Naumann et al. (2006) showed that circulating lathosterol and sitosterol were reduced in subjects supplemented with a fruit drink containing oat β-glucan (5 g β-glucan/day), which suggests less cholesterol absorption. Andersson et al. (2002) measured serum 7 α-hydroxy-4-cholesten-3-one levels as a marker of bile acid synthesis and found that the concentration was almost double at 8 and 12 h after ingestion of oat bran (11 g β-glucan/day), compared to wheat bran. This implies that cholesterol is being diverted to bile acid synthesis and/or secretion, and therefore less cholesterol enters the circulation.

Additionally, fermentation in the large intestine increases plasma SCFAs such as acetate and propionate, which may inhibit hepatic cholesterol synthesis and promote healthy intestinal flora

(Bridges et al. 1992, Wolever et al. 1996, Naruszewicz et al. 2002, Wong et al. 2006). SCFAs are the products of bacterial fermentation of fibers, proteins, and glycoproteins in the colon (Cummings and Macfarlane 1991). Certain fibers such as lignins, cellulose, and hemicelluloses are poorly fermented, while others such as pectins, gums, and mucilages undergo substantial fermentation (Cummings and Englyst 1987, Cummings and Macfarlane 1991). Fermentation of prebiotics such as inulin and oligofructose (polyfructans) by *Lactobacillus* and *Bifidobacterium* species has been associated with not only LDL-C lowering but also with TG lowering (Delzenne et al. 2002). As Wong et al. (2006) explain in their review, fibers that have been beneficial in lowering circulating lipids seem to lower the acetate:proprionate ratio. Acetate is the main SCFA present in the colon and once absorbed and transported to the liver, is the primary substrate for cholesterol synthesis (Wolever et al. 1996, Cook and Sellin 1998). Proprionate may inhibit cholesterol synthesis by inhibiting 3-hydroxy-3-methyl-glutaryl-coA synthase and reductase (Rodwell et al. 1976, Venter et al. 1990). Also, SCFAs may decrease expression of hepatic enzymes involved in lipogenesis, such as fatty acid synthase (FAS), and LDL receptor, as demonstrated in rat models (Roberfroid and Delzenne 1998, Fukushima et al. 2001). Ranganna et al. (2007) have demonstrated a very specific role for butyrate in the activation of the glutathione/glutathione-*S*-transferase antioxidant system and the inhibition of smooth muscle cell proliferation and thus atherosclerosis.

The mechanisms for LDL-C lowering may also explain the lower circulating apoB observed in some clinical studies on fiber (discussed in Section 10.9.2.6). ApoB is an atherogenic lipoprotein found in chylomicrons, chylomicron remnants, VLDL, IDL, and LDL. The fact that it is reduced by fiber in some trials without affecting apoAI, an antiatherogenic lipoprotein associated with HDL, is beneficial to CVD risk. In fact, some have shown that apoB predicts CVD risk better than LDL-C (Grundy 2002). In rats fed atherogenic diets, supplementation of "Fibernat" (fenugreek seed powder, guar gum, and wheat bran 70:15:15) reduced liver cholesterol concentrations, attenuated circulating VLDL and LDL-C, and upregulated the hepatic apoB/E (LDL) receptors (Venkatesan et al. 2003).

In summary, fiber intake appears to have multiple mechanisms of action within the body, including effects on digestion as well as central and peripheral metabolism, many of which infer benefit for CVD prevention.

10.11 FIBER–GENE INTERACTIONS

CVD is a polygenic disease, that is, a wide variety of gene variations contribute to its development and severity. An exciting new focus of nutrition research involves taking a closer look at the interplay between specific nutrients and genetic variations or gene expression. Nutrigenetics examines how gene variations modify an individual's response to diet, while nutrigenomics looks at how nutrients affect gene expression (Ryan-Harshman and Vogel, 2009). While it is generally agreed that it is too early to make specific diet or nutrient recommendations based on genetic makeup and gene expression in individuals, there are examples of how people may respond differently to dietary fiber.

From a nutrigenetics point of view, a study of adult obese women ($n = 549$) showed that there was a fiber × genotype interaction with the -514 C > T polymorphism of the hepatic lipase C gene (Santos et al. 2006). The main function of hepatic lipase is to convert IDL to LDL. While the authors acknowledge some limitations in this report, the results suggest that further investigation is warranted to see if obese subjects with this polymorphism may respond differently to the effects of fiber on bile and cholesterol metabolism, the biochemical pathways where this particular lipase is involved. Wu et al. (2007) did not show that ApoE variations contribute to the positive effects of fiber on plasma cholesterol levels in 22,915 men and women aged between 45 and 75 taking part in the European Prospective Investigation of Cancer. An important point that these authors have made is that the mechanisms for the effects of fiber may be outside of a relationship with ApoE and thus would not be expected to show any interactions.

From a nutrigenomics standpoint, fibers may influence the expression of a number of genes based on experimental data in animals, some already described in Section 10.10, including FAS and LDL receptors. Additionally, it was shown that, in pigs, insoluble fiber sources differentially affected gut mRNA levels of nuclear factor-KB, tumor necrosis factor-α, and other genes involved in the inflammatory or cell cycle process (Schedle et al. 2008). Likewise in weanling rats, a high-fiber diet downregulated hepatic FAS mRNA compared to the control diet (Maurer et al. 2009). As well, mice fed isolated rhubarb fiber showed increased cholesterol 7 α-hydroxylase mRNA levels and activity (Goel et al. 1999).

Given that there are still undetermined numbers of genes involved in CVD, there is no doubt that further research will elucidate the role of nutrigenetics and nutrigenomics, including the interplay of fiber in CVD. These fields of study are expected to flourish, particularly once the mechanisms of action are fully understood and the relevant methodology improves to the point that accurate targeting of specific genes becomes possible (Kaput et al. 2005). Studies to date have used traditional, isolated approaches to test specific genes. Microarrays may be a useful screening tool to identify multiple gene targets of fiber treatment.

10.12   HIGH-FIBER DIET PATTERNS

As mentioned earlier, national consumer guidance from MyPyramid (USDA 2009a) and Canada's Food Guide (Health Canada 2007a) should lead to adequate dietary fiber intake among individuals. There are also other dietary patterns, including the Portfolio, Mediterranean, DASH, and OmniHeart diets reported in the literature, that have the capacity to provide the AI for dietary fiber.

The Portfolio diet, as described by Jenkins et al. (2005a,b), consists of 10 g viscous fibers/1000 kcal/day from oats, barley, psyllium, vegetables, and a daily serving of almonds. It also provides margarine with plant sterol esters (see Chapter 6 for an in-depth discussion on plant sterols) and uses strictly vegetarian sources of protein including soy. The Portfolio diet was found to reduce LDL-C, 10 year CHD risk, and cholesterol concentration in the smallest subclass of LDL particles in hypercholesterolemic adults to the same extent as statins, which are cholesterol-lowering, HMG-CoA reductase inhibitor drugs (Jenkins et al. 2005a,b).

Mediterranean-type dietary patterns provide whole grains, fruits, vegetables, legumes, nuts, fish, olive oil, and/or small amounts of red wine, and therefore emphasize sources of dietary fiber, as well as unsaturated fatty acids and several micronutrients and phytochemicals (Keys 1980, Willett 2006). This type of dietary pattern can meet the DRI for fiber, depending on total energy intake (de Souza et al. 2008, Shai et al. 2008). Using the definition above, Sofi et al. (2008) have shown through meta-analysis a 0.91 relative risk for CVD for adults with greater adherence to a Mediterranean diet (Knoops et al. 2004, Mitrou et al. 2007, Trichopoulou et al. 2008). In clinical trials, this type of diet, over varying time frames, reduced body weight, fat mass, inflammation (CRP, interleukin-6), IR, and plasma fibrinogen, as well as improved endothelial function score (Esposito et al. 2004b, Rallidis et al. 2009).

The DASH (Sacks et al. 1995) and OmniHeart (Appel et al. 2005, Carey et al. 2005) diets emphasize whole grains, fruits, and vegetables, as well as nuts, seeds, and dried beans 4–5 times per week, along with restricted sodium intake. These dietary patterns can provide the AI for dietary fiber. For example, it has been shown that a DASH diet provided 29 ± 1 g dietary fiber/2000 kcal (de Souza et al. 2008). These patterns reduce the estimated risk of heart disease according to the Framingham criteria, including beneficial effects on lowering LDL-C and blood pressure (Appel et al. 2005, Lin et al. 2007, Swain et al. 2008).

10.13   FIBER-RELATED HEALTH CLAIMS

10.13.1   CURRENT HEALTH CLAIMS

The US Food and Drug Administration (USFDA 2009a) have approved health claims related to dietary fiber and CVD (Table 10.5). Health claims regarding fiber intake and heart disease must

TABLE 10.5

Dietary Fiber and Cardiovascular Disease Health Claims

Claim	Model Statements
101.77 Health claims: fruits, vegetables, and grain products that contain fiber, particularly soluble fiber, and risk of coronary heart disease.	1. Diets low in saturated fat and cholesterol and rich in fruits, vegetables, and grain products that contain some types of dietary fiber, particularly soluble fiber, may reduce the risk of heart disease, a disease associated with many factors. 2. Development of heart disease depends on many factors. Eating a diet low in saturated fat and cholesterol and high in fruits, vegetables, and grain products that contain fiber may lower blood cholesterol levels and reduce your risk of heart disease.

101.81 Health claims: Soluble fiber from certain foods and risk of coronary heart disease.	1. Soluble fiber from foods such as [name of soluble fiber source], as part of a diet low in saturated fat and cholesterol, may reduce the risk of heart disease. A serving of [name of food] supplies____ grams of the [grams of soluble fiber] soluble fiber from [name of the soluble fiber source] necessary per day to have this effect.
	  • 3 g or more per day of beta-glucan soluble fiber from either whole oats or barley, or a combination of whole oats and barley
	  • 7 g or more per day of soluble fiber from psyllium seed husk
	2. Diets low in saturated fat and cholesterol that include____ grams of soluble fiber per day from [name of soluble fiber and, if desired, the name of the food product] may reduce the risk of heart disease. One serving of [name of food] provides____ grams of this soluble fiber.

Source: United States Food and Drug Administration (USFDA). 2009b. *Department of Health and Human Services. Guidance for Industry: Evidence-Based Review Systems for the Scientific Evaluation of Health Claims.* Available at: http://www.fda.gov/Food/GuidanceComplianceRegulatoryInformation/GuidanceDocuments/FoodLabelingNutrition/ucm073332.htm

acknowledge the role of diets low in saturated fat and cholesterol. Additionally, the focus is on soluble fiber within the model statements including products containing β-glucan (e.g., oats, barley) or psyllium.

Health Canada currently has approved four health claims, none of which are specific to dietary fiber. The Canadian Food Inspection Agency (CFIA) states that "the use of heart symbols and heart healthy claims to describe a food or food choice (whether on labels, menus or in advertising) are generally not acceptable. They may give an erroneous impression that consuming a single food or menu selection will provide heart health or prevent heart disease" (CFIA 2009).

10.13.2 QUALITY OF DATA: CURRENT AND FUTURE REQUIREMENTS

Investigations on the health benefits of fibers aim to provide the consumers with facts that allow them to make well-informed choices regarding the foods they eat. At the same time, these studies are laying the foundation for the preparation of health claims that will help the marketing of food products to the consumers. The quality of the studies is therefore an important factor in determining whether the claims are accurate and appropriate.

Health claims are considered disease *reduction* claims by the USFDA and Health Canada, and are not to be confused with claims of disease *prevention*. Clinical studies typically use individuals who have been diagnosed with a specific disease and thus only demonstrate disease reduction. Consequently, before such studies can be included in a health claim for disease prevention, there must be evidence that the effects attributed to the intervention can be extrapolated to individuals who are disease-free. The latter requirement establishes why epidemiological studies (discussed in Section 10.9.1), are considered to be significantly weaker than most other clinical studies. In fact, the USFDA guidance document, the interim evidence-based ranking system for scientific data, places the descriptive epidemiological study eighth of the nine human trial designations, with only case reports considered to be weaker (USFDA 2009b). There are two explanations for the low confidence of epidemiological studies. First, an epidemiological study is unable to ascertain with confidence the actual intake of a specific food component in the population being investigated. Second, epidemiological studies are an excellent approach for determining disease incidence and distribution, but they cannot evaluate cause and effect, which is an important element of determining efficacy (Lewis and Yetley 1999). Furthermore, these studies are not capable of examining the potential negative effects of consumption (Lichtenstein and Russell 2005). With respect to fiber, a significant number of the supporting studies are epidemiological (discussed in Section 10.9.1). However, even though they are considered weaker than interventional studies, the ability to examine long-term exposure has enabled these types of studies to look at the clinical endpoints which most strongly define efficacy, specifically mortality and morbidity.

The FDA-preferred clinical study design is that of a randomized, controlled interventional trial, since it can determine both safety and efficacy. The key component of such trials is the selection of the final endpoint for the study, since it must effectively predict the presence of a disease or health-related condition. In the case of CVD, events such as mortality, stroke, and heart attacks serve as the best endpoints. At the same time, obtaining significant differences in these parameters entails long-term trials with a large patient cohort. These types of investigations are therefore not feasible in many cases, particularly for food-based interventions, usually because of their prohibitive costs. Consequently, interventional trials have usually elected to monitor one of the risk factors that has been linked to CVD.

Interventional studies examining the benefits of consuming fiber have primarily emphasized serum lipid levels (discussed in Section 10.9.2.5), with only a few utilizing endpoints that monitor atherosclerotic disease directly. There are two reasons for being concerned with studies that utilize an endpoint that examines only a single parameter of CVD risk. First, there are multiple risk factors for CVD, and altering one of these may be insufficient to produce a beneficial effect. Likewise, the pathology of atherosclerotic disease, the disease that is responsible for the majority of cardiovascular-related deaths, is very complex. Thus, choosing a single risk factor or pathological marker for observation may not provide the necessary power to make an accurate determination regarding the presence or severity of CVD. Second, concerns regarding the validity of the endpoints being used to monitor CVD, whether they are total serum cholesterol, LDL-C, or more recently introduced imaging techniques and functional measurements (Fleming and DeMets 1996, Stein 2008, Schoenhagen and Tuzcu 2008, Wang et al. 2008) have been raised (Ravnskov 2008, Rosch 2008, 2003, Rasnake et al. 2008).

What are the reasons for this controversy about endpoints? It is generally accepted that secondary and surrogate markers of a disease should be objective predictors of the presence of the disease and not simply be associated with the disease. Even so, Fleming and DeMets (1996) have suggested caution whenever a primary endpoint (death or disease-related event) is not employed in a clinical trial. This point is extremely important since it is assumed that the results of these trials will be used to make decisions about patient care. A topical example of a surrogate endpoint now being reexamined is serum cholesterol levels. With respect to CVD, it has long been held that high circulating levels of cholesterol are responsible for onset and progression of atherosclerotic disease, the primary cause of heart attacks, stroke, and peripheral artery disease (Levine et al. 1995). Not only is there associative support for this view through the Framingham study (Feinleib et al. 1979) and the high CVD mortality due to familial hypercholesterolemia, there exists a direct relationship between LDL-C lowering by statins and life expectancy (Mehta et al. 2006) as well. This causal relationship between serum cholesterol levels (total and LDL) and CVD has led to its acceptance as a clinical study endpoint alongside blood pressure, in accordance with the definition above (Rasnake et al.

2008). Nevertheless, recent studies have raised doubts about the robustness of this association. First, Kressel et al. (2009) conducted a study of more than 150 individuals in which they examined the correlation between CVD risk and specific risk factors. Upon completion of the study, the authors found no significant differences in assessments of total and LDL-C, metabolic syndrome, IR, and traditional CVD risk factors. Interestingly, these were the only traditional risk factors that failed to correlate with CVD. Likewise, it was recently shown that a significant reduction in serum cholesterol levels did not affect blood vessel function (Raitakari et al. 2008), and in one case was shown to be detrimental (Weingartner et al. 2008). Consequently, it is logical to assume that serum cholesterol may not have as great an effect on CVD risk as was originally viewed. Second, similar conclusions have now been reached with several intervention studies. The primary example is the ENHANCE study, which was designed to examine the additive effects of a statin with a nonstatin (Drazen et al. 2008, Kastelein et al. 2008, Smith 2008). In this trial, the combination of ezetimibe, which inhibits cholesterol absorption, and simvastatin resulted in a 56% reduction in LDL-C versus 39% with simvastatin alone. This higher potency combination, however, did not translate to improvements in the IMT of the carotid artery, an index directly related to the severity of atherosclerosis. Third, it is now being recognized that the beneficial actions of statins may be more accurately linked to mechanisms that operate independent of cholesterol (Calabro and Yeh 2005, Lahera et al. 2007, Wang et al. 2008, Rashid et al. 2009, Rikitake and Hirata 2009). Indeed, it is now recognized that the improvement in CVD outcomes achieved with statins cannot be duplicated with any other agent that can solely lowers LDL-C levels. Consequently, it is now presumed that the beneficial effects of HMG-CoA reductase inhibitors (statins) occur by enhancing the release of the cardioprotective agent nitric oxide (Zhou and Liao 2009).

So how will these considerations affect the current and pending health claims for fiber? The use of cholesterol as a target may be more appropriate in the case of genetic disorders where cholesterol levels greatly exceed the normal range (Pullinger et al. 2003), and which may promote CVD via a mechanism of action that is distinct from those currently in vogue. Unlike stanols, however, which are solely intended for lowering LDL-C levels (Abumweis et al. 2008), fibers likely affect other processes associated with CVD progression, and it is these effects that have led to the epidemiological association between fiber consumption and cardiovascular health. At the same time, health claims now in preparation are primarily based on the cholesterol-lowering properties of fiber.

So, while there is excellent evidence from various studies that fiber consumption does reduce the risk of CVD, given the ongoing debate, inclusion of additional endpoints that measure the vascular function directly might be advised for future studies. This approach would ensure that revisiting certain health claims is not necessary, since proof of effectiveness will have been obtained with studies of proper design that used evidence-based clinical endpoints, even if selection of the best endpoint is still underway. By addressing these issues, health claim applications for fibers will remain valid even if the cholesterol standard is eventually shown to be unreliable.

Additionally, decisions will have to be made regarding the targets of health claims. In most cases, claims that fiber is capable of reducing the risk of CVD would be of greatest benefit to industry and, of course, help with disease management. In large part, while the wording would be fairly vague in terms of the specific target, in reality, evidence that shows atherosclerotic disease is blocked or reversed would be required. At this point of time, cholesterol is the most often utilized endpoint in trials, but the limitations that have been observed suggest that other endpoints should be employed. The general principles for selecting these endpoints were originally articulated by Wilson (1968) and applied to cancer, but are equally applicable to other diseases, including CVD (Greenland and Lloyd-Jones 2008). Indeed, a variety of alternative screening tools have been proposed by Duprez and Cohn (2008) due to their ability to detect asymptomatic disease. One of these, IMT, is increasingly being used in conjunction with serum lipid since it is a legitimate measure of disease extent, and because carotid artery blockage prevents blood flow to the brain. As described in Section 10.9.2.7, IMT has been used to validate the positive actions of fiber on CVD (Wu et al. 2003, Erkkila et al. 2005, Buil-Cosiales et al. 2009), but there is concern that the application of IMT as an endpoint marker will be limited to long-term trials since it measures a vascular property that does not change rapidly. A similar endpoint would be coronary angiography, which defines the degree of blockage of the coronary arteries that feed the heart. On the contrary, arterial compliance (elasticity of blood vessels) and flow-mediated dilatation (measure of endothelial dysfunction) can be monitored with instruments that provide rapid results with high sensitivity. Furthermore, it is generally agreed that these and related methods are capable of monitoring changes in vascular properties which become compromised early in the atherogenic process (Cohn et al. 2005, Lane et al. 2006, Simon et al. 2007, Al-Qaisi et al. 2008, Wang et al. 2008) and that they are appropriate for examining the changes that occur during short-term dietary interventions (Stamatelopoulos et al. 2009). Nevertheless, even with the evidence showing that arterial stiffness and endothelial dysfunction are correlated with CVD risk, these methods have yet to be completely accepted (Greenland and Lloyd-Jones 2008). In large part, this is an issue of validation. However, it has also been argued that the various noninvasive methods now being developed can only identify changes in a single property of a blood vessel (Al-Qaisi et al. 2008). At the same time, the reverse argument with respect to risk factor modification is also valid. Thus, the application of techniques that can detect disease prior to the emergence of symptoms (Eijgelaar et al. 2009) may be most appropriate. In parallel, screening for circulating biomarkers that better represent the disease state as opposed to risk factors (Hurks et al. 2009) could be used to assist in confirming the existence of CVD. A panel of measurements that adequately covers the spectrum of changes associated with CVD, as advocated by Cohn and Duprez (2008), and may therefore represent the best option rather than trying to select a single endpoint. The end result would be the ability to treat the disease of patients based on their individual results rather than in comparison to the norm of a broad population (Plicht et al. 2009).

10.14   LIMITATIONS

Fiber is generally thought to be beneficial for all individuals with CVD and there are very few patient populations that should restrict their fiber intake. Fiber may be limited during CVD if acute gastrointestinal disease is present as a comorbidity (e.g., in acute Crohn's disease, ulcerative colitis, or diverticulitis). However, in the quiescent stages of these diseases, a high-fiber intake is often also therapeutic (Razack and Seidner 2007). Some work shows that subjects with functional bowel disorders such as irritable bowel syndrome and/or fructose malabsorption may also be beneficial in restricting inulin and FOSs, along with certain fruits and vegetables that are sources of fiber but have a high ratio of fructose:glucose or contain fructans, for example, apples, pears, guava, honeydew melon, papaya, quince, star fruit, watermelon, artichokes, asparagus, leeks, and onion (Shepherd and Gibson 2006).

Fiber may reduce the absorption of certain medications by up to 30% (Schmidt and Dalhoff 2002). Such medications relevant to a population with CVD may include cholesterol-lowering medications such as cholestyramine, colestipol, and statins, as well as the cardiac glycoside, digoxin. Because fiber is beneficial to the populations taking these medications, fiber intakes should not be restricted. Rather, they should be maintained at a consistent level. Any changes in fiber intake should be introduced slowly and patients may be advised not to take their medications with a high-fiber meal or supplement.

10.15   FUTURE DEVELOPMENTS

Developments will likely continue through the marketing of functional/novel fibers as supplements or their incorporation into food products. For example, inulin is now added to many products in the United States or Canada, such as breads, cereals, snack bars, and yogurts. Novel fiber sources, such as inulin, appear to be acceptable when incorporated into foods such as baked products and ice cream (Peressin and Sensidoni 2009, Vitali et al. 2009). There are also emerging, but understudied, fiber supplements such as PolyGlycopleX® (PGX®) on the market. PGX is made up of three fibers:

konjac powder, sodium alginate, and xanthan gum. One study has shown reductions of 14% and 16% in TC and LDL-C, respectively, when healthy participants were supplemented with 5–10 g/day for 3 weeks (Carabin et al. 2009). The participants consuming the control product, skim milk powder, had a nonsignificant 8% reduction in both TC and LDL-C at the end of the study period. Other extracts or by-products from various sources are also currently being investigated as possible functional fibers, including those from kiwicha, maize, asparagus, mango peel, date, cauliflower and soybean seeds (Ajila et al. 2008, Elleuch et al. 2008, Kendall et al. 2008, Redondo-Cuenca et al. 2008, Stojceska et al. 2008, Fuentes-Alventosa et al. 2009, Repo-Carrasco-Velencia et al. 2009). It will be critical to ensure that the emerging functional foods or supplements are beneficial to the consumer through quality research. Given the synergistic effects of foods that are still unknown, nutrition education should focus primarily on overall healthy diet patterns that include sources of dietary fiber.

10.16 SUMMARY AND CONCLUSIONS

Epidemiological studies have provided evidence that dietary fiber is beneficial for reducing the risk of CVD. There have also been several studies showing positive effects of fiber on a number of CVD risk factors. The observational data suggest that high total fiber intake can prevent obesity, IR, and inflammation. The clinical data show that viscous fiber sources such as oats/β-glucan, psyllium, pectin, or guar gum, as well as inulin may reduce hypertension modestly, and serum LDL-C and apoB of the order of ~5–15% in adults. The mechanisms for these modifications may be multifactorial and related to effects on digestion, and central and peripheral metabolism. The DRI for fiber is not met by most adults in North America and therefore applications such as MyPyramid, Canada's Food Guide, and the Portfolio, Mediterranean, DASH, or OmniHeart diets that emphasize whole grains, fruits, vegetables, nuts and legumes may prove useful in assisting public compliance to recommendations for dietary fiber and risk reduction for CVD. Several functional/novel fibers are under investigation for their health benefits and they may also help people meet these fiber requirements. Additional clinical data examining the effects of fiber on traditional and emerging CVD risk factors, as well as direct assessments of blood vessel function, are required.

REFERENCES

Abumweis, S.S., Barake, R. and Jones, P.J. 2008. Plant sterols/stanols as cholesterol lowering agents: A meta-analysis of randomized controlled trials. *Food Nutr. Res.* **52**, 10.3402/fnr.v52i0.1811. Epub 2008 Aug. 18.

Ajila, C.M., Leelavathi, K. and Prasada Rao, J.J.S. 2008. Improvement of dietary fiber content and antioxidant properties in soft dough biscuits with the incorporation of mango peel powder. *J. Cereal Sci.* **48**(2): 319–326.

Alberti, K.G., Zimmet, P. and Shaw, J. 2006. Metabolic syndrome—A new world-wide definition. A Consensus Statement from the International Diabetes Federation. *Diabet. Med.* **23**(5): 469–480.

ALINORM 09/32/26 2009, *Report of the 30th Session of the Codex Committee on Nutrition and Foods for Special Dietary Use.* Available at https://www.ccnfsdu.de/.

Al-Qaisi, M., Kharbanda, R.K., Mittal, T.K. and Donald, A.E. 2008. Measurement of endothelial function and its clinical utility for cardiovascular risk. *Vasc. Health Risk Manag.* **4**(3): 647–652.

American Association of Cereal Chemists (AACC). 2001. The definition of dietary fiber. *Cereal Foods World* **46**(3): 112–126.

American Association of Cereal Chemists (AACC). 2008. Definitions/Reports. Available at http://www.aaccnet.org/definitions/labeling.asp

American Heart Association (AHA) 2009. *Statistics.* Available at http://www.americanheart.org/presenter.jhtml?identifier=1200026.

Ames, N.P. and Rhymer, C.R. 2008. Issues surrounding health claims for barley. *J. Nutr.* **138**(6): 1237S–1243S.

Anderson, J.W., Allgood, L.D., Lawrence, A., Altringer, L.A., Jerdack, G.R., Hengehold, D.A. and Morel, J.G. 2000. Cholesterol-lowering effects of psyllium intake adjunctive to diet therapy in men and women with hypercholesterolemia: Meta-analysis of 8 controlled trials. *Am. J. Clin. Nutr.* **71**(2): 472–479.

Anderson, J.W. and Bridges, S.R. 1984. Short-chain fatty acid fermentation products of plant fiber affect glucose metabolism of isolated rat hepatocytes. *Proc. Soc. Exp. Biol Med.* **177**(2): 372–376.

Anderson, J.W., Davidson, M.H., Blonde, L., Brown, W.V., Howard, W.J., Ginsberg, H., Allgood, L.D. and Weingand, K.W. 2000. Long-term cholesterol-lowering effects of psyllium as an adjunct to diet therapy in the treatment of hypercholesterolemia. *Am. J. Clin. Nutr.* **71**(6): 1433–1438.

Anderson, J.W., Deakins, D.A., Floore, T.L., Smith, B.M. and Whitis, S.E. 1990. Dietary fiber and coronary heart disease. *Crit. Rev. Food Sci. Nutr.* **29**(2): 95–147.

Anderson, J.W., Gilinsky, N.H., Deakins, D.A., Smith, S.F., O'Neal, D.S., Dillon, D.W. and Oeltgen, P.R. 1991. Lipid responses of hypercholesterolemic men to oat-bran and wheat-bran intake. *Am. J. Clin. Nutr.* **54**(4): 678–683.

Anderson, J.W., Randles, K.M., Kendall, C.W. and Jenkins, D.J. 2004. Carbohydrate and fiber recommendations for individuals with diabetes: A quantitative assessment and meta-analysis of the evidence. *J. Am. Coll. Nutr.* **23**(1): 5–17.

Anderson, J.W., Spencer, D.B., Hamilton, C.C., Smith, S.F., Tietyen, J., Bryant, C.A. and Oeltgen, P. 1990. Oat-bran cereal lowers serum total and LDL cholesterol in hypercholesterolemic men. *Am. J. Clin. Nutr.* **52**(3): 495–499.

Andersson, M., Ellegard, L. and Andersson, H. 2002. Oat bran stimulates bile acid synthesis within 8 h as measured by 7alpha-hydroxy-4-cholesten-3-one. *Am. J. Clin. Nutr.* **76**(5): 1111–1116.

Appel, L.J., Sacks, F.M., Carey, V.J., Obarzanek, E., Swain, J.F., Miller, E.R., 3rd, Conlin, P.R. et al. 2005. Effects of protein, monounsaturated fat, and carbohydrate intake on blood pressure and serum lipids: Results of the OmniHeart randomized trial. *JAMA.* **294**(19): 2455–2464.

Appleby, P.N., Thorogood, M., Mann, J.I. and Key, T.J. 1998. Low body mass index in non-meat eaters: The possible roles of animal fat, dietary fibre and alcohol. *Int. J. Obes.* **22**(5): 454–460.

Association of Analytical Communities (AOAC). 2009. *Official Methods of Analysis: Fiber*. Available at http://www.eoma.aoac.org/methods/result.asp?string=b.

Bazzano, L.A., He, J., Ogden, L.G., Loria, C.M., Whelton, P.K. and National Health and Nutrition Examination Survey I Epidemiologic Follow-up Study. 2003. Dietary fiber intake and reduced risk of coronary heart disease in US men and women: The National Health and Nutrition Examination Survey I Epidemiologic Follow-up Study. *Arch. Intern. Med.* **163**(16): 1897–1904.

Behall, K.M., Scholfield, D.J. and Hallfrisch, J. 2004a. Diets containing barley significantly reduce lipids in mildly hypercholesterolemic men and women. *Am. J. Clin. Nutr.* **80**(5): 1185–1193.

Behall, K.M., Scholfield, D.J. and Hallfrisch, J. 2004b. Lipids significantly reduced by diets containing barley in moderately hypercholesterolemic men. *J. Am. Coll. Nutr.* **23**(1): 55–62.

Betteridge, V. 2009. Dietary Fibre: An evolving definition. *Nutr. Bull.* **34**: 122–125.

Biorklund, M., van Rees, A., Mensink, R.P. and Onning, G. 2005, Changes in serum lipids and postprandial glucose and insulin concentrations after consumption of beverages with beta-glucans from oats or barley: A randomised dose-controlled trial. *Eur. J. Clin. Nutr.* **59**(11): 1272–1281.

Blake, D.E., Hamblett, C.J., Frost, P.G., Judd, P.A. and Ellis, P.R. 1997. Wheat bread supplemented with depolymerized guar gum reduces the plasma cholesterol concentration in hypercholestrerolemic human subjects. *Am. J. Clin. Nutr.* **65**(1): 107–113.

Bloedon, L.T., Balikai, S., Chittams, J., Cunnane, S.C., Berlin, J.A., Rader, D.J. and Szapary, P.O. 2008. Flaxseed and cardiovascular risk factors: Results from a double blind, randomized, controlled clinical trial. *J. Am. Coll. Nutr.* **27**(1): 65–74.

Bourdon, I., Yokoyama, W., Davis, P., Hudson, C., Backus, R., Richter, D., Knuckles, B. and Schneeman, B.O. 1999. Postprandial lipid, glucose, insulin, and cholecystokinin responses in men fed barley pasta enriched with beta-glucan. *Am. J. Clin. Nutr.* **69**(1): 55–63.

Brand-Miller, J., Dickinson, S., Barclay, A. and Celermajer, D. 2007. The glycemic index and cardiovascular disease risk. *Curr. Atheroscler. Rep.* **9**(6): 479–485.

Bridges, S.R., Anderson, J.W., Deakins, D.A., Dillon, D.W. and Wood, C.L. 1992. Oat bran increases serum acetate of hypercholesterolemic men. *Am. J. Clin. Nutr.* **56**(2): 455–459.

Brighenti, F., Casiraghi, M.C., Canzi, E. and Ferrari, A. 1999. Effect of consumption of a ready-to-eat breakfast cereal containing inulin on the intestinal milieu and blood lipids in healthy male volunteers. *Eur. J. Clin. Nutr.* **53**(9): 726–733.

Brown, L., Rosner, B., Willett, W.W. and Sacks, F.M. 1999. Cholesterol-lowering effects of dietary fiber: A meta-analysis. *Am. J. Clin. Nutr.* **69**(1): 30–42.

Buil-Cosiales, P., Irimia, P., Ros, E., Riverol, M., Gilabert, R., Martinez-Vila, E., Nunez, I., Diez-Espino, J., Martinez-Gonzalez, M.A. and Serrano-Martinez, M. 2009. Dietary fibre intake is inversely associated with carotid intima-media thickness: A cross-sectional assessment in the PREDIMED study. *Eur. J. Clin. Nutr.* **33**(10): 1213–1219.

Buttriss, J.L. and Stokes, C.S. 2008. Dietary fibre and health: An overview. *Nutr. Bull.* **33**: 186–200.

Calabro, P. and Yeh, E.T. 2005. The pleiotropic effects of statins. *Curr. Opin. Cardiol.* **20**(6): 541–546.

Cani, P.D., Dewever, C. and Delzenne, N.M. 2004. Inulin-type fructans modulate gastrointestinal peptides involved in appetite regulation (glucagon-like peptide-1 and ghrelin) in rats. *Br. J. Nutr.* **92**(3): 521–526.

Carabin, I.G., Lyon, M.R., Wood, S., Pelletier, X., Donazzolo, Y. and Burdock, G.A. 2009. Supplementation of the diet with the functional fiber PolyGlycoplex is well tolerated by healthy subjects in a clinical trial. *Nutr. J.* **8**: 9.

Carey, V.J., Bishop, L., Charleston, J., Conlin, P., Erlinger, T., Laranjo, N., McCarron, P. et al. 2005. Rationale and design of the Optimal Macro-Nutrient Intake Heart Trial to Prevent Heart Disease (OMNI-Heart). *Clin. Trials.* **2**(6): 529–537.

Cavalot, F., Petrelli, A., Traversa, M., Bonomo, K., Fiora, E., Conti, M., Anfossi, G., Costa, G. and Trovati, M. 2006. Postprandial blood glucose is a stronger predictor of cardiovascular events than fasting blood glucose in type 2 diabetes mellitus, particularly in women: Lessons from the San Luigi Gonzaga Diabetes Study. *J. Clin. Endocrinol. Metab.* **91**(3): 813–819.

Centers for Disease Control and Prevention (CDC) 2009. *National Health and Nutrition Examination Survey.* Available at http://www.cdc.gov. proxy2.lib.umanitoba.ca/ nchs/ nhanes.htm.

Canadian Food Inspection Agency (CFIA). 2009. *Guide to Food Labelling and Advertising. Chapter 8—Diet-Related Health Claims.* Available at http://www.inspection.gc.ca/english/fssa/labeti/guide/ch8ae.shtml.

Chang, L.C., Huang, K.C., Wu, Y.W., Kao, H.L., Chen, C.L., Lai, L.P., Hwang, J.J. and Yang, W.S. 2009, The clinical implications of blood adiponectin in cardiometabolic disorders, *J. Formos. Med. Assoc.* **108**(5): 353–366.

Chiasson, J.L., Josse, R.G., Gomis, R., Hanefeld, M., Karasik, A., Laakso, M. and STOP-NIDDM Trial Research Group. 2003. Acarbose treatment and the risk of cardiovascular disease and hypertension in patients with impaired glucose tolerance: The STOP-NIDDM trial. *JAMA.* **290**(4): 486–494.

Cicero, A.F., Derosa, G., Manca, M., Bove, M., Borghi, C. and Gaddi, A.V. 2007. Different effect of psyllium and guar dietary supplementation on blood pressure control in hypertensive overweight patients: A six-month, randomized clinical trial. *Clin. Exp. Hypertens.* **29**(6): 383–394.

Cohn, J.N. and Duprez, D.A. 2008. Time to foster a rational approach to preventing cardiovascular morbid events. *J. Am. Coll. Cardiol.* **52**(5): 327–329.

Cohn, J.N., Duprez, D.A. and Grandits, G.A. 2005. Arterial elasticity as part of a comprehensive assessment of cardiovascular risk and drug treatment. *Hypertension.* **46**(1): 217–220.

Combs, T.P., Berg, A.H., Obici, S., Scherer, P.E. and Rossetti, L. 2001. Endogenous glucose production is inhibited by the adipose-derived protein Acrp30. *J. Clin. Invest.* **108**(12): 1875–1881.

Cook, S.I. and Sellin, J.H. 1998. Review article: Short chain fatty acids in health and disease. *Aliment. Pharmacol. Ther.* **12**(6): 499–507.

Cummings, J.H. and Englyst, H.N. 1987. Fermentation in the human large intestine and the available substrates. *Am. J. Clin. Nutr.* **45**(5 Suppl.): 1243–1255.

Cummings, J.H. and Macfarlane, G.T. 1991. The control and consequences of bacterial fermentation in the human colon. *J. Appl. Bacteriol.* **70**(6): 443–459.

Davidson, M.H., Dugan, L.D., Burns, J.H., Bova, J., Story, K. and Drennan, K.B. 1991. The hypocholesterolemic effects of beta-glucan in oatmeal and oat bran. A dose-controlled study. *JAMA.* **265**(14): 1833–1839.

Davidson, M.H. and Maki, K.C. 1999. Effects of dietary inulin on serum lipids. *J. Nutr.* **129**(7 Suppl.): 1474S–1477S.

De Groot, A., Luyken, R. and Pikaar, N.A. 1963. Cholesterol-lowering effect of rolled oats. *Lancet.* **2**(7302): 303–304.

De Souza, R.J., Swain, J.F., Appel, L.J. and Sacks, F.M. 2008. Alternatives for macronutrient intake and chronic disease: A comparison of the OmniHeart diets with popular diets and with dietary recommendations. *Am. J. Clin. Nutr.* **88**(1): 1–11.

DeClercq, V., Taylor, C. and Zahradka, P. 2008. Adipose tissue: The link between obesity and cardiovascular disease. *Cardiovasc. Hematol. Disord. Drug Targets.* **8**(3): 228–237.

Delzenne, N.M., Daubioul, C., Neyrinck, A., Lasa, M. and Taper, H.S. 2002. Inulin and oligofructose modulate lipid metabolism in animals: Review of biochemical events and future prospects. *Br. J. Nutr.* **87**(Suppl. 2): S255–S259.

Dhaliwal, S.S. and Welborn, T.A. 2009. Central obesity and multivariable cardiovascular risk as assessed by the Framingham prediction scores. *Am. J. Cardiol.* **103**(10): 1403–1407.

Djousse, L., Ellison, R.C., Zhang, Y., Arnett, D.K., Sholinsky, P. and Borecki, I. 1998. Relation between dietary fiber consumption and fibrinogen and plasminogen activator inhibitor type 1: The National Heart, Lung, and Blood Institute Family Heart Study. *Am. J. Clin. Nutr.* **68**(3): 568–575.

Dodin, S., Cunnane, S.C., Masse, B., Lemay, A., Jacques, H., Asselin, G., Tremblay-Mercier, J. et al. 2008. Flaxseed on cardiovascular disease markers in healthy menopausal women: A randomized, double-blind, placebo-controlled trial. *Nutrition.* **24**(1): 23–30.

Drazen, J.M., Jarcho, J.A., Morrissey, S. and Curfman, G.D. 2008. Cholesterol lowering and ezetimibe. *N. Engl. J. Med.* **358**(14): 1507–1508.

Dubois, C., Armand, M., Senft, M., Portugal, H., Pauli, A.M., Bernard, P.M., Lafont, H. and Lairon, D. 1995. Chronic oat bran intake alters postprandial lipemia and lipoproteins in healthy adults. *Am. J. Clin. Nutr.* **61**(2): 325–333.

Duprez, D.A. and Cohn, J.N. 2008. Identifying early cardiovascular disease to target candidates for treatment. *J. Clin. Hypertens.* **10**(3): 226–231.

Eijgelaar, W.J., Heeneman, S. and Daemen, M.J. 2009. The vulnerable patient: Refocusing on the plaque? *Thromb. Haemost.* **102**(2): 231–239.

Elleuch, M., Besbes, S., Roiseux, O., Blecker, C., Deroanne, C., Drira, N. and Attia, H. 2008. Date flesh: Chemical composition and characteristics of the dietary fibre. *Food Chem.* **111**(3): 676–682.

Erkkila, A.T., Herrington, D.M., Mozaffarian, D. and Lichtenstein, A.H. 2005. Cereal fiber and whole-grain intake are associated with reduced progression of coronary-artery atherosclerosis in postmenopausal women with coronary artery disease. *Am. Heart J.* **150**(1): 94–101.

Esposito, K., Giugliano, D., Nappo, F., Marfella, R. and Campanian Postprandial Hyperglycemia Study Group. 2004a. Regression of carotid atherosclerosis by control of postprandial hyperglycemia in type 2 diabetes mellitus. *Circulation.* **110**(2): 214–219.

Esposito, K., Marfella, R., Ciotola, M., Di Palo, C., Giugliano, F., Giugliano, G., D'Armiento, M., D'Andrea, F. and Giugliano, D. 2004b. Effect of a Mediterranean-style diet on endothelial dysfunction and markers of vascular inflammation in the metabolic syndrome: A randomized trial. *JAMA.* **292**(12): 1440–1446.

Esposito, K., Nappo, F., Giugliano, F., Di Palo, C., Ciotola, M., Barbieri, M., Paolisso, G. and Giugliano, D. 2003. Meal modulation of circulating interleukin 18 and adiponectin concentrations in healthy subjects and in patients with type 2 diabetes mellitus. *Am. J. Clin. Nutr.* **78**(6): 1135–1140.

Fehily, A.M., Burr, M.L., Butland, B.K. and Eastham, R.D. 1986. A randomised controlled trial to investigate the effect of a high fibre diet on blood pressure and plasma fibrinogen. *J. Epidemiol. Community Health.* **40**(4): 334–337.

Feinleib, M., Kannel, W.B., Tedeschi, C.G., Landau, T.K. and Garrison, R.J. 1979. The relation of antemortem characteristics to cardiovascular findings at necropsy—The Framingham Study. *Atherosclerosis.* **34**(2): 145–157.

Fleming, T.R. and DeMets, D.L. 1996. Surrogate end points in clinical trials: Are we being misled? *Ann. Intern. Med.* **125**(7): 605–613.

Forcheron, F. and Beylot, M. 2007. Long-term administration of inulin-type fructans has no significant lipid-lowering effect in normolipidemic humans. *Metabolism.* **56**(8): 1093–1098.

Fuentes-Alventosa, J.M., Rodriguez-Gutierrez, G., Jaramillo-Carmona, S., Espejo-Calvo, J.A., Rodriguez-Arcos, R., Fernandez-Bolanos, J., Guillen-Bejarano, R. and Jimeniz-Araujo, A. 2009. Effect of extraction method on chemical composition and functional characteristics of high dietary fibre powders obtained from aparagus by-products. *Food Chem.* **113**(2): 665–671.

Fukushima, M., Ohashi, T., Fujiwara, Y., Sonoyama, K. and Nakano, M. 2001. Cholesterol-lowering effects of maitake (*Grifola frondosa*) fiber, shiitake (*Lentinus edodes*) fiber, and enokitake (*Flammulina velutipes*) fiber in rats. *Exp. Biol. Med.* **226**(8): 758–765.

Galisteo, M., Duarte, J. and Zarzuelo, A. 2008. Effects of dietary fibers on disturbances clustered in the metabolic syndrome. *J. Nutr. Biochem.* 19(2): 71–84.

Genest, J., McPherson, R., Frohlich, J., Anderson, T., Campbell, N., Carpentier, A., Couture, P. et al. 2009. 2009 Canadian Cardiovascular Society/Canadian guidelines for the diagnosis and treatment of dyslipidemia and prevention of cardiovascular disease in the adult—2009 recommendations. *Can. J. Cardiol.* **25**(10): 567–579.

Gerhardt, A.L. and Gallo, N.B. 1998. Full-fat rice bran and oat bran similarly reduce hypercholesterolemia in humans. *J. Nutr.* **128**(5): 865–869.

Giannessi, D., Maltinti, M. and Del Ry, S. 2007. Adiponectin circulating levels: A new emerging biomarker of cardiovascular risk. *Pharmacol. Res.* **56**(6): 459–467.

Goel, V., Cheema, S.K., Agellon, L.B., Ooraikul, B. and Basu, T.K. 1999. Dietary rhubarb (*Rheum rhaponticum*) stalk fibre stimulates cholesterol 7 alpha-hydroxylase gene expression and bile acid excretion in cholesterol-fed C57BL/6J mice. *Br. J. Nutr.* **81**(1): 65–71.

Greenland, P. and Lloyd-Jones, D. 2008. Defining a rational approach to screening for cardiovascular risk in asymptomatic patients. *J. Am. Coll. Cardiol.* **52**(5): 330–332.

Grundy, S.M. 2002. Low-density lipoprotein, non-high-density lipoprotein, and apolipoprotein B as targets of lipid-lowering therapy. *Circulation.* **106**(20): 2526–2529.

Hamsten, A., de Faire, U., Walldius, G., Dahlen, G., Szamosi, A., Landou, C., Blomback, M. and Wiman, B. 1987. Plasminogen activator inhibitor in plasma: Risk factor for recurrent myocardial infarction. *Lancet.* **2**(8549): 3–9.

Han, S.H., Quon, M.J., Kim, J.A. and Koh, K.K. 2007. Adiponectin and cardiovascular disease: Response to therapeutic interventions. *J. Am. Coll. Cardiol.* **49**(5): 531–538.

Hanefeld, M., Fischer, S., Julius, U., Schulze, J., Schwanebeck, U., Schmechel, H., Ziegelasch, H.J. and Lindner, J. 1996a. Risk factors for myocardial infarction and death in newly detected NIDDM: The Diabetes Intervention Study, 11-year follow-up. *Diabetologia.* **39**(12): 1577–1583.

Hanefeld, M., Schmechel, H., Julius, U. and Schwanebeck, U. 1996b. Determinants for coronary heart disease in non-insulin-dependent diabetes mellitus: Lessons from the diabetes intervention study. *Diabetes Res. Clin. Pract.* **30**(Suppl.): 67–70.

Hanefeld, M. and Schaper, F. 2004. Postprandial hyperglycemia as a risk factor for cardiovascular disease. Therapy improves prognosis. *Herz.* **29**(5): 480–487.

Health Canada 2009, *Food Label Claims.* Available at http://www.hc-sc.gc.ca. proxy2. lib. umanitoba.ca/fn-an/label-etiquet/claims-reclam/qa-qr_claims-allegations-eng.php.

Health Canada 2007a, *Eating Well with Canada's Food Guide.* Available at http://www.hc-sc.gc.ca/fn-an/food-guide-aliment/index-eng.php

Health Canada 2007b, *Canadian Nutrient File.* Available at http://webprod.hc-sc.gc.ca.proxy2.lib.umanitoba.ca/cnf-fce/index-eng.jsp.

Health Canada 1985. *Expert Advisory Committee on Dietary Fibre.* Available at http://www.inspection.gc.ca/english/fssa/labeti/guide/ch6ae.shtml.

Heart and Stroke Foundation of Canada (HSFC) 2005. *Heart Disease.* Available at http://www.heartandstroke.mb.ca/site/c.lgLSIVOyGpF/b.3661119/k.7E59/Heart_Disease.htm.

Holt, S., Brand, J., Soveny, C. and Hansky, J. 1992. Relationship of satiety to postprandial glycaemic, insulin and cholecystokinin responses. *Appetite.* **18**(2): 129–141.

Howarth, N.C., Saltzman, E. and Roberts, S.B. 2001. Dietary fiber and weight regulation. *Nutr. Rev.* **59**(5): 129–139.

Hurks, R., Peeters, W., Derksen, W.J., Hellings, W.E., Hoefer, I.E., Moll, F.L., de Kleijn, D.P. and Pasterkamp, G. 2009. Biobanks and the search for predictive biomarkers of local and systemic outcome in atherosclerotic disease. *Thromb. Haemost.* **101**(1): 48–54.

Institute of Medicine (IOM) (eds). 2006. *Dietary Reference Intakes: The Essential Guide to Nutrient Requirements,* The National Academies Press, Washington, D.C.

Institute of Medicine (IOM). 2001. *Dietary Reference Intakes: Proposed Definition of Dietary Fiber,* The National Academies Press, Washington, D.C.

Jackson, K.G., Taylor, G.R., Clohessy, A.M. and Williams, C.M. 1999. The effect of the daily intake of inulin on fasting lipid, insulin and glucose concentrations in middle-aged men and women. *Br. J. Nutr.* **82**(1): 23–30.

Jenkins, D.J., Kendall, C.W., Marchic, A., Faulkner, D.A., Josse, A.R., Wong, J.M., de Souza, R. et al. 2005a. Direct comparison of dietary portfolio vs statin on C-reactive protein. *Eur. J. Clin. Nutr.* **59**(7): 851–860.

Jenkins, D.J., Kendall, C.W., Marchie, A., Faulkner, D.A., Wong, J.M., de Souza, R., Emam, A. et al. 2005b. Direct comparison of a dietary portfolio of cholesterol-lowering foods with a statin in hypercholesterolemic participants. *Am. J. Clin. Nutr.* **81**(2): 380–387.

Jenkins, D.J., Kendall, C.W., Vidgen, E., Agarwal, S., Rao, A.V., Rosenberg, R.S., Diamandis, E.P. et al. 1999. Health aspects of partially defatted flaxseed, including effects on serum lipids, oxidative measures, and *ex vivo* androgen and progestin activity: A controlled crossover trial. *Am. J. Clin. Nutr.* **69**(3): 395–402.

Jenkins, D.J., Kendall, C.W., Vuksan, V., Vidgen, E., Parker, T., Faulkner, D., Mehling, C.C. et al. 2002. Soluble fiber intake at a dose approved by the US Food and Drug Administration for a claim of health benefits: Serum lipid risk factors for cardiovascular disease assessed in a randomized controlled crossover trial. *Am. J. Clin. Nutr.* **75**(5): 834–839.

Jenkins, D.J., Wolever, T.M., Taylor, R.H., Barker, H., Fielden, H., Baldwin, J.M., Bowling, A.C., Newman, H.C., Jenkins, A.L. and Goff, D.V. 1981. Glycemic index of foods: A physiological basis for carbohydrate exchange. *Am. J. Clin. Nutr.* **34**(3): 362–366.

Jiamsripong, P., Mookadam, M., Alharthi, M.S., Khandheria, B.K. and Mookadam, F. 2008. The metabolic syndrome and cardiovascular disease: Part 2. *Prev. Cardiol.* **11**(4): 223–229.

Jimenez, J.P., Serrano, J., Tabernero, M., Arranz, S., Diaz-Rubio, M.E., Garcia-Diz, L., Goni, I. and Saura-Calixto, F. 2008. Effects of grape antioxidant dietary fiber in cardiovascular disease risk factors. *Nutrition.* **24**(7–8): 646–653.

Kadowaki, T. and Yamauchi, T. 2005. Adiponectin and adiponectin receptors. *Endocr. Rev.* 26(3): 439–451.

Kadowaki, T., Yamauchi, T., Kubota, N., Hara, K., Ueki, K. and Tobe, K. 2006. Adiponectin and adiponectin receptors in insulin resistance, diabetes, and the metabolic syndrome. *J. Clin. Invest.* 116(7): 1784–1792.

Kannel, W.B. 2009. Hypertension: Reflections on risks and prognostication. *The Med. Clin. North Am.* 93(3): 541–558.

Kaput, J., Ordovas, J.M., Ferguson, L., van Ommen, B., Rodriguez, R.L., Allen, L., Ames, B.N. et al. 2005. The case for strategic international alliances to harness nutritional genomics for public and personal health. *Br. J. Nutr.* 94(5): 623–632.

Karmally, W., Montez, M.G., Palmas, W., Martinez, W., Branstetter, A., Ramakrishnan, R., Holleran, S.F., Haffner, S.M. and Ginsberg, H.N. 2005. Cholesterol-lowering benefits of oat-containing cereal in Hispanic Americans. *J. Am. Diet. Assoc.* 105(6): 967–970.

Kastelein, J.J., Akdim, F., Stroes, E.S., Zwinderman, A.H., Bots, M.L., Stalenhoef, A.F., Visseren, F.L. et al. 2008. Simvastatin with or without ezetimibe in familial hypercholesterolemia. *N. Eng. J. Med.* 358(14): 1431–1443.

Katsoulis, K., Blaudeau, T.E., Roy, J.P. and Hunter, G.R. 2009. Diet-induced changes in intra-abdominal adipose tissue and CVD risk in American women. *Obesity (Silver Spring).* 17(12): 2169–2167.

Keenan, J.M., Goulson, M., Shamliyan, T., Knutson, N., Kolberg, L. and Curry, L. 2007. The effects of concentrated barley beta-glucan on blood lipids in a population of hypercholesterolaemic men and women. *Br. J. Nutr.* 97(6): 1162–1168.

Kendall, C.W., Esfahani, A., Hoffman, A.J., Evans, A., Sanders, L.M., Josse, A.R., Vidgen, E. and Potter, S.M. 2008. Effect of novel maize-based dietary fibers on postprandial glycemia and insulinemia. *J. Am. Coll. Nutr.* 27(6): 711–718.

Keogh, G.F., Cooper, G.J., Mulvey, T.B., McArdle, B.H., Coles, G.D., Monro, J.A. and Poppitt, S.D. 2003. Randomized controlled crossover study of the effect of a highly beta-glucan-enriched barley on cardiovascular disease risk factors in mildly hypercholesterolemic men. *Am. J. Clin. Nutr.* 78(4): 711–718.

Kerckhoffs, D.A., Hornstra, G. and Mensink, R.P. 2003. Cholesterol-lowering effect of beta-glucan from oat bran in mildly hypercholesterolemic subjects may decrease when beta-glucan is incorporated into bread and cookies. *Am. J. Clin. Nutr.* 78(2): 221–227.

Kestin, M., Moss, R., Clifton, P.M. and Nestel, P.J. 1990. Comparative effects of three cereal brans on plasma lipids, blood pressure, and glucose metabolism in mildly hypercholesterolemic men. *Am. J. Clin. Nutr.* 52(4): 661–666.

Keys, A. 1980. Coronary heart disease, serum cholesterol, and the diet. *Acta Medica Scand.* 207(3): 153–160.

King, D.E., Egan, B.M., Woolson, R.F., Mainous, A.G., 3rd, Al-Solaiman, Y. and Jesri, A. 2007. Effect of a high-fiber diet vs a fiber-supplemented diet on C-reactive protein level. *Arch. Int. Med.* 167(5): 502–506.

Kirby, R.W., Anderson, J.W., Sieling, B., Rees, E.D., Chen, W.J., Miller, R.E. and Kay, R.M. 1981. Oat-bran intake selectively lowers serum low-density lipoprotein cholesterol concentrations of hypercholesterolemic men. *Am. J. Clin. Nutr.* 34(5): 824–829.

Knoops, K.T., de Groot, L.C., Kromhout, D., Perrin, A.E., Moreiras-Varela, O., Menotti, A. and van Staveren, W.A. 2004. Mediterranean diet, lifestyle factors, and 10-year mortality in elderly European men and women: The HALE project. *JAMA.* 292(12): 1433–1439.

Koh-Banerjee, P., Franz, M., Sampson, L., Liu, S., Jacobs, D.R., Jr., Spiegelman, D., Willett, W. and Rimm, E. 2004. Changes in whole-grain, bran, and cereal fiber consumption in relation to 8-y weight gain among men. *Am. J. Clin. Nutr.* 80(5): 1237–1245.

Kressel, G., Trunz, B., Bub, A., Hulsmann, O., Wolters, M., Lichtinghagen, R., Stichtenoth, D.O. and Hahn, A. 2009. Systemic and vascular markers of inflammation in relation to metabolic syndrome and insulin resistance in adults with elevated atherosclerosis risk. *Atherosclerosis.* 202(1): 263–271.

Lahera, V., Goicoechea, M., de Vinuesa, S.G., Miana, M., de las Heras, N., Cachofeiro, V. and Luno, J. 2007. Endothelial dysfunction, oxidative stress and inflammation in atherosclerosis: Beneficial effects of statins. *Curr. Med. Chem.* 14(2): 243–248.

Lairon, D., Arnault, N., Bertrais, S., Planells, R., Clero, E., Hercberg, S. and Boutron-Ruault, M.C. 2005. Dietary fiber intake and risk factors for cardiovascular disease in French adults. *Am. J. Clin. Nutr.* 82(6): 1185–1194.

Landin, K., Holm, G., Tengborn, L. and Smith, U. 1992. Guar gum improves insulin sensitivity, blood lipids, blood pressure, and fibrinolysis in healthy men. *Am. J. Clin. Nutr.* 56(6): 1061–1065.

Lane, H.A., Smith, J.C. and Davies, J.S. 2006. Noninvasive assessment of preclinical atherosclerosis. *Vasc. Health Risk Manag.* 2(1): 19–30.

Leadbetter, J., Ball, M.J. and Mann, J.I. 1991. Effects of increasing quantities of oat bran in hypercholesterol-emic people. *Am. J. Clin. Nutr.* 54(5): 841–845.

Letexier, D., Diraison, F. and Beylot, M. 2003. Addition of inulin to a moderately high-carbohydrate diet reduces hepatic lipogenesis and plasma triacylglycerol concentrations in humans. *Am. J. Clin. Nutr.* 77(3): 559–564.

Levine, G.N., Keaney, J.F., Jr. and Vita, J.A. 1995. Cholesterol reduction in cardiovascular disease. Clinical benefits and possible mechanisms. *N. Engl. J. Med.* 332(8): 512–521.

Lewis, C.J. and Yetley, E.A. 1999. Health claims and observational human data: Relation between dietary fat and cancer. *Am. J. Clin. Nutr.* 69(6): 1357S–1364S.

Li, J., Kaneko, T., Qin, L.Q., Wang, J. and Wang, Y. 2003. Effects of barley intake on glucose tolerance, lipid metabolism, and bowel function in women. *Nutrition.* 19(11–12): 926–929.

Lichtenstein, A.H. and Russell, R.M. 2005. Essential nutrients: Food or supplements? Where should the empha-sis be? *JAMA.* 294(3): 351–358.

Liddle, R.A. 1997. Cholecystokinin cells. *Annu. Rev. Physiol.* 59: 221–242.

Lin, P.H., Appel, L.J., Funk, K., Craddick, S., Chen, C., Elmer, P., McBurnie, M.A. and Champagne, C. 2007. The PREMIER intervention helps participants follow the dietary approaches to stop hypertension dietary pattern and the current Dietary Reference Intakes recommendations. *J. Am. Diet. Assoc.* 107(9): 1541–1551.

Liu, S., Stampfer, M.J., Hu, F.B., Giovannucci, E., Rimm, E., Manson, J.E., Hennekens, C.H. and Willett, W.C. 1999. Whole-grain consumption and risk of coronary heart disease: Results from the Nurses' Health Study. *Am. J. Clin. Nutr.*, 70(3), 412–419.

Liu, S., Willett, W.C., Manson, J.E., Hu, F.B., Rosner, B. and Colditz, G. 2003. Relation between changes in intakes of dietary fiber and grain products and changes in weight and development of obesity among middle-aged women. *Am. J. Clin. Nutr.* 78(5): 920–927.

Lovegrove, J.A., Clohessy, A., Milon, H. and Williams, C.M. 2000. Modest doses of beta-glucan do not reduce concentrations of potentially atherogenic lipoproteins. *Am. J. Clin. Nutr.* 72(1): 49–55.

Lupton, J.R., Robinson, M.C. and Morin, J.L. 1994. Cholesterol-lowering effect of barley bran flour and oil. *J. Am. Diet. Assoc.* 94(1): 65–70.

Ma, Y., Griffith, J.A., Chasan-Taber, L., Olendzki, B.C., Jackson, E., Stanek, E.J., 3rd, Li, W., Pagoto, S.L., Hafner, A.R. and Ockene, I.S. 2006. Association between dietary fiber and serum C-reactive protein. *Am. J. Clin. Nutr.* 83(4): 760–766.

Maki, K.C., Galant, R., Samuel, P., Tesser, J., Witchger, M.S., Ribaya-Mercado, J.D., Blumberg, J.B. and Geohas, J. 2007. Effects of consuming foods containing oat beta-glucan on blood pressure, carbohydrate metabolism and biomarkers of oxidative stress in men and women with elevated blood pressure. *Eur. J. Clin. Nutr.* 61(6): 786–795.

Mantzoros, C.S., Li, T., Manson, J.E., Meigs, J.B. and Hu, F.B. 2005. Circulating adiponectin levels are associated with better glycemic control, more favorable lipid profile, and reduced inflammation in women with type 2 diabetes. *J. Clin. Endocrinol. Metab.* 90(8): 4542–4548.

Marlett, J.A., McBurney, M.I., Slavin, J.L. and American Dietetic Association 2002. Position of the American Dietetic Association: Health implications of dietary fiber. *J. Am. Diet. Assoc.* 102(7): 993–1000.

Massimino, S.P., McBurney, M.I., Field, C.J., Thomson, A.B., Keelan, M., Hayek, M.G. and Sunvold, G.D. 1998. Fermentable dietary fiber increases GLP-1 secretion and improves glucose homeostasis despite increased intestinal glucose transport capacity in healthy dogs. *J. Nutr.* 128(10): 1786–1793.

Maurer, A.D., Chen, Q., McPherson, C. and Reimer, R.A. 2009. Changes in satiety hormones and expression of genes involved in glucose and lipid metabolism in rats weaned onto diets high in fibre or protein reflect susceptibility to increased fat mass in adulthood. *J. Physiol.* 587(Part 3): 679–691.

McCleary, B.V. 2007. An integrated procedure for the measurement of total dietary fibre (including resistant starch), non-digestible oligosaccharides and available carbohydrates. *Anal. Bioanal. Chem.* 389(1): 291–308.

McIntosh, G.H., Whyte, J., McArthur, R. and Nestel, P.J. 1991. Barley and wheat foods: Influence on plasma cholesterol concentrations in hypercholesterolemic men. *Am. J. Clin. Nutr.* 53(5): 1205–1209.

McKeown, N.M., Meigs, J.B., Liu, S., Wilson, P.W. and Jacques, P.F. 2002. Whole-grain intake is favorably associated with metabolic risk factors for type 2 diabetes and cardiovascular disease in the Framingham Offspring Study. *Am. J. Clin. Nutr.* 76(2): 390–398.

Meade, T.W., Ruddock, V., Stirling, Y., Chakrabarti, R. and Miller, G.J. 1993. Fibrinolytic activity, clotting fac-tors, and long-term incidence of ischaemic heart disease in the Northwick Park Heart Study. *Lancet.* 342(8879): 1076–1079.

Mehta, J.L., Bursac, Z., Hauer-Jensen, M., Fort, C. and Fink, L.M. 2006. Comparison of mortality rates in statin users versus nonstatin users in a United States veteran population. *Am. J. Cardiol.* 98(7): 923–928.

Mellen, P.B., Liese, A.D., Tooze, J.A., Vitolins, M.Z., Wagenknecht, L.E. and Herrington, D.M. 2007. Whole-grain intake and carotid artery atherosclerosis in a multiethnic cohort: The Insulin Resistance Atherosclerosis Study. *Am. J. Clin. Nutr.* **85**(6): 1495–1502.

Meyer, K.A., Kushi, L.H., Jacobs, D.R., Jr., Slavin, J., Sellers, T.A. and Folsom, A.R. 2000. Carbohydrates, dietary fiber, and incident type 2 diabetes in older women. *Am. J. Clin. Nutr.* **71**(4): 921–930.

Mitrou, P.N., Kipnis, V., Thiebaut, A.C., Reedy, J., Subar, A.F., Wirfalt, E., Flood, A. et al. 2007. Mediterranean dietary pattern and prediction of all-cause mortality in a US population: Results from the NIH-AARP Diet and Health Study. *Arch. Int. Med.* **167**(22): 2461–2468.

Mozaffarian, D., Kumanyika, S.K., Lemaitre, R.N., Olson, J.L., Burke, G.L. and Siscovick, D.S. 2003. Cereal, fruit, and vegetable fiber intake and the risk of cardiovascular disease in elderly individuals. *JAMA.* **289**(13): 1659–1666.

Naruszewicz, M., Johansson, M.L., Zapolska-Downar, D. and Bukowska, H. 2002. Effect of Lactobacillus plantarum 299 v on cardiovascular disease risk factors in smokers. *Am. J. Clin. Nutr.* **76**(6): 1249–1255.

National Cholesterol Education Program (NCEP) Expert Panel on Detection, Evaluation, and Treatment of High Blood Cholesterol in Adults (Adult Treatment Panel III) 2002. Third Report of the National Cholesterol Education Program (NCEP) expert panel on detection, evaluation, and treatment of high blood cholesterol in adults (Adult Treatment Panel III) final report. *Circulation.* **106**(25): 3143–3421.

Naumann, E., van Rees, A.B., Onning, G., Oste, R., Wydra, M. and Mensink, R.P. 2006. Beta-glucan incorporated into a fruit drink effectively lowers serum LDL-cholesterol concentrations. *Am. J. Clin. Nutr.* **83**(3): 601–605.

Nelson, L.H. and Tucker, L.A. 1996. Diet composition related to body fat in a multivariate study of 203 men. *J. Am. Diet. Assoc.* **96**(8): 771–777.

Newman, R.K., Newman, C.W., Hofer, P.J. and Barnes, A.E. 1991. Growth and lipid metabolism as affected by feeding of hull-less barleys with and without supplemental beta-glucanase. *Plant Foods Hum. Nutr.* **41**(4): 371–380.

Nicolosi, R., Bell, S.J., Bistrian, B.R., Greenberg, I., Forse, R.A. and Blackburn, G.L. 1999. Plasma lipid changes after supplementation with beta-glucan fiber from yeast. *Am. J. Clin. Nutr.* **70**(2): 208–212.

Niemi, M.K., Keinanen-Kiukaanniemi, S.M. and Salmela, P.I. 1988. Long-term effects of guar gum and microcrystalline cellulose on glycaemic control and serum lipids in type 2 diabetes. *Eur. J. Clin. Pharmacol.* 34(4): 427–429.

Nilsson, A.C., Ostman, E.M., Holst, J.J. and Bjorck, I.M. 2008. Including indigestible carbohydrates in the evening meal of healthy subjects improves glucose tolerance, lowers inflammatory markers, and increases satiety after a subsequent standardized breakfast. *J. Nutr.* **138**(4): 732–739.

Nugent, A. 2005. Health properties of resistant starch. *Nutr. Bull.* **30**: 27–55.

Onning, G., Wallmark, A., Persson, M., Akesson, B., Elmstahl, S. and Oste, R. 1999. Consumption of oat milk for 5 weeks lowers serum cholesterol and LDL cholesterol in free-living men with moderate hypercholesterolemia. *Ann. Nutr. Metab.* **43**(5): 301–309.

Panahi, S., Ezatagha, A., Temelli, F., Vasanthan, T. and Vuksan, V. 2007. Beta-glucan from two sources of oat concentrates affect postprandial glycemia in relation to the level of viscosity. *J. Am. Coll. Nutr.* **26**(6): 639–644.

Pedersen, A., Sandstrom, B. and Van Amelsvoort, J.M. 1997. The effect of ingestion of inulin on blood lipids and gastrointestinal symptoms in healthy females. *Br. J. Nutr.* **78**(2): 215–222.

Pencina, M.J., D'Agostino RB, S., Larson, M.G., Massaro, J.M. and Vasan, R.S. 2009. Predicting the 30-year risk of cardiovascular disease: The Framingham Heart Study. *Circulation.* **119**(24): 3078–3084.

Pereira, M.A. and Ludwig, D.S. 2001. Dietary fiber and body-weight regulation. Observations and mechanisms. *Pediatr. Clin. North Am.* **48**(4): 969–980.

Peressin, D. and Sensidoni, A. 2009. Effect of soluble fibre addition on rheological and breadmaking properties of wheat doughs. *J. Cereal Sci.* **49**(2): 190–201.

Philippou, E., McGowan, B.M., Brynes, A.E., Dornhorst, A., Leeds, A.R. and Frost, G.S. 2008. The effect of a 12-week low glycaemic index diet on heart disease risk factors and 24 h glycaemic response in healthy middle-aged volunteers at risk of heart disease: A pilot study. *Eur. J. Clin. Nutr.* **62**(1): 145–149.

Pietinen, P., Rimm, E.B., Korhonen, P., Hartman, A.M., Willett, W.C., Albanes, D. and Virtamo, J. 1996. Intake of dietary fiber and risk of coronary heart disease in a cohort of Finnish men. The Alpha-Tocopherol, Beta-Carotene Cancer Prevention Study. *Circulation.* **94**(11): 2720–2727.

Pins, J.J., Geleva, D., Keenan, J.M., Frazel, C., O'Connor, P.J. and Cherney, L.M. 2002. Do whole-grain oat cereals reduce the need for antihypertensive medications and improve blood pressure control? *J. Fam. Pract.* **51**(4): 353–359.

Plicht, B., Erbel, R. and Mohlenkamp, S. 2009. Is there a preventive value in non-invasive cardiac imaging? Debate on the case of a marathon runner. *Dtsch. Med. Wochenschr.* **134**(40): e1–e5, 1990-4.

Prosky, L., Asp, N.G., Furda, I., DeVries, J.W., Schweizer, T.F. and Harland, B.F. 1985. Determination of total dietary fiber in foods and food products: Collaborative study. *J. Assoc Off. Anal. Chem.* 68(4): 677–679.

Pullinger, C.R., Kane, J.P. and Malloy, M.J. 2003. Primary hypercholesterolemia: Genetic causes and treatment of five monogenic disorders. *Expert Rev. Cardiovasc.Ther.* 1(1): 107–119.

Qi, L., Meigs, J.B., Liu, S., Manson, J.E., Mantzoros, C. and Hu, F.B. 2006. Dietary fibers and glycemic load, obesity, and plasma adiponectin levels in women with type 2 diabetes. *Diabetes Care.* 29(7): 1501–1505.

Qi, L., Rimm, E., Liu, S., Rifai, N. and Hu, F.B. 2005. Dietary glycemic index, glycemic load, cereal fiber, and plasma adiponectin concentration in diabetic men. *Diabetes Care.* 28(5): 1022–1028.

Queenan, K.M., Stewart, M.L., Smith, K.N., Thomas, W., Fulcher, R.G. and Slavin, J.L. 2007. Concentrated oat beta-glucan, a fermentable fiber, lowers serum cholesterol in hypercholesterolemic adults in a randomized controlled trial. *Nutr. J.* 6: 6.

Raitakari, O.T., Juonala, M., Ronnemaa, T., Keltikangas-Jarvinen, L., Rasanen, L., Pietikainen, M., Hutri-Kahonen, N. et al. 2008. Cohort profile: The cardiovascular risk in Young Finns Study. *Intern. J. Epidemiol.* 37(6): 1220–1226.

Rallidis, L.S., Lekakis, J., Kolomvotsou, A., Zampelas, A., Vamvakou, G., Efstathiou, S., Dimitriadis, G., Raptis, S.A. and Kremastinos, D.T. 2009. Close adherence to a Mediterranean diet improves endothelial function in subjects with abdominal obesity. *Am. J. Clin. Nutr.* 90(2):263–268.

Ranganna, K., Mathew, O.P., Yatsu, F.M., Yousefipour, Z., Hayes, B.E. and Milton, S.G. 2007. Involvement of glutathione/glutathione *S*-transferase antioxidant system in butyrate-inhibited vascular smooth muscle cell proliferation. *FEBS J.* 274(22): 5962–5978.

Rashid, M., Tawara, S., Fukumoto, Y., Seto, M., Yano, K. and Shimokawa, H. 2009. Importance of Rac1 signaling pathway inhibition in the pleiotropic effects of HMG-CoA reductase inhibitors. *Circ. J.* 73(2): 361–370.

Rasnake, C.M., Trumbo, P.R. and Heinonen, T.M. 2008. Surrogate endpoints and emerging surrogate endpoints for risk reduction of cardiovascular disease. *Nutr. Rev.* 66(2): 76–81.

Ravnskov, U. 2008. The fallacies of the lipid hypothesis. *Scand. Cardiovasc. J.* 42(4): 236–239.

Razack, R. and Seidner, D.L. 2007. Nutrition in inflammatory bowel disease. *Curr. Opin. Gaststroentol.* 23(4): 400–405.

Redondo-Cuenca, A., Villanueva-Suarex, M.J. and Mateos-Aparicio, I. 2008. Soybean seeds and its by-product okara as sources of dietary fibre. *Food Chem.* 108(3): 1099–1105.

Repo-Carrasco-Velencia, R., Pena, J., Kallio, H. and Salminen, S. 2009. Dietary fiber and other functional components in two varieties of crude and extruded kiwicha (*Amaranthus caudatus*). *J. Cereal Sci.* 49(2): 219–224.

Reyna-Villasmil, N., Bermudez-Pirela, V., Mengual-Moreno, E., Arias, N., Cano-Ponce, C., Leal-Gonzalez, E., Souki, A. et al. 2007. Oat-derived beta-glucan significantly improves HDLC and diminishes LDLC and non-HDL cholesterol in overweight individuals with mild hypercholesterolemia. *Am. J. Ther.* 14(2): 203–212.

Rikitake, Y. and Hirata, K. 2009. Inhibition of RhoA or Rac1? Mechanism of cholesterol-independent beneficial effects of statins. *Circ. J.* 73(2): 231–232.

Rimm, E.B., Ascherio, A., Giovannucci, E., Spiegelman, D., Stampfer, M.J. and Willett, W.C. 1996. Vegetable, fruit, and cereal fiber intake and risk of coronary heart disease among men. *JAMA.* 275(6): 447–451.

Ripsin, C.M., Keenan, J.M., Jacobs, D.R., Jr., Elmer, P.J., Welch, R.R., Van Horn, L., Liu, K., Turnbull, W.H., Thye, F.W. and Kestin, M. 1992. Oat products and lipid lowering. A meta-analysis. *JAMA.* 267(24): 3317–3325.

Roberfroid, M.B. and Delzenne, N.M. 1998. Dietary fructans. *Annu. Rev. Nutr.* 18: 117–143.

Roberts, C.K., Ng, C., Hama, S., Eliseo, A.J. and Barnard, R.J. 2006. Effect of a short-term diet and exercise intervention on inflammatory/anti-inflammatory properties of HDL in overweight/obese men with cardiovascular risk factors. *J. Appl. Physiol.* 101(6): 1727–1732.

Rodwell, V.W., Nordstrom, J.L. and Mitschelen, J.J. 1976. Regulation of HMG-CoA reductase. *Adv. Lipid Res.* 14: 1–74.

Rosch, P.J. 2008. Cholesterol does not cause coronary heart disease in contrast to stress. *Scand. Cardiovasc. J.* 42(4): 244–249.

Rosch, P.J. 2003. Lipoproteins and cardiovascular risk. *Lancet.* 361(9373): 1988; 1989.

Ryan-Harshman, M. and Vogel, E. Jan 12, 2009. Nutritional genomics—A new frontier in nutrition. *Dietitians of Canada Current Issues.* pp. 1–4.

Sacks, F.M., Obarzanek, E., Windhauser, M.M., Svetkey, L.P., Vollmer, W.M., McCullough, M., Karanja, N., Lin, P.H., Steele, P. and Proschan, M.A. 1995. Rationale and design of the Dietary Approaches to Stop Hypertension trial (DASH). A multicenter controlled-feeding study of dietary patterns to lower blood pressure. *Ann. Epidemiol.* 5(2): 108–118.

Saemann, M.D., Böhmig, G.A., Zlabinger, G.J. 2002. Short-chain fatty acids: Bacterial mediators of a balanced host-microbial relationship in the human gut. *Wien Kin Wochenschr* **114**(8–9): 289–300.

Salas-Salvado, J., Bullo, M., Perez-Heras, A. and Ros, E. 2006. Dietary fibre, nuts and cardiovascular diseases. *Br. J. Nutr.* **96**(Suppl. 2): S46–S51.

Salenius, J.P., Harju, E., Jokela, H., Riekkinen, H. and Silvasti, M. 1995. Long term effects of guar gum on lipid metabolism after carotid endarterectomy. *BMJ.* **310**(6972): 95–96.

Salmeron, J., Ascherio, A., Rimm, E.B., Colditz, G.A., Spiegelman, D., Jenkins, D.J., Stampfer, M.J., Wing, A.L. and Willett, W.C. 1997. Dietary fiber, glycemic load, and risk of NIDDM in men. *Diabetes Care.* **20**(4): 545–550.

Saltzman, E., Das, S.K., Lichtenstein, A.H., Dallal, G.E., Corrales, A., Schaefer, E.J., Greenberg, A.S. and Roberts, S.B. 2001. An oat-containing hypocaloric diet reduces systolic blood pressure and improves lipid profile beyond effects of weight loss in men and women. *J. Nutr.* **131**(5): 1465–1470.

Santos, J.L., Boutin, P., Verdich, C., Holst, C., Larsen, L.H., Toubro, S., Dina, C. et al. 2006. Genotype-by-nutrient interactions assessed in European obese women. A case-only study. *Eur. J. Nutr.* **45**(8): 454–462.

Schedle, K., Pfaffl, M.W., Plitzner, C., Meyer, H.H. and Windisch, W. 2008, Effect of insoluble fibre on intestinal morphology and mRNA expression pattern of inflammatory, cell cycle and growth marker genes in a piglet model. *Arch. Anim. Nutr.* **62**(6): 427–438.

Scherer, P.E., Williams, S., Fogliano, M., Baldini, G. and Lodish, H.F. 1995. A novel serum protein similar to C1q, produced exclusively in adipocytes. *J. Biol. Chem.* **270**(45): 26746–26749.

Schmidt, L.E. and Dalhoff, K. 2002. Food–drug interactions. *Drugs.* **62**(10): 1481–1502.

Schoenhagen, P. and Tuzcu, E.M. 2008. Atherosclerosis imaging in progression/regression trials: surrogate marker or direct window into the atherosclerotic disease process? *Arq. Bras. Cardiol.* **91**(6): 385–398.

Schulze, M.B., Liu, S., Rimm, E.B., Manson, J.E., Willett, W.C. and Hu, F.B. 2004. Glycemic index, glycemic load, and dietary fiber intake and incidence of type 2 diabetes in younger and middle-aged women. *Am. J. Clin. Nutr.* **80**(2): 348–356.

Schwab, U., Louheranta, A., Torronen, A. and Uusitupa, M. 2006. Impact of sugar beet pectin and polydextrose on fasting and postprandial glycemia and fasting concentrations of serum total and lipoprotein lipids in middle-aged subjects with abnormal glucose metabolism. *Eur. J. Clin, Nutr.* **60**(9): 1073–1080.

Shai, I., Schwarzfuchs, D., Henkin, Y., Shahar, D.R., Witkow, S., Greenberg, I., Golan, R. et al. 2008. Weight loss with a low-carbohydrate, Mediterranean, or low-fat diet. *N. Engl. J. Med.* **359**(3): 229–241.

Shepherd, S.J.and Gibson, P.R. 2006. Fructose malabsorption and symptoms of irritable bowel syndrome: Guidelines for effective dietary management. *J. Am. Diet. Assoc.* **106**(10): 1631–1639.

Shin, M.S., Lee, S., Lee, K.Y. and Lee, H.G. 2005. Structural and biological characterization of aminated-derivatized oat beta-glucan. *J. Agric. Food Chem.* **53**(14): 5554–5558.

Simon, A., Chironi, G. and Levenson, J. 2007. Comparative performance of subclinical atherosclerosis tests in predicting coronary heart disease in asymptomatic individuals. *Eur. J. Heart J.* **28**(24): 2967–2971.

Slavin, J.L. 2008. Position of the American Dietetic Association: Health implications of dietary fiber. *J. Am. Diet. Assoc.* **108**(10): 1716–1731.

Smith, D. 2008, Making sense of ENHANCE: Ezetimibe (Zetia) lowers LDL cholesterol but doesn't decrease carotid intima-media thickness. *Mt. Sinai J. Med.* **75**(2): 143–147.

Sofi, F., Cesari, F., Abbate, R., Gensini, G.F. and Casini, A. 2008. Adherence to Mediterranean diet and health status: Meta-analysis. *BMJ.* **337**: a1344.

Sola, R., Godas, G., Ribalta, J., Vallve, J.C., Girona, J., Anguera, A., Ostos, M. et al. 2007. Effects of soluble fiber (*Plantago ovata* husk) on plasma lipids, lipoproteins, and apolipoproteins in men with ischemic heart disease. *Am. J. Clin. Nutr.* **85**(4): 1157–1163.

Song, Y.J., Sawamura, M., Ikeda, K., Igawa, S. and Yamori, Y. 2000. Soluble dietary fibre improves insulin sensitivity by increasing muscle GLUT-4 content in stroke-prone spontaneously hypertensive rats. *Clin. Exp. Pharmacol. Physiol.* **27**(1–2): 41–45.

Spiller, R.C. 1994, Pharmacology of dietary fibre. *Pharmacol. Ther.* **62**(3): 407–427.

Stamatelopoulos, K., Karatzi, K. and Sidossis, L.S. 2009. Noninvasive methods for assessing early markers of atherosclerosis: The role of body composition and nutrition. *Curr. Opin. Clin. Nutr. Met. Care.* **12**(5): 467–473.

Statistics Canada *Canadian Community Health Survey (CCHS) (Cycle 4.1)*. 2007. Available at http://www.statcan.gc.ca/cgi-bin/imdb/p2SV.pl?Function=getSurvey&SurvId=3226&SurvVer=1&InstaId=15282&InstaVer=4&SDDS=3226&lang=en&db=imdb&adm=8&dis=2.

Stein, E.A. 2008. Additional lipid lowering trials using surrogate measurements of atherosclerosis by carotid intima-media thickness: More clarity or confusion? *J. Am. Coll. Cardiol.* **52**(25): 2206–2209.

Stevens, J., Ahn, K., Juhaeri, j., Houston, D., Steffan, L. and Couper, D. 2002, Dietary fiber intake and glycemic index and incidence of diabetes in African-American and white adults: The ARIC study. *Diabetes Care.* **25**(10): 1715–1721.

Stojceska, V., Ainsworth, P., Plunkett, A., Ibanoglu, E. and Ibanoglu, S. 2008. Cauliflower by-products as a new source of dietary fibre, antioxidants and proteins in cereal based ready-to-eat expanded snacks. *J. Food Eng.* **87**(4): 554–563.

Streppel, M.T., Ocke, M.C., Boshuizen, H.C., Kok, F.J. and Kromhout, D. 2008. Dietary fiber intake in relation to coronary heart disease and all-cause mortality over 40 y: The Zutphen Study. *Am. J. Clin. Nutr.* **88**(4): 1119–1125.

Sun, Y., Xun, K., Wang, C., Zhao, H., Bi, H., Chen, X. and Wang, Y. 2009. Adiponectin, an unlocking adipocytokine. *Cardiovasc. Therap.* **27**(1): 59–75.

Suter, P.M. 2005. Carbohydrates and dietary fiber. *Handbook Exp. Pharmacol.* **170**:231–261.

Swain, J.F., McCarron, P.B., Hamilton, E.F., Sacks, F.M. and Appel, L.J. 2008, Characteristics of the diet patterns tested in the optimal macronutrient intake trial to prevent heart disease (OmniHeart): Options for a heart-healthy diet, *J. Am. Diet. Assoc.* **108**(2): 257–265.

Swain, J.F., Rouse, I.L., Curley, C.B. an Sacks, F.M. 1990. Comparison of the effects of oat bran and low-fiber wheat on serum lipoprotein levels and blood pressure. *N. Eng. J. Med.* **322**(3): 147–152.

Taylor, C.G., Noto, A., Stringer, D.M., Froese, S. and Malcomson, L. 2010. Dietary milled flaxseed and flaxseed oil improve n-3 fatty acid status and do not affect glycemic control in individuals with well-controlled type 2 diabetes, *J. Am. Coll. Nutr.* **29**(2): 72–80.

Theuwissen, E. and Mensink, R.P. 2007. Simultaneous intake of beta-glucan and plant stanol esters affects lipid metabolism in slightly hypercholesterolemic subjects. *J. Nutr.* **137**(3): 583–588.

Trichopoulou, A., Yiannakouris, N., Bamia, C., Benetou, V., Trichopoulos, D. and Ordovas, J.M. 2008. Genetic predisposition, nongenetic risk factors, and coronary infarct. *Arch. Intern. Med.* **168**(8): 891–896.

Turner, P.R., Tuomilehto, J., Happonen, P., La Ville, A.E., Shaikh, M. and Lewis, B. 1990. Metabolic studies on the hypolipidaemic effect of guar gum. *Atherosclerosis.* **81**(2): 145–150.

United States Department of Agriculture (USDA). 2009a, *MyPyramid.* Available at http://www.mypyramid.gov/.

United States Department of Agriculture (USDA). 2009b. Agricultural Research Service, *Nutrient Data Laboratory. USDA National Nutrient Database for Standard Reference, Release 21. Content of Selected Foods per Common Fiber, Total Dietary g, Measure, Sorted by Nutrient Content.* Available at http://www. nal.usda.gove/fnic/foodcomp/Data/SR21/nutrlist/sr21w291.pdf.

United States Food and Drug Administration (USFDA). 2009a. *Center for Food Safety and Applied Nutrition. Label Claims.* Available at http://www.cfsan.fda.gov/~dms/lab-ssa.html.

United States Food and Drug Administration (USFDA). 2009b. *Department of Health and Human Services. Guidance for Industry: Evidence-Based Review Systems for the Scientific Evaluation of Health Claims.* Available at http://www.fda.gov/Food/GuidanceCompliance RegulatoryInformation/GuidanceDocuments/ FoodLabelingNutrition/ucm073332.htm.

Uusitupa, M., Tuomilehto, J., Karttunen, P. and Wolf, E. 1984, Long term effects of guar gum on metabolic control, serum cholesterol and blood pressure levels in type 2 (non-insulin-dependent) diabetic patients with high blood pressure. *Ann. Clin. Res.* **16**(Suppl. 43): 126–131.

Van Horn, L., Moag-Stahlberg, A., Liu, K.A., Ballew, C., Ruth, K., Hughes, R. and Stamler, J. 1991. Effects on serum lipids of adding instant oats to usual American diets. *Am. J. Public Health.* **81**(2): 183–188.

Venkatesan, N., Devaraj, S.N. and Devaraj, H. 2003. Increased binding of LDL and VLDL to apo B,E receptors of hepatic plasma membrane of rats treated with Fibernat. *Eur. J. Nutr.* **42**(5): 262–271.

Venter, C.S., Vorster, H.H. and Cummings, J.H. 1990. Effects of dietary propionate on carbohydrate and lipid metabolism in healthy volunteers. *Am. J. Gastroenterol.* **85**(5): 549–553.

Ventura, E.E., Davis, J.N., Alexander, K.E., Shaibi, G.Q., Lee, W., Byrd-Williams, C.E., Toledo-Corral, C.M. et al. 2008. Dietary intake and the metabolic syndrome in overweight Latino children. *J. Am. Diet. Assoc.* **108**(8): 1355–1359.

Vitali, D., Vedrina, D.I. and Sebecic, B. 2009. Effects of incorporation of integral raw materials and dietary fibre on the selected nutritional and functional properties of biscuits. *Food Chem.* **114**(4): 1462–1469.

Wang, C.Y., Liu, P.Y. and Liao, J.K. 2008. Pleiotropic effects of statin therapy: Molecular mechanisms and clinical results. *Trends Mol. Med.* **14**(1): 37–44.

Wang, X., Keith, J.C., Jr., Struthers, A.D. and Feuerstein, G.Z. 2008. Assessment of arterial stiffness, a translational medicine biomarker system for evaluation of vascular risk. *Cardiovasc. Ther.* **26**(3): 214–223.

Weickert, M.O., Mohlig, M., Schofl, C., Arafat, A.M., Otto, B., Viehoff, H., Koebnick, C., Kohl, A., Spranger, J. and Pfeiffer, A.F. 2006. Cereal fiber improves whole-body insulin sensitivity in overweight and obese women. *Diabetes Care.* **29**(4): 775–780.

Weingartner, O., Lutjohann, D., Ji, S., Weisshoff, N., List, F., Sudhop, T., von Bergmann, K. et al. 2008. Vascular effects of diet supplementation with plant sterols, *J. Am. Coll. Cardiol.* **51**(16): 1553–1561.

Willett, W.C. 2006. The Mediterranean diet: Science and practice. *Public Health Nutr.* 9(1A): 105–110.

Wilson, J.M.G. 1968. The evaluation of the worth of early disease detection. *J. R. Coll. Gen. Pract.* **16**(Suppl. 2): 48–57.

Wolever, T.M., Fernandes, J. and Rao, A.V. 1996. Serum acetate:propionate ratio is related to serum cholesterol in men but not women. *J. Nutr.* **126**(11): 2790–2797.

Wolever, T.M., Jenkins, D.J., Mueller, S., Boctor, D.L., Ransom, T.P., Patten, R., Chao, E.S., McMillan, K. and Fulgoni, V., 3rd. 1994. Method of administration influences the serum cholesterol-lowering effect of psyllium. *Am. J. Clin. Nutr.* **59**(5): 1055–1059.

Wolk, R., Cobbe, S.M., Hicks, M.N. and Kane, K.A. 1999. Functional, structural, and dynamic basis of electrical heterogeneity in healthy and diseased cardiac muscle: Implications for arrhythmogenesis and anti-arrhythmic drug therapy. *Pharmacol. Ther.* **84**(2): 207–231.

Wong, J.M., de Souza, R., Kendall, C.W., Emam, A. and Jenkins, D.J. 2006. Colonic health: Fermentation and short chain fatty acids. *J. Clin. Gastroenterol.* **40**(3): 235–243.

World Health Organization /Food and Agriculture Organization of the United Nations (WHO/FAO). 2003, *Diet, Nutrition and the Prevention of Chronic Diseases*, Geneva. Available at http://www.who.int/diet-physicalactivity/publications/trs916/en/.

Wu, H., Dwyer, K.M., Fan, Z., Shircore, A., Fan, J. and Dwyer, J.H. 2003. Dietary fiber and progression of atherosclerosis: The Los Angeles Atherosclerosis Study. *Am. J. Clin. Nutr.* **78**(6): 1085–1091.

Wu, K., Bowman, R., Welch, A.A., Luben, R.N., Wareham, N., Khaw, K.T. and Bingham, S.A. 2007. Apolipoprotein E polymorphisms, dietary fat and fibre, and serum lipids: The EPIC Norfolk study. *Eur. Heart J.* **28**(23): 2930–2936.

Ylonen, K., Saloranta, C., Kronberg-Kippila, C., Groop, L., Aro, A., Virtanen, S.M. and Botnia Dietary Study 2003. Associations of dietary fiber with glucose metabolism in nondiabetic relatives of subjects with type 2 diabetes: The Botnia Dietary Study. *Diabetes Care.* 26(7): 1979–1985.

Zapolska-Downar, D., Siennicka, A., Kaczmarczyk, M., Kolodziej, B. and Naruszewicz, M. 2004. Butyrate inhibits cytokine-induced VCAM-1 and ICAM-1 expression in cultured endothelial cells: The role of NF-kappaB and PPARalpha. *J. Nutr. Biochem.* **15**(4): 220–228.

Zeymer, U., Schwarzmaier-D'assie, A., Petzinna, D., Chiasson, J.L. and STOP-NIDDM Trial Research Group. 2004. Effect of acarbose treatment on the risk of silent myocardial infarctions in patients with impaired glucose tolerance: Results of the randomised STOP-NIDDM trial electrocardiography substudy. *Eur. J. Cardiovasc. Prev. Rehabil.* **11**(5): 412–415.

Zhou, Q. and Liao, J.K. 2009. Rho kinase: An important mediator of atherosclerosis and vascular disease. *Curr. Pharm. Des.* 15(27): 3108–3115.

Zhu, W., Cheng, K.K., Vanhoutte, P.M., Lam, K.S. and Xu, A. 2008. Vascular effects of adiponectin: Molecular mechanisms and potential therapeutic intervention. *Clin. Sci. (Lond).* 114(5): 361–374.

11 Chocolate and Cocoa
A Comprehensive Review on Cardiovascular Benefits

*Ayyappan Appukuttan Aachary, Usha Thiyam,
and N. A. Michael Eskin*
University of Manitoba

CONTENTS

11.1   INTRODUCTION

Cacao is the unprocessed cocoa bean from the cacao tree which originated deep in the equatorial rain forests of the Americas. In 1753, the noted naturalist Carl Linnaeus named it *Theobroma cacao*—"food of the Gods" (Wilson, 2010). Over the centuries, the use of cacao has evolved to what we now know as chocolate (processed bean in solid or liquid form containing varying percentages of cocoa liquor, cocoa butter, sugar, and milk) while cultivation is also found in equatorial regions of Africa and Asia. Indeed, few natural products such as chocolate have been claimed to effectively treat a wide variety of disorders. Historically, cacao was viewed as magical and mystical with the chocolate's medicinal benefits traceable as far back as Aztec medical practice. The use of either cocoa or chocolate in medicine and suggestions about its possible cocoa-dependent health benefits is not a new concept. This "food of the gods" was enobled by many cultures as a curative drug, a culinary delight, and even a source of currency for commodity trading. It has still retained its appeal over the centuries but its medical uses progressively disappeared. In contrast, recent studies demonstrated a potential and a somewhat unexpected role for cacao in "promoting health" (Dillinger et al., 2000; Ding et al., 2006; Grassi et al., 2006). At least on one level, our continued craving to uncover chocolate's medicinal benefits represents good taste in therapeutic choice.

Because of the continued interest in health promotion and bioactive phytochemicals in foods, health educators continue to reassess and evaluate traditional views on foods and their contribution to health. Scientific evidence supports the hypothesis that a variety of plant-based foods in the diet can provide a wealth of potentially beneficial phytochemicals and other components that contribute to reducing cardiovascular disease (CVD) risk. Most of the cardiovascular health benefits of cocoa and chocolate are attributed to its flavonoids. Recent reports indicate that the main flavonoids found in cocoa, flavan-3-ols and their oligomeric derivatives, procyanidins, have a variety of beneficial actions, including antioxidant protection and modulation of vascular homeostasis. The lipid content of chocolate is relatively high; however, one-third of the lipid in cocoa butter is composed of the fat stearic acid, which exerts a neutral cholesterolemic response in humans. Cocoa and chocolate contribute to trace mineral intake, which is necessary for optimum functioning of all biological systems and for vascular tone. Thus, multiple components in chocolate, particularly flavonoids, contribute to the complex interplay of nutrition and health.

Epidemiological studies reported an inverse relationship between polyphenol-rich cocoa and the reduced risk of CVD. Data from experimental and clinical studies suggest consumption of flavanol-rich cocoa and chocolate, as well as other flavanol-rich foods can reduce cardiovascular risk by improving endothelial function (EF) and decreasing blood pressure (BP). Interest in the biological activities of cocoa flavonoids is steadily increasing. This chapter offers a review of current research perspective regarding the potential cardiovascular health benefits of flavonoids found in cocoa and chocolate.

11.2 CARDIOVASCULAR DISEASES AND FLAVONOIDS

CVDs remain the principal cause of death in both developed and developing countries, accounting for roughly 20% of mortality (Coady et al., 2001). The common environment of CVDs, for example, atherosclerosis, coronary heart disease (CHD), arterial hypertension, and heart failure, is the presence of oxidative stress. Oxidative stress is a condition of imbalance between endogenous antioxidants and reactive oxygen/nitrogen species (RONS) with the predominance of the latter (Halliwell and Gutteridge, 1999). In principle, RONS can be generated enzymatically by a few of enzymes such as nicotinamide adenosine dinucleotide phosphate (NADPH) oxidase, xanthine oxidase, and lipoxygenases and further multiplied by the catalytic role of the transient metals iron and copper. The dominant features of the pathogenesis of atherosclerosis include the modification of LDL particles by oxidative stress with the successive induction of inflammation from increased leukocyte adherence and attenuation of endothelial protective properties (Kuhn et al., 1994; Ozaki et al., 2002; Cheng and Li, 2007; Ogura et al., 2009; Huang, 2009). The severest form of CHD, acute myocardial infarction (AMI), is usually caused by a thrombosis as a result of increased procoagulation facilitated by endothelial dysfunction with increased platelet aggregation.

Chemically, flavonoids are benzopyrone derivatives that are ubiquitous in photosynthesizing cells (Chen et al., 1990) and are the most abundant antioxidants found in common diets. The total number of flavonoids exceeds over 4000 different types in the foods we eat, with a spectrum of sources such as apples, onions, mulberries, bilberries, chocolate, red fruits, citrus fruits, nuts, tea, beer, and wine (Russo et al., 2000). The daily intake of flavonoids has been determined to range between 3 and 70 mg depending mainly on dietary habits of a person or the country they live in (Hertog et al., 1993; Russo et al., 2000; Geleijnse et al., 2002). Flavonoids are divided according to their chemical structure into several classes. The structural requirements for the antioxidant and free radical scavenging functions of flavonoids are a hydroxyl group in carbon position three, a double bond between carbon positions two and three, a carbonyl group in carbon position four, and polyhydroxylation of the A and B aromatic rings.

Evidence from epidemiological studies indicated that long-term administration of flavonoids can reduce, or at least, tend to decrease the incidence of CVD and their consequences (Hertog et al., 1993; Geleijnse et al., 2002; Knekt et al., 2002). However, results from such studies must be interpreted with caution. This is especially true if there is some form therapy, such as pharmacotherapy or additional factors such as the intake of vitamins, concomitant diseases, or smoking.

Peroral (p.o.) administration of flavonoids has been shown to improve health status in a mouse model of atherosclerosis and a lipoprotein spectrum of diabetic rats without affecting blood glucose levels (Cayatte et al., 2001; Xiao et al., 2009). Similarly, a few reports demonstrated a significant reduction of myocardial or cerebral infarction consequences after the administration of various flavonoids (van Jaarsveld et al., 1996; Ralay Ranaivo et al., 2004; Krishna et al., 2005). Other studies showed a positive influence of p.o. administration of some flavonoids on catecholamine-based model of AMI, but aggravated by rutin (Karthick and Prince, 2006; Rajadurai and Prince, 2007). Peroral administration of flavonoids was found to reduce BP in hypertensive animal models but did not affect the BP of healthy animals (Sanchez et al., 2006; Jackman et al., 2007; Mladenka et al., 2009). The beneficial effects of flavonoids on elevated BP observed in animals may not always be found in humans (Jackman et al., 2007). However, some positive effects of flavonoids in heart failure and in the reduction of arrhythmias in a few animal and human studies have been reported (Duan et al., 2000; Vianna et al., 2006). It has been documented that doxorubicin cardiotoxicity in rat cardiomyocytes can be reduced by certain flavonoids and such positive results have also been reported in a few *in vivo* studies (Psotova et al., 2004, Kaiserova et al., 2007). The inference of these studies is that most flavonoids have some potential positive effects on the cardiovascular system, although the final pharmacological targets differ markedly among various flavonoids. Apart from direct scavenging activity and transient metal chelation, different flavonoids possess a complex range of useful activities such as inhibition of reactive oxygen species (ROS)-forming enzymes,antiplatelet activity, inhibition of leukocyte activation, and vasodilatory properties to combat the diseases of the cardiovascular system (Mladenka et al., 2010).

11.3 COCOA FLAVONOIDS AND BIOAVAILABILITY

Polyphenols in cocoa beans are stored in the pigment cells of the cotyledons. Depending on the amount of anthocyanins, those pigment cells are also called polyphenol-storage cells, and range in color from white to deep purple. Flavonoids are the major polyphenolics present in cocoa bean and especially in cocoa powder. Structurally, a flavonoid consists of two aromatic rings linked through an oxygenated heterocyclic ring. Generally, food flavonoids have a glycosidic moiety attached to it. Based on the degree of hydroxylation and oxidation of the rings, the flavonoids are subdivided into 13 classes of which flavonols are very important with respect to cocoa (Harbone, 1989). The primary flavonoids in cocoa and chocolate are the flavan-3-ols catechin and epicatechin (monomeric units) (Figure 11.1) and proanthocyanidins (also termed as procyanidins), which are polymeric compounds comprised of catechin and epicatechin subunits (Harbone, 1989). The main catechin is (−)-epicatechin which accounts for up to 35% of polyphenol content (Wollgast and Anklam, 2000). Phenolic compounds make up 12–18% of the total weight of dried cocoa nibs (i.e., roasted cocoa beans) (Bravo, 1998). Approximately 35% of the total content of polyphenols in nonfermented cocoa nibs belonging to the Forastero variety is epicatechin. The epicatechin content in nonfermented cocoa nibs of different varieties range between 34.65 and 43.27 mg/g (defatted sample). This amount

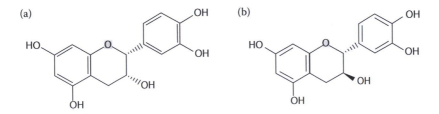

FIGURE 11.1 Chemical structure of the major cocoa monomeric flavanols, (a) (−)-epicatechin and (b) (+)-catechin.

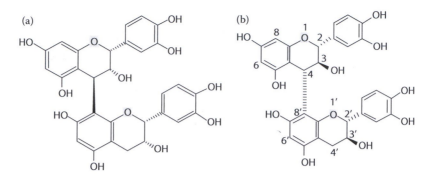

FIGURE 11.2 Chemical structures of (a) procyanidin dimer B2 and (b) procyanidin dimer B3 identified from cocoa.

decreases during the process of fermentation and drying. Depending on the place of production, the epicatechin content may decrease between 2.66 and 16.5 mg/g of the defatted sample (Forsyth and Quesnel, 1952, 1957; Kim and Keeney, 1984; Wollgast and Anklam, 2000), while the amount of catechin increases (Porter et al., 1991).

Procyanidins with as many as 10 subunits have been identified in chocolate with the procyanidin oligomers accounting for 12–48% of the dry weight of the cocoa bean (Bravo, 1998), while tea and wine consist mainly of the monomeric flavonoids. Procyanidin B1 and procyanidin B2 are dimers of flavan-3-ols monomeric units (Figure 11.2). Procyanidins form complexes with salivary proteins and is responsible for the bitterness of cocoa. Chocolate products have a higher total flavan-3-ol concentration on a per weight basis than is found in most plant-based foods and beverages that contain flavan-3-ols (Lazarus et al., 1999; Hammerstone and Lazurus, 2000; Hammerstone et al., 2000).

The following polyphenols have been identified and quantified in cocoa beans or cocoa products: procyanidin B3 (catechin-(4$\alpha \rightarrow$ 8)-catechin), procyanidin B4 (catechin-(4$\alpha \rightarrow$ 8)-epicatechin), procyanidin B5 (epicatechin-(4$\beta \rightarrow$ 6)-epicatechin), procyanidin C1 (epicatechin-(4$\beta \rightarrow$ 8)-epicatechin-(4$\beta \rightarrow$ 8)-epicatechin), procyanidin D (epicatechin-(4$\beta \rightarrow$ 8)-epicatechin-(4$\beta \rightarrow$ 8)-epicatechin), higher oligo- and polymers, mostly homologs of epicatechin with 2–18 monomeric units, as well the following flavanols: quercetin, quercetin-3-O-glucoside (isoquercitin), quercetin-3-O-galactoside (hyperoside), quercetin-3-O-arabinoside. Moreover, following flavones have been detected (Figure 11.3): apigenin, apigenin-8-C-glucoside (vitexin), apigenin-6-C-glucoside (isovitexin), luteolin and luteolin-7-Oglucoside, dihydroquercetin, dihydroxykaempferol, kaempferolrutinoside, naringenin, naringenin-glucoside, myricetin-glucoside. The following phenolic compounds were also identified: caffeic acid, chlorogenic acid, coumaric acid, ferulic acid, phenylacetic acid, phloretic acid, protocatechuic acid, syringic acid, vanillic acid, clovamide, and dideoxyclovamide (Borchers et al., 2000; Wollgast and Anklam, 2000, Sanchez-Rabaneda et al., 2003; Ortega et al., 2008).

The flavonoid content in chocolate depends on many processing parameters, such as time, temperature, and the alkalization process. Substantial amounts of these potentially beneficial compounds can be retained from the cocoa bean by adopting proper processing and manufacturing controls (Meursing, 1994). An efficient processing method will result in a cocoa powder with as much as 10% flavonoids on a dry weight basis. Not all chocolates are equal sources of flavonoids as studies showed dark chocolate contains greater amounts of flavonoids as it is formulated with a higher percentage of cocoa bean liquor compared to milk chocolate.

Flavanols are distinct from other flavonoid classes; instead of appearing as glycosides, flavanols are present in the aglycone form, as oligomers, or esterified with gallic acid (Kuhnau, 1976). In order to establish a causal relationship between the consumption of cocoa flavanols and specific

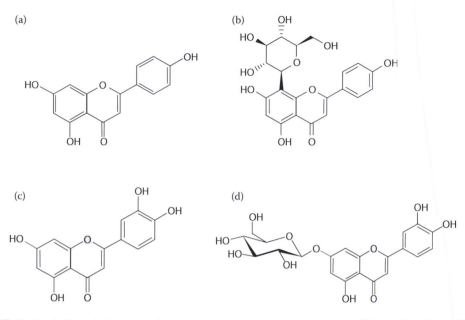

FIGURE 11.3 A few of the minor flavones present in cocoa: (a) apigenin, (b) vitexin, (c) luteolin, and (d) luteolin-7-O-glucoside.

physiological effects, it is critical not only to establish that the food product contains cocoa flavanols, but it is also important to ensure that these compounds are absorbed into the circulation.

Spencer et al. (2000) assumed that procyanidins were degraded under the acidic conditions of the stomach. However, the stability of flavanols and procyanidins during gastric transit was later confirmed by Rios et al. (2002). Once in the mesenteric circulation, flavanols exist predominately in a conjugated form. Generally, the flavanols are absorbed from the jejunal lumen into the epithelial cell layer and are further methylated and glucuronidated before reaching the blood stream (Donovan et al., 2001; Spencer, 2003). Additional glucuronidation, methylation, and sulfation of these flavonoids will take place in the liver (Donovan et al., 2001; Spencer, 2003). Flavanol conjugates have been mainly detected in the plasma and urine of experimental animals and human subjects (Baba et al., 2000, 2002; Donovan et al., 2002). Their presence has also been confirmed in rat bile (Donovan et al., 2002) and brain (Abd El Mohsen et al., 2002). A few of the colonic microflora can degrade the flavan structure of flavonoids to form simple phenolic and ring-fission metabolites that may be physiologically important (Rechner et al., 2002; Unno et al., 2003). Rios et al. (2003) showed an increase in urinary excretion of *m*-hydroxyphenylpropionic acid, 3,4-dihydroxyphenylacetic acid, *m*-hydroxybenzoic acid, and *m*-hydroxylphenylacetic acid in human subjects, 9–48 h after cocoa consumption. The authors suggested that these phenolic compounds are possible products of the colonic microbial degradation of the procyanidins (Rios et al., 2003). Consequently, these products of colonic metabolism must be considered when examining the potential biological effects of cocoa and chocolate, as well as other flavanol- and procyanidin-rich foods.

Nonmethylated epicatechin in the micromolar range has been detected in plasma as early as 1 h after cocoa consumption by human subjects (Baba et al., 2000; Holt et al., 2002; Steinberg et al., 2002). The major metabolites identified were epicatechin-7-β-D-glucuronide and epicatechin-7-sulfate. Baba et al. (2000) also confirmed the presence of 3'-O-methylepicatechin, a methylated epicatechin form in the plasma in the micromolar range. They showed this molecule, like the rest of the metabolites, was rapidly excreted. There is some evidence that certain flavanols are better absorbed than others. After human subjects were given a cocoa beverage containing epicatechin and catechin in a 1:1 ratio, peak plasma catechin concentrations were <10% of the peak epicatechin concentrations (Holt et al., 2002). Dimer cleavage can be one of the reasons for the difference in plasma concentrations between epicatechin and catechin (Spencer et al., 2001; Baba et al., 2002).

The bioavailability of the monomeric flavanols has been well established while there is only limited information on the metabolism of the procyanidins. Various studies indicated the presence of epicatechin-(4β-8)-epicatechin and epicatechin-(4β-6)-epicatechin in the plasma of humans and rats (Baba et al., 2002; Holt et al., 2002; Steinberg et al., 2002; Zhu et al., 2002). Other procyanidins, such as catechin-(4α-8)-catechin (Gonthier et al., 2003) and catechin-(4α-8)-catechin-(4α-8)-catechin (Gonthier et al., 2003), could not be detected. It is important to note that the oligomers found in the plasma consisted of epicatechin and not catechin subunits. It is assumed that the observed differences between the plasma concentrations of epicatechin and catechin, and their oligomers, might be due to stereochemical differences resulting in differences in hydrophobicity and some biological properties, such as antioxidant activity (Rice-Evans et al., 1996; Haslam, 1998; Schroeder et al., 2003).

The nature of the food matrix can affect the bioavailability and potential biological activity of cocoa flavanols and procyanidins. Schroeter et al. (2003) observed no differences in either antioxidant capacity or epicatechin bioavailability when cocoa was provided with or without milk, under isocaloric and isolipidemic conditions, to healthy human subjects. The observed differences in antioxidant activity and bioavailability between dark chocolate and milk chocolate (Serafini et al., 2003) were the result of the food matrix altering the kinetics of absorption and were likely not attributable to flavanol–milk protein interactions.

11.4   EFFECTS OF COCOA FLAVONOIDS ON CARDIOVASCULAR HEALTH

Numerous epidemiological studies indicated an inverse association between high fruit and vegetable intakes and the risk of CVD mortality (Renaud and de Lorgeril, 1992; Hertog et al., 1993, 1995; Knekt et al., 1996; Rimm et al., 1996). These results led to many hypotheses regarding the physiological role of flavonoids. Cocoa, tea, and wine are increasingly viewed as sources of dietary components with potentially beneficial functional activities (Visioli et al., 2000; Kris-Etherton and Keen, 2002). The chemical structure of flavonoids in cocoa suggests that they have the ability to scavenge free radicals, and chelate redox active metal ions (Rice-Evans et al., 1995) and therefore, function as antioxidants. These bioactive compounds can contribute to the maintenance of the integrated network of cellular and plasma oxidant defense mechanisms, to vascular wall tone, and to a reduction in platelet reactivity with a subsequent reduction in the risk for clot formation. In order to establish the physiological significance of dietary flavonoids, their metabolism and mechanisms of action should be elucidated. Most of the clinical evidence demonstrated a beneficial effect of cocoa on BP, insulin resistance, and vascular and platelet function. A number of mechanisms through which cocoa might produce these benefits have been proposed and debated, including activation of nitric oxide (NO) and antioxidant and anti-inflammatory effects (Corti et al., 2009) (Table 11.1).

11.5   COCOA FLAVANOLS AND INHIBITION OF LDL OXIDATION

Because of its high saturated fat content, chocolate is often postulated to have a hypercholesterolemic effect. In contrast to this assumption, clinical trials have shown that chocolate consumption has a neutral effect on serum total and LDL cholesterol (Kris-Etherton and Mustad, 1994). This is attributed to the high content of stearic acid in cocoa (~30% of fatty acids), which is considered to be neutral with respect to total and LDL cholesterol. Consumption of cocoa or dark chocolate may actually have a beneficial effect on serum lipids. In a study by Wan et al. (2001), consumption of cocoa with dark chocolate increased the serum concentration of HDL cholesterol by 4%.

Most epidemiological studies have associated a high intake of dietary flavonoids with a reduction in CHD risk. Perhaps, this protective effect is attributed to the antioxidant properties of flavonoids (Fuhrman and Aviram, 2001). The oxidative modification of LDL plays an important role in

TABLE 11.1

Significant Studies on Various Cardiovascular Effects of Cocoa and Chocolate

No	Study	References
	EF	
1	Cocoa induces vasodilatation via an NO-dependent mechanism	Fisher et al. (2003)
2	Improvement in vascular function in humans 2 h after flavanol-rich cocoa consumption	Schroeter et al. (2006)
3	Acute consumption of dark chocolate by healthy volunteers increased acute dilatation of muscular arteries and a decreased wave deflection	Vlachopoulos et al. (2005)
4	An increase in the circulating NO pool in plasma by approximately 50% after acute consumption of a flavanol-rich cocoa beverage	Heiss et al. (2005)
5	Ingestion of sugar-free and sugar-sweetened cocoa beverages improved EF compared to placebo	Njike et al. (2009)
	Antioxidant Activity and Inhibition of LDL Oxidation	
6	Antioxidant activity of procyanidins with biological substrates is not attributable to chain length or charge delocalization through polymeric linkages, but primarily on ring structures and catechol groups	Steinberg et al. (2002)
7	Long-term consumption of cocoa polyphenols increases the antioxidative capacity of plasma and inhibits LDL oxidation *ex vivo*	Osakabe et al. (2001)
8	Cocoa polyphenols increase the concentration of HDL cholesterol, while chocolate fatty acids modify the fatty acid composition of LDL and make it more resistant to oxidative damage	Mursu et al. (2004)
	Hypercholesterolemic Effect and Antiobesity Effects	
9	Consumption of cocoa with dark chocolate increased serum concentration of HDL cholesterol by 4%	Wan et al. (2001)
10	LDL cholesterol level lowered significantly (~5%) after 4 weeks of a dietary intervention with cocoa powder in hypercholesterolemic subjects	Baba et al. (2007)
11	LDL cholesterol level was reduced by 15% reduction after 14 days of a daily consumption of flavanol-containing milk chocolate in normo-cholesterolemic young subjects	Fraga et al. (2005)
12	An 11% decrease in LDL cholesterol was observed in patients with essential hypertension after 15 days receiving 100 g/day dark chocolate	Grassi et al. (2005)
13	A 27.5% decrease in LDL cholesterol was observed in patients with glucose-intolerant hypertension after chocolate consumption	Grassi et al. (2008)
14	Consumption of chocolate and almonds for 6 weeks led to favorable dietary changes and showed no harmful effects on healthy women's weights, serum lipids, and inflammatory markers	Kurlandsky and Stote (2006)
15	In diabetic rats, with enhanced serum TG and cholesterol concentrations, intake of a cocoa extract also increased HDL cholesterol and decreased TG and total and LDL cholesterol concentrations	Ruzaidi et al. (2005)
16	A mechanism has been postulated for the anti-obesity effects of cocoa in which ingestion effectively prevented TG accumulation by modulating lipid metabolism	Matsui et al. (2005)
	Effects on Coronary Circulation	
17	Dark chocolate consumption improved endothelium-dependent FMD of the brachial artery	Vlachopoulos et al. (2005)
18	Flavonoid-rich dark chocolate intake significantly improved coronary circulation in healthy adults, independent of changes in oxidative stress parameters, BP and lipid profile, whereas nonflavonoid white chocolate had no such effects	Shiina et al. (2009)
19	Chocolate consumption is inversely associated with prevalent CAC in a dose–response manner	Djoussé et al. (2011)

continued

TABLE 11.1   (continued)
Significant Studies on Various Cardiovascular Effects of Cocoa and Chocolate

No	Study	References
	Antihypertensive Effects	
20	24 h ambulatory BP levels decreased while insulin sensitivity improved in healthy and hypertensive volunteers after the acute intake of dark chocolate	Grassi et al. (2005)
21	In a cohort study, the Zutphen Elderly Study, cocoa intake was inversely related to BP levels	Buijsse et al. (2006)
22	Consumption of foods rich in cocoa may reduce BP as shown by a meta-analysis of five randomized, small, short-term, controlled trials	Taubert et al. (2007a,b)
23	A decrease of 4.5 mmHg in systolic and 2.5 mmHg in diastolic BP was observed in a meta-analysis of randomized controlled trials involving dark chocolate and cocoa beverages	Desch et al. (2010)
24	A higher cocoa intake was an independent determinant of low arterial stiffiness and wave reflection indexes and was also independently assocoated with significantly lower central (aortic) pulse pressure	Vlachopoulos et al (2007)
25	Chocolate intake was more frequent among normotensive (80.7%) than preeclamptic (62.5%) or gestational hypertensive women (75.8%), and associated with reduced risks of preeclampsia	Saftlas et al. (2010)
	Effects on Platelet Aggregation	
26	Consumption of flavanol-rich cocoa products inhibited epinephrine- and ADP-induced expression of specific glycoproteins and selectins thus ultimately reducing platelet activation	Pearson and Holt (2008)
27	Acute exposure to flavanol-rich cocoa could modulate the formation of platelet microparticles as markers of platelet activation	Howard et al. (1988)
28	Long-term cocoa supplementation was shown to reduce platelet aggregation to a degree comparable to acetylsalicylic acid	Murphy et al. (2003)
29	Platelet clotting function was significantly increased with casual cocoa intake	Bordeaux et al. (2007)
30	Cocoa flavanols failed to show an additive effect on platelet aggregation in human subjects when combined with acetylsalicylic acid	Heptinstall et al. (2006)
31	Cocoa reduced ADP/collagen- and adrenaline/collagen-activated, platelet related, primary hemostasis within hours after subjects consumed high or moderate amounts of cocoa flavanols	Rein et al. (2000); Holt et al. (2002); Pearson et al. (2002)
32	Cocoa flavanols and procyanidins inhibit human platelet 12-lipoxygenase and 5-lipoxygenase	Schewe et al. (2001) and Schewe et al. (2002)
	Other Cardiovascular Effects	
33	Long-term cocoa supplementation resulted in lowering of BP which is mediated by NO	Fisher et al. (2003)
34	Reduced insulin resistance was observed in patients with essential hypertension after a 15-day diet with 100 g flavonoid-rich chocolate daily	Grassi et al. (2005)
35	Cocoa dose dependently prevents hyperglycemia in obese diabetic mice	Tomaru et al. (2007)

atherogenesis (Steinberg et al., 1989; Salonen et al., 1992; Salonen et al., 1997), and agents capable of preventing LDL oxidation in the arterial wall might delay the onset of atherosclerosis. The antioxidant potential of cocoa powder and chocolate and its *in vitro* ability to inhibit LDL oxidation have been clearly demonstrated (Kondo et al., 1996; Waterhouse et al., 1996; Vinson et al., 1999; Serafini et al., 2003). An increase in the antioxidant capacity of plasma (Rein et al., 2000; Wang et al., 2000; Wan et al., 2001; Serafini et al., 2003), a decrease in the formation of plasma 2-thiobarbituric acid–reactive substances (Rein et al., 2000; Wang et al., 2000), and inhibition of LDL oxidation *ex vivo* (Kondo et al., 1996) have been observed following the ingestion of a single bolus of cocoa or chocolate.

Examining *in vitro* or *ex vivo* LDL oxidation susceptibility in response to dietary flavonoids can provide useful information regarding their influence on cardiovascular health. There are a few reports on the *in vitro* antioxidant action of purified cocoa procyanidins oligomers using synthetic liposomes and LDL (Lotito et al., 2000; Pearson et al., 2001), and some data exist on the effectiveness of cocoa procyanidins consumption to delay *ex vivo* human LDL oxidation susceptibility (Waterhouse et al., 1996; Osakabe et al., 2001; Wan et al., 2001). However, the effect of chain length on the efficiency of these compounds to prevent LDL oxidation has not been fully investigated. Steinberg et al. (2002) tested cocoa flavan-3-ols (catechin, epicatechin and oligomeric procyanidins) for their ability to decrease LDL oxidative susceptibility and spare α-tocopherol *in vitro*. Although procyanidins decreased LDL oxidative susceptibility with increasing chain length, it inhibited LDL oxidation to a similar extent when based on equivalent amounts of monomeric units. This suggested that the antioxidant activity of procyanidins with biological substrates is not attributable to chain length or charge delocalization through polymeric linkages, but primarily on ring structures and catechol groups (Steinberg et al., 2002). Procyanidin dimers were detected in plasma concordant with the appearance of monomeric flavanols at 2 h following consumption. Research carried out by Steinberg et al. (2002) confirmed the presence of procyanidins in human plasma, and extends previous structure–function observations regarding flavonoid protection of LDL.

A few studies suggest that long-term consumption of cocoa polyphenols also increases the antioxidative capacity of plasma and inhibits LDL oxidation *ex vivo* (Osakabe et al., 2001; Wan et al., 2001). However, studies dealing with the effects of long-term consumption of chocolate on lipid peroxidation *in vivo* are scarce (Mathur et al., 2002; Mursu et al., 2004). Mathur et al. (2002) demonstrated in human subjects that cocoa products affected LDL oxidizability, but not urinary F2 isoprostanes or markers of inflammation. The authors attributed the lack of effects on biomarkers of inflammation and F2 isoprostanes to the short biological half-life of flavonoids from cocoa products. Consequently, this result may indicate a decreased risk of CVD when changes in susceptibility and extent of LDL oxidation are implicated as important causative factors. Similarly, Mursu et al. (2004) studied the effects of long-term ingestion of chocolate, with differing amounts of polyphenols, on serum lipids and lipid peroxidation *ex vivo* and *in vivo* (45 nonsmoking, healthy volunteers). The concentration of serum LDL diene conjugates, a marker of lipid peroxidation *in vivo*, decreased 11.9% in all study groups. No changes were seen in the total antioxidant capacity of plasma, in the oxidation susceptibility of serum lipids or in the concentration of plasma F2-isoprostanes or hydroxy fatty acids. Mursu et al. (2004) concluded that cocoa polyphenols may increase the concentration of HDL cholesterol, while chocolate fatty acids may modify the fatty acid composition of LDL and make it more resistant to oxidative damage.

11.6 EFFECTS OF COCOA FLAVANOLS ON LIPID METABOLISM AND ATHEROSCLEROSIS

Alterations in plasma cholesterol concentration, especially increased levels of LDL cholesterol and decreased levels of HDL cholesterol, are associated with the development of atherosclerosis (Stamler et al., 1986; Shepherd et al., 1995) and CVD. Reductions in LDL cholesterol plasma levels have been reported after treatment with polyphenols from different sources (Ikeda et al., 1992; Wilcox et al., 2001; Borradaile et al., 2002; Pal et al., 2003). Regarding the action of cocoa, mild hypercholesterolemic subjects lowered significantly (~5%) their LDL cholesterol level after 4 weeks of a dietary intervention with cocoa powder (81–163 mg/day of (−)-epicatechin (EC) + (+)-catechin (CT)) (Baba et al., 2007). Even in normo-cholesterolemic young subjects, a 15% reduction was observed in LDL cholesterol level after 14 days of a daily consumption of 105 g of flavanol-containing milk chocolate (168 mg of flavanols) (Fraga et al., 2005). Patients with essential hypertension showed an 11% decrease in LDL cholesterol after 15 days of receiving 100 g/day dark chocolate (88 mg of flavanols) (Grassi et al., 2005). Under an equivalent protocol, similar results were observed in patients with glucose-intolerant hypertension (27.5%) (Grassi et al., 2008).

Although the above studies did not investigate potential mechanisms, other researches have proposed that the decrease in LDL cholesterol was associated with flavonoids consumption from different sources include (1) inhibition of cholesterol absorption in the digestive tract (Ikeda et al., 1992), (2) inhibition of LDL biosynthesis in the liver (Wilcox et al., 2001), (3) suppression of the hepatic secretion of apolipoprotein B100 (Borradaile et al., 2002), and/or (4) increased expression of LDL receptors in the liver (Pal et al., 2003). All these mechanisms were attributed to interactions between flavanols and membranes, as whole structures, or with particular lipids or proteins. An increase in HDL cholesterol was also demonstrated in normo-cholesterolemic and mildly hypercholesterolemic subjects after dark chocolate or cocoa powder supplementation (Mursu et al., 2004; Baba et al., 2007). The mechanisms responsible for these effects on HDL cholesterol, however, remain unclear. It is generally accepted that oxidized LDL has a role in the development of atherosclerosis (Steinberg et al., 1989). A large number of studies in animals and humans showed that isolated LDLs were more resistant to *in vitro* oxidation after the consumption of cocoa products (Kondo et al., 1996; Rein et al., 2000; Osakabe et al., 2001; Wan et al., 2001; Mathur et al., 2002; Baba et al., 2007). One particular study showed a decrease in plasma levels of oxidized LDL plasma levels after dietary cocoa powder supplementation (Baba et al., 2007). All these studies suggest a role for cocoa components in the *in vivo* protection of LDL. These effects have been mostly ascribed to the scavenging of oxidants formed in the surface of the LDL and to the chelation of metals that are catalysts for free radical formation. However, they could also be the result of changes in the LDL surface rendering LDL less susceptible to oxidation.

Kurlandsky and Stote (2006) reported that consumption of chocolate and almonds for 6 weeks led to favorable dietary changes and showed no harmful effects on healthy women's weights, serum lipids, and inflammatory markers. The beneficial effects of chocolate consumption on circulating intercellular adhesion molecule (an important inflammatory marker) levels and serum triacylglycerols warranted further investigation using a larger sample size.

As for the effect of cocoa products on serum lipid levels, there is a dearth of information on this subject. Several investigators reported increased HDL cholesterol levels in healthy humans consuming dark chocolate (Wan et al., 2001; Mursu et al., 2004). In diabetic rats, with enhanced serum TG and cholesterol concentrations, intake of a cocoa extract also increased HDL cholesterol and decreased TG and total and LDL cholesterol concentrations (Ruzaidi et al., 2005). This is in agreement with the observed effects elicited by cocoa fiber in an animal model of dietary-induced hyperlipidemia investigated by Lecumberri et al. (2007).

Other favorable effects of cocoa have been reported including antibacterial effects (Sato et al., 1999), neutralization of lipopolysaccharides (Ono et al., 2003), improvements in bowel movement and reduction of stool odor (Mato et al., 1999), enhancement of wound healing (Inokuchi, 2002), and mitigation of peripheral intolerance to cold (Kamei et al., 2003). While studying these effects, these authors found that visceral adipose tissue weight tended to be lower in rats fed a cocoa-containing diet compared to those fed a cocoa-free diet. Matsui et al. (2005) postulated a mechanism for the antiobesity effects of cocoa in which ingestion effectively prevented TG accumulation by modulating lipid metabolism. Further studies are needed to elucidate the molecular mechanisms underlying such effects.

11.7 EFFECTS OF COCOA FLAVANOLS ON CORONARY CIRCULATION

Although dark chocolate consumption has been reported to improve endothelium-dependent flow-mediated dilation (FMD) of the brachial artery (Vlachopoulos et al., 2005), no reports have directly proved the acute effects of the oral intake of flavonoid-rich dark chocolate on coronary circulation. Recently, Shiina et al. (2009) assessed the effects of the oral intake of flavonoid-rich dark chocolate on coronary circulation by measuring coronary flow velocity reserve by noninvasive transthoracic Doppler echocardiography in healthy adult subjects. Their results indicated that flavonoid-rich dark chocolate intake significantly improved coronary circulation in healthy adults, independent of changes in oxidative stress parameters, BP and lipid profile, whereas nonflavonoid white chocolate had no such effects. However, this study had some limitations as the authors measured coronary flow velocity not coronary flow volume, while changes in the coronary diameter were not assessed. However, it has been reported that changes in coronary flow velocities during drug-induced hyperemia closely reflect changes in coronary blood flow (Wilson et al., 1985).

While a diet rich in antioxidants has been favorably associated with coronary disease and hypertension, limited data are available on the influence of such diet on subclinical disease. It was previously shown that the extent of calcified atherosclerotic plaque in the coronary arteries (CAC) was highly correlated with total burden of atherosclerotic plaques (Sangiorgi et al., 1998; Rumberger et al., 1995). The degree of CAC, measured by cardiac CT, provides more prognostic information on CHD incidence (Haberl et al., 2001; Park et al., 2002; Greenland et al., 2004) and CHD mortality (Shaw et al., 2003; Raggi et al., 2004). Djoussé et al. (2011) recently examined whether chocolate consumption was associated with CAC. In this study, the authors demonstrated that chocolate consumption was inversely associated with the prevalence of CAC in a dose–response manner. Calcium deposition in the arterial walls occurs in the early stages of atherosclerosis just after fatty streak formation (Wexler et al., 1996) and has been shown to correlate closely with the total burden of atheroma (Rumberger et al., 1995; Sangiorgi et al., 1998). In sensitivity analyses, Djoussé et al. (2011) observed an inverse association between chocolate intake and CAC using Agatston scores other than 0 to define the prevalence of CAC. It is likely that with a lower Agatston score cut point such as 0, cardiac CT might not have been able to accurately discriminate the presence or absence of clinically relevant CAC.

11.8   EFFECTS OF COCOA FLAVANOLS ON ENDOTHELIAL FUNCTION

The vascular endothelium regulates hemostasis through maintenance of vasomotor tone and through its influence on platelet function and leukocyte adherence. Under normal physiological conditions, several mediators are released from the endothelium, such as endothelin, prostacylin, leukotrienes, NO, and adenosine (Becker et al., 2000). Impaired arterial EF has been shown to be a significant early event in atherogenesis and has been associated with an increased cardiovascular risk. Shear stress, ischemia and reperfusion, inflammation, and disease states, such as atherosclerosis, diabetes mellitus, and hypertension, can disrupt EF, which is associated with alterations in endothelium-derived regulatory mediators, an inability to regulate vascular tone, and an overall shift toward the prothrombotic state. As a result, a dysfunctional endothelium may lose its protective effects on the vascular system with reduced antiatherosclerotic and antithrombotic activities (Perticone et al., 2001). It is possible that flavanols, by functioning as antioxidants in addition to modulating prostacylin and leukotriene concentrations (Schramm et al., 2001), can improve EF through the prevention and possible reduction of oxidative damage. However, other mechanisms involved are yet to be elucidated.

The evaluation of EF can be done by observing the degree of FMD. FMD is dependent predominantly on NO release by the endothelium. Therefore, reduced bioactivity of NO and impaired FMD can be used to estimate endothelial dysfunction. Data obtained from studies evaluating the acute consumption of dark chocolate by healthy volunteers have shown the acute dilatation of muscular arteries and a decreased wave deflection (an indication of increased arterial elasticity) (Vlachopoulos et al., 2005). Studies by Schroeter et al. (2006) showed that the peak in plasma epicatechin concentration 2 h after flavanol-rich cocoa consumption paralleled an improvement in vascular function in humans. These investigators confirmed their results by demonstrating the complete reversal of the effects *in vivo* and *ex vivo* after NO synthase (NOS) inhibition. These findings were extended to other *in vivo* studies with healthy humans (Bayard et al., 2007). Fisher et al. (2003) showed that cocoa-induced vasodilatation was achieved via an NO-dependent mechanism by abolishing vasodilatation completely with intravenous administration of L-NAME (an inhibitor of NOS). The aforementioned vascular effects were further supported by Heiss et al. (2005)

in a study on a population in which smoking was the only cardiovascular risk factor. They found an increase in the circulating NO pool in plasma and FMD response by approximately 50% after acute consumption of a flavanol-rich cocoa beverage. In addition, a more recent study found that the vascular effects occurred in a sustained (up to 7 days) and dose-dependent manner (Heiss et al., 2007).

While evidence indicates that cocoa improves EF, it is possible that sugar may adversely affect cardiovascular risk by increasing blood glucose, lipid levels, and body weight (Hermann et al., 2006). In fact, one study reported impairment of EF with acute glucose loading (Akbari et al., 1998). The effects of daily intake of sugar-free and sugar-sweetened cocoa beverages on EF are yet to be established. A more recent study by Njike et al. (2009) found that cocoa ingestion improved EF measured as FMD compared to placebo. The magnitude of improvement in FMD after consumption of sugar-free versus sugar-sweetened cocoa was greater, but not significant. Other biomarkers of cardiac risk did not change appreciably from baseline while BMI remained stable throughout the study. The authors suggested that daily cocoa ingestion improved EF independently of other biomarkers of cardiac risk, and did not cause weight gain. Sugar-free preparations may further augment EF. This trial suggested, but did not conclusively establish, that the cardioprotective influence of cocoa ingestion was attenuated by the sugar content of cocoa-containing beverages, and accentuated by the removal of sugar.

11.9 COCOA FLAVANOLS AND ANTIHYPERTENSIVE EFFECTS

Studies conducted by Grassi et al. (2005) on healthy subjects and later on hypertensive subjects showed the possible benefits of cocoa in lowering BP. In both studies, 24 h ambulatory BP levels decreased while insulin sensitivity improved in healthy and hypertensive volunteers after the acute intake of dark, but not white chocolate. There is also some experimental evidence that flavanol-rich foods reduced angiotensin-converting enzyme (ACE) activity. In vitro studies have demonstrated ACE inhibition by flavanol-rich foods (Actis-Goretta et al., 2006). However, the presence of ACE inhibition needs to be determined in vivo as no studies have been conducted on the effect of cocoa flavanols on ACE activity.

Studies have also examined the effects of flavanols in cocoa products on morbidity and mortality. In a cohort study, the Zutphen Elderly Study, cocoa intake was inversely related to BP levels and 15-year cardiovascular and all-cause mortality (Buijsse et al., 2006). The findings of a meta-analysis of five randomized, small, short-term, controlled trials suggested that consumption of foods rich in cocoa may reduce BP in contrast to tea, which had no effect (Taubert et al., 2007a,b). The magnitude of the hypotensive effects of cocoa were comparable to that observed with a β-blocker or ACE inhibitor monotherapy.

Desch et al. (2010) recently performed a meta-analysis of randomized controlled trials assessing the antihypertensive effects of flavanol-rich cocoa products. The primary outcome measure was the change in systolic and diastolic BP between intervention and control groups. The principal finding of this meta-analysis of randomized clinical trials was the antihypertensive effects of cocoa products such as dark chocolate and cocoa beverages, which resulted in a decrease of 4.5 mmHg in systolic and 2.5 mmHg in diastolic BP. The precise mechanisms responsible for the presumed BP-lowering effect of cocoa-containing foods are not fully understood. However, an increase in vasodilating NO bioavailability possibly caused, in part, by an enhanced NOS activity is considered a likely pathway (Fisher et al., 2003; Heiss et al., 2003, 2005; Taubert et al., 2007a,b). Other mechanisms such as the inhibition of ACE activity by flavanols (Actis-Goretta et al., 2006) or theobromine (Kelly, 2005) may also contribute to the antihypertensive effect. The meta-analysis conducted by Desch et al. (2010) confirms the BP-lowering capacity of flavanol-rich cocoa products. However, several questions such as the most appropriate dose and the long-term side-effect profile remain to be answered before cocoa products can be recommended as a treatment option for hypertension. A large-scale, well-controlled trial preferably with clinical end points appears warranted.

The effect of habitual cocoa consumption on arterial stiffness and wave reflection indexes, as well as on peripheral and central BP, was assessed in 198 healthy subjects by Vlachopoulos et al. (2007). These authors concluded that a higher cocoa intake was an independent determinant of low arterial stiffness and wave reflection indexes and was also independently associated with significantly lower central (aortic) pulse pressure.

Accumulating evidence from long-term follow-up studies showed that women with a history of preeclampsia faced an increased risk of developing chronic hypertension, insulin resistance, and lipid abnormalities later in life (Irgens et al., 2001; Wilson et al., 2003; Lykke et al., 2009). Chocolate consumption is associated with favorable levels of BP and other CVD risk markers. To date, two published studies in which the authors used theobromine as a biomarker of chocolate intake have tested this hypothesis but reported conflicting findings (Triche et al., 2008; Klebanoff et al., 2009). Triche et al. (2008) found that regular chocolate consumption and greater levels of theobromine in cord blood had a protective effect against preeclampsia. In contrast, Klebanoff et al. (2009) observed no protective effect of increased theobromine in maternal serum collected after 26 weeks, but did not assess dietary chocolate consumption. Recently, Saftlas et al. (2010) analyzed a prospective cohort study to determine whether regular chocolate intake during pregnancy is associated with reduced risks of preeclampsia and gestational hypertension (GH). Their results indicated that chocolate intake was more frequent among normotensive (80.7%) than preeclamptic (62.5%) or GH women (75.8%), and associated with reduced odds of preeclampsia. These findings provide additional evidence for the benefits of chocolate. However, prospective studies are needed to confirm and delineate protective effects of chocolate intake on the risk of preeclampsia.

11.10   EFFECTS OF COCOA FLAVANOLS ON PLATELETS AGGREGATION

Thromboxanes (Tx) derived from the arachidonic acid metabolism are greatly involved at different levels in the inflammatory pathogenesis of atherosclerosis and coronary artery disease (CAD) through vascular changes (Homaidan et al., 2002). Platelet aggregation starts when the damaged endothelium becomes exposed to circulating platelets, which adhere to the matrix and secrete adenosine diphosphate (ADP) and Tx. This initiates the thrombosis cascade with erythrocytes and lymphocytes (Cooper et al., 2008). Platelet activation also contributes to the development of the atherosclerotic plaque and is currently being evaluated as a promising therapeutic target (Lindemann et al., 2007).

The effects of flavanol-rich cocoa on platelet activation and function in healthy human subjects have been extensively documented. Pearson and Holt (2008) demonstrated that the consumption of flavanol-rich cocoa products inhibited epinephrine- and ADP-induced expression of specific glycoproteins and selectins thus reducing platelet activation. The inhibitory effect ensued 6 h after consumption (Rein et al., 2000a) induced mainly by trimers and pentamers of flavanols (Rein et al., 2000b) and paralleled by coronary artery diameter increase (Flammer et al., 2007). In addition, Howard et al. (1988) demonstrated that acute exposure to flavanol-rich cocoa could also modulate the formation of platelet microparticles as markers of platelet activation. Long-term cocoa supplementation was shown to reduce platelet aggregation (Murphy et al., 2003) to a degree comparable to acetylsalicylic acid (Pearson et al., 2002) while platelet clotting function was significantly increased also with casual cocoa intake (Bordeaux et al., 2007). However, cocoa flavanols failed to show an additive effect in human subjects when combined with acetylsalicylic acid (Heptinstall et al., 2006) and was more prominent in subjects with an active lifestyle compared to sedentary controls (Singh et al., 2006).

Several antiplatelet strategies have been developed to prevent secondary events because of the major role of platelets in the development and manifestation of AMI, stroke, and venous thromboembolism. Cocoa was shown to reduce ADP/collagen- and adrenaline/collagen-activated, platelet-related, primary hemostasis within hours after subjects consumed high (897 mg) or moderate (220 mg) amounts of cocoa flavanols (Rein et al., 2000; Holt et al., 2002; Pearson et al., 2002). These antiaggregatory effects observed with cocoa were shown to be attributable, in part, to a reduction in the ADP- and adrenaline-induced expression of the activated conformation of the GPIIa/IIIb surface protein (Rein et al., 2000; Pearson et al., 2002). In addition, cocoa was able to reduce GPIIa/IIIb expression to an extent that was only slightly less than that achieved with low-dose aspirin (81 mg) (Pearson et al., 2002). The effects observed in these short-term studies were extended to a 4-week study, during which subjects consumed moderate amounts of cocoa flavanols. As a result, decreases in P-selectin expression, ADP-induced platelet aggregation, and platelet volume (marker of lowered activation status) were observed (Murphy et al., 2003).

It is possible that flavanols may mediate their activity through antioxidant and NO-related mechanisms, and such mechanisms can be implicated in platelet function. Superoxide anion is known to enhance platelet aggregation and can bind to NO to form peroxynitrite. Freedman et al. (2001) observed that purple grape juice consumption reduced platelet superoxide release, with a corresponding increase in platelet NO production and a reduction in platelet aggregation. In addition, catechin was shown to reduce platelet aggregation and hydrogen peroxide production *in vitro* (Pignatelli et al., 2000). These studies suggest that flavanols may exert their antioxidant effects through their well-described antioxidant activities, although it should be emphasized that flavanols may act through nonantioxidant mechanisms. For example, purple grape juice has been reported to reduce platelet protein kinase C activity (Freedman et al., 2001), whereas dimer B2 has been shown to inhibit platelet Tx production (Chang and Hsu, 1989). In addition, cocoa flavanols and procyanidins have been reported to inhibit human platelet 12- lipoxygenase (Schewe et al., 2001) and 5-lipoxygenase (Schewe et al., 2002). Inhibition of 5- and 12-lipoxygenase could partly explain the observations by Schramm et al. (2001) and Holt et al. (2002) that the ratio of plasma prostacyclin and leukotriene concentrations increased among human subjects after the consumption of flavanol-rich chocolate.

11.11   COCOA FLAVANOLS AND NO-BASED MECHANISMS

Recent studies indicate that one of the principal mechanisms of action responsible for the reduced risk of vascular disease associated with the consumption of diets rich in cocoa and its flavanols is the regulation of NO in the blood stream (Wallace et al., 2009). NO has multiple roles in the regulation of the cardiovascular system. The differences in their functional effects and the subcellular impact of different NOS (NOS) isoforms are attributed to their mode of actions in a constitutive (endothelial NOS) or inducible fashion (Andrew and Mayer, 1999; Li and Forstermann, 2000). However, the effect of the neuronal form NOS remains poorly understood in cardiovascular health. Huang et al. (1995) postulated that NO is a potent vasodilator and maintains vascular tone, as shown in animal models lacking specific NOS isoforms. Further, endothelium-derived NO also counteracts leukocyte recruitment and platelet aggregation to the site of inflammation (Kubes et al., 1991; Achike and Kwan, 2003), thus exerting a significant anti-inflammatory effect while the attracted leukocytes stimulate local NO production (Achike and Kwan, 2003). NO is critical in determining the oxidative stress in several conditions by reacting with the superoxide to produce more reactive oxygen species. Further, studies by Mann et al. (2007) indicated that NO and reactive oxygen species may mediate the flavanol-induced activation of the antioxidant response element-driven transcription of phase II detoxifying and antioxidant defense enzymes in the endothelium.

The multiple effects of cocoa flavanols on NO-mediated pathways are sometimes inferred from the observed endothelial changes in which their impact was assessed from the circulating levels of nitrosylated species and taken as a marker of EF (Balzer et al., 2006). Heiss et al. (2003) investigated the effects of a single dose of a cocoa-rich drink in human subjects and the results indicated a significant amelioration of the endothelial dysfunction in patients with at least one cardiovascular risk factor. On the other hand, longer periods of supplementation led to significant lowering of BP. Previously, a longer cocoa supplementation resulted in similar observations and further demonstrated that the effects were mediated by NO (Fisher et al., 2003). From an epidemiological standpoint, data from a study by Bayard et al. (2007) in San Blas, Panama, suggested that the high cocoa intake in this population might lead to significantly reduced incidence rates for cardiovascular and neoplastic diseases. Karim et al. (2000) suggested that larger flavanol molecules appear to be more active in this scenario compared to smaller ones. When the NO-based oxidative stress changes were utilized as endpoints, flavanols elicited a significant benefit in an experimental model mainly by enhancing the antioxidant mechanisms (Arteel and Sies, 1999; Arteel et al., 2000; Klotz and Sies, 2003). In this later evidence, however, tetramers appeared to be the most active flavanol molecules. Finally, it is noteworthy that macrophages challenged by bacterial stimuli produced lower amounts of NO in the presence of cocoa extract (Ono et al., 2003). The mechanisms of flavanol action on NO-mediated pathways appear to be mediated by NADPH in the case of mono-O-methylated flavanols (Steffen et al., 2008).

11.12   COCOA FLAVANOLS AND INSULIN RESISTANCE

Insulin sensitivity is partly dependent on insulin-mediated NO release (Zeng et al., 2000). Thus, flavanols and dietary antioxidants may decrease insulin resistance by ameliorating NO bioavailability. In line with this concept, Grassi et al. (2005) reported reduced insulin resistance in patients with essential hypertension after a 15-day diet with 100 g flavonoid-rich chocolate daily. Moreover, in hypertensive patients with impaired glucose tolerance, flavonoid-rich dark chocolate not only reduced BP and improved EF but also ameliorated insulin sensitivity and β-cell function (Grassi et al., 2005). As intravenous infusion of ascorbic acid improves not only FMD but also insulin sensitivity in subjects with impaired glucose tolerance and in smokers (Hirai et al., 2000), the antioxidant properties of flavanols might also contribute to these beneficial effects of cocoa on insulin sensitivity. However, because studies with cocoa in diabetics are scarce and because diabetics tend to be obese, recommending cocoa or flavonoid-rich chocolate consumption to such patients should be done cautiously. Nevertheless, experimental evidence in obese diabetic mice suggests that cocoa dose dependently prevents hyperglycemia (Tomaru et al., 2007).

11.13   OTHER COMPOUNDS OF COCOA AND CARDIOVASCULAR EFFECTS

Theobromine, the primary active ingredient in chocolate, is a methylxanthine that could alter cardiac conduction or inotropic state (Bender et al., 1997; Donnerstein et al., 1998; Vassallo and Lipsky, 1998). Baron et al. (1999) conducted a study to determine, via a double-blind, placebo controlled, randomized, crossover method, the hemodynamic and electrophysiologic effects of chocolate on the heart of young adults. Under an approved protocol, subjects, aged 21–33 years, without detectable heart disease were selected. The primary echocardiographic finding of this study is that chocolate, and hence, theobromine, does not cause any acute hemodynamic changes in the hearts of young adults. Theobromine is known to be considerably weaker than caffeine and theophylline, and has only 1/10th the cardiac effects of the other methylxanthines (Horton, 1993). This report possibly offers an explanation for the hemodynamic trends seen in this study. Since caffeine was shown to increase cardiac contractility significantly, it can be theorized that because theobromine is only 1/10th as effective, its inotropic effects would likewise be approximately 1/10 that of caffeine. Hence, the upward trends seen in the velocity of circumferential fiber shortening corrected for heart rate, shortening fraction, and left ventricular posterior wall thickening immediately after chocolate ingestion did not reach the same level of effect shown in a previous caffeine study.

Chocolate has methylxanthine alkaloids theobromine and caffeine (Smit and Blackburn, 2005). Caffeine is a methylxanthine whose primary biological effect is the competitive antagonism of the adenosine receptor (Chou and Benowitz, 1994). Normal consumption of caffeine was not associated with risk of atrial fibrillation or flutter (Frost and Vestergaard, 2005). Patanè et al. (2010) presented a case of atrial fibrillation associated with chocolate intake abuse in a 19-year-old Italian woman with chronic salbutamol inhalation abuse. This case focused attention on chocolate intake abuse associated with chronic salbutamol abuse as the substrate for atrial fibrillation.

Theobromine, 3,7 dimethylxanthine is a purine-derived alkaloid that is widely consumed in cocoa beverages (Eteng et al., 1997). There has been considerable interest in the possible beneficial or adverse effects of theobromine consumption on human health. For instance, theobromine at the therapeutic dose of 500 mg/kg has been used in the treatment of cardiac edema and angina pectoralis, and its analogs pentoxyfylline, suramin-theobromine, and lisophylline are currently being exploited in cancer chemotherapy (Chang et al., 1993; Gil et al., 1993; Clark et al., 1996). However, sudden death in laboratory animals exposed to cocoa-based meals containing moderate-to-high amounts of theobromine has been attributed to cardiac failure (Soffietti et al., 1989). Although there appears to be no direct link between theobromine and hypercholesterolemia, it is well known that an elevated blood lipid, particularly hypercholesterolemia, is a risk factor for heart failure. The effects of theobromine and an extract of cocoa seeds on lipid parameters were compared in rats (Eteng and Ettarh, 2000). Theobromine (700 mg/kg) and cocoa extract were administered orally on four consecutive days and serum obtained for lipid analysis. The results suggest that the hypercholesterolemic effect observed with cocoa extract is not due to the alkaloid theobromine but may rather be caused by some other constituent of the extract.

11.14   SUMMARY AND CONCLUSION

Epidemiological studies reported an inverse relationship between polyphenol-rich cocoa and reduced risk of CVD. Data from most recent investigations confirms that cocoa flavanols and procyanidins have the ability to act as *in vivo* antioxidants. The cocoa flavanols provide cardiovascular protection by affecting numerous intracellular signaling cascades and thereby influencing the cardiovascular system by enhancing vascular function and decreasing platelet reactivity. Significantly, *in vitro* studies with highly purified flavanols and procyanidins support the hypothesis that many of the biological effects observed with flavonoid-rich foods can be directly attributed to the flavonoids. There is only limited information on the intracellular metabolism of these compounds and on the bioactivity of the different metabolites. Although several short-term clinical trials have been reported, the health effects of cocoa flavanols will best be determined by long-term, randomized, and clinical trials. Further rigorous, prospective studies are needed. These should involve large patient populations with outcomes of cocoa intervention that include not only CVD biomarkers, but also metabolic endpoints. In addition, comparative human intervention studies should address the effects of chocolate and cocoa powder versus purified cocoa flavanols, and any potential synergistic actions with other nutrients or medications.

REFERENCES

Abd El Mohsen, M. M., Kuhnle, G., Rechner, A. R., Schroeter, H., Rose, S., Jenner, P., and Rice-Evans, C. A. 2002. Uptake and metabolism of epicatechin and its access to the brain after oral ingestion. *Free Radic. Biol. Med.* **33**: 1693–1702.

Achike, F. I. and Kwan, C. Y. 2003. Nitric oxide, human diseases and the herbal products that affect the nitric oxide signalling pathway. *Clin. Exp. Pharmacol. Physiol.* **30**: 605–615.

Actis-Goretta, L., Ottaviani, J. I., and Fraga, C. G. 2006. Inhibition of angiotensin converting enzyme activity by flavanol-rich foods. *J. Agric. Food Chem.* **54**: 229–234.

Akbari, C. M., Saouaf, R., Barnhill, D. F., Newman, P. A., LoGerfo, F. W., and Veves, A. 1998. Endotheliumdependent vasodilatation is impaired in both microcirculation and macrocirculation during acute hyperglycemia. *J. Vasc. Surg.* **28**: 687–694.

Andrew, P. J. and Mayer, B. 1999. Enzymatic function of nitric oxide synthases. *Cardiovasc. Res.* **43**: 521–531.

Arteel, G. E., Schroeder, P., and Sies, H. 2000. Reactions of peroxynitrite with cocoa procyanidin oligomers. *J. Nutr.* **130**: 2100S–2104S.

Arteel, G. E. and Sies, H. 1999. Protection against peroxynitrite by cocoa polyphenol oligomers. *FEBS Lett.* **462**: 167–170.

Baba, S., Natsume, M., Yasuda, A., Nakamura, Y., Tamura, T., Osakabe, N., Kanegae, N., and Kondo, K. 2007. Plasma LDL and HDL cholesterol and oxidized LDL concentrations are altered in normo- and hypercholesterolemic humans after intake of different levels of cocoa powder. *J. Nutr.* **137**: 1436–1441.

Baba, S., Osakabe, N., Kato, Y., Natsume, M., Yasuda, A., Kido, T., Fukuda, K., Muto, Y., and Kondo, K. 2007. Continuous intake of polyphenolic compounds containing cocoa powder reduces LDL oxidative susceptibility and has beneficial effects on plasma HDL-cholesterol concentrations in humans. *Am. J. Clin. Nutr.* **85**: 709–717.

Baba, S., Osakabe, N., Natsume, M., and Terao J. 2002. Absorption and urinary excretion of procyanidin B2 [epicatechin-(4β-8)-epicatechin] in rats. *Free Radic. Biol. Med.* **33**: 142–148.

Baba, S., Osakabe, N., Yasuda, A., Natsume, M., Takizawa, T., Nakamura, T., and Terao, J. 2000. Bioavailability of (_)-epicatechin upon intake of chocolate and cocoa in human volunteers. *Free Radic Res.* **33**: 635–641.

Balzer, J., Heiss, C., Schroeter, H., Brouzos, P., Kleinbongard, P., Matern, S., Lauer, T., Rassaf, T., and Kelm, M. 2006. Flavanols and cardiovascular health: Effects on the circulating NO pool in humans. *J. Cardiovasc. Pharmacol.* **47**(Suppl. 2): S122–S127; discussion S172–S126.

Baron, A. M., Donnerstein, R. L., Samson, R. A., Baron, J. A., Padnick, J. N., and Goldberg, S. J. 1999. Hemodynamic and electrophysiologic effects of acute chocolate ingestion in young adults. *Am. J. Cardiol.* **84**: 370–373.

Bayard, V., Chamorro, F., Motta, J., and Hollenberg, N. K. 2007. Does flavanol intake influence mortality from nitric oxide-dependent processes? Ischemic heart disease, stroke, diabetes mellitus, and cancer in Panama. *Int. J. Med. Sci.* **4**: 53–58.

Becker, B., Heindl, B., Kupatt, C., and Zahler, S. 2000. Endothelial function and hemostasis. *Z. Kardiol.* **89**: 160–167.

Bender, A. M., Donnerstein, R. L., Samson, R. A., Zhu, D., and Goldberg, S. J. 1997 Hemodynamic effects of acute caffeine ingestion in young adults. *Am. J. Cardiol.* **79**: 696–699.

Borchers, A. T., Keen, C. L., Hannum, S. M., and Gershwin, M. E. 2000. Cocoa and chocolate: Composition, bioavailability, and health implications. *J. Med. Food.* **3**: 77–105.

Bordeaux, B., Yanek, L. R., Moy, T. F., White, L. W., Becker, L. C., Faraday, N., and Becker, D. M. 2007. Casual chocolate consumption and inhibition of platelet function. *Prev. Cardiol.* **10**: 175–180.

Borradaile, N. M., de Dreu, L. E., Wilcox, L. J., Edwards, J. Y., and Huff, M. W. 2002. Soya phytoestrogens, genistein and daidzein, decrease apolipoprotein B secretion from HepG2 cells through multiple mechanisms. *Biochem. J.* **366**: 531–539.

Bravo L. 1998. Polyphenols: Chemistry, dietary sources, metabolism and nutritional significance. *Nutr Rev.* **56**: 317–333.

Buijsse, B., Feskens, E. J., Kok, F. J., and Krumhout, D. 2006. Cocoa intake, blood pressure, and cardiovascular mortality: The Zutphen Elderly Study. *Arch. Intern. Med.* **166**: 411–417.

Cayatte, A. J., Rupin, A., Oliver-Krasinsi, J., Maitland, K., Sansilvestri-Morel, P., Boussard, M. F., Wierzbicki, M., Verbeuren, T. J., and Cohen, R. A. 2001. S17834, a new inhibitor of cell adhesion and atherosclerosis that targets NADPH- oxidase. *Arterioscler. Thromb. Vasc.* Biol. **21**: 1577–1584.

Chang, C. C., Chang, T. C., Kao, S. C., Kuo, Y. F., and Chien, C. F. 1993. Pentoxyfylline inhibits the proliferation and glycosaminoglycan synthesis of cultured fibroblasts derived from patients with Grave's ophthalmopathy and pretibial myoedema. *Acta Endocrinol. Copehn.* **129**: 322–327.

Chang, W.-C. and Hsu, F.-L.1989. Inhibition of platelet aggregation and arachidonate metabolism in platelets by procyanidins. *Prostaglandins Leukot. Essent. Fatty Acids* **38**: 181–188.

Chen, Y. T., Zheng, R. L., Jia, Z. J., and Ju, Y. 1990. Flavonoids as superoxide scavengers and antioxidants. *Free Radic. Biol. Med.* **9**: 19–21.

Cheng, Z. and Li, Y. 2007. What is responsible for the initiating chemistry of iron-mediated lipid peroxidation: An update. *Chem. Rev.* **107**: 748–766.

Chou, T. M. and Benowitz, N. L.1994. Caffeine and coffee: Effects on health and cardiovascular disease. *Comp. Biochem. Physiol. C Pharmacol. Toxicol. Endocrinol.* **109**(2): 173–189.

Clark, E., Rice, G. C., Weeks, R. S., Jenkins, N., Nelson, R., Bianco, J. A., and Singer, J. W. 1996. Lisofylline inhibits transforming growth factor beta release and enhances trilineage hematopoietic recovery after 5-fluorouracil. *Cancer Res. J.* **56**(1): 105–112.

Coady, S. A., Sorlie, P. D., Cooper, L. S., Folsom, A. R., Rosamond, W. D., and Conwill, D. E. 2001. Validation of death certificate diagnosis for coronary heart disease: The Atherosclerosis Risk in Communities (ARIC) Study. *J. Clin. Epidemiol.* **54**: 40–50.

Cooper, K. A., Donovan, J. L., Waterhouse, A. L., and Williamson, G. 2008. Cocoa and health: A decade of research. *Br. J. Nutr.* **99**: 1–11.

Corti, R., Flammer, A. J., Hollenberg, N. K., and Lüscher, T. F. 2009. Cocoa and cardiovascular health. *Circulation* **119**: 1433–1441.

Desch, S., Kobler, D., and Schmidt, J., 2010. Low vs. higher-dose dark chocolate and blood pressure in cardiovascular high-risk patients. *Am. J. Hypertension.* **23**(6): 694–700.

Dillinger, T. L. P., Barriga, S., Escarcega, M., Jimenez, D. S., Lowe, L. E., and Grivetti, J. 2000. Foods for the Gods: Cure for humanity? A cultural history of the medicinal and ritual use of chocolate. *Nutr.* **130**: 2057S–2072S.

Ding, E. L., Hutfless, S. M., Ding, X., and Girotra, S. 2006. Chocolate and prevention of cardiovascular disease: A systematic review. *Nutr. Metab.* **3**(2006): 2.

Djoussé, L., Hopkins, P. N., Arnett, D. K., Pankowe, J. S, Borecki, I., North, K. E., and Curtis Ellison, C. R. 2011. Chocolate consumption is inversely associated with calcified atherosclerotic plaque in the coronary arteries: The NHLBI Family Heart Study. *Clin. Nutr.* **30**: 38–43.

Donnerstein, R. L., Zhu, D., Samson, R. A., Bender, A. M., and Goldberg, S. J. 1998. Acute effects of caffeine ingestion on signal-averaged electrocardiograms. *Am. Heart J.* **136**: 643–646.

Donovan, J. L., Crespy, V., Manach, C., Morand, C., Besson, C., Scalbert, A., and Remesy, Y. 2001. Catechin is metabolized by both the small intestine and liver of rats. *J. Nutr.* **131**: 1753–1757.

Donovan, J. L., Kasim-Karakas, S., German, J. B., and Waterhouse, A. L. 2002. Urinary excretion of catechin metabolites by human subjects after red wine consumption. *Br. J. Nutr.* **87**: 31–37.

Duan, S., Li, Y. F., and Luo, X. L. 2000. Effect of puerarin on heart function and serum oxidized-LDL in the patients with chronic cardiac failure. *Hunan Yi Ke Da Xue Xue Bao* **25**: 176–178, abstract.

Eteng, M. U., Eyong, E. U., Akpanyung, E. O., Agiang, M. A., and Aremu, C. Y. 1997. Recent advances in caffeine and theobromine toxicities: A review. *Plant Foods Hum. Nutr.* **11**: 231–243.

Eteng, M. U. and Ettarh, R. R. 2000. Comparative effects of theobromine and cocoa extract on lipid profile in rats. *Nutr. Res.* **20**(10): 1513–1517.

Fisher, N. D., Hughes, M., Gerhard-Herman, M., and Hollenberg, N. K. 2003. Flavanol-rich cocoa induces nitric-oxide-dependent vasodilation in healthy humans. *J. Hypertens.* **221**: 2281–2286.

Flammer, A. J., Hermann, F., Sudano, I., Spieker, L., Hermann, M., Cooper, J. A., Serafini, M. et al. 2007. Dark chocolate improves coronary vasomotion and reduces platelet reactivity. *Circulation* **116**: 2376–2382.

Forsyth, W. G. C. and Quesnel, V. C. 1957. Cacao glycosidase and colour changes during fermentation. *J. Sci. Food Agric.* **8**: 505–509.

Forsyth, W. G. C. 1952. Cacao polyphenolic substances II. Changes during fermentation. *Biochem. J.* **51**: 516–520.

Fraga, C. G., Actis-Goretta, L., Ottaviani, J. I., Carrasquedo, F., Lotito, S. B., Lazarus, S., Schmitz, H. H., and Keen, C. L. 2005. Regular consumption of a flavanol-rich chocolate can improve oxidant stress in young soccer players. *Clin. Dev. Immunol.* **12**: 11–17.

Freedman, J. E., Parker, C. III., Liquing, L., Perlman, J. A., Frei, B., Ivanov, V., Deak, L. R., Iafrati, M. D., and Folts, J. D. 2001. Select flavonoids and whole juice from purple grapes inhibit platelet function and enhance nitric oxide release. *Circulation* **103**: 2792–2798.

Frost, L. and Vestergaard, P. 2005. Caffeine and risk of atrial fibrillation or flutter: The Danish Diet, Cancer, and Health Study. *Am. J. Clin. Nutr.* **81**(3): 578–582.

Fuhrman, B. and Aviram, M. 2001. Flavonoids protect LDL from oxidation and attenuate atherosclerosis. *Curr. Opin. Lipidol.* **12**: 41–48.

Geleijnse, J. M., Launer, L. J., Van der Kuip, D. A., Hofman, A., and Witteman, J. C., 2002. Inverse association of tea and flavonoid intakes with incident myocardial infarction: The Rotterdam study. *Am. J. Clin. Nutr.* **75**: 880–886.

Gil, M., Skopinska, R. E., Radomska, D., Demkon, U., Skurzak, H., Rochowska, M., Beauth, J., and Roszkowski, K. 1993. Effect of purinergic receptor antagonists, suramin and theobromine on tumour-induced angiogenesis in BALB/C mice. *Folia Biol.* (Praha) **39**(2): 63–68.

Gonthier, M.-P., Donovan, J. L., Texier, O., Felgines, C., Remesy, C., and Scalbert, A. 2003. Metabolism of dietary procyanidins in rats. *Free Radic. Biol. Med.* **35**: 837–844.

Grassi, D., Desideri, G., Necozione, S., Lippi, C., Casale, R., Properzi, G., Blumberg, J. B., and Ferri, C. 2008. Blood pressure is reduced and insulin sensitivity increased in glucose-intolerant, hypertensive subjects after 15 days of consuming high-polyphenol dark chocolate. *J. Nutr.* **138**: 1671–1676.

Grassi, D., Lippi, C., Necozione, S., Desideri, G., and Ferri, C. 2005. Short-term administration of dark chocolate is followed by a significant increase in insulin sensitivity and a decrease in blood pressure in healthy persons. *Am. J. Clin. Nutr.* **81**(3): 611–614.

Grassi, D., Aggio, A., Onori, L., Croce, G., Tiberti, S., Ferri, C., Ferri, L., and Desideri, G. 2008. Tea flavonoids and nitric-oxide mediated vascular activity. *J. Nutr.* **138**: 1554S–1560S.

Grassi, D., Desideri, G., Croce, G., Pasqualetti, P., Lippi, C., and Ferri, C. 2006. Cocoa and cardiovascular disease. The sweet heart connection. *Agro Food Ind. Hi-Tech.* **17**(1): XIII–XVI.

Grassi, D., Mulder, T. P., Draijer, R., Desideri, G., Molhuizen, H. O., and Ferri, C. 2009. Black tea consumption dose-dependently improves flow-mediated dilation in healthy men. *J. Hypertens.* **27**: 774–781.

Greenland, P., LaBree, L., Azen, S. P., Doherty, T. M., and Detrano, R. C. 2004. Coronary artery calcium score combined with Framingham score for risk prediction in asymptomatic individuals. *JAMA* **291**: 210e5.

Haberl, R., Becker, A., Leber, A., Knez, A., Becker, C., Lang, C., Bruning, R., Reiser, M., and Steinbeck, G. 2001. Correlation of coronary calcification and angiographically documented stenoses in patients with suspected coronary artery disease: Results of 1764 patients. *J. Am. Coll. Cardiol.* **37**: 451–457.

Halliwell, B. and Gutteridge, J. 1999. *Free Radicals in Biology and Medicine* (3rd edition). New York: Oxford University Press.

Hammerstone, J. F., Lazarus, S. A., and Schmitz, H. H. 2000. Procyanidin content and variation in some commonly consumed foods. *J. Nutr.* **130**: 2086S–2092S.

Hammerstone, J. F. and Lazurus, S. A. 2000. HPLC-MS analysis of flavonoids in foods and beverages. In *Caffeinated Beverages: Health Benefits, Physiological Effects, and Chemistry*, Parliament, T. H., Ho, C., and Schieberle, P. (eds). Washington, DC: Oxford University Press, pp. 374–384.

Harbone, J. B. 1989. *Methods in Plant Biochemistry: Plant Phenolics.* London: Academic Press.

Haslam, E. 1998. *Practical Polyphenolics: from Structure to Molecular Recognition and Physiological Action.* New York: Cambridge University Press.

Heiss, C., Dejam, A., Kleinbongard, P., Schewe, T., Sies, H., and Kelm, M. 2003. Vascular effects of cocoa rich in flavan-3-ols. *JAMA* **290**: 1030–1031.

Heiss, C., Finis, D., Kleinbongard, P., Hoffmann, A., Rassaf, T., Kelm, M., and Sies, H. 2007. Sustained increase in flow-mediated dilation after daily intake of high-flavanol cocoa drink over 1 week. *J. Cardiovasc. Pharmacol.* **49**: 74–80.

Heiss, C., Kleinbongard, P., Dejam, A., Perré, S., Schroeter, H., Sies, H., and Kelm, M. 2005. Acute consumption of flavanol-rich cocoa and the reversal of endothelial dysfunction in smokers. *J. Am. Coll. Cardiol.* **46**: 1276–1283.

Heptinstall, S., May, J., Fox, S., Kwik-Uribe, C., and Zhao, L. 2006. Cocoa flavanols and platelet and leukocyte function: Recent *in vitro* and *ex vivo* studies in healthy adults. *J. Cardiovasc. Pharmacol.* **47**(Suppl. 2): S197–S205.

Hermann, F., Spieker, L. E., Ruschitzka, F., Sudano, I., Hermann, M., Binggeli, C., Luscher, T. F., Riesen, W., Noll, G., and Corti, R. 2006. Dark chocolate improves endothelial and platelet function. *Heart* **92**: 119–120.

Hertog, M. G., Feskens, E. M., Hollman, P. C., Katan, M. B., and Kromhout, D. 1993. Dietary anitoxidant flavonoids and risk of coronary heart disease: The Zutphen Elderly Study. *Lancet* **342**: 1007–1011.

Hertog, M. G., Kromhout, D., Aravanis, C., Blackburn, H., Buzina, R., Fidanza, F., Gioampaoli, S. et al. 1995. Flavonoid intake and longterm risk of coronary heart disease and cancer in the Seven Countries Study. *Arch. Intern. Med.* **155**: 381–386.

Hirai, N., Kawano, H., Hirashima, O., Motoyama, T., Moriyama, Y., Sakamoto, T., Kugiyama, K., Ogawa, H., Nakao, K., and Yasue, H. 2000. Insulin resistance and endothelial dysfunction in smokers: Effects of vitamin C. *Am. J. Physiol. Heart Circ. Physiol.* **279**: H1172–H1178.

Holt, R. R., Lazarus, S. A., Sullards, M., Zhu, Q. Y., Schramm, D. D., Hammerstone, J. F., Fraga, C. G., Schmitz, H. H., and Keen, C. L. 2002. Procyanidin dimer B2 (epicatechin-(4β-8)-epicatechin) in human plasma after the consumption of a flavanol-rich cocoa. *Am. J. Clin. Nutr.* **76**: 798–804.

Holt, R. R., Schramm, D. D., Keen, C. L., Lazarus, S. A., and Schmitz, H. 2002. Flavonoid rich chocolate and platelet function. *JAMA* **287**: 2212–2213.

Homaidan, F. R., Chakroun, I., Haidar, H. A., and El-Sabban, M. E., 2002. Protein regulators of eicosanoid synthesis: Role of inflammation. *Curr. Protein Pept. Sci.* **3**: 467–484.

Horton, H. R. 1993. *Principles of Biochemistry.* Englewood Cliffs, NJ: Patterson Publishers.

Howard, M. A., Coghlan, M., David, R., and Pfueller, S. L. 1988. Coagulation activities of plasma microparticles. *Thromb. Res.* **50**: 145–156.

Huang, P. L. 2009. eNOS, metabolic syndrome and cardiovascular disease. *Trends Endocrinol. Metab.* **20**: 295–302.

Huang, P. L., Huang, Z., Mashimo, H., Bloch, K. D., Moskowitz, M. A., Bevan, J. A., and Fishman, M. C. 1995. Hypertension in mice lacking the gene for endothelial nitric oxide synthase. *Nature* **377**: 239–242.

Ikeda, I., Imasato, Y., Sasaki, E., Nakayama, M., Nagao, H., Takeo, T., Yayabe, F., and Sugano, F. 1992. Tea catechins decrease micellar solubility and intestinal absorption of cholesterol in rats. *Biochim. Biophys. Acta* **1127**: 141–146.

Inokuchi, K. 2002. Ingestion of cacao mass enhances wound healing of skin. In: The various effects of chocolate & cocoa. *Proceedings of the International Symposium of Chocolate & Cocoa Nutrition* (in Japanese). Tokyo: Chocolate & Cocoa Association of Japan. pp.196–199.

Irgens, H. U., Reisater, L., Irgens, L. M., and Lie, R. T. 2001. Long term mortality of mothers and fathers after preeclampsia: Population based Cohort Study. *BMJ* **323**: 1213–1217.

Jackman, K. A., Woodman, O. L., and Sobey, C. G. 2007. Isoflavones, equol and cardiovascular disease: Pharmacological and therapeutic insights. *Curr. Med. Chem.* **14**: 2824–2830.

Kaiserova, H., Simunek, T., van der Vijgh, W. J., Bast, A., and Kvasnickova, E. 2007. Flavonoids as protectors against doxorubicin cardiotoxicity: Role of iron chelation, antioxidant activity and inhibition of carbonyl reductase. *Biochim. Biophys. Acta* **1772**: 1065–1074.

Kamei, M., Yoshikawa, M., and Hashizume, S. 2003. New application of cocoa to mitigation of peripheral intolerance to cold (in Japanese). *Food Ind. Food Sci. J.* **300**: 4–13.

Karim, M., McCormick, K., and Kappagoda, C. T. 2000. Effects of cocoa extracts on endothelium-dependent relaxation. *J. Nutr.* **130**: 2105S–2108S.

Karthick, M. and Stanely Mainzen Prince, P. 2006. Preventive effect of rutin, a bioflavonoid, on lipid peroxides and antioxidants in isoproterenol-induced myocardial infarction in rats. *J. Pharm. Pharmacol.* **58**: 701–707.

Kelly, C. J. 2005. Effects of theobromine should be considered in future studies. *Am. J. Clin. Nutr.* **82**: 486–487.

Kim, H. and Keeney, P. G. 1984. (−)-Epicatechin content in fermented and unfermented cocoa beans. *J. Food Sci.* **49**: 1090–1092.

Klebanoff, M. A., Zhang, J., Zhang, C., and Levine, R. J. 2009. Maternal serum theobromine and the development of preeclampsia. *Epidemiology* **20**: 727–732.

Klotz, L. O. and Sies, H. 2003. Defenses against peroxynitrite: Selenocompounds and flavonoids. *Toxicol. Lett.* **140–141**: 125–132.

Knekt, P., Jarvinen, F., Reunanen, A., and Maatela, J. 1996. Flavonoid intake and coronary mortality in Finland: A Cohort Study. *BMJ* **312**: 478–481.

Knekt, P., Kumpulainen, J., Jarvinen, R., Rissanen, H., Heliovaara, M., Reunanen, A., Hakulinen, T., and Aromaa, A., 2002. Favonoid intakes and risk of chronic diseases. *Am. J. Clin. Nutr.* **76**: 560–568.

Kondo, K., Hirano, R., Matsumoto, A. Igarashi, O., and Itakura, H. 1996. Inhibition of LDL oxidation by cocoa. *Lancet* **348**: 1514.

Kris-Etherton, P. and Keen, C. L. 2002. Evidence that the antioxidant flavonoids in tea and cocoa are beneficial for cardiovascular health. *Curr. Opin. Lipidol.* **13**: 41–49.

Kris-Etherton, P. M. and Mustad, V. A. 1994. Hocolate feeding studies: A novel approach for evaluating the plasma lipid effects of stearic acid. *Am. J. Clin. Nutr.* **60**: 1029–1036.

Krishna, K. M., Annapurna, A., Gopal, G. S., Chalam, C. R., Madan, K., Kumar, V. K., and Prakash, G. J. 2005. Partial reversal by rutin and quercetin of impaired cardiac function in streptozotocin-induced diabetic rats. *Can. J. Physiol. Pharmacol.* **83**: 343–355.

Kubes, P., Suzuki, M., and Granger, D. N. 1991. Nitric oxide. An endogenous modulator of leukocyte adhesion. *Proc. Natl. Acad. Sci.* USA **88**: 4651–4655.

Kuhn, H., Belkner, J., Suzuki, H., and Yamamoto, S. 1994. Oxidative modification of human lipoproteins by lipoxygenases of different positional specificities. *J. Lipid Res.* **35**: 1749–1759.

Kuhnau, J. 1976. The flavonoids: A class of semi-essential food components: Their role in human nutrition. *World Rev. Nutr. Diet.* **24**: 117–191.

Kurlandsky, S. B. and Stote, K. S. 2006. Cardioprotective effects of chocolate and almond consumption in healthy women. *Nutr. Res.* **26**: 509–516.

Lazarus, S. A., Adamson, G. E., Hammerstone, J. F., and Schmitz, H. H. 1999. High-performance liquid chromatography/mass spectrometry analysis of proanthocyanidins in foods and beverages. *J. Agric. Food Chem.* **47**: 3693–3701.

Lecumberri, E., Goya, L., Mateos, R., Alía, M., Ramos, S., Izquierdo-Pulido, M., and Bravo, L. 2007. A diet rich in dietary fiber from cocoa improves lipid profile and reduces malondialdehyde in hypercholesterolemic rats. *Nutrition* **23**: 332–341.

Li, H. and Forstermann, U. 2000. Nitric oxide in the pathogenesis of vascular disease. *J. Pathol.* **190**: 244–254.

Lindemann, S., Kramer, B., Seizer, P., and Gawaz, M. 2007. Platelets, inflammation and atherosclerosis. *J. Thromb. Haemost.* **5**(Suppl. 1): 203–211.

Lotito, S. B., Actis-Goretta, L., Renart, M. L., Caligiuri, M., Rein, D., Schmitz, H. H., Steinberg, F. M., Keen, C. L., and Fraga, C. G. 2000. Influence of oligomer chain length on the antioxidant activity of procyanidins. *Biochem. Biophys. Res. Commun.* **276**: 945–951.

Lykke, J. A., Langhoff-Roos, J., Sibai, B. M., Funai, E. F., Triche, E. W., and Paidas, M. J. 2009. Hypertensive pregnancy disorders and subsequent cardiovascular morbidity and type 2 diabetes mellitus in the mother. *Hypertension* **53**: 944–951.

Mann, G. E., Rowlands, D. J., Li, F. Y., deWinter, P., and Siow, R. C. 2007. Activation of endothelial nitric oxide synthase by dietary isoflavones: Role of NO in Nrf2-mediated antioxidant gene expression. *Cardiovasc. Res.* **75**: 261–274.

Mathur, S., Devaraj, S., Grundy, S. M., and Jialal, I. 2002. Cocoa products decrease low density lipoprotein oxidative susceptibility but do not affect biomarkers of inflammation in humans. *J. Nutr.* **132**: 3663–3667.

Mato, T., Tsutsumi, H., Kamei, M., Ito, R., and Hashizume, S. 1999. New application of cocoa to enteral feeding in intensive care patients (in Japanese). *Bio Industry* **16**: 49–56.

Matsui, N., Ito, R., Nishimura, E., Yoshikawa, M., Kato, M., Kamei, M., Shibata, H., Matsumoto, I., Abe, K., and Hashizume, S. 2005. Ingested cocoa can prevent high-fat diet-induced obesity by regulating the expression of genes for fatty acid metabolism. *Nutr.* javascript:AL_get(this, 'jour', 'Nutrition.') **21**(5): 594–601.

Meursing, E. H. 1994. Cocoa mass, cocoa butter, cocoa powder. In *Industrial Chocolate Manufacturing and Use*, Becket, S. T., (ed.). Glasgow, United Kingdom: Blackie Academic & Professional.

Mladenka, P., Zatloukalová, L., Filipský, T., and Hrdina, R. 2010. Cardiovascular effects of flavonoids are not caused only by direct antioxidant activity. *Free Radic. Biol. Med.* **49**: 963–975.

Mladenka, P., Zatloukalova, L., Simunek, T., Bobrovova, Z., Semecky, V., Nachtigal, P., Haskova, P. et al. 2009. Direct administration of rutin does not protect against catecholamine cardiotoxicity. *Toxicology* **255**: 25–32.

Murphy, K. J., Chronopoulos, A. K., Singh, I., Francis, M. A., Moriarty, H., Pike, M. J., Turner, M. H., Mann, N. J., and Sinclair, A. J. 2003. Dietary flavanols and procyanidin oligomers from cocoa (*Theobroma cacao*) inhibit platelet function. *Am. J. Clin. Nutr.* **77Z**: 1466–1473.

Mursu, J., Voutilainen, S., Nurmi, T., Rissanen, T. H., Virtanen, J. K., Kaikkonen, J., Nyysonen, K., and Salonen, J. T. 2004. Dark chocolate consumption increases HDL cholesterol concentration and chocolate fatty acids may inhibit lipid peroxidation in healthy humans. *Free Radic. Biol. Med.* **37**: 1351–1359.

Njike, V. Y., Faridi, Z., Shuval, K., Dutta, S., Kay, C. D., West, S. G., Kris-Etherton, P. M., and Katz, D. L. 2009. Effects of sugar-sweetened and sugar-free cocoa on endothelial function in overweight adults. *Int. J. Cardiol.*, **147**(1): 83–88.

Ogura, S., Kakino, A., Sato, Y., Fujita, Y., Iwamoto, S., Otsui, K., Yoshimoto, R., and Sawamura, T. 2009. Lox-1: The multifunctional receptor underlying cardiovascular dysfunction. *Circ. J.* **73**: 1993–1999.

Ono, K., Takahashi, T., Kamei, M., Mato, T., Hashizume, S., Kamiya, S., and Tsutsumi, H. 2003. Effects of aqueous extract of cocoa on nitric oxide production of macrophages activated by lipopolysaccharide and interferon-gamma. *Nutr.* **19**: 681–685.

Ortega, N., Romero, M.P., Macia, A., Reguant, J., Angles, N., Morello, J. R., and Motilva, M. J. 2008. Obtention and characterisation of phenolic extracts from different cocoa sources. *J. Agric. Food Chem.* **56**: 9621–9627.

Osakabe, N., Baba, S., Yasuda, A., Iwamoto, T., Kamiyama, M., Takizawa, T., Itakura, H., and Kondo, K. 2001. Daily cocoa intake reduces the susceptibility of low-density lipoprotein to oxidation as demonstrated in healthy human volunteers. *Free Radic. Res.* **34**: 93–99.

Ozaki, M., Kawashima, S., Yamashita, T., Hirase, T., Namiki, M., Inoue, N., Hirata, K. et al. 2002. Overexpression of endothelial nitric oxide synthase accelerates atherosclerotic lesion formation in apoE-deficient mice. *J. Clin. Invest.* **110**: 331–340.

Pal, S., Ho, N., Santos, C., Dubois, P., Mamo, J., Kroft, K., and Allister, E. 2003. Red wine polyphenolics increase LDL receptor expression and activity and suppress the secretion of ApoB100 from human HepG2 cells. *J. Nutr.* **133**: 700–706.

Park, R., Detrano, R., Xiang, M., Fu, P., Ibrahim, Y., LaBree, L., and Azen, S. 2002. Combined use of computed tomography coronary calcium scores and C-reactive protein levels in predicting cardiovascular events in nondiabetic individuals. *Circulation* **106**: 2073–2077.

Patanè, S., Marte, F., Carmelo La Rosa, F., and La Rocca, R. 2010. Atrial fibrillation associated with chocolate intake abuse and chronic salbutamol inhalation abuse. *Int. J. Cardiol.* **145**: e74–e76.

Pearson, D. A., Paglieroni, T. G, Rein, D., Wun, T., Schramm, D. D., Wang, J. F., Holt, R. R., Gosselin, R., Schmidtz, H. H., and Keen, C. L. 2002. The effects of flavanol-rich cocoa and aspirin on *ex vivo* platelet function. *Thromb. Res.* **106**: 191–197.

Pearson, D. A., Schmitz, H. H., Lazarus, S. A., and Keen, C. J. 2001. Inhibition of *in vitro* low-density lipoprotein oxidation by oligomeric procyanidins present in chocolate and cocoas. *Methods Enzymol.* **335**: 350–360.

Perticone, F., Ceravolo, R., Pujia, A., Ventura, G., Iacopino, S., ScozZafava, A., Ferraro, A. et al. 2001. Prognostic significance of endothelial dysfunction in hypertensive patients. *Circulation* **104**: 191–196.

Pignatelli, P., Pulcinelli, F. M., Celestini, A., Lenti, L., Ghiselli, A., Gazzaniga, P. P., and Violi, F. 2000. The flavonoids quercetin and catechin synergistically inhibit platelet function by antagonizing the intracellular production of hydrogen peroxide. *Am. J. Clin. Nutr.* **72**: 1150–1155.

Porter, L. J., Ma, Z., and Chan, B. 1991. Cacao procyanidins: Major flavonoids and identification of some minor metabolites. *Phytochemistry* **30**: 1657–1663.

Psotova, J., Chlopcikova, S., Miketova, P., Hrbac, J., and Simanek, V. 2004. Chemoprotective effect of plant phenolics against anthracycline-induced toxicity on rat cardiomyocytes. Part III. Apigenin, baicalelin, kaempherol, luteolin and quercetin. *Phytother. Res.* **18**: 516–521.

Raggi, P., Shaw, L. J., Berman, D. S., and Callister, T. Q. 2004. Gender-based differences in the prognostic value of coronary calcification. *J. Womens Health* (Larchmt) **13**: 273–283.

Rajadurai, M. and Prince, P. S. 2007. Preventive effect of naringin on isoproterenol-induced cardiotoxicity in Wistar rats: An *in vivo* and *in vitro* study. *Toxicology* **232**: 216–225.

Ralay Ranaivo, H., Diebolt, M., and Andriantsitohaina, R. 2004. Wine polyphenols induce hypotension, and decrease cardiac reactivity and infarct size in rats: Involvement of nitric oxide. *Br. J. Pharmacol.* **142**: 671–678.

Rechner, A. R., Kuhnle, G., Bremner, P., Hubbard, G. P., Moore, K. P., and Rice-Evans, C. 2002. The metabolic fate of dietary polyphenols in humans. *Free Radic. Biol. Med.* **33**: 220–235.

Rein, D., Lotito, S., Holt, R. R., Keen, C. L., Schmitz, H. H., and Fraga, G. G., 2002b. Epicatechin in human plasma: *In vivo* determination and effect of chocolate consumption on plasma oxidation status. *J. Nutr.* **130**: 2109S–2114S.

Rein, D., Paglieroni, T. G., Pearson, D. A., Wun, T., Schmitz, H. H., Gosselin, R., and Keen, C. L. 2000a. Cocoa and wine polyphenols modulate platelet activation and function. *J. Nutr.* **130**: 2120S–2126S.

Rein, D., Lotito, S., Holt, R. R., Keen, C. L., Schmitz, H. H., Fraga, C. G., and Gosselin, R. 2000. Epicatechin in human plasma: *In vivo* determination and effect of chocolate consumption on plasma oxidation status. *J. Nutr.* **130**: 2109–2114.

Renaud, S. and de Lorgeril, M. 1992. Wine, alcohol, platelets and the French paradox for coronary heart disease. *Lancet* **339**: 1523–1526.

Rice-Evans, C. A., Miller, N. J., Bolwell, P. G., Bramley, P. M., and Pridham, J. B. 1995. The relative antioxidant activities of plant-derived polyphenolic flavonoids. *Free Radic. Res.* **22**: 375–383.

Rice-Evans, C. A., Miller, N. J., and Paganga, G. 1996. Structure-antioxidant activity relationships of flavonoids and phenolic acids. *Free Radic. Biol. Med.* **20**: 933–956.

Rimm, E. B., Katan, M. B., Ascherio, A., Stampfer, M. J., and Willett, W. C. 1996. Relation between intake of flavonoids and risk for coronary heart disease in male health professionals. *Ann. Intern. Med.* **125**: 384–389.

Rios, L., Bennett, R., Lazarus, S., Remesy, C., Scalbert, A., and Williamson, G. 2002. Cocoa procyanidins are stable during gastric transit in humans. *Am. J. Clin. Nutr.* **76**:1106–1110.

Rios, L. Y., Gonthier, M.-P., Remesy, C., Mila, I., Lapierre, C., Lazarus, S. A., Williamson, G., and Scalbert, A. 2003. Chocolate intake increases urinary excretion of polyphenol-derived phenolic acids in healthy human subjects. *Am. J. Clin. Nutr.* **77**: 912–918.

Rumberger, J. A., Simons, D. B., Fitzpatrick, L. A., Sheedy, P. F., and Schwartz, R. S. 1995. Coronary artery calcium area by electron-beam computed tomography and coronary atherosclerotic plaque area. A Histopathologic Correlative Study. *Circulation* **92**: 2157–2162.

Russo, A., Acquaviva, R., Campisi, A., Sorrenti, V., Di Giacomo, C., Virgata, G., Barcellona, M. L., and Vanella, A. 2000. Bioflavonoids as antiradicals, antioxidants and DNA cleavage protectors. *Cell Biol. Toxicol.* **16**: 91–98.

Ruzaidi, A., Amin, I., Nawalyah, A. G., Hamid, M., and Faizul, H. A. 2005. The effect of Malaysian cocoa extract on glucose levels and lipid profiles in diabetic rats. *J. Ethnopharmacol.* **98**: 55–60.

Saftlas, A. F., Triche, E. W., Beydoun, H., and Bracken, M. B. 2010. Does chocolate intake during pregnancy reduce the risks of preeclampsia and gestational hypertension? *Ann. Epidemiol.* **20**: 584–591.

Salonen, J. T., Nyyssfnen, K., Salonen, R., Porkkala-Sarataho, E., Tuomainen, T. P., Diczfalusy, U., and Bjorkhem, I. 1997. Lipoprotein oxidation and progression of carotid atherosclerosis. *Circulation* **95**: 840–845.

Salonen, J. T., Yl7-Herttuala, S., Yamamoto, R., Butler, S., Korpela, H., Salonen, R., Nyyssonen, K., Palinski, W., and Witztum, J. L. 1992. Autoantibody against oxidised LDL and progression of carotid atherosclerosis. *Lancet* **339**: 883–887.

Sanchez, M., Galisteo, M., Vera, R., Villar, I. C., Zarzuelo, A., Tamargo, J., Perez-Vizcaino, F., and Duarte, J. 2006. Quercetin downregulates NADPH oxidase, increases eNOS activity and prevents endothelial dysfunction in spontaneously hypertensive rats. *J. Hypertens.* **24**: 75–84.

Sanchez-Rabaneda, F., Jaurequi, O., Casals, I., Andres-Lacueva, C., Izquierdo-Pulido, M., and Lamuela-Raventos, R. M. 2003. Liquid chromatographic/electron spray ionisation tandem mass spectrometric study of the phenolic composition of cocoa (*Theobroma cacao*). *J. Mass Spectrom.* **38**: 35–42.

Sangiorgi, G., Rumberger, J. A., Severson, A., Edwards, W. D., Gregoire, J., Fitzpatrick, L. A., and Schwartz, R. S. 1998. Arterial calcification and not lumen stenosis is highly correlated with atherosclerotic plaque burden in humans: A histologic study of 723 coronary artery segments using nondecalcifying methodology. *J. Am. Coll. Cardiol.* **31**: 126–133.

Sato, S., Takahashi, T., Kamei, M., and Hashizume, S. 1999. New functions of cocoa (cacao) (in Japanese). *Foods Food Ingredients J. Japan* **180**: 71–76.

Schewe, T., Kuhn, H., and Sies, H. 2002. Flavonoids of cocoa inhibit recombinant human 5-lipoxygenase. *J. Nutr.* **132**: 1825–1829.

Schewe, T., Sadik, C., Klotz, L-O., Yoshimoto, T., Kuhn, H., and Sies, H. 2001. Polyphenols of cocoa: inhibition of mammalian 15-lipoxygenase. *Biol. Chem.* **382**: 1687–1696.

Schramm, D. D., Wang, J. F., Holt, R. R., Ensuna, J. L., Gonsalves, J. L., Lazarus, S. A., Schmitz, H. H., German, J. B., and Keen, C. L. 2001. Chocolate procyanidins decrease the leukotriene-prostacyclin ratio in humans and human aortic endothelial cells. *Am. J. Clin. Nutr.* **73**: 36–40.

Schroeder, P., Klotz, L-O., and Sies, H. 2003. Amphiphilic properties of (-)-epicatechin and their significance for protection of cells against peroxynitrite. *Biochem. Biophys. Res. Commun.* **307**: 69–73.

Schroeter, H., Heiss, C., Balzer, J., Kleinbongard, P., Keen, C. L., Hollenberg, N. K., Sies, H., Kwik-Uribe, C., Schmitz, H. H., and Kelm, H. 2006. (-)-Epicatechin mediates beneficial effects of flavanol-rich cocoa on vascular function in humans. *Proc. Natl. Acad. Sci. USA.* **103**: 1024–1029.

Schroeter, H., Holt, R. R., Orozco, T. J., Schmitz, H. H., and Keen, C. L. 2003. Milk and absorption of dietary flavanols. *Nature* **426**: 787–788.

Serafini, M., Bugianesi, R., Maiani, G., Valtuena, S., DeSantis, S., and Crozier, A. 2003. Plasma antioxidants from chocolate. *Nature* **424**: 1013.

Shaw, L. J., Raggi, P., Schisterman, E., Berman, D. S., and Callister, T. Q. 2003. Prognostic value of cardiac risk factors and coronary artery calcium screening for all-cause mortality. *Radiology* **228**: 826–833.

Shepherd, J., Cobbe, S. M., Ford, I., Isles, C. G., Lorimer, A. S., Mcfarlane, P. W., McKillop, J. H., and Packard, C. J. 1995. Prevention of coronary heart disease with pravastatin in men with hypercholesterolemia. West of Scotland Coronary Prevention Study Group. *N. Engl. J. Med.* **333**: 1301–1307.

Shiina, Y., Funabashi, N., Lee, K., Murayama, T., Nakamura, K., Wakatsuki, Y., Daimon, W., and Komuro, I. 2009. Acute effect of oral flavonoid-rich dark chocolate intake on oronary circulation, as compared with non-flavonoid white chocolate, by transthoracic Doppler echocardiography in healthy adults. *Int. J. Cardiol.* **131**(3): 424–429.

Singh, I., Quinn, H., Mok, M., Southgate, R. J., Turner, A. H., Li, D., Sinclair, J., and Hawley, J. A. 2006. The effect of exercise and training status on platelet activation: Do cocoa polyphenols play a role? *Platelets.* **17**: 361–367.

Smith, J. and Blackburn, R. J. 2005. Enforcing effects of caffeine and theobromine as found in chocolate. *Psychopharmacology* (Berl) **181**(1): 101–106.

Soffietti, M. G., Nebbia, C., Valenza, F., Amedeo, S., and Re, G. 1989. Effects of theobromine in mature and immature rabbits. *J. Comp. Pathol.* **100**: 47–68.

Spencer, J. P., Chaudry, F., Pannala, A. S., Srai, S. K., Debnam, E., and Rice-Evans, C. 2000. Decomposition of cocoa procyanidins in the gastric milieu. *Biochem. Biophys. Res. Commun.* **272**: 236–241.

Spencer, J. P., Schroeter, H., Shenoy, B., Srai, S. K., Debnam, E., and Rice-Evans, C. 2001. Epicatechin is the primary bioavailable form of the procyanidin dimmers B2 and B5 after transfer across the small intestine. *Biochem. Biophys. Res. Commun.* **285**: 588–593.

Spencer, J. P. 2003. Metabolism of tea flavonoids in the gastrointestinal tract. *J. Nutr.* **133**: 3255S–3261S.

Stamler, J., Wentworth, D., and Neaton, J. D. 1986. Is relationship between serum cholesterol and risk of premature death from coronary heart disease continuous and graded? Findings in 356,222 primary screenees of the Multiple Risk Factor Intervention Trial (MRFIT). *J. Am. Med. Assoc.* **256**: 2823–2828.

Steffen, Y., Gruber, C., Schewe, T., and Sies, H. 2008. Mono-O-methylated flavanols and other flavonoids as inhibitors of endothelial NADPH oxidase, *Arch. Biochem. Biophys.* **469**: 209–219.

Steinberg, D., Parthasarathy, S., Carew, T. E., Khoo, J. C., and Witztum, J. L. 1989. Beyond cholesterol. Modifications of low-density lipoprotein that increase its atherogenicity. *N. Engl. J. Med.* **320**: 915–924.

Steinberg, F. M., Holt, R. R., Schmitz, H. H., and Keen, C. L. 2002. Cocoa procyanidin chain length does not determine ability to protect LDL from oxidation when monomer units are controlled. *J. Nutr. Biochem.* **13**(11): 645–652.

Steinberg, D., Parthasarathy, S., Carew, T. E., and Witztum, J. L. 1989. Modifications of low-density lipoprotein that increase its atherogenecity. *N. Engl. J. Med.* **320**: 915–924.

Taubert, D., Roesen, R., Lehmann, C., Jung, N., and Schömig, E. 2007a. Effects of low habitual cocoa intake on blood pressure and bioactive nitric oxide: A randomized controlled trial. *JAMA* **298**: 49–60.

Taubert, D., Roesen, R., and Schomig, E. 2007b. Effect of cocoa and tea intake on blood pressure. A meta-analysis. *Arch. Intern. Med.* **167**: 626–634..

Tomaru, M., Takano, H., Osakabe, N., Yasuda, A., Inoue, K., Yanagisawa, R., Ohwatari, T., and Uematsu, H. 2007. Dietary supplementation with cacao liquor proanthocyanidins prevents elevation of blood glucose levels in diabetic obese mice. *Nutr.* **23**: 351–355.

Triche, E. W., Grosso, L. M., Belanger, K., Darefsky, A. S., Benowitz, N. L., and Bracken, M. B. 2008. Chocolate consumption in pregnancy and reduced likelihood of preeclampsia. *Epidemiology* **19**: 459–464.

Unno, T., Tamemoto, K., Yayabe, F., and Kakuda, T. 2003. Urinary excretion of 5-(3',4'-dihydroxyphenyl)-gamma-valerolactone, a ring-fission metabolite of (-)-epicatechin, in rats and its *in vitro* antioxidant activity. *J. Agric. Food Chem.* **51**: 6893–6898.

van Jaarsveld, H., Kuyl, J. M., Schulenburg, D. H., and Wiid, N. M. 1996. Effect of flavonoids on the outcome of myocardial mitochondrial ischemia/reperfusion injury. *Res. Commun. Mol. Pathol. Pharmacol.* **91**: 65–75.

Vassallo, R. and Lipsky, J. J. 1998. Theophylline: Recent advances in the understanding of its mode of action and uses in clinical practice. *Mayo Clin. Proc.* **73**: 346–354.

Vianna, H. R., Cortes, S. F., Ferreira, A. J., Capettini, L. S., Schmitt, M., Almeida, A. P., Massensini, A. R., and Lemos, V. S. 2006. Antiarrhythmogenic and antioxidant effect of the flavonoid dioclein in a model of cardiac ischemia/reperfusion. *Planta Med.* **72**: 300–303.

Vinson, J. A., Proch, J., and Zubik, L. 1999. Phenol antioxidant quantity and quality in foods: Cocoa, dark chocolate, and milk chocolate. *J. Agric. Food Chem.* **47**: 4821–4824.

Visioli, F., Borsani, L., and Galli, C. 2000. Diet and prevention of coronary heart disease: The potential role of phytochemicals. *Cardiovasc. Res.* **47**: 419–425.

Vlachopoulos, C., Aznaouridis, K., Alexopoulos, N., Economou, E., Andreadou, I., and Stefanadis, C. 2005. Effect of dark chocolate on arterial function in healthy individuals. *Am. J. Hypertens.* **18**: 785–791.

Vlachopoulos, C. V., Alexopoulos, N. A., Aznaouridis, K. A., Ioakeimidis, N. C., Dima, I. A., Dagre, A., Vasiliadou, C., Stefanadi, E. C., and Stefanadis, C. I. 2007. Relation of habitual cocoa consumption to aortic stiffness and wave reflections, and to central hemodynamics in healthy individuals. *Am. J. Cardiol.* **90**: 1473–1475.

Wallace, T. C., Wagner, M., Leveille, G., Keen, C. L., Woteki, C. E., Manley, C., Rizk, S. W., Heber, D., and Shrikhande, A. J. 2009. Unlocking the Benefits of Cocoa Flavanols. *Food Technol.* **63**(10): 34–41.

Wan, Y., Vinson, J. A., Etherton, T. D., Proch, J., Lazarus, S. A., and Kris-Etherton, P. M. 2001. Effects of cocoa powder and dark chocolate on LDL oxidative susceptibility and prostaglandin concentrations in humans. *Am. J. Clin. Nutr.* **74**: 596–602.

Wang, J. F., Schramm, D. D., Holt, R. R., Ensunsa, J. L., Fraga, C. G., Schmitz, H. H., and Keen, C. L. 2000. A dose-dependent effect from chocolate consumption on plasma epicatechin and oxidative damage. *J. Nutr.* **130**: 2115–2119.

Waterhouse, A. L., Shirley, J. R., and Donovan, J. L. 1996. Antioxidants in chocolate. *Lancet* **348**: 834.

Wexler, L., Brundage, B., Crouse, J., Detrano, R., Fuster, V., Maddahi, J., Rumberger, J., Stanford, W., White, R., and Taubert, K. 1996. Coronary artery calcification: Pathophysiology, epidemiology, imaging methods, and clinical implications. A statement for health professionals from the American Heart Association. *Circulation* **94**: 1175–1192.

Wilcox, L. J, Borradaile, N. M., de Dreu, L. E., and Huff, M. W. 2001. Secretion of hepatocyte apoB is inhibited by the flavonoids, naringenin and hesperetin, via reduced activity and expression of $ACAT_2$ and MTP. *J. Lipid Res.* **42**: 725–734.

Wilson, B. J., Watson, M. S., Prescott, G. J., Sunderland, S., Campbell, D. M., Hannaford, P., Cairns, W., and Smith, S. 2003. Hypertensive diseases of pregnancy and risk of hypertension and stroke in later life: Results from Cohort Study. *BMJ* **326**: 845–849.

Wilson, P. K. 2010. Centuries of seeking chocolate's medicinal benefits. *Lancet* **376**(9736): 158–159.

Wilson, R. F., Laughlin, D. E., Ackell, P. H., Chilian, W. M., Holida, M. D., Hartley, C. J., Armstrong, M. L., Marcus, M. L., and White, C. W. 1985. Transluminal subselective measurement of coronary artery blood flow velocity and vasodilator reserve in man. *Circulation* **72**: 82–92.

Wollgast, J. and Anklam, E. 2000. Review on polyphenols in Theobroma cacao: Changes in composition during the manufacture of chocolate and methodology for identification and quantification. *Food Res. Int.* **33**: 423–447.

Xiao, J., Cao, H., Wang, Y., Zhao, J., and Wei, X., 2009. Glycosylation of dietary flavonoids decreases the affinities for plasma protein. *J. Agric. Food Chem.* **57**: 6642–6648.

Zeng, G., Nystrom, F. H., Ravichandran, L. V., Cong, L. N., Kirby, M., Mostowski, H., and Quon, M. J. 2000. Roles for insulin receptor, PI3-kinase, and Akt in insulin-signaling pathways related to production of nitric oxide in human vascular endothelial cells. *Circulation* **101**: 1539–1545.

Zhu, Q. Y., Holt, R. R., Lazarus, S. A., Orozco, T., and Keen, C. L. 2002. Inhibitory effects of cocoa flavanols and procyanidin oligomers on free radical-induced erythrocyte hemolysis. *Exp. Biol. Med.* **227**: 321–329.

12 Tea and Coffee
A Concise Review of Effects on Cardiovascular Risk Factors

Ayyappan Appukuttan Aachary, Usha Thiyam,
and N. A. Michael Eskin
University of Manitoba

CONTENTS

12.1 INTRODUCTION

Coffee and tea are consumed in most countries (Grigg, 2002). Worldwide, approximately three cups of tea are drunk for every cup of coffee. Between 1994 and 1996, 76.6% of tea consumption took place in developing countries with tea drinking dominating throughout Asia, the former Soviet Union, and Africa. In contrast, 71.5% of coffee consumption took place in developed countries (Grigg, 2002). There has been considerable interest in investigating the health effects of tea and coffee. While the majority of evidence comes from epidemiological studies, they are backed up by animal studies, *in vitro* studies, and some human interventions using biomarkers or other interim end points.

12.2 TEA AND BIOACTIVE MOLECULES FOR CVD PREVENTION

The term "tea" refers to the plant *Camellia sinensis*, its leaves and infusions derived from them. Worldwide, the consumption of tea is second only to water and, therefore, any physiological effects of tea could be important. Tea is classified based on the manner in which the leaves are processed.

The three main types are fermented black tea, partially fermented Oolong tea, and nonfermented green tea. Of these, black tea accounts for almost 80% of the tea consumed followed by green tea at 20% and Oolong tea at 2% (International Tea Committee, 2002). This chapter focuses on the potential cardiovascular benefits of black and green tea.

Black teas are produced by promoting the enzymatic oxidation of tea flavonoids while the enzymes involved in flavonoid oxidation are inactivated in the production of green tea. Both black and green teas can be major contributors to total flavonoid intake. Approximately 35–40% of the weight of the tea leaf, both black and green, is flavonoids. The processing of black tea results in many changes to the chemical composition of the tea leaf. The most prominent is oxidation of the catechins, the main class of flavonoids in tea, which results in a significant reduction in catechin concentration. This is often reduced to less than 10% in the black tea leaf. However, black tea is rich in flavonoid oxidation products derived from the enzymatic oxidation of catechins. Monomeric catechins undergo enzymatic polymerization, which leads to the formation of condensation compounds such as theaflavins and thearubigens (Harbowy and Ballentine, 1997). These differences in flavonoid composition between black and green tea may result in differences in physiological effects. Tea is an ideal vehicle to investigate the effects of dietary flavonoids on cardiovascular disease-related end-points in intervention studies. The flavonoids are provided in the form in which they occur in the diet. Within many populations, tea provides approximately half the total flavonoid intake. Dietary intake of flavonoids has been estimated at 1000 mg/day. One cup of tea provides 150–300 mg flavonoids (Hodgson et al., 1999). Finally, tea provides almost no energy and, therefore, in an intervention study, no other aspect of the diet needs to be changed to maintain an isoenergetic diet.

Tea polyphenols are comprised largely of the epicatechin group of flavanols, which differ from catechins in the spatial orientation of the hydroxyl group on the pyran ring. Gallocatechins are characterized by the presence of three hydroxyl groups on the B ring, and catechin gallates are gallic acid esters of the hydroxyl group on the pyran ring (Graham, 1992). Six catechins occur in significant quantities in green tea leaves: (+)-catechin, (−)-epicatechin, (+)-gallocatechin, (−)-epigallocatechin, (−)-epicatechin gallate, and (−)-epigallocatechin gallate (Figure 12.1). Overall, levels of catechins vary with leaf age, tending to be higher in young leaves. During the manufacture of black tea, enzyme-catalyzed oxidation of the catechins leads to the formation of catechin quinones, which subsequently react to form the more complexly structured pigmented theaflavins and thearubigens. Compositionally, the main difference between green and black tea lies in the relative levels of epicatechins and their oxidized condensation products (Table 12.1).

12.3   COFFEE AND BIOACTIVE MOLECULES FOR CVD PREVENTION

Coffee contains several biologically active substances that may have either beneficial or harmful effects on the cardiovascular system (Spiller, 1998). Cafestol and kahweol are diterpenoid alcohols that occur naturally in coffee beans and have been identified as hypercholesterolemic compounds (Urgert and Katan, 1997). They are released from roasted and ground coffee beans by hot water but are largely trapped by the use of a paper filter during coffee preparation (Viani, 1993). The cholesterol-raising factors, first isolated in coffee oil, were later found to be the diterpenes, cafestol, and kahweol (Figure 12.2) (Urgert and Katan, 1997). Scandinavian boiled coffee, Turkish coffee, and French press (cafetiere) coffee contain relatively high levels of cafestol and kahweol (6–12 mg/cup), while filtered coffee, percolated coffee, and instant coffee contain low levels of cafestol and kahweol (0.2–0.6 mg/cup) (Gross et al., 1997; Urgert et al., 1995). The mechanisms for the effects of these diterpenes on lipoprotein metabolism are not yet clear, but consumption of cafestol and kahweol in French press coffee has been found to result in persistent increases in cholesterol ester transfer protein activity in humans, which may contribute to increases in LDL cholesterol (De Roos et al., 2000).

Coffee also contains chlorogenic acid, flavonoids, melanoidins, and various lipid-soluble compounds such as furans, pyrroles, and maltol (Spiller, 1998; Yanagimoto et al., 2004). Many of these compounds are efficiently absorbed, have relatively high bioavailability, and have been shown to

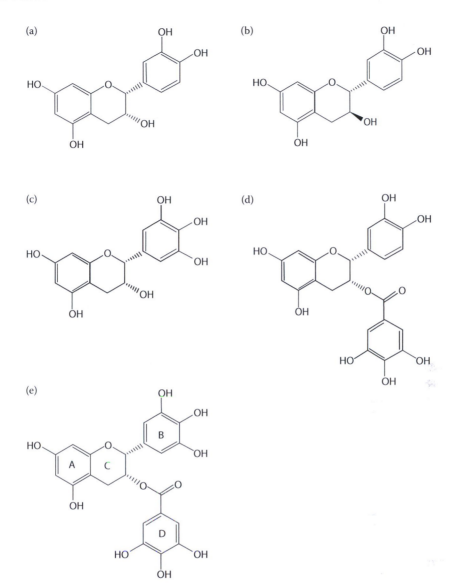

FIGURE 12.1 Major flavan-3-ols found in green tea infusions: (a) (−)-epicatechin; (b) (+)-catechin; (c) (−)-epigallocatechin; (d) (−)-epicatechin gallate; (e) (−)-epigallocatechin gallate. (Adapted from Moore, R.J. et al., 2009. *Br. J. Nutr.* **102**: 1790–1802.)

have antioxidant properties (Borrelli et al., 2002; Daglia et al., 2000; Olthof et al., 2001b; Pellegrini et al., 2003; Yanagimoto et al., 2004). Chlorogenic acids are a family of esters formed between quinic and *trans*-cinnamic acids, which are an important group of dietary phenols (Figure 12.3a). The most common individual chlorogenic acid is 5-*O*-caffeoylquinic acid, which is still often called chlorogenic acid. For those who drink it, coffee represents the richest dietary source of chlorogenic acids and cinnamic acids (caffeic acid). The chlorogenic acid content of a 200 mL (7-oz) cup of coffee has been reported to range from 70 to 350 mg, which would provide about 35–175 mg of caffeic acid (Clifford, 1999).

Indeed, coffee has been identified as a major contributor to the total antioxidant capacity of the diet of some populations because of its widespread use (Pulido et al., 2003; Svilaas et al., 2004). Caffeine (1,3,7-trimethylxanthine), the best characterized compound in coffee, is a purine alkaloid

TABLE 12.1

Phenolic Constituents (% Dry Solids) in Green and Black Tea Beverages

Constituents	Green Tea	Black Tea
Flavanols	30–40	5–10
Epigallocatechin gallate	10–15	4–5
Epicatechin gallate	3–10	3–4
Epigallocatechin	3–10	1–2
Epicatechin	1–5	1–2
Flavandiols	2–3	
Flavonols[a]	5–10	6–8
Phenolic acids and depsides[b]	3–5	10–12
Theaflavins		3–6
Thearubigen		10–30

Source: Adapted from Dreosti, I.E. 1996. *Nutr. Rev.* **54**: S51–S58.

[a]   Flavonols include kaempferol, quercetin, and myricetin.

[b]   Phenolic acids and depside include gallic acid and theogallin.

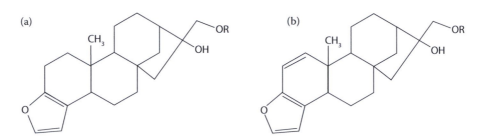

FIGURE 12.2   Chemical structures of diterpenes in coffee (a) cafestol and (b) kahweol. R = H:free diterpene; R = fatty acid:diterpene ester. (Adapted from Higdon, J.V. and Frei, B. 2006. *Crit. Rev. Food Sci. Nutr.* **46**: 101–123.)

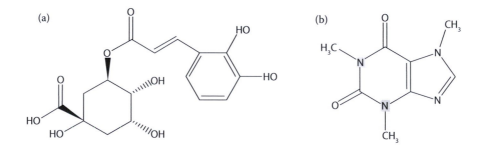

FIGURE 12.3   Chemical structures of (a) chlorogenic acid and (b) caffeine.

that occurs naturally in coffee beans (Figure 12.3b) (Spiller, 1998). At intake levels associated with coffee consumption, caffeine appears to exert most of its biological effects through the antagonism of the A1 and A2A subtypes of the adenosine receptor (James, 2004). Some physiological effects associated with caffeine administration include central nervous system stimulation, acute elevation of blood pressure, increased metabolic rate, and diuresis (Carrillo and

Benitez, 2000). Caffeine is rapidly and almost completely absorbed in the stomach and small intestine and distributed to all tissues, including the brain. Caffeine concentrations in coffee beverages can be quite variable. A standard cup of coffee is often assumed to provide 100 mg of caffeine, but an analysis of 14 different specialty coffees purchased at coffee shops in the United States found that the amount of caffeine in 8 oz (~240 mL) of brewed coffee ranged from 72 to 130 mg (McCusker et al., 2003).

12.4   CARDIOVASCULAR DISEASE: RESULTS OF POPULATION STUDIES

Evidence from population studies suggests that tea and coffee consumption and a higher flavonoid intake may reduce the risk for CVD. A few of the studies conducted among Asian populations established a positive correlation between green tea consumption and cardioprotective effect (Iwai et al., 2002; Kuriyama, 2008; Nakachi et al., 2000; Sato et al., 1989). A meta-analysis (10 cohort and seven case–control studies) on the effect of tea consumption on CVD by Peters et al. (2001) indicated an 11% reduction in the incidence rate of myocardial infarction (MI) with an increase in tea consumption of three cups per day. The authors also established that these observations were not specific to green or black tea. However, extra care is needed to interpret these results because of evidence for a publication bias and geographic heterogeneity. A parallel meta-analysis by Arab et al. (2009) demonstrated that daily consumption of either green or black tea (3 cups/day) was associated with reduced risk of ischemic stroke. Since tea is often the main contributor to flavonol intake in populations, Huxley and Neil (2003) assessed the association of dietary flavonol intake with the subsequent risk of coronary heart disease mortality. The analysis clearly indicated a decreased risk of CVD with higher tea consumption.

In the largest epidemiological study carried out to-date, long-term habitual coffee consumption was followed for 16–20 years in over 44,000 men and 85,000 women free of CHD to assess heart disease risk in the US Physician's and Nurses Health Study (Lopez-Garcia et al., 2006) and the results indicated that there was no effect of coffee on risk even at >6 cups/day. The data did not provide any evidence that coffee consumption increased the risk of CHD. However, the study had certain drawbacks as there was no separation of caffeinated and decaffeinated coffee drinkers. A meta-analysis which included 13 case–control and 10 cohort studies followed from 3 to 44 years concluded that "despite a significant association between high consumption of coffee and CHD reported among case-control studies, no significant association between daily coffee consumption and CHD emerged from long-term follow-up prospective cohort studies" (Sofi et al., 2007, p. 209). Interestingly, a study conducted by Andersen et al. (2006) over 40,000 postmenopausal US women (examined healthy subjects for 15 years) concluded that the consumption of coffee may inhibit inflammation and thus reduce the risk of cardiovascular and other inflammatory diseases in postmenopausal women. Epidemiological investigations of the effects of coffee consumption on MI were carried out by Baylin et al. (2006) and Martinez-Ortiz et al. (2006). Baylin et al. (2006) examined the population in Costa Rican, known to have a very high intake of saturated fats from tropical oils with an overall low HDL and an increased risk for MI. They showed that the risk of MI decreased with increasing coffee consumption in Costa Rican population. An inception cohort study by Mukamal and coworkers (2004) on 1935 patients with a confirmed acute MI between 1989 and 1994 showed no association between coffee or cola consumption and survival. These results further supported the hypothesis that coffee posed little cardiovascular risk to patients suffering from acute MI.

Overall studies, predominantly epidemiological, together with animal and *in vitro* studies, indicate that coffee and tea are both safe beverages. There are no comparative studies to ascertain the efficiency of tea over coffee or coffee over tea. However, tea seems to be the healthier option because it has a possible role in the prevention of several cancers and CVD. While the evidence for such relationships is far from definitive, nevertheless, the perceived benefits will encourage the public to continue to drink both tea and coffee until more definitive results are forthcoming.

12.5 EFFECTS OF TEA AND COFFEE ON CVD RISK FACTORS

12.5.1 ATHEROSCLEROSIS

Few human studies have investigated the relationship between tea or flavonoid intake and atherosclerosis. Debette et al. (2008) showed that carotid plaques were less frequent with increasing tea consumption in women. Mursu et al. (2007) showed that high intake of flavonoids was associated with decreased carotid atherosclerosis in middle-aged Finnish men. In contrast there is a significant literature describing studies using animal models to investigate the effects of flavonoid-rich foods or extracts on the development of atherosclerosis. The apo E-deficient mouse and hamsters have been used as animal models to investigate the effects of flavonoid-rich foods or extracts on the development of atherosclerosis (Hodgson and Croft, 2006). In the apo E-deficient mouse inhibition of atherosclerotic lesion development has been demonstrated with teaand tea-derived flavonoids, red wine-derived flavonoids, isolated quercetin or catechin, and a pure phenolic acid derivative from honey. Similar inhibition has been found with red grape extracts in the cholesterol-fed hamster (Auger et al., 2004). More recently, Loke et al. (2010) showed that isolated quercetin, found in both green and black tea, as well as theaflavin, an important black tea flavonoid, can inhibit the development of atherosclerosis in the apo E-deficient mouse. Overall, the results of studies using animal models clearly show that flavonoids present in tea can inhibit the development of atherosclerosis. Further human studies, however, are needed.

Using male Wistar rats, Sakamoto et al. (2005) investigated the relationship of coffee consumption with risk factors of atherosclerosis and found that coffee diets increased serum caffeine in a dose–response manner, although caffeine in serum was not detected in rats fed the control diet. It also led to slightly increased total serum levels of homocysteine and cholesterol, but no significant differences were found between the control and coffee groups. From these results, the authors concluded that moderate coffee intake is not a risk factor for atherogenesis. Comparable results were obtained using Hamster models (Auger et al., 2004).

12.5.2 ENDOTHELIAL FUNCTION AND INFLAMMATION

The development of endothelial dysfunction is considered as an early biomarker for the development of CVD (Schroeder et al., 1999) and cardiovascular events (Schächinger et al., 2000). The loss of normal endothelium-dependent and NO-mediated vasodilation in the artery is the major event in endothelial dysfunction and in the normal conditions, NO released by the endothelium functions as a regulator of arterial wall tone. Several *in vitro* studies indicated that tea and tea flavonoids cause vasorelaxation of rat aortic rings which is NO and endothelium-dependent (Hodgson et al., 2006). In humans, a number of studies have now investigated the effects of black or green tea, or tea flavonoids on flow-mediated dilatation of the brachial artery. A significant improvement in flow-mediated dilatation by green and black teas has been reported in a few human trials, in healthy and diabetic subjects, after acute and chronic tea consumption (Alexopoulos et al., 2008; Duffy et al., 2001; Jochmann et al., 2008; Kim et al., 2006; Nagaya et al., 2004). Interestingly, Grassi et al. (2009) reported a dose–response of improved endothelial function in healthy male subjects to black tea polyphenols. Experimental studies have also demonstrated that isolated flavonoids found in tea can enhance NO status. Dietary flavonoids of green tea (quercetin and epicatechin) could augment NO status and reduce endothelin-1 concentrations (a potent vasoconstrictor) (Loke et al., 2008). Data from these randomized controlled trials thus indicated that endothelial function could be improved by consumption of black and green tea.

Inflammation is thought to play a significant role in the initiation and progression of vascular disease. Inflammatory processes in the vascular wall may be mediated by a range of factors, such as cytokines, eicosanoids, and NO, which in turn modulate cellular signaling, cell growth and differentiation, and a variety of other cellular processes. Results obtained from *in vitro* studies suggested that flavonoids present in tea and other foods have effects on inflammatory mediators consistent with anti-inflammatory effects (Sies et al., 2005). However, to date there is little support for anti-inflammatory effects in randomized controlled trials. Several studies have shown no effect of regular ingestion of tea for up to 8 weeks on circulating C-reactive protein concentrations, a nonspecific marker of inflammation (Hodgson, 2008; Lee et al., 2005). Effects of tea on other inflammatory markers remain less clear.

With respect to coffee, Zampelas et al. (2004) showed that boiled coffee consumed at moderate to high doses increased C-reactive protein, an inflammatory marker. Homocysteine is another risk factor for heart disease and a study of 12,000 heavy coffee-drinking men indicated that coffee consumption is a major lifestyle determinant of plasma homocysteine in a healthy population (Refsum et al., 2006). Chrysohoou et al. (2004) reached the same conclusion in another study. Lopez-Garcia et al. (2006) observed a significant correlation between high coffee consumption and lower plasma concentrations of E-selectin and C-reactive protein in women with type 2 diabetes. Interestingly, in healthy women, no appreciable differences in plasma concentrations of the markers were found across categories of caffeinated coffee intake. However, the consumption of decaffeinated coffee lowered plasma concentrations of E-selectin and C-reactive protein only in healthy women. An observation can be made from these studies that neither caffeinated nor decaffeinated filtered coffee has a detrimental effect on endothelial function. However, more specific human intervention studies are warranted to definitively conclude the benefits of coffee and tea in healthy and diabetic men and women.

12.5.3 Blood Pressure

Hypertension is a major risk factor for CHD, stroke, and congestive heart failure (Flebach et al., 1989; Vasan and Levy, 1996). A few of the animal studies resulted in inconsistent data with respect to tea flavonoids and their association of blood pressure. However, a long-term daily consumption of tea may reduce blood pressure as suggested by certain population studies (Hodgson and Croft, 2006). Nevertheless, controlled trials are needed to address the question because a large number of other life style factors are associated with tea intake and all these factors together contribute to CVD risk and pathogenesis. Acutely, tea can increase blood pressure. Both flavonoids and caffeine, present in tea cause a transient increase in blood pressure in subjects who avoided caffeine for 12 h or more (Hodgson et al., 2005; Pincomb et al., 1996; Quinlan et al., 1997). The relevance of these acute effects to any longer term effects of regular consumption is uncertain. In controlled trials, the short-term regular ingestion of tea for up to 8 weeks has not been found to alter blood pressure in largely normotensive individuals (Hodgson, 2006; Hodgson and Croft, 2006). A recent meta-analysis of these trials found no overall effect on systolic or diastolic blood pressure, whereas analysis of a similar number of trials using flavonoid-rich dark chocolate showed significant blood pressure lowering (Taubert et al., 2007). It is possible that longer term effects on vasodilator function may be required to alter vascular tone and blood pressure. There have been no controlled trials investigating the longer term effects of regular ingestion of tea. Therefore, there is some support for the idea that tea and tea flavonoids can attenuate the development of hypertension. Results of population studies suggest reduced risk of hypertension and lower blood pressure. However, further trials are needed to establish the effect of tea on blood pressure.

Increased levels of stress hormones such as epinephrine, norepinephrine and cortisol could lead to increased blood pressure. Caffeine can raise plasma levels of these stress hormones and hence theoretically coffee consumption may lead to raised blood pressure (Lane et al., 1990; Robertson et al., 1978). Interestingly, there were no effects of coffee on hypertension. On the other hand, consumption of sugared colas led to hypertension. This difference between coffee with no hypertension risk and cola with risk is attributed to the lack of polyphenols in the colas and their presence in the coffee (Vinson, 2006). These results indicate that high consumption of caffeine with no antioxidants could lead to hypertension.

Chlorogenic acid (CGA) was examined in human studies for blood pressure and vasoreactivity effects. A double-blind placebo-controlled study, which included hypertensive subjects, showed that CGA administration had no effect on normal serum or cell biochemistry (Watanabe et al., 2006). The result indicated a reduced blood pressure with the authors speculating that the mechanism of CGA effect is an increase in the level of nitric oxide (NO). Normotensive subjects with reduced vasoreactivity were also studied with the CGA green coffee bean extract (Ochiai et al., 2004). A significant decrease in plasma homocysteine compared with the baseline value for the CGA group was observed which indicated a decreased risk of CHD. In addition, a positive benefit was noted in the vasodilation responses to ischemic reactive hyperemia in the CGA group indicating improved vasoreactivity, a surrogate for endothelial function.

The effects of caffeine have also been studied (Nurminen et al., 1999; Umemura et al., 2006). Umemura et al. (2006) examined the effect of acute administration of caffeine on vascular function and observed that the blood pressure was increased by the caffeine but heart rate and forearm blood flow were unchanged. It was suggested that caffeine improved endothelium-dependent vasodilation by a mechanism which increased the release of nitric oxide. An increase in systolic pressure was reported earlier by Nurminen et al. (1999) in normotensive subjects who received a single dose of caffeine. A meta-analysis of a few selected clinical trials of coffee or caffeine (median trial duration of 56 days) indicated increased systolic pressure and diastolic pressure with coffee compared with control (Lee et al., 1999). The effect was more prominent in subjects falling within a young age group. The meta-analysis also concluded that the blood pressure-raising effects are due to caffeine rather than other ingredients. Noordzij et al. (2005) carried out a meta-analysis from 1966 to 2003 data and emphasized that regular caffeine consumption significantly increased blood pressure. However these effects were small when caffeine was ingested in coffee. Normotensive subjects switching from caffeinated to decaffeinated coffee would experience a small but real decrease in blood pressure as shown by van Dusseldorp et al. (1989) in a group of Dutch subjects (45 male and female subjects with a habitual intake of 4–6 cups of coffee per day). In this study the subjects received five cups of caffeinated coffee (445 mg dose of caffeine) for 6 weeks or five cups of decaffeinated coffee (40 mg dose of caffeine) for 6 weeks then switched to the other form of coffee for 6 weeks. Even though, chronic alcohol consumption increases blood pressure (Klatsky et al., 2006), a few weeks of moderate coffee consumption by hypertensive or prehypertensive subjects, who also were heavy alcohol drinkers, caused a significant decrease in systolic and diastolic blood pressure.

12.5.4 OXIDATIVE STRESS

The antioxidant property of tea flavonoids is the major factor which reduces the CVD risk on tea consumption. The antioxidant potency of tea flavonoids have been experimentally proven in many *in vitro* studies, but the *in vivo* data are very limited (Halliwell et al., 2005; Manach et al., 2005). This is mainly attributed to their poor bioavailability and changes in antioxidant activity due to metabolic transformation. Good support for a lack of systemic antioxidant activity of flavonoids *in vivo* comes from studies showing that inhibition of atherosclerosis in animal models is not associated with markers of change in oxidative damage (Auger et al., 2004; Waddington et al., 2004). Thus, it is possible that antioxidant activity is not an important mechanism for beneficial effects of tea flavonoids on endothelial function, atherosclerosis, and CVD risk.

12.5.5 CHOLESTEROL REDUCTION

In vitro studies suggested that flavonoids could reduce blood cholesterol concentrations (Hodgson, 2008). With respect to increased flavonoid intake from black tea, most human intervention studies indicated no change in blood cholesterol concentrations (Hodgson, 2000, 2008; Manach et al., 2005). Similar observations were made for green tea (Tsubono and Tsugane, 1997; Unno et al., 2005; Van het hof et al., 1997). But these effects are not prominent in human trials. The discrepancies between experimental and clinical data may be explained by the fact that most animal studies were performed with high doses of tea and tea components. In the context of lipid-lowering effects with respect to coffee consumption, the two compounds—cafestol and kahweol are of special interest. These two diterpene molecules cause the elevation of serum cholesterol. *In vitro* cellular study by Rustan et al. (1997) showed that the diterpenes reduced the activity of LDL receptors thus causing extracellular accumulation of LDL.

12.5.6 PLATELET FUNCTION

Increased susceptibility to aggregation and clotting are the major effects of platelet activation which in turn leads to thrombosis, MI, and stroke. High physiological concentrations of flavonoids can reduce platelet aggregation and markers of platelet activation (Rein et al., 2000). Studies investigating the effects of tea on platelet function were inconsistent and most of them showed no effect (Hodgson, 2008). However, studies by Hodgson et al. (2001) and Lee et al. (2005) reported that regular ingestion of tea for 4 weeks resulted in a reduction in circulating p-selectin concentrations, which is a marker of platelet activation. In order to establish the effects of tea on platelet function additional trials are needed.

12.5.7 HOMOCYSTEINE LEVELS

An increased total homocysteine (tHcy) level in plasma is associated with an enhanced risk for CVD. Homocysteine is an intermediate metabolite of methionine and its metabolism can be influenced by several dietary factors including polyphenols and caffeine (Hodgson et al., 2003; Olthof et al., 2001). Studies by Olthof et al. (2001) and Verhoef et al. (2002) suggested that polyphenols and caffeine could enhance homocysteine levels. However, it has also been shown in population studies that a higher intake of tea is associated with lower tHcy (Hodgson et al., 2006; de Bree et al., 2001; Nygard et al., 1997). Contradictory tresults were obtained from a controlled intervention study in which high doses of tea solids found that tea solids increased tHcy (Olthof et al., 2001). Thus, any acute effects of tea polyphenols and caffeine to elevate homocysteine acutely do not appear to translate into effects following regular consumption. Coffee consumption has been positively associated with tHcy concentrations in a dose-dependent manner in numerous cross-sectional studies conducted in Europe, Scandinavia, and the United States (Husemoen et al., 2004; de Bree et al., 2001; Mennen et al., 2002; Nygard et al., 1997; Stolzenberg-Solomon and Miller, 1999). Controlled clinical trials have confirmed the homocysteine-raising effect of relatively high intakes of coffee (Christensen et al., 2001; Grubben et al., 2000; Urgert et al., 2000). The results of controlled clinical trials suggest that caffeine and chlorogenic acid contribute to the homocysteine-raising effect of coffee (Verhoef et al., 2002; Olthof et al., 2001).

12.5.8 BODY WEIGHT, BODY COMPOSITION, AND VISCERAL FATNESS

Abdominal obesity and percentage body fat, which are independent risk factors for CVD, have also been parameters of interest for researchers in green tea intervention. There is no real data to support an effect of black tea on body weight and composition, however, green tea is thought to exert a beneficial effect. Regular consumption of green tea is thought to increase energy expenditure and reduce body fatness. This is supported by a number of studies that reported increased energy expenditure after consumption of green tea/green tea flavonoids and caffeine (Dulloo et al., 1999; Rumpler et al., 2001; Westerterp-Plantenga et al., 2006). Catechin appears to have a major role, as a few acute and long-term studies showed green tea catechin ingestion increased fat oxidation during exercise (Takashima et al., 2004; Venables et al., 2008). Tea flavonoids and caffeine synergistically cause the increase in energy (Dulloo et al., 1999; Rumpler et al., 2001). Unfortunately, we do not have any data on their relative contributions for this effect. But the effect of caffeine alone is dose dependent as low doses of caffeine was not found to significantly alter energy expenditure (Dulloo et al., 1999; Rumpler et al., 2001). An increase in fat oxidation by high catechin green tea could be contributed to the longer term beneficial effects on body weight and composition. Two recent meta-analyses of results from human intervention studies suggested that green tea flavonoids with caffeine significantly reduced a portion of body weight (Hursel et al., 2009; Phung et al., 2010). While the results of randomized controlled trials suggested green tea could reduce visceral fat during medium-term consumption, the effects of black tea remain unclear.

Caffeine increases circulating catecholamine levels and, partially, through this mechanism increases the basal metabolic rate. Lipolysis releases free fatty acids resulting in free-fatty acid levels of serum rising to 50–100% above normal. This is most likely a consequence of systemic catecholamines and/or antagonism of adenosine-mediated inhibition of lipolysis. The effect of caffeine on blood sugar has been the subject of some debate. Most studies have shown that caffeine does not appreciably increase blood glucose in normal healthy people (Chou and Benowitz, 1994).

12.5.9 TYPE 2 DIABETES

Another contributing factor to increased risk of CVD is the development of type 2 diabetes. Tea consumption is associated with a decreased risk of diabetes and a reduced level of fasting blood glucose in nonobese people as per the data obtained in selected epidemiological studies (Iso et al., 2006; Panagiotakos et al., 2009; Polychronopoulos et al., 2008; Song et al., 2005). However, additional prospective population studies are needed to investigate the relationship of tea consumption with risk of type 2 diabetes. Moreover, the results of studies with animal models (Wu et al., 2004) and human intervention studies (Fukino et al., 2005; Mackenzie et al., 2007; Ryu et al., 2006) do not provide evidence to clearly support any benefits of tea consumption on glucose and insulin metabolism. Further human studies are needed before drawing any conclusion on the effects of tea on blood glucose control and type 2 diabetes.

A few cohort studies, however, found a significant inverse association between the risk of type 2 diabetes mellitus (DM) and coffee intake (Carlsson et al., 2004; Rosengren et al., 2004; Tuomilehto et al., 2004; van Dam and Feskens et al., 2002). van Dam and Feskens et al. (2002) in a prospective study of Dutch men and women found that the risk of developing type 2 DM was 50% lower in those who consumed at least 7 cups of coffee daily. Similar observation was made by Tuomilehto et al. (2004) with Finnish people where 10 cups of coffee daily resulted in a 55% lower risk of developing type 2 DM. However the reduction of CVD was only 35% when Finnish twins consumed at least seven cups of coffee daily (Carlsson et al., 2004). van Dam and Hu (2005) also showed a 35% reduction in risk of CVD in subjects who consumed at least six cups of coffee daily. However, not all prospective cohort studies have observed significant inverse associations between coffee consumption and type 2 DM risk (Reunanen et al., 2003). Prospective studies in two smaller cohorts did not observe significant associations between coffee consumption and type 2 DM diagnosed by oral glucose tolerance testing (OGTT) instead of self-reporting (Saremi et al., 2003; van Dam et al., 2004). Although short-term clinical trials found caffeine administration impaired glucose tolerance and decreased insulin sensitivity, limited data from epidemiological studies suggest that habitual coffee consumption was inversely associated with impaired glucose tolerance. Until the relationship between long-term coffee consumption and type 2 DM risk is better understood, it is premature to recommend coffee consumption as a means of preventing type 2 DM.

12.6   CONCLUSIONS

Available data suggest that tea and coffee are likely to provide protection against CVD. Tea flavonoids are mainly responsible for reducing the risk of CVD which is attributed to their ability to enhance nitric oxide status and improve endothelial function. There is accumulated knowledge on the benefit of regular consumption of green tea on body fatness and the development of obesity.

However, its hypocholesterolemic effects have not been demonstrated convincingly in humans, so that further studies are warranted. Although there have been numerous *in vitro* studies, cell-culture studies, animal studies, and epidemiology investigations on the effects of coffee and its bioactive components on CVD, there has been a paucity of human trials. The effects of chlorogenic acid on blood pressure and endothelial function are intriguing. More long-term interventional studies are needed with caffeinated and decaffeinated coffees in different human populations and pathological conditions. Nevertheless, the current epidemiological studies combined with animal and *in vitro* studies, support coffee and tea as safe beverages. However, there are no comparative studies to ascertain the efficiency of tea over coffee or coffee over tea. Nevertheless, a diet rich in functional foods containing antioxidant polyphenols, such as in black and green tea beverages and coffee, combined with physical activity and lifestyle changes, offer a potential strategy for reducing the risk of CVD.

REFERENCES

Alexopoulos, N., Vlachopoulos, C., Aznaouridis, K., Baou, K., Vasiliadou, C., Pietri, P., Xaplanteris, P., Stefanadi, E., and Stefanadis, C., 2008. The acute effect of green tea consumption on endothelial function in healthy individuals. *Eur. J. Cardiovasc. Prev. Rehabil.* **15**: 300–305.

Andersen, L.F., Jacobs Jr., D.R., Carlsen, M.H., and Blomhoff, R. 2006. Consumption of coffee is associated with reduced risk of death attributed to inflammatory and cardiovascular diseases in the Iowa Women's Health Study. *Am. J. Clin. Nutr.* **83**:1039–1046.

Arab, L., Liu, W., and Elashoff, D. 2009. Green and black tea consumption and risk of stroke: A meta-analysis. *Stroke.* **40**: 1786–1792.

Auger, C., Laurent, N., Laurent, C., Besancon, P., Caporiccio, B., Teissedre, P.L., and Rouasnet, J.M. 2004. Hydroxycinnamic acids do not prevent aortic atherosclerosis in hypercholesterolemic golden Syrian hamsters. *Life Sci.* **74**: 2365–2377.

Auger, C., Gerain, P., Laurent-Bichon, F., Portet, K., Bornet, A., Caporiccio, B., Cros, G., Teissedre, P.L., and Rouanet, J.M., 2004. Phenolics from commercialized grape extracts prevent early atherosclerotic lesions in hamsters by mechanisms other than antioxidant effect. *J. Agric. Food. Chem.* **52**: 5297–5302.

Baylin A., Hernandez-Diaz, S., Kabagambe, E.K., Siles X., and Campos H. 2006. Transient exposure to coffee as a trigger of a first nonfatal myocardial infarction. *Epidemiology* **7**: 506–511.

Borrelli, R.C., Visconti, A., Mennela, C., Anese, M., and Fogliano, V. 2002. Chemical characterization and antioxidant properties of coffee melanoidins. *J. Agric. Food. Chem.* **50**: 6527–6533.

Carlsson, S., Hammar, N., Grill, V., and Kaprio, J. 2004. Coffee consumption and risk of type 2 diabetes in Finnish twins. *Int. J. Epidemiol.* **33**: 616–617.

Carrillo, J.A. and Benitez, J. 2000. Clinically significant pharmacokinetic interactions between dietary caffeine and medications. *Clin. Pharmacokinet* **39**:127–153.

Chou, T.M. and Benowitzt, N.L. 1994. Caffeine and coffee: Effects on health and cardiovascular disease *Comp. Biochem. Physiol. C Pharmacol. Toxicol. Endocrinol.* **109**: 173–189.

Christensen, B., Mosdol, A., Retterstol, L., Landaas, S., and Thelle, D.S. 2001. Abstention from filtered coffee reduces the concentrations of plasma homocysteine and serum cholesterol—A randomized controlled trial. *Am. J. Clin. Nutr.* **74**:302–307.

Chrysohoou, C., Panagiotakos, D.B., Pitsavos, C., Zeimbekis, A., Zampelas, A., Papademetriou, L., Masoura, C., and Stefandis, C. 2004. The associations between smoking, physical activity, dietary habits and plasma homocysteine levels in cardiovascular disease-free people: The 'ATTICA' study. *Vasc. Med.* **9**: 117–123.

Clifford, M.N. 1999. Chlorogenic acids and other cinnamates—Nature occurrence and dietary burden. *J. Sci. Food Agric.* **79**: 362–372.

Daglia, M., Papetti, A., Gregotti, C., Berte, F., and Gazzani, G. 2000. *In vitro* antioxidant and *ex vivo* protective activities of green and roasted coffee. *J. Agric. Food Chem.* **48**: 1449–1454.

de Bree, A., Verschuren, W.M., Blom, H.J., and Kromhout, D., 2001. Lifestyle factors and plasma homocysteine concentrations in a general population sample. *Am. J. Epidemiol.* **154**: 150–154.

De Roos, B., Van Tol, A., Urgert, R., Scheek, L.M., Van Gent, T., Buytenhek, R., Princen, H.M.G., and Katan, M.B., 2000. Consumption of French-press coffee raises cholesteryl ester transfer protein activity levels before LDL cholesterol in normolipidaemic subjects. *J. Intern. Med.* **248**: 211–216.

Debette, S., Courbon, D., Leone, N., Gariepy, J., Tzourio, C., Dartigues, J.F., Barberger-Gateau, P., Ritchie, K., Alperovitch, A., Amouyel, P., Ducimetiere, P. and Zureik, M., 2008. Tea consumption is inversely associated with carotid plaques in women. *Arterioscler. Thromb. Vasc. Biol.* **28**: 353–359.

Dreosti, I.E. 1996. Bioactive ingredients: Antioxidants and polyphenols in tea. *Nutr. Rev.* **54**: S51–S58.

Duffy, S.J., Keaney, J.F., Holbrook, M., Gokce, N., Swerdloff, P.L., Frei, B., and Vita, J.A., 2001. Short and long term black tea consumption reverses endothelial dysfunction in patients with coronary artery disease. *Circulation* **104**: 151–156.

Dulloo, A.G., Duret, C., Rohrer, D., Girardier, L., Mensi, N., Fathi, M., Chantre, P., and Vandermander, J., 1999. Efficacy of a green tea extract rich in catechin polyphenols and caffeine in increasing 24-h energy expenditure and fat oxidation in humans. *Am. J. Clin. Nutr.* **70**: 1040–1045.

Flebach, N.H., Hebert, P.R., Stampfer, M.J., Colditz, G.A., Willett, W.C., Rosner, B.Spelzer, F.E., and Hennekens, C.H. 1989. A prospective study of high blood pressure and cardiovascular disease in women. *Am. J. Epidemiol.* **130**: 646–654.

Fukino, Y., Shimbo, M., Aoki, N., Okubo, T., and Iso, H., 2005. Randomized controlled trial for an effect of green tea consumption on insulin resistance and inflammation markers. *J. Nutr. Sci. Vitaminol.* **51**: 335–342.

Graham, H.N. 1992. Green tea composition, consumption and polyphenol chemistry. *Prev. Med.* **21**: 334–350.

Grassi, D., Mulder, T.P.J., Draijer, R., Desideri, G., Molhuizen, H.O.F., Ferri, C., 2009. Black tea consumption dose-dependently improves flow-mediated dilation in healthy males. *J. Hypertens.* 27: 774–781.

Grigg, D. 2002 The worlds of tea and coffee: Patterns of consumption. *GeoJournal* 57: 283–294.

Gross, G., Jaccaud, E., and Huggett, A.C. 1997. Analysis of the content of the diterpenes cafestol and kahweol in coffee brews. *Food Chem. Toxicol.* **35**: 547–554.

Grubben, M.J., Boers, G.H., Blom, H.J., Broekhuizen, R., de Long, R., van Rijt, L., de Ruijter, E., Swinkels, D.W., Nagengast, F.N., and Katan, M.B. 2000. Unfiltered coffee increases plasma homocysteine concentrations in healthy volunteers: A randomized trial. *Am. J. Clin Nutr.* **71**: 480–484.

Halliwell, B., Rafter, J., and Jenner, A., 2005. Health promotion by flavonoids, tocopherols, tocotrienols, and other phenols: Direct or indirect effects? Antioxidant or not? *Am. J. Clin. Nutr.* **81**: 268S–276S.

Harbowy, M.E. and Ballentine, D.A. 1997. Tea chemistry. *Crit. Rev. Plant Sci.* **16**: 415–480.

Higdon, J.V. and Frei, B. 2006. Coffee and health: A review of recent human research. *Crit. Rev. Food Sci. Nutr.* **46**: 101–123.

Higdon, J.V. and Frei, B. 2003. Tea catechins and polyphenols: Health effects, metabolism, and antioxidant functions. *Crit. Rev. Food Sci. Nutr.* **43**: 89–143.

Hodgson, J.M. 2000. Tea and cardiovascular disease: A review. *Proc. Nutr. Soc. Austr.* **24**: 241–249.

Hodgson, J.M. 2006. Effects of tea and tea flavonoids on endothelial function and blood pressure: A brief review. *Clin. Exp. Pharmacol. Physiol.* **33**: 838–841.

Hodgson, J.M. 2008. Tea flavonoids and cardiovascular disease. *Asia Pacific J. Clin. Nutr.* **17**: S288–S290.

Hodgson, J.M., Burke, V., Beilin, L.J., Croft, K.D., Puddey, I.B., 2003. Can black tea influence plasma total homocysteine concentrations?. *Am. J. Clin. Nutr.* **77**: 907–911.

Hodgson, J.M., Burke, V., and Puddey, I.B. 2005. Acute effects of tea on fasting and postprandial vascular function and blood pressure in humans. *J. Hypertens.* **23**: 47–54.

Hodgson, J.M. and Croft, K.D., 2006. Dietary flavonoids: Effects on endothelial function and blood pressure. *J. Sci. Food Agric.* **86**: 2492–2498.

Hodgson, J.M., Devine, A., Puddey, I.B., Beilby, J., and Prince, R.L., 2006. Drinking tea is associated with lower plasma total homocysteine in older women. *Asia Pacific J. Clin. Nutr.* **15**(2): 253–258.

Hodgson, J.M., Proudfoot, J.M., Croft, K.D., Puddey, I.B., Mori, T.A., and, Beilin, L.J. 1999. Comparison of the effects of black and green tea on *in vitro* lipoprotein oxidation in human serum. *J. Sci. Food Agric.* **79**: 561–566.

Hodgson, J.M., Puddey, I.B., Burke, V., Beilin, L.J., Mori, T.A., and Chan, S.Y. 2002. Acute effects of ingestion of black tea on postprandial platelet aggregation in humans. *Br. J. Nutr.* **87**: 141–145.

Hodgson, J.M., Puddey, I.B., Mori, T.A., Burke, V., Baker, R., and Beilin, L.J. 2001. Effects of regular ingestion of black tea on haemostasis and cell adhesion molecules in humans. *Eur. J. Clin. Nutr.* **55**: 881–886.

Hursel, R., Viechtbauer, W., and Westerterp-Plantenga, M.S. 2009. The effects of green tea on weight loss and weight maintenance: A meta-analysis. *J. Obes.* **33**: 956–961.

Husemoen, L.L., Thomsen, T.F., Fenger, M., and Jorgensen, T. 2004. Effect of lifestyle factors on plasma total homocysteine concentrations in relation to MTHFR(C677T) genotype. Inter99 (7). *Eur. J. Clin. Nutr.* **58**: 1142–1150.

Huxley, R.R., and Neil, H.A. 2003. The relation between dietary flavonol intake and coronary heart disease mortality: A meta-analysis of prospective cohort studies. *Eur. J. Clin. Nutr.* **57**: 904–908.

International Tea Committee. 2002. *Annual Bulletin of Statistics*, ITC.

Iso, H., Date, C., Wakai, K., Fukui, M., and Tamakoshi, A. 2006. JACC Study Group. The relationship between green tea and total caffeine intake and risk for self reported type 2 diabetes among Japanese adults. *Ann. Intern. Med.* **144**: 554–562.

Iwai, N., Ohshiro, H., Kurozawa, Y., Hosoda, T., Morita, H., Funakawa, K., Okamoto, M., and Nose, T., 2002. Relationship between coffee and green tea consumption and all-cause mortality in a cohort of a rural Japanese population. *J. Epidemiol.* **12**: 191–198.

James, J.E. 2004. Critical review of dietary caffeine and blood pressure: A relationship that should be taken more seriously. *Psychosom. Med.* **66**: 63–71.

Jochmann, N., Lorenz, M., von Krosigk, A., Martus, P., Böhm, V., G, Baumann, Stangl, K., and Stangl, V., 2008. The efficacy of black tea in ameliorating endothelial function is equivalent to that of green tea. *Br. J. Nutr.* **99**: 863–868.

Kim, W., Jeong, M.H., Cho, S.H., Yun, J.H., Chae, H.J., Ahn, Y.K., Lee, M.C. and Cheng, X., Kondo, T., Murohara, T., Kang, J.C., 2006. Effect of green tea consumption on endothelial function and circulating endothelial progenitor cells in chronic smokers. *Circ. J.* **70**: 1052–1057.

Klatsky, A.L., Koplik, S., Gunderson, E., Kipp, H., and Friedman, G.D. 2006. Sequelae of systemic hypertension in alcohol abstainers, light drinkers, and heavy drinkers. *Am. J. Cardiol.* **98**: 1063–1068.

Kuriyama, S. 2008. The relation between green tea consumption and cardiovascular disease as evidenced by epidemiological studies. *J. Nutr.* **138**: 1548S–1553S.

Lane, J.D., Adcock, R.A., Williams, R.B., and Kuhn, C.M. 1990. Caffeine effects on cardiovascular and neuro-endocrine responses to acute psychosocial stress and their relationship to level of habitual caffeine consumption. *Psychosom. Med.* 152: 320–336.

Lee, S.H., He, J., Whelton, P.K., Suh, I., and Klag, M.J. 1999. The effect of chronic coffee drinking on blood pressure: A meta-analysis of controlled clinical trials. *Hypertension* 33: 647–652.

Lee, W., Min, W.K., Chun, S., Lee, Y.W., Park, H., Lee, D.H., Lee, Y.K., Son, J.E., 2005. Long-term effects of green tea ingestion on atherosclerotic biological markers in smokers. *Clin. Biochem.* **38**: 84–87.

Loke, W.M., Hodgson, J.M., Proudfoot, J.M., McKinley, A.J., Puddey, I.B., and Croft, K.D. 2008. Pure dietary flavonoids, quercetin and (-)-epicatechin augment nitric oxide products and reduce endothelin-1 acutely in healthy human volunteers. *Am. J. Clin. Nutr.* **88**: 1018–1025.

Loke, W.M., Proudfoot, J.M., McKinley, A.J., Hodgson, J.M., and Croft, K.D. 2010. Pure dietary polyphenols attenuate atherosclerosis in apo E knockout mice via alleviating oxidative stress, inflammation and endothelial dysfunction. *Arterioscl. Thrombos. Vasc. Biol.* **30**: 749–757.

Lopez-Garcia E, van Dam, R.M., Qi, L., and Hu, F.B. 2006. Coffee consumption and markers of inflammation and endothelial dysfunction in healthy and diabetic women. *Am. J. Clin. Nutr.* **84**: 888–893.

Lopez-Garcia, E., van Dam, R.M., Willett, W.C., Rimm, E.B., Manson, J.E., Stampfer, M.J., Rexrode, K.M., and Hu, F.B. 2006. Coffee consumption and coronary heart disease in men and women: a prospective cohort study. *Circulation* **13**: 2045–2053.

Mackenzie, T., Leary, L., and Brooks, W.B. 2007. The effect of an extract of green and black tea on glucose control in adults with type 2 diabetes mellitus: Double blind randomized study. *Metabolism* **56**: 1340–1344.

Manach, C., Mazur, A., and Scalbert, A. 2005. Polyphenols and prevention of cardiovascular disease. *Curr. Opin. Lipidol.* **16**: 77–84.

Martinez-Ortiz, J.A., Fung, T.T., Baylin, A., Hu, F.B., and Campos, H. 2006. Dietary patterns and risk of nonfatal acute myocardial infarction in Costa Rican adults. *Eur. J. Clin. Nutr.* **60**: 770–777.

McCusker, R.R., Goldberger, B.A., and Cone, E.J. 2003. Caffeine content of specialty coffees. *J. Anal. Toxicol.* **27**: 520–522.

Mennen, L.I., de Courcy, G.P., Guilland, J.C., Ducros, V., Bertrais, S., Nicolas, J-P., Maurel, M., Zarebska, M., Favier, A., Franchisseur, C., Hercberg, S. and Galan, P. 2002. Homocysteine, cardiovascular disease risk factors, and habitual diet in the French Supplementation with Antioxidant Vitamins and Minerals Study. *Am. J. Clin. Nutr.* **76**: 1279–1289.

Moore, R.J., Kim, G., Jackson, K.G., and Minihane, A.M. 2009. Green tea (*Camellia sinensis*) catechins and vascular function. *Br. J. Nut.* **102**: 1790–1802.

Mukamal, K.J., Maclure, M., Muller, J.E., Sherwood, J.B., and Mittleman, M.A. 2004. Caffeinated coffee consumption and mortality after acute myocardial infarction. *Am. Heart J.* **147**: 999–1004.

Mursu, J., Nurmi, T., Tuomainen, T.P., Ruusunen, A., Salonen, J.T., and Voutilainen, S. 2007. The intake of flavonoids and carotid atherosclerosis: The Kuopio ischaemic heart disease risk factor study. *Br. J. Nutr.* **98**: 814–818.

Nagaya, N., Yamamoto, H., Uematsu, M., Itoh, T., Nakagawa, K., Miyazawa, T., Kangawa, K., Miyatake, K. 2004. Green tea reverses endothelial dysfunction in healthy smokers. *Heart* **90**: 1485–1486.

Nakachi, K., Matsuyama, S., Miyake, S., Suganuma, M., and Imai, K. 2000. Preventive effects of drinking green tea on cancer and cardiovascular disease: Epidemiological evidence for multiple targeting prevention. *Biofactors* **13**: 49–54.

Noordzij, M., Uiterwaal, C.S., Arends, L.R., Kok, F.J., Grobbee, D.E., and Geleijnse, J.M. 2005. Blood pressure response to chronic intake of coffee and caffeine: A meta-analysis of randomized controlled trials. *J. Hypertens.* **23**: 921–928.

Nurminen, M.L., Nittynen, L., Korpela, R., and Vapaatalo, H. 1999. Coffee, caffeine and blood pressure: A critical review. *Eur. J. Clin. Nutr.* **53**: 891–899.

Nygard, O., Refsum, H., Ueland, P.M., Sternsvold, I., Nordrehaug, J.E., Kvale, G., and Vollset, S.E. 1997. Coffee consumption and plasma total homocysteine: The Hordal and homocysteine study. *Am. J. Clin. Nutr.* **65**: 136–143.

Ochiai, R., Jokura, H., Suzuki, A., Tokimutsu, I., Ohish,i M., Komai, N., Rakugi, H., and Ogihara, T. 2004. Green coffee bean extract improves human vasoreactivity. *Hypertens. Res.* **27**: 731–737.

Olthof, M.R., Hollman, P.C., and Katan, M.B. 2001a. Chlorogenic acid and caffeic acid are absorbed in humans. *J. Nutr.* **131**:66–71.

Olthof, M.R., Hollman, P.C., Zock, P.L., and Katan, M.B. 2001b. Consumption of high doses of chlorogenic acid, present in coffee, or of black tea increases plasma total homocysteine concentrations in humans. *Am. J. Clin. Nutr.* **73**: 532–538.

Panagiotakos, D.B., Lionis, C., Zeimbekis, A., Gelastopoulou, K., Papairakleous, N., Das, U.N., and Polychronopoulos, E., 2009. Long-term tea intake is associated with reduced prevalence of (type 2) diabetes mellitus among elderly people from Mediterranean islands: MEDIS epidemiological study. *Yonsei Med. J.* **50**: 31–38.

Pellegrini, N., Serafini, M., Colombi, B., Del Rio, D. Salvatore, S., Bianchi, M., and Brighenti, F. 2003. Total antioxidant capacity of plant foods, beverages and oils consumed in Italy assessed by three different *in vitro* assays. *J. Nutr.* **133**: 2812–2819.

Peters, U., Poole, C., and Arab, L., 2001. Does tea affect cardiovascular disease? A meta-analysis. *Am. J. Epidemiol.* **154**: 495–503.

Phung, O.J., Baker, W.L., Matthews, L.J., Lanosa, M., Thorne, A., and Coleman, C.I. 2010. Effect of green tea catechins with or without caffeine on anthropometric measures: A systematic review and meta-analysis. *Am. J. Clin. Nutr.* **91**: 73–81.

Pincomb, G.A., Lovallo, W.R., McKey, B.S., Sung, B.H., Passey, R.B., Everson, S.A., and Wilson, M.F. 1996. Acute blood pressure elevations with caffeine in men with borderline systemic hypertension. *Am. J. Cardiol.* **77**: 270–274.

Polychronopoulos, E., Zeimbekis, A., Kastorini, C.M., Papairakleous, N., Vlachou, I., Bountziouka, V., and Panagiotakos, D.B. 2008. Effects of black and green tea consumption on blood glucose levels in non-obese elderly men and women from Mediterranean islands (MEDIS epidemiological study). *Eur. J. Nutr.* **47**: 10–16.

Pulido, R., Hernandez-Garcia, M., and Saura-Calixto F. 2003. Contribution of beverages to the intake of lipophillic and hydrophillic antioxidants in the Spanish diet. *Eur. J. Clin. Nutr.* **57**: 1275–1282.

Quinlan, P., Lane, J., and Aspinall, L., 1997. Effects of hot tea, coffee and water ingestion on physiological responses and mood: The role of caffeine, water and beverage type. *Psychopharmacology* **134**: 164–173.

Refsum, H., Nurk, E., Smith, A.D., Ueland, P.M., Gjesdal, C.G. Bjelland I, Tverdal, A., Tell, G.S., Nygard, O., and Vollset, S.E. 2006. The Hordaland Homocysteine Study: A community-based study of homocysteine, its determinants, and associations with disease. *J. Nutr.* **136**: 1731S–1740S.

Rein, D., Paglieroni, T.G., Pearson, D.A., Wun, T., Schmitz, H.H., Gosselin, R., and Keen, C.L., 2000. Cocoa and wine polyphenols modulate platelet activation and function. *J. Nutr.* **130**: 2120S–2126S.

Reunanen, A., Heliovaara, M., and Aho, K. 2003. Coffee consumption and risk of type 2 diabetes mellitus. *Lancet* **361**: 702–703.

Robertson, D., Frolich, J.C., Carr, R.K., Watson, J.T., Hollifield, J.W., Shand, D.G., and Oates, J.A. 1978. Effects of caffeine on plasma rennin activity, catecholamines and blood pressure. *N. Engl. J. Med.* **298**: 181–186.

Rosengren, A., Dotevall, A., Wilhelmsen, L., Thelle, D., and Johansson, S. 2004. Coffee and incidence of diabetes in Swedish women: A prospective 18-year follow-up study. *J. Intern. Med.* **255**: 89–95.

Rumpler, W., Seale, J., Clevidence, B., Judd, J., Wiley, E., Yamamoto, S., Komatsu, T., Sawaki, T., Ishikura, Y., and Hosoda, K. 2001. Oolong tea increases metabolic rate and fat oxidation in men. *J. Nutr.* **131**: 2848–2858.

Rustan, A.C., Halvorsen, B., Huggett, A.C., Ranheim, T., and Drevon CA. 1997. Effect of coffee lipids (cafestol and kahweol) on regulation of cholesterol metabolism in HepG2 cells. *Arterioscler. Thromb. Vasc. Biol.* **17**: 2140–2139.

Ryu, O.H., Lee, J., Lee, K.W., Kim, H.Y., Seo, J.A., Kim, S.G., Kim, N.H., Baik, S.H., Choi, D.S., and Choi, K.M., 2006. Effects of green tea consumption on inflammation, insulin resistance and pulse wave velocity in type 2 diabetes patients. *Diabetes Res. Clin. Pract.* **71**: 356–358.

Sakamoto, W., Isomura, H., Fujie, K., Takahashi, K., Nakao, K., and Izumi, H. 2005. Relationship of coffee consumption with risk factors of atherosclerosis in rats. *Ann. Nutr. Metab.* **49**: 149–154.

Saremi, A., Tulloch-Reid, M., and Knowler, W.C. 2003. Coffee consumption and the incidence of type 2 diabetes. *Diabetes Care* **26**:2211–2212.

Sato, Y., Nakatsuka, H., Watanabe, T., Hisamichi, S., Shimizu, H., Fujisaku, S., Ichinowatari, Y. Ida, Y., Suda, S., Kato, et al. 1989. Possible contribution of green tea drinking habits to the prevention of stroke. *Tohoku J. Exp. Med.* **157**: 337–343.

Schächinger, V., Britten, M.B., and Zeiher, A.M. 2000. Prognostic impact of coronary vasodilator dysfunction on adverse long-term outcome of coronary heart disease. *Circulation* 101: 1899–1906.

Schroeder, S., Enderle, M.D., Ossen, R., Meisner, C., Baumbach, A., Pfohl, M., Oberhoff, M., Haering, H.U., and Karsch, K.R. 1999. Noninvasive determination of endothelium-mediated vasodilation as a screening test for coronary artery disease: Pilot study to assess the predictive value in comparison with angina pectoris, exercise electrocardiography, and myocardial perfusion imaging. *Am. Heart J.* **138**: 731–739.

Sies, H., Schewe, T., Heiss, C., and Kelm, M., 2005. Cocoa polyphenols and inflammatory mediators. *Am. J. Clin. Nutr.* **81**: 304S–312S.

Sofi, F., Conti, A.A., Gori, A.M., Eliana Luisi, M.L., Casini, A., Abbate, R., and Gensini, G.F. 2007. Coffee consumption and risk of coronary heart disease: A meta-analysis. *Nutr. Metab. Cardiovasc. Dis.* **17**:209–223.

Song, Y., Manson, J.E., Buring, J.E., Sesso, H.D., and Liu, S. 2005. Associations of dietary flavonoids with risk of type 2 diabetes, and markers of insulin resistance and systemic inflammation in women: a prospective study and cross-sectional analysis. *J. Am. Coll. Nutr.* 24:376–384.

Spiller, M.A. 1998. The chemical components of coffee. In: *Caffeine*, pp. 97–161. Spiller, G. A., Ed., CRC Press, Boca Raton.

Stolzenberg-Solomon, R.Z., Miller, E.R., 3rd, Maguire, M.G., Selhub, J., and Appel, M.J. 1999. Association of dietary protein intake and coffee consumption with serum homocysteine concentrations in an older population. *Am. J. Clin. Nutr.* **69**: 467–475.

Svilaas, A., Sakhi, A.K., Andersen, L.F., Svilaas, T., Strom, E.C., Jacobs, D.R. Jr., Ose, L., and Blomhoff, R. 2004. Intakes of antioxidants in coffee, wine, and vegetables are correlated with plasma carotenoids in humans. *J. Nutr.* **134**: 562–567.

Takashima, S., Kataoka, K., Shibata, E., Hoshino, E. 2004. The long term intake of catechins improves lipid catabolism during exercise. *Prog. Med.* **24**: 3371–3379.

Taubert, D., Roesen, R., and Schomig, E. 2007. Effect of cocoa and tea intake on blood pressure: A meta-analysis. *Arch. Intern. Med.* **167**: 626–634.

Tsubono, Y. and Tsugane, S. 1997. Green tea intake in relation to serum lipid levels in middle-aged Japanese men and women. *Ann. Epidemiol.* **7**: 280–284.

Tuomilehto, J., Hu, G., and Bidel, S. 2004. Coffee consumption and risk of type 2 diabetes mellitus among middle-aged Finnish men and women. *JAMA* **291**: 1213–1219.

Umemura, T., Ueda, K., Nishioka, K., Hidaka, T., Takemoto, H., Nakamura, S., Jitsuki, D., Soga, J., Goto, C., Chayama, K., Yoshizumi, M. and Higachi, Y. 2006. Effects of acute administration of caffeine on vascular function. *Am. J. Cardiol.* **98**: 1538–1541.

Unno, T., Tago, M., Suzuki, Y., Nozawa, A., Sagesaka, Y.M., Kakuda, T., Egawa, K., and Kondo, K., 2005. Effect of tea catechins on postprandial plasma lipid responses in human subjects. *Br. J. Nutr.* **93**: 543–547.

Urgert, R. and Katan, M.B. 1997. The cholesterol-raising factor from coffee beans. *Ann. Rev. Nutr.* **17**: 305–324.

Urgert, R., van derWeg, G., Kosmeijer-Schuil, T.G., van de Bovenkamp, P.,Hovenier, R., and Katan, M.B. 1995. Levels of the cholesterol-elevating diterpenes cafestol and kahweol in various coffee brews. *J. Agric. Food Chem.* **43**: 2167–2172.

Urgert, R., van Vliet, T., Zock, P. L., and Katan, M. B. 2000. Heavy coffee consumption and plasma homocysteine: A randomized controlled trial in healthy volunteers. *Am. J. Clin Nutr.* **72**: 1107–1110.

van Dam, R.M., and Feskens, E.J. 2002. Coffee consumption and risk of type 2 diabetes mellitus. *Lancet* **360**: 1477–1478.

van Dam, R.M., and Hu, F.B., 2005. Coffee consumption and risk of type 2 diabetes: A systematic Review. *JAMA*, **294**(1): 97–104.

van Dam, R.M., Dekker, J.M., Nijpels, G., Stehouwer, C.D.A., Bouter, L.M., and Heine, R.J. 2004. Coffee consumption and incidence of impaired fasting glucose, impaired glucose tolerance, and type 2 diabetes: The Hoorn Study. *Diabetologia* **47**: 2152–2159.

van Dusseldorp, M., Smits, P., Thien, T., and Katan, M.B. 1989. Effect of decaffeinated versus regular coffee on blood pressure. A 12-week, double-blind trial. *Hypertension* **14**: 563–569.

Van het Hof, K.H., deBoer, H.S.M., Wiseman, S.A., Lien, N., Weststrate, J.A., and Tijburg, L.B.M. 1997. Consumption of green or black tea does not increase resistance of low-density lipoprotein to oxidation in humans. *Am. J. Clin. Nutr.* **66**: 1125–1132.

Vasan, R.S. and Levy, D. 1996. The role of hypertension in the pathogenesis of heart failure. A clinical mechanistic overview. *Arch. Intern. Med.* **156**: 1789–1796.

Venables, M.C., Hulston, C.J., Cox, H.R., and Jeukendrup, A.E., 2008. Green tea extract ingestion, fat oxidation, and glucose tolerance in healthy humans. *Am. J. Clin. Nutr.* **87**: 778–784.

Verhoef, P., Pasman, W.J., van Vliet, T., Urgert, R., and Katan, M.B., 2002. Contribution of caffeine to the homocysteine-raising effect of coffee: A randomized controlled trial in humans. *Am. J. Clin. Nutr.* **76**: 1244–1248.

Viani, R. 1993. Composition of coffee. In *Caffeine, Coffee and Health*, ed. Garattini, S. Raven Press. New York: pp. 17–41.

Vinson, J.A.2006. Caffeine and incident hypertension in women. *JAMA* **295**: 2135.

Waddington, E., Puddey, I.B., and Croft, K.D. 2004. Red wine polyphenolic compounds inhibit atherosclerosis in apolipoprotein E-deficient mice independently of effects on lipid peroxidation. *Am. J. Clin. Nutr.* **79**: 54–61.

Watanabe, T., Arai, Y., Mitsui, Y., Kusaura, T., Okawa, W., Kajihara, Y., and Saito, I. 2006. The blood pressure-lowering effect and safety of chlorogenic acid from green coffee bean extract in essential hypertension. *Clin. Exp. Hyperten.* **28**: 439–449.

Westerterp-Plantenga, M., Dieprens, K., Joosen, A.M., Berube-Parent, S., and Tremblay, A. 2006. Metabolic effects of spices, teas, and caffeine. *Physiol. Behav.* **89**: 85–91.

Wu, L.Y., Juan, C.C., Ho, L.T., Hsu, Y.P., and Hwang, L.S. 2004. Effect of green tea supplementation on insulin sensitivity in Sprague–Dawley rats. *J. Agric. Food Chem.* **52**: 643–648.

Yanagimoto, K., Ochi, H., Lee, K.G., and Shibamoto, T. 2004. Antioxidative activities of fractions obtained from brewed coffee. *J. Agric. Food Chem.* **52**: 592–596.

Zampelas, A., Panagiotakos, D.B., Pitsavos, C., Chrysohoou, C., and Stefanadis C. 2004. Associations between coffee consumption and inflammatory markers in healthy persons: The ATTICA study. *Am. J. Clin. Nutr.* **80**: 862–867.

Index

Note: n = Footnote

A

AA. *See* Arachidonic acid (AA)
AACC. *See* American Association of Cereal Chemists (AACC)
ABC. *See* ATP-binding cassette (ABC)
ABCG5. *See* ATP-binding cassette G5 (ABCG5)
ACB test. *See* Albumin cobalt binding test (ACB test)
ACE. *See* Angiotensin-converting enzyme (ACE)
Acrp30. *See* Adiponectin (Acrp30)
Activated protein C resistance (APC™ resistance), 81
Acute myocardial infarction (AMI), 234
    flavonoid effects, 235
    platelet effects, 245
Adaptive immune system, 4. *See also* Innate immune system
Adenosine diphosphate (ADP), 245
    platelet aggregation, 172, 246
Adequate intake (AI), 186, 200
    choline, 187, 189–190
ADH1C. *See* Alcohol dehydrogenase type 1C (ADH1C)
ADH3. *See* Alcohol dehydrogenase type 1C (ADH1C)
Adipocytes, 6. *See also* Adipose tissue; Resistin
    CRP, 11
    in fatty acid metabolism, 7
    infiltration, 7
    TNF-α secretion, 10–11
Adipokines, 6. *See also* Adipose tissue
    coronary artery disease, 6
    expression, 6–7
    and inflammatory markers, 208–209
Adiponectin (Acrp30), 8–9, 11, 208
    hypertension, 214
    on inflammatory profile, 189
    resveratrol stimulation, 151
Adipose tissue, 6. *See also* Adipocytes; Adipokines; Adiponectin (Acrp30)
    alpha-linolenic acid, 74, 81
    atherogenic factors, 8
    CRP, 11
    endocrine function, 208
    fatty acids, 7
    leptin, 9–10
    resistin, 10
    TNF-α, 10–11
    white, 6–7
ADP. *See* Adenosine diphosphate (ADP)
AFSA. *See* Aortic fatty streak area (AFSA)
Aged garlic extracts (AGEs), 168. *See also* Garlic (*Allium sativum*)
Age-related diseases, 79
Age-related macular degeneration (AMD), 190
    cost benefit of egg diet, 192
AGEs. *See* Aged garlic extracts (AGEs)

AHA. *See* American Heart Association (AHA)
AI. *See* Adequate intake (AI)
Ajoenes, 168. *See also* Garlic (*Allium sativum*)
ALA. *See* Alpha-linolenic acid (ALA)
Albumin cobalt binding test (ACB test), 15
Alcohol. *See also* Wine
    and all-cause mortality, 146
    blood pressure, 266
    cardiovascular risk reduction, 142, 146, 147, 148
    on cellmediated oxidation of lipids, 150
    CHD risk, 149
    consumption, 145, 148
    MI risk, 149
Alcohol dehydrogenase type 1C (ADH1C), 147–148
Allium sativum. *See* Garlic (*Allium sativum*)
Alpha-linolenic acid (ALA), 31, 71. *See also* Omega-3 fatty acid; Omega-6 fatty acid
    anti-inflammatory effects, 79–81
    conversion into LCPUFA, 74–77
    and CVD, 77–79, 81–82. *See also* Cardiovascular disease (CVD)
    dietary omega-6 to omega-3 FA ratio, 82
    eicosanoids, 80
    enriched meat and eggs, 32, 191
    health claims, 85, 87
    market products containing, 83–84
    metabolism, 72–74
    nutrient content claims, 85, 86
    regulations, 85–87
    structure/function claims, 85
AMD. *See* Age-related macular degeneration (AMD)
American Association of Cereal Chemists (AACC), 200
American Heart Association (AHA), 13
AMI. *See* Acute myocardial infarction (AMI)
Angiotensin-converting enzyme (ACE), 244
    blood pressure reduction, 173
Anthocyanins, 30, 142. *See also* Proacyanidins
    and CHD, 141
    in cocoa beans, 235
    enrichment of tomato, 31
    structure, 143
Antioxidant enzymes, 126
AOAC. *See* Association of Analytical Communities (AOAC)
Aortic fatty streak area (AFSA), 152
APC™ resistance. *See* Activated protein C resistance (APC™ resistance)
apoA. *See* Apolipoprotein A (apoA)
apoA-I. *See* Apolipoprotien A-I (apoA-I)
apoB. *See* Apolipoprotein B (apoB)
Apolipoprotein A (apoA), 211
Apolipoprotein B (apoB), 58, 111, 211
Apolipoprotien A-I (apoA-I), 17
Arachidonic acid (AA), 73
Area under the curve (AUC), 208

275

9 781420 071108

An environmentally friendly book printed and bound in England by www.printondemand-worldwide.com

PEFC Certified

This product is
from sustainably
managed forests
and controlled
sources

www.pefc.org

PEFC/16-33-415

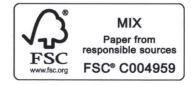

MIX
Paper from
responsible sources
FSC® C004959

This book is made entirely of sustainable materials; FSC paper for the cover and PEFC paper for the text pages.

Reprint of # - C0 - 254/178/16 - CB - Lamination Gloss - Printed on 26-Jan-16 08:42